Family-Centered
Maternity and
Newborn Care

Family-Centered Maternity and Newborn Care

A BASIC TEXT

Celeste R. Phillips, RN, EdD

Maternity Instructor,
Cabrillo College, Aptos, California
President, Phillips and Fenwick, Inc.

FOURTH EDITION
with 212 illustrations

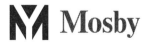

Mosby

St. Louis Baltimore Boston Carlsbad Chicago Naples New York Philadelphia Portland
London Madrid Mexico City Singapore Sydney Tokyo Toronto Wiesbaden

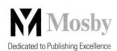

Mosby
Dedicated to Publishing Excellence

A Times Mirror Company

Vice-President and Publisher: Nancy L. Coon
Senior Editor: Susan R. Epstein
Associate Developmental Editor: Laurie K. Muench
Project Manager: John Rogers
Production Editor: Cheryl Abbott Bozzay
Designer: Renée Duenow
Cover design: Elizabeth Rohne Rudder
Manufacturing Manager: Theresa Fuchs
Chapter Opener Photography: Marjorie Pyle, RNC,
    Lifecircle, Costa Mesa, California

FOURTH EDITION

Copyright © 1996 Mosby–Year Book, Inc.

Printed in the United States of America
Composition by the Clarinda Company
Printing/binding by W.C. Brown

Mosby–Year Book, Inc.
11830 Westline Industrial Drive
St. Louis, Missouri 63146

Library of Congress Cataloging in Publication Data

Phillips, Celeste R., 1933-
    Family-centered maternity and newborn care : a basic text /
Celeste R. Phillips.--4th ed.
    p.   cm.
    Includes bibliographical references and index.
    ISBN 0-8151-6794-6
    1. Maternity nursing.   2. Neonatology.   I. Title.
RG951.P63   1996
610.73'678--dc20   95-33554
                                                                CIP

95 96 97 98 99 / 9 8 7 6 5 4 3 2 1

To
my mother
Catherine M. Nagel,
the strongest woman I have ever known.

February 23, 1908–June 22, 1994

REVIEWERS

Sandra R. DeStaffany, BS, ICCE

President, International Childbirth Education Association
Minneapolis, Minnesota

Patricia M. Jacobson, RN, BSN, MSN

Nursing Instructor
Bullard Havens Regional Vocational-Technical School
Bridgeport, Connecticut

Mona L. White, RN, BSN, MSN, CNS

Assistant Professor
Delta College
University Center, Michigan

PREFACE

Revolutionary changes are occurring in the provision of maternity care in today's dynamic health care environment. The lengths of inpatient stays for maternity care are becoming shorter and shorter. Antepartum and postpartum home care programs are rapidly growing in number. Maternity department job descriptions are expanding, and staff members are being fully cross trained to meet these expanded job descriptions. Maternity staff may include CNMs, RNs, LPNs/LVNs, advanced practice nurses, nurse extenders/technicians, childbirth and family educators, doulas, monitrices, home health workers, patient care technicians, and patient service associates (expanded housekeeper roles). The focus is on a multidisciplinary approach to care with new expanded roles for all members of the multidisciplinary team. This text has been designed for use by the beginning health care students who will function in these new roles.

This fourth edition of *Family-Centered Maternity and Newborn Care* has been revised, expanded, and updated to provide the latest basic information on care of childbearing families. Each chapter begins with goals and student objectives, so the direction of study is clear. An extensive, current bibliography, self-assessment exercises (with answers provided at the end of the text), learning activities, suggested audiovisual materials, and in-depth study activities are provided at the end of each chapter. Through completion of the self-assessment exercises the student receives immediate feedback on attainment of objectives.

Although this book is chronologically organized for clarity (antepartum, intrapartum, postpartum, and newborn), the theme of family care is woven into each chapter. Every attempt was made not to compartmentalize the childbearing experience. Throughout the text there is an emphasis on the normalcy of pregnancy and birth and on individualized care for the family unit.

A new chapter on continuity of care focuses on home care for childbearing families. Case management and program development for short-stay maternity programs are discussed.

At the end of the text, clinical learning objectives and learning activities are included for students and instructors to use where and when appropriate. Extensive appendices are also included.

In appreciation . . .

Thanks and appreciation to family members and colleagues who contributed photographs used in this edition. Special thanks to Jeffrey A. Nagel, who prepared new illustrations for edition 4. For manuscript preparation for all four editions, Ann Bennett gets the credit and sincere thanks for her excellent work. Laurie Muench, Associate Developmental Editor, Nursing Editorial at Mosby, encouraged and assisted in the preparation and production of this text. Suzi Epstein, Managing Editor, "kept the faith" when I needed it most. Laurie and Suzi have my special thanks.

I also extend appreciation to the reviewers who provided valuable feedback in their evaluation of the manuscript. And to the nursing students, colleagues, and childbearing families who have inspired me through the years, I owe a special debt of gratitude.

As always, to my husband Roger Phillips goes extra special thanks for his love and support. Each day he grows more precious to me.

Celeste R. Phillips

CONTENTS

Family-Centered Maternity and Newborn Care

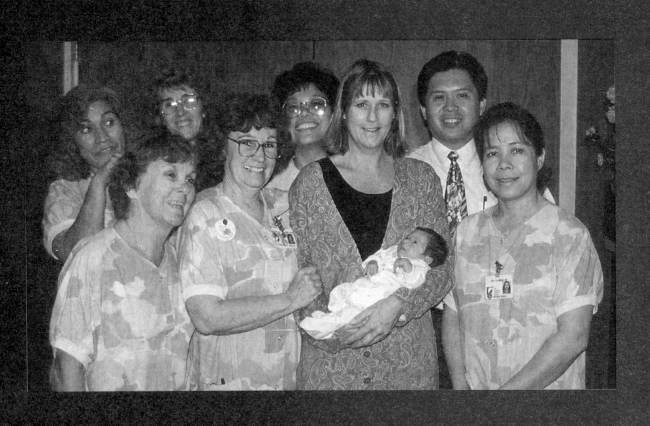

1

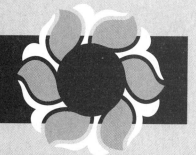

INTRODUCTION AND OVERVIEW

GOALS

This chapter is designed to provide information that will help the reader to develop:

- a background for the study of family-centered maternity and newborn care.
- awareness of parenting processes: mothering and fathering.
- appreciation for variations influencing the parenting process.
- awareness of contemporary trends in maternity care.
- understanding of team practice in maternity care.

STUDENT OBJECTIVES

After studying this chapter, you should be able to:

1. Differentiate between the key components of conventional and family-centered models of maternity care.
2. Describe historical trends influencing American maternity care.
3. Identify the numerical position of the U.S. infant mortality rate in the world.
4. Describe factors contributing to poor pregnancy outcome.
5. Discuss the concept of family and explain how pregnancy and birth can affect family members.
6. Indicate several ways in which fathers may be helped to adapt to pregnancy.
7. Discuss at least two basic differences in attitudes toward childbearing and birth.
8. Identify three emotional phases for men and three for women to experience during pregnancy to begin bonding with their unborn baby.
9. Identify four experiences that could interfere with the parent-infant relationship and result in bonding difficulty.
10. Discuss the concept of team as applied to maternity care.
11. Describe programs that seek to meet the needs of today's childbearing families.
12. Discuss culture and its implications for provision of maternity care.

INTRODUCTION

The U.S. health care system has been undergoing rapid and dramatic change since the introduction of a prospective payment system for Medicare recipients in October 1983. No longer working on a cost-plus basis, hospitals have had to reduce costs. This need for cost control has led to more efficiency, shorter hospital stays, home health care programs, wellness and fitness programs, and innovative care options both outside and within hospitals.

The conventional obstetric multitransfer system of hospital maternity care is not cost effective. In addition, it is not marketable. The issue of marketability will become more important as the health care industry becomes more competitive, price sensitive, and economically driven. A combination of increased competition and pressure for cost reduction will continue to influence the ways in which maternity care is delivered in the United States well into the twenty-first century.

Maternity Nursing

The nursing care of pregnant families is changing from obstetric nursing to maternity nursing.

Obstetrics is that branch of medicine defined as the art and science of caring for the childbearing woman and her unborn baby. The term *obstetrics* was derived from the Latin verb *obstare,* "to stand before." From this point, whenever possible we will purposely omit the terms *obstetrics, obstetric nurse,* and *obstetric personnel* because these old terms pertain to standing before the mother and concentrating on adapting care around her medical treatment.

The obstetric model is the conventional model of care, which treats pregnancy and birth as an illness that requires professional medical intervention. The patient's role is not active, and medical and nursing personnel who are in a position of authority and control make decisions about treatment. The mother and infant are considered independent patients and are served by medical and nursing personnel with different specialties (obstetricians/pediatricians and labor and delivery, postpartum, and nursery nurses, respectively). Labor and delivery often take place in separate locations. After the birth, the mother and infant may be separated at any time for routine medical and nursing procedures. Infants may be cared for primarily in a nursery, and may be taken to the mother's room only for feedings. In addition, restrictive visiting hours may be designated for the father and for other visitors.

This book is titled *Family-Centered Maternity and Newborn Care* because it focuses on a family-centered model of care and not the obstetric medical model. The term *maternity nursing* will be used. Maternity nursing is a system of care in which the nurse collaborates with the childbearing family and health care team to optimize the childbearing experience.

Nursing Process and Maternity Care

Nursing is the art and science of caring. The scope of nursing practice deals with physiologic, psychologic, and social responses of people. The nursing process is the framework upon which the maternity nursing care of the childbearing family is based. The nursing process is a dynamic, logical, problem-solving process composed of five separate but interrelated stages: assessment, diagnosis, planning, implementation, and evaluation.

The use of nursing process in maternity care benefits families by enhancing goal-directed interventions that meet family needs during the entire childbearing year.

Assessment

Assessment begins when the nurse is alerted to the needs or problems of a childbearing woman and her family. Assessment involves data collection and interpretation. Observations involve the collection of both objective and subjective data from many sources, including the woman and her family, other members of the health care team, the woman's previous records and chart, interviews, and examinations.

Nursing diagnosis

Based on the nursing assessment, the nurse develops an appropriate nursing diagnosis. Individualized nursing diagnoses are particularly helpful because they identify the woman's unique problems. Nursing diagnoses are concerned with all types of responses to childbearing and parenting and do not concentrate only on medical conditions.

Planning

Following the assessment and diagnosis steps of the nursing process, the nurse formulates a plan of care. By collaborating with the woman and her family and using physicians' orders and recommendations, together with the information obtained during the nursing assessment, the nurse can develop a nursing care plan. When planning, the nurse sets goals in family-centered terms, prioritizes these goals, and selects nursing actions to help the woman meet the goals. The goals are stated as expected outcomes for the woman and her family.

Implementation (or intervention)

Nursing interventions are the nursing actions selected to assist the woman to achieve the expected outcomes. The implementation phase includes referral to other health care team members as appropriate and co-ordination of care with all team members. To implement the nursing care plan, the nurse may perform a nursing procedure, counsel, support, administer medications, teach, or offer physical or emotional care.

Evaluation

The evaluation phase is a team process between the nurse and the family and other health care professionals, as appropriate. The purpose is to evaluate the effectiveness of the interventions and determine whether the identified goals or outcomes have been met. If goals have not been met, reassessment and modification of the plan of care is necessary.

FAMILY-CENTERED MATERNITY AND NEWBORN CARE

Family-centered maternity and newborn care (FCMNC) is a philosophy of care that focuses on the physical, social, psychological, spiritual, and economic needs of the total family unit, however the family may be defined. The family is included in decision making and planning, and its individual needs and responsibilities are recognized. FCMNC respects diversity in family structures, cultural backgrounds, choices, strengths, weaknesses, and needs. The philosophy of family-centered care requires partnerships between the childbearing woman, her family, and health care professionals.

In 1978 a joint position statement titled "The Development of Family-Centered Maternity/Newborn Care in Hospitals" was approved by the American College of Obstetricians and Gynecologists, the American Academy of Pediatrics, the American College of Nurse-Midwives, the American Nurses' Association, and the Nurses' Association of the American College of Obstetricians and Gynecologists. In this position paper, the following family-centered childbirth policies were recommended.

1. Hospitals offer preparation for birth classes for both mothers and fathers, including instruction on the role of men at birth.
2. Fathers be permitted to accompany women giving birth during the entire process, including being present in the delivery room and helping at the birth itself.
3. Hospitals offer the option of using a homelike "birthing room" rather than a standard delivery room. The birthing room would contain informal furnishings and bear little resemblance to a surgical facility, as delivery rooms presently resemble.
4. Hospitals consider an end to restrictions (some spelled out by state law or health department regulation) on young children visiting their mothers and newborn siblings in the hospital.
5. Hospitals develop programs for early discharge of mothers after birth so that the family can quickly move back into the more psychologically secure atmosphere of the home. (To do this, hospitals would probably have to develop programs in which health professionals make home visits.)

Before listing these possible physical and functional changes, the position statement emphasized that the major change in maternity care needed to make family-centered care work was *attitudinal*.

Over the years that have followed publication of this joint position statement, American maternity care has changed to become more family centered. Childbirth education, prenatal care that includes the father and other family members, 24-hour visitation for fathers in the hospital at the time of birth, sibling visitation policies, and extended visiting hours for other family members are some examples of practices that have become increasingly commonplace. However, in some hospitals medical professionals still "take over" and control the birth experience and also separate mother and infant in the first hours of life. In these instances attitudes of providers may be the stumbling blocks to achieving family-centered care.

For effective and meaningful change to occur in childbearing, FCMNC must become the norm. In FCMNC, health care personnel offer support during the childbearing year and emphasize the individual needs of the mother and family. FCMNC involves caring for not one but all family members—mother, father, infant, siblings, grandparents, and significant others. At no time during the childbearing experience should any person in this multifaceted unit be neglected because exclusion of one member of the family can have serious consequences for all members.

A team of health care professionals cooperates with family members to provide FCMNC. In this way both the physical and psychosocial needs of the family are met. This model is medically supervised but family centered. It actively involves the family and mother in what is considered a normal process (birth). The medical staff, providing unbiased information, uses their expertise to educate the family about options so that they can make decisions about treatment. The family is treated as a unit that is not separated during the hospital stay. Whenever possible, the entire birth process of labor, delivery, recovery, postpartum, and neonatal care takes place in one location, which is a homelike environment.

TABLE 1-1
Key Components of Conventional and Family-Centered Care

Conventional model	Family-centered model
Childbirth education provided simply describes hospital program.	Prepared childbirth education provides freedom of choice based on knowledge of alternatives. Pre-conception and parenting education are offered.
Pregnancy, labor, and delivery considered an illness.	Pregnancy, labor, and delivery considered a normal time of emotional, social, and physical change and stress.
Staff, in position of authority, makes treatment decisions.	Staff uses expertise to inform family of options; family makes decision; family and staff create team for treatment.
Care is routinized and rigid: governed by tradition, committees, protocols.	Care is individualized and flexible: readiness to change and depart from tradition.
Mother and infant considered separate patients.	Mother and infant served as a unit with mother-baby nursing.
Labor, delivery, recovery, postpartum, and neonatal care occur in different locations.	Labor, delivery, recovery, postpartum, and neonatal care occur in one location.
Infant cared for primarily in nursery.	Infant cared for primarily in mother's room.
Visiting hours prescribed for fathers and others.	Family and friends are encouraged to be present at any time mother wishes.
Father or supportive person(s) informed of labor progress and birth.	Father or support person(s) present, actively involved in labor, delivery, postpartum, and neonatal care.

Family and friends may visit at the mother's discretion. Table 1-1 compares characteristics of the conventional model and family-centered model of maternity care.

HISTORICAL BACKGROUND

Early Times

Until the eighteenth century, few people, including physicians, were concerned with providing women in childbirth with attendants other than untrained women. The first services provided to women at childbirth really were maternal, with mothers helping their own daughters give birth at home. However, even in these early times, women with special skills were recognized as midwives who would assist at deliveries outside their own families. The midwives concentrated on the labor and delivery; physicians were called only when there were medical complications. Even in these problem cases, however, the physician would usually only supervise or give advice while the midwife assisted the delivery.

Seventeenth Century to Nineteenth Century

Milestones in obstetric care occurred in this period: discovery of fetal heart tones and fetal circulation in the

seventeenth century, release of the Chamberlen family secret of obstetric forceps in 1813, calculation of expected date of confinement (EDC) in the early *nineteenth century,* and measurement of the female pelvis to determine the eventual course of labor. In the *eighteenth century* the use of male physicians as obstetricians came into vogue. When many of these physicians chose to deliver babies in hospitals, a new scourge, known as *puerperal sepsis* or "childbed fever," claimed the lives of many previously healthy mothers. Dr. Oliver Wendell Holmes in the United States and Dr. Ignaz Semmelweis in Vienna published papers warning of the contagiousness of puerperal fever and outlining the steps necessary (e.g., careful handwashing) to reduce the mortality from the disease. Although many physicians laughed at the simple practice of handwashing by those attending a birth, maternal mortality in hospitals declined significantly when this practice was enforced. In 1860 Louis Pasteur discovered the organism causing puerperal fever—*Streptococcus*—and thus provided the scientific rationale for the theories of Holmes and Semmelweis.

In 1853 Simpson introduced chloroform as an anesthetic in obstetrics. Although anesthetics had been used for surgery before this time, they were not used in obstetrics because it was believed that God meant for women to bring forth children in pain and suffering.

Twentieth Century

Within little more than 100 years, childbirth in the United States was dramatically transformed from a normal life event that was the province of women and took place in their homes to a medical procedure preferably attended by an obstetric specialist in a hospital.

The Industrial Revolution and its attendant impact on technology filtered through all levels of Western society and in the process significantly altered the course of childbirth. Families moved from the farms to cities and left behind many of their support structures. They also became exposed to a whole new set of dangers: poor sanitation, overcrowded living conditions, inadequate nutrition, and the poor working conditions of the newly industrialized society. A result of this dramatic social upheaval was an increase in maternal and infant mortality. As a result, public health in general and the well-being of mothers and infants in particular became new priorities.

Antepartal and postpartal care were finally seen as important parts of the care of pregnant women when the U.S. Congress established a Children's Bureau in 1912 to educate the public on the need for prenatal care. Advances in general medicine and surgical knowledge, discovery and use of antibiotics, and advances in anesthesia and analgesia all served to make giant strides in improving maternity care in the twentieth century.

In a sincere attempt to improve the lot of the childbearing family, these modern miracles led to the complete medicalization of childbirth. Leading physicians of the time considered pregnancy a disease and childbirth a surgical procedure to be managed according to the practices of general surgery. The design of hospital maternity units was identical to that of surgical suites.

The medical literature of the day contained many articles and editorials on ways to improve the care of hospitalized childbearing women. Most reinforced the belief that safety could only be assured through strict control. As a result, controlling practices proliferated, and the form of the obstetric system—the policies, procedures, and physical structure—grew to reinforce the practice of control.

Before 1900 only poor and unwed mothers gave birth in hospitals. By the 1930s it had become fashionable in American to give birth in a hospital with a male physician in attendance instead of giving birth at home with a female midwife in attendance. The percentage of American babies born in hospitals had grown to 50% by 1940 and to 99.2% by 1975.

Within a relatively short period of time, women were relegated from being the most important participant in the childbirth process to the status of the acted-upon. At this time maternal and infant mortality had improved dramatically. However, with the danger to mother and baby now under control other problems with the system surfaced. In focusing on the medical needs of the family important psychosocial needs were being neglected. Couples were undergoing a major life experience without the preparation, support, or satisfaction important to the healthy beginning of a new family.

Also, the childbearing process had become routinized at the level of maximum need; all women experienced the same, and often the maximum, amount of medical care possible. This had the effect of increasing the number of procedures, the need for nursing care, the length of stay, and the overall high cost of maternity care.

Today many childbearing families expect excellent outcomes in humanized environments with family-centered care. While increased litigation has created a defensive posture among physicians and nurses and driven up the cost of maternity care, the need for cost containment has reduced the average length of stay (ALOS) for childbirth to 24 hours post vaginal birth. To provide quality maternity care in a cost-effective manner is maternity nursing's challenge. As numerous changes continue to occur in the delivery of maternity care, nurses will continue to adjust to change while improving the quality of maternity care.

THE PLACES OF BIRTH

In the United States today families can choose where to give birth.

Alternative Birth Center

An alternative birth center (ABC) or birthing room offers a homelike environment in a hospital, usually in the maternity unit, with immediate access to emergency intervention and all of the tools that modern medicine has to offer (Fig. 1-1). These birthing rooms are cheerfully and comfortably furnished in homelike fashion. The mother is admitted to this room where she labors, gives birth and from where she may be discharged if time and requirements for room utilization permit. Sometimes she may be required to transfer to a standard postpartum room if the birthing room is needed by another family.

A birthing room is a private space designed for only low-risk childbearing families to stay in throughout their birth experience and until they are ready to go home. All medicines and equipment that may be needed are stored out of sight in a cabinet in the room. The mother gives birth, positioning herself to meet her own comfort needs (Fig. 1-2). After the birth the infant remains with the family (Fig. 1-3). Ideally one nurse stays

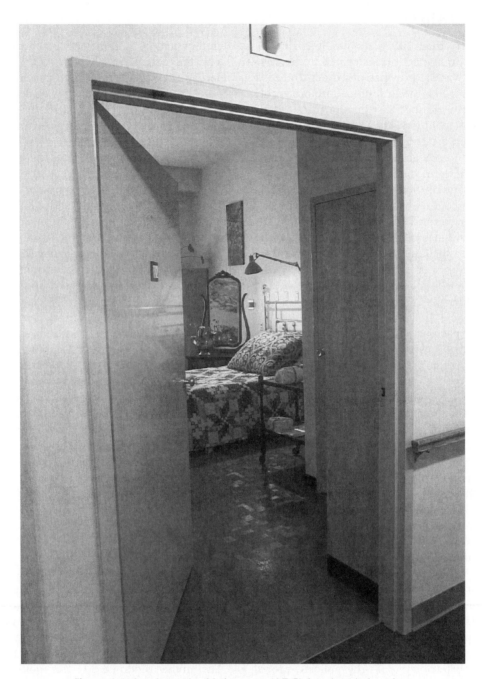

Figure 1-1 An alternative birth center (ABC) in a hospital setting.

with the family throughout labor, birth, and the immediate postpartum period, thus providing continuity of care. Within a 24- to 72-hour period after discharge, home visits to the family may be made by this nurse to check the mother and baby and to provide support for the family.

Most U.S. hospital birthing rooms were planned and designed in the early to middle 1970s to provide a viable alternative to the conventional obstetric unit in response to changing consumer desires. Utilization of ABCs varied dramatically because of diverse "risking

out criteria" and because nurses often were busy in the conventional labor and delivery rooms and could not (or would not) be spared to staff an isolated ABC. Also, low room utilization rates, extra supplies, and staffing requirements to operate two parallel systems proved to be very costly.

However, parents liked birthing rooms for the "intimate" birth experience they provided, with partner and family sharing the event. Elimination of the transfer from the labor room to the delivery suite was often singled out as the best feature of the ABC.

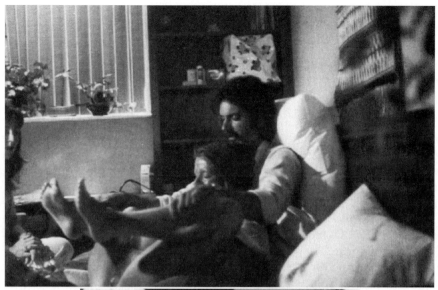

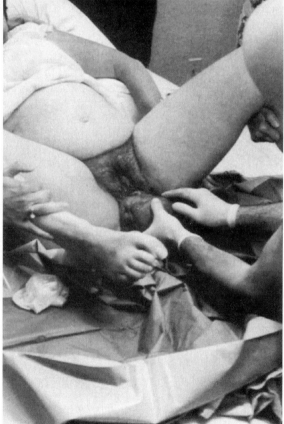

Figure 1-2 Birth.

Labor, Delivery, and Recovery Room

Clinical experience in alternative birth centers or birthing rooms proved these settings to be safe and satisfactory for many health care providers and families. Evaluation of these changes in clinical practice led to new obstetric unit designs. The combination labor, delivery, and recovery (LDR) room was designed by Ross Planning Associates (Fig. 1-4). This room was designed to eliminate transfer from labor to delivery to recovery. It is sized to accommodate up to eight persons during the birth process and equipped to provide care for all births other than cesarean births. There is no need for risk criteria or transfer to a delivery room to cope with problems. Clinical care in LDRs has proved to be safe, satisfying, and marketable.

Single Room Maternity Care

Experience in LDR rooms proved that using a single room, rather than separate rooms for labor and birth, could provide greater safety for all mothers. However, the LDR system requires a separate postpartum area and two separate nursing staffs to handle the normal childbirth process. Therefore, although LDRs are more marketable than multitransfer programs, they are no more cost efficient.

Single room maternity care (SRMC) consolidates all aspects of maternal and newborn care (labor, delivery, recovery, postpartum, and healthy newborn care) in a system of multipurpose labor/delivery/recovery/postpartum (LDRP) rooms. The SRMC system was developed to provide more cost-effective operation in the era of shorter and shorter lengths of stay and to accommodate contemporary clinical practices. (See box). It was also designed to meet the needs of parents seeking safe, quality, family-centered care in a comfortable setting

(Fig. 1-5). Unlike the birthing room, SRMC is not an alternative to low-risk maternity care. Instead it is a comprehensive replacement for the conventional multitransfer system. SRMC can be configured for Level I, II, or III maternity services in hospitals with annual birth volumes ranging from a low of 365 to a high of 8000-10,000 births per year.

In SRMC well babies are cared for along with their mothers in the LDRP rooms (mother-baby nursing). In mother-baby nursing the nursery for healthy babies is replaced by a baby "holding area" or "respite area" and a procedure room, which are part of the nursing station. The SRMC system includes operating rooms for cesarean delivery and special care nurseries (Level II and/or Neonatal Intensive Care Units) for babies in need of medical care.

The SRMC system was designed to improve high-risk care and it uses the same layout as the modern cardiac intensive care unit. Ideally, the LDRP rooms are clustered around a central service core. Equipment for labor and birth is not kept in the room but is stored within the core. The mother is not moved to special rooms for each stage of childbirth, as in the multitransfer system. All procedures, including those that deal

---

 Advantages of single room maternity care

For the physicians
Increased patient load and revenue
Less time required to make rounds on all patients clustered in one place
Greater involvement with the family
Decreased potential for liability from patient injury or infection
Positive family feedback
Opportunities to educate patients and help parents increase their skills and confidence
More cost-effective care

For the family
Decreased disruption of the physical and emotional aspects of childbirth
Safe, positive environment conducive to a sense of well-being
Opportunity for more physiological labor and delivery
Reduced risk of injury/infection by avoiding multiple transfers
No separation of the mother from her support person
No separation of the parents and the baby
Greater opportunity to increase parenting skills and confidence through shared responsibility of the baby's care
Reduced hospital cost
Increased opportunity to establish rapport with nursing personnel

For the nursing staff
Elimination of multiple transfers and the related duplication of paperwork
Fewer opportunities for communication breakdown with decreased transfer of information from one special area to another
Closer and more continuous contact improves recognition skills of potential problems
Greater involvement with the family in the childbearing process
Increased job satisfaction
More time available for nursing care and family education; less time required for multiple cleanups
Rewarding primary care nursing role
Special training in obstetrics, pediatrics and postpartum care

For the hospital
Increased savings through increased staff productivity
Increased utilization through consumer response
Increased efficiency through elimination of unnecessary tasks
Decreased risk of injury to mother by elimination of multiple transfers
Reduced space requirements
Reduced staff turnover because of greater job satisfaction
Heightened community image and visibility
More flexible utilization of staff, cross-trained in perinatal areas

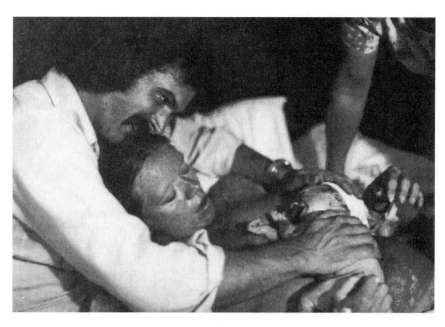

Figure 1-3 A family.

with complications and emergencies, are handled immediately in the LDRP room. Instead of moving the mother to special beds, stretchers, and tables, all-purpose birthing beds are used for both normal and complicated obstetric procedures.

Nursing care provided in LDRP rooms is truly family-centered and requires nurses capable of caring for families in all phases of the childbearing experience. These nurses are not limited in skills by functioning in only one subspecialty, that is, only the nursery, only postpartum, or only labor and delivery. They are prepared to provide care for mother and baby together in mother-baby nursing and often provide this mother-baby care to the same couple they supported during labor and birth. Instead of providing the old impersonal, fragmented, and compartmentalized care, today's nurses can put the pieces of families together in comprehensive care. Obviously rooms do not provide humanized care, people do (Fig. 1-6, *A* and *B*). However, contemporary settings such as LDR and LDRP rooms provide the environment in which maternity care can become more humane, productive, cost-effective, and marketable.

Freestanding Birth Centers

Although most ABCs or birthing rooms are located within existing hospitals, there are also freestanding birth centers. These units are outside of but often close to a hospital so that quick transport to that institution is possible if necessary. The Maternity Center Association in New York City pioneered operating a center in a homelike setting designed to serve families in the childbearing experience when it opened the first urban birth

center in New York City in 1975. Since opening day, families are accommodated in the center for prenatal care, classes in preparation for childbirth and infant care, labor and delivery, pediatric examination, and postpartum care. The environment is personalized and homelike, emphasizing family involvement and parental responsibility. The mother and baby are discharged within 12 hours of delivery and follow-up care is provided at home. As with hospital birth centers, careful prenatal screening is done and only well mothers without complications are accepted.

Most states now regulate and license birth centers and most insurance plans cover their services. Maternity care in some birth centers is one third to one half of the cost of maternity care in a hospital. Reasons for this cost reduction include the provision of few invasive procedures and the fact that supportive care occurs in a residential rather than a hospital space. There is no need for cost shifting of other hospital services, such as laboratories, laundries, and diet kitchens, to the maternity fees. As a result, overhead is kept to a minimum and consists of only the costs of operating the birth center. An additional important factor is that much of the care is provided by nurse-midwives, which means savings in staff salaries and a family-centered approach to care that supports physiologic childbirth.

The National Birth Center Study published in December 1989 dealt with questions of safety in a study of 11,814 women admitted for labor and birth in 84 freestanding birth centers in the United States. The findings showed a cesarean rate of 4.4%, no maternal mortality, and an infant mortality rate of 1.3 per 1000 births. These findings are significantly lower than hospital statistics. One woman in six (15.8%) was transferred

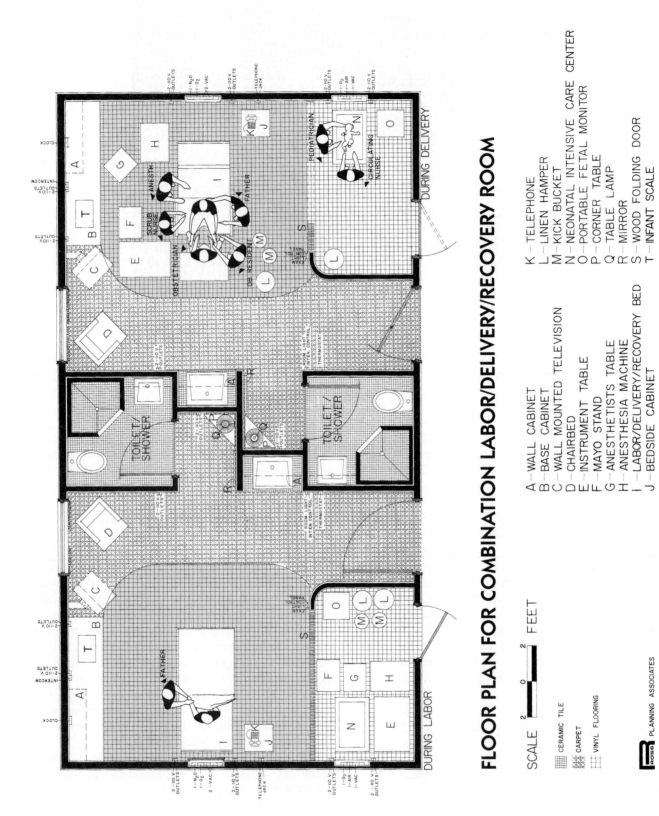

FLOOR PLAN FOR COMBINATION LABOR/DELIVERY/RECOVERY ROOM

SCALE

FEET

CERAMIC TILE
CARPET
VINYL FLOORING

ROSS PLANNING ASSOCIATES

A—WALL CABINET
B—BASE CABINET
C—WALL MOUNTED TELEVISION
D—CHAIRBED
E—INSTRUMENT TABLE
F—MAYO STAND
G—ANESTHETISTS TABLE
H—ANESTHESIA MACHINE
I—LABOR/DELIVERY/RECOVERY BED
J—BEDSIDE CABINET

K—TELEPHONE
L—LINEN HAMPER
M—KICK BUCKET
N—NEONATAL INTENSIVE CARE CENTER
O—PORTABLE FETAL MONITOR
P—CORNER TABLE
Q—TABLE LAMP
R—MIRROR
S—WOOD FOLDING DOOR
T—INFANT SCALE

Figure 1-4 The combination labor, delivery, and recovery room (LDR).

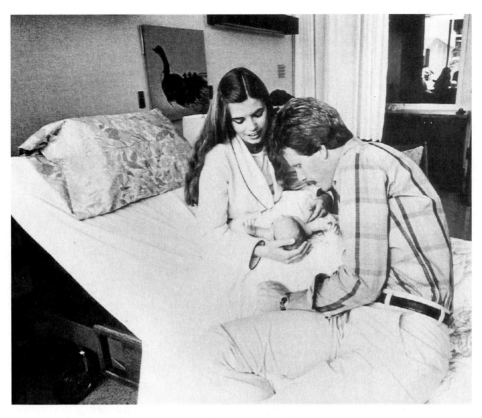

Figure 1-5 A family in SRMC.

to a hospital; 2.4% had emergency transfers. There was a savings in cost and a high degree of consumer satisfaction. The study concluded that birth centers offer a safe and acceptable alternative to hospital care for selected pregnant women, particularly multigravidas.

Despite the safety, satisfaction, and savings offered by birth centers, their future depends on health care coverage plans and liability insurance. Along with medical malpractice insurance costs for all maternity care, insurance costs for birth centers have increased. In order for birth centers to pay the high costs, charges must be adequate and the volume of births must be high enough to cover the costs of operation.

No matter what happens to the reimbursement and liability issue, however, birth centers have had a positive influence on hospital maternity care. Much of what has been learned about the normalcy of childbirth in birth centers can be utilized in all maternity care.

Home Birth

In 1989 almost all infants (98.8%) in the United States were born in hospitals, whereas 26,648 (0.7%) were born at home and 14,273 (0.4%) were born in freestanding birth centers. When births occurred in hospitals, 99.5% were attended by MDs, DOs, or certified nurse-midwives; however, doctors attended less than one fourth of home births and nurse-midwives attended

only about one eighth. Direct-entry, lay midwives, and not yet certified nurse-midwives attended 29.4% of these home births, and "others" attended 36.6%.

The literature on childbirth contains excellent statistics on medically directed home birth services with skilled nurse-midwives and medical backup. The Chicago Maternity Center, with 12,000 home births without a single maternal death from 1950 to 1960, and the Frontier Nursing Service in Appalachia, whose home delivery statistics show 23 years without a single maternal death, are two examples of such home birth services. In the United States today there are reports of very low-risk home delivery populations who have very low levels of difficulty and consequently have excellent statistics. However, there is danger in taking these data on very select populations and applying them to the total population. It must be recognized that even though labor and delivery are normal physiological events, they do present potential hazards to the mother and fetus both before and after birth. These hazards require provisions for emergency intervention and medical backup that are available in hospitals and birthing homes or in freestanding birth centers.

People who choose home birth are often very sincere and concerned about their own safety and the health and safety of their unborn child. In fact there are probably as many sincere and well-considered reasons for choosing home birth as there are home births. For many

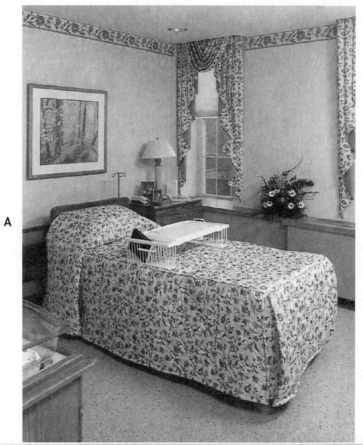

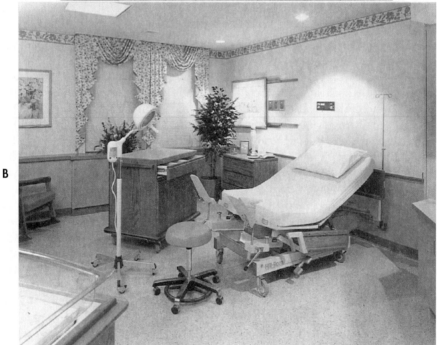

Figure 1-6 A, The LDRP Suite, Salem Hospital, Salem, Mass **B,** Working LDRP Suite, Salem Hospital, Salem, Mass. *(Photos by Robert E Mikrut. Courtesy Architects: TRO/The Ritchie Organization, Newton, Mass.)*

people, birth is a very special, intensely personal event to be shared only with family and friends and not with assorted hospital personnel who are strangers. For many others, birth is an intensely spiritual experience for which a hospital setting is totally inappropriate. Still others do not relish giving up responsibility for their births to hospital personnel. Most people choosing home birth fully understand the risks involved but also understand that there are risks in hospital birth.

In this time of rapid change, the day is probably coming when home birth will be provided with all of the necessary emergency standards and medical backup. In the meantime, health professionals have the urgent and immediate responsibility to develop hospital environments or freestanding birth center environments that provide the highest possible standards in maternity care in a family-centered environment.

NURSE PRACTITIONERS

Nursing today is dynamic—changing to include more sophisticated care requiring a substantial amount of knowledge or technical skill. Nurses are prodding the conscience of health professionals, legislatures, the government, and the public alike in their determination to improve health care. A nursing role designed to bridge the gap in the delivery of primary health care is the role of nurse practitioner, in which the nurse is prepared to practice in an expanded role. The term *nurse practitioner* originated in 1965 with the establishment of a Pediatric Nurse Practitioner program at the University of Colorado.

Important functions of nurse practitioners as members of health teams include health maintenance and preventive care. Depending on where nurse practitioners function, their duties may range from history taking and physical assessment to ordering laboratory tests and writing prescriptions for medications approved as appropriate by the physician in charge. More than half of the nurse practitioners are employed by private physicians with the remainder being employed in clinics and community agencies.

In the era of cost containment, it has become clear that many physician services can be provided by advanced practice nurses at lower cost and with equal patient satisfaction. Nurse practitioners in perinatal care are providing patient care in diverse settings such as nurse-run clinics, mobile vans, and patients' homes in addition to the traditional acute-care delivery system. Advanced practice nurses are joining in partnerships with physicians to provide quality care and balance costs.

Maternal-Child Nurse Practitioner

Nurse practitioners prepared in the specialty area of maternal and child health provide continuity of care for the mother and child throughout pregnancy and then focus on child health and development. Although they may function during the prenatal period much like nurse-midwives, maternal-child nurse practitioners do not deliver the baby.

Pediatric Nurse Practitioner

Nurse practitioners prepared in the specialty area of pediatrics provide care for infants and children in clinic settings, physicians' offices, community agencies, and hospitals. They serve a very important function in well baby care and in teaching and counseling of families with infants and children.

CHILDBIRTH EDUCATORS

Childbirth educators may be registered nurses, paraprofessionals, or laypersons with special preparation in childbirth education. The International Childbirth Education Association (ICEA) and the American Society for Psychoprophylaxis in Obstetrics (ASPO) are examples of groups that have national teacher-training and certification programs. (See Appendix H for a list of childbirth education associations).

Currently standards for childbirth educators depend on the association to which they belong, and there are no generally accepted national standards for their education. There are also no national standards for the education of nurse practitioners.

Clinical Nurse Specialists

The *clinical nurse specialist* functions in an expanded nursing role, providing direct patient care, staff education and development, and conducting research. Master's level preparation is required, and many clinical nurse specialists in maternity care have skills and preparation that cover the entire scope of perinatal care.

MIDWIFERY

The term *midwife* literally means "a helping woman." Every culture has had its midwives. American midwifery was given professional status when the first school of nurse-midwifery was started in 1932. In 1989 there were 27 educational programs in the United States and approximately 4000 certified nurse-midwives (CNMs); 200 to 250 nurse-midwives have been certified each year since 1970. Today the nurse-midwife in the United States is licensed as a registered nurse and is certified by the American College of Nurse Midwives (ACNM). The practice of nurse-midwifery has achieved separate legal recognition in a number of states, and nurse-midwives are practicing in all 50 states and Washington, D.C. In 1991 CNMs attended 158,068 hospital births, accounting for almost 4% of the total in-hospital births in the United States. A decade ago CNMs attended 55,537 or 1.5% of total hospital births.

The economic realities of managed care are creating demand for CNMs. In a capitated health care plan, providers receive a fixed amount of money to care for each individual enrolled. Certified nurse-midwives, who typically use less medical intervention than physicians and have low cesarean rates, can deliver cost-effective, quality care.

Nurse-midwives practice true FCMNC as interdependent health professionals, whether working in maternity centers, hospitals and community agencies, or with physicians in private practice. Nurse-midwives focus on the complete maternity cycle: ensuring health and growth, preventing illness, fostering family life, and helping families take responsibility for their health care while providing care for pregnancy, labor, and birth. In fact, nurse-midwives have provided many of the models for viable alternatives to conventional maternity care.

Despite an increasing awareness among consumers and health professionals that CNMs are valuable and often essential members of the health team, there are a number of lay midwives (empirical or direct-entry midwives) in this country. A lay midwife may be exceptionally well prepared for practice through self-study, apprenticeship, formal study in the basic sciences, and teaching from sympathetic health professionals. In some states lay midwives may become licensed. Conversely, a lay midwife may have very little preparation or education. Because there is no formal licensing of lay midwifery practice, a wide range of skills can be found.

OTHER TEAM MEMBERS

There are innovative programs in the United States preparing valuable maternity team members in paraprofessional roles, that is, the obstetrical technician and home health aide. The obstetric technician may be a licensed vocational nurse (LVN) or a licensed practical nurse (LPN) with intensive preparation in maternity nursing over and above the basic education program. This team member is prepared to give supportive care to well families in the childbearing cycle within hospitals or birth centers.

The home health aide is usually a high-school graduate who receives special preparation in the home care of mothers and babies. This health care team member can provide valuable assistance to the new family as they make the transition from hospital to home when there is no extended family to help.

In addition to the roles of obstetric technician and home health aide, new multiskilled patient care technicians are being developed to assume basic tasks traditionally performed by registered nurses. Selected technical tasks are assigned to nonprofessional staff. As a result it is possible to decrease the amount of time nurses spend on nonnursing tasks and "extend" the nurse.

DEFINITIONS

At the end of each chapter is a vocabulary list for the major terms in that chapter. However, a few key terms will be defined here because they are basic to understanding today's maternity care.

neonatal period the period extending from birth through the first 28 days of life. During this period the infant is referred to as a *neonate,* also called a *newborn.*

perinatal period the period extending from the 28th week of gestation through the 28th day after birth.

neonatologist a pediatrician with special training in the care of the infant in the neonatal period (neonate).

perinatologist an obstetrician with special interest in the perinatal period and particular interest in high-risk mothers and infants.

birth rate the number of live births per 1000 in population.

infant mortality rate the number of deaths of liveborn infants per 1000 live births either within the first 28 days (neonatal) or from 28 days to one year (postneonatal) in a specified geographic area or institution.

fetal mortality rate the number of deaths per 1000 births during the period from the 20th week of gestation to delivery.

perinatal mortality rate usually the sum of stillbirths and neonatal deaths per 1000 live births in a specified geographic area or institution in a given period of time.

preterm delivery birth before the 37th week of gestation.

low birth weight weight less than 2500 grams because of either prematurity or growth retardation.

morbidity condition of being diseased; number of cases of diseased or sick persons in relationship to a specific population.

maternal mortality rate the number of maternal deaths per 100,000 live births.

neonatal mortality rate the number of deaths per 1000 live births during the first 28 days of life in a specified geographic area or institution in a given time.

In maternity care, statistics such as birth rate, birth weight, and maternal and infant mortality are indicators of pregnancy outcome.

Note that infant mortality is listed in rates per 1000, whereas maternal mortality is listed in rates per 100,000. This higher base for reporting maternal mortality denotes the significant improvements in these rates.

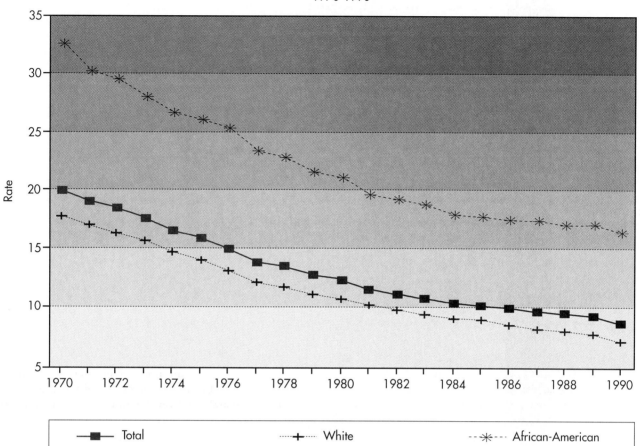

Figure 1-7 U.S. infant mortality rate by race, 1970-1990. *(From National Commission to Prevent Infant Mortality, Washington, DC.)*

CURRENT PROBLEMS AND TRENDS

Infant Mortality Rate

A common indicator of the adequacy of prenatal care is the infant mortality rate. In the United States the infant mortality rate in 1990 was 9.9 per 1000 live births, the lowest level ever recorded in this country (Fig. 1-7). However, the difference between black infant mortality, particularly in the neonatal period, was more than two times that for whites (Table 1-2).

Despite advances in health and technology, the United States tied for 21st place in infant mortality in a ranking of 28 countries with populations of more than 2,500,000 and infant mortality rates of less than 15 in 1987 (Table 1-3). Of the 28 countries reporting, 19 had rates less than 10; Japan continued to top the list, reporting a provisional rate for 1988 of an incredible 4.8.

Factors Contributing to Poor Pregnancy Outcomes

Of all the factors associated with higher infant mortality in the United States, low birth weight is cited most often. Low-birth-weight infants can be divided into two groups: preterm (about 70%) and term but growth retarded (about 30%). Infant mortality is primarily a problem of prematurity. Most deaths of premature infants are caused by:

1. Respiratory distress syndrome
2. Intraventricular hemorrhage
3. Necrotizing enterocolitis
4. Sepsis

The cause of growth retardation is unclear, but factors that have been suggested include:

1. Maternal hypotension or renal disease
2. Placental abnormalities
3. Nutritional disturbance

TABLE 1-2
Infant Mortality Rates and Black to White Ratios for Major Cause Groups

	ICD codes†	1988‡ Rate	1987‡ Rate	Total no. of deaths	1987 Rate Total	1987 Rate White	1987 Rate Black	B/W Ratio	1979	Reduction 1979 to 1987 (%)
All causes		992.9	997.0	38 408	1 008.2	862.5	1 786.4	2.07	1 296.7	22.2
Certain perinatal conditions	760-4, 766, 770-9	273.2	277.9	10 394	272.9	235.6	549.9	2.33	317.3	14.0
Congenital anomalies	740-759	207.2	207.0	7 884	207.0	206.2	226.5	1.10	257.7	19.7
Sudden infant death syndrome	798.0	117.4	116.1	5 230	137.3	120.5	225.5	1.87	142.8	3.9
Respiratory distress syndrome	769	80.4	86.4	3 283	86.2	76.5	145.6	1.90	155.8	44.7
Short gestation and low birth weight	765	90.9	84.8	3 354	88.0	59.4	233.2	3.93	100.5	12.4
Intrauterine hypoxia–birth asphyxia	768	20.3	25.5	791	20.8	16.8	41.9	2.49	48.4	57.0
Pneumonia and influenza	480-487	14.4	17.6	674	17.7	13.8	35.4	2.57	33.1	46.5
Birth trauma	767	4.6	5.0	248	6.5	5.3	12.8	2.42	31.7	79.5
Certain gastrointestinal diseases	008-9, 535, 555-8	4.4	5.0	203	5.3	3.7	13.5	3.65	10.7	50.5
Human immunovirus infection	*042-*044§	‖	‖	87	2.3	1.1	8.4	7.63		
All other causes	Residual	180.1	172.1	6 260	166.5	124.7	302.1	2.42	199.0	16.3

International Classification of Diseases (ICD), 9th revision.
†Provisonal data.
‡This category was added by National Center for Health Statistics in 1987. Categories *042 to *044 are not part of ICD.
§Data not available.
Data from National Center for Health Statistics.[2,6] Rates per 100,000 live births.

TABLE 1-3
Births and Infant Mortality Rates, 28 Countries with Population More than 2,500,000 and Infant Mortality Rate Less than 15 in 1987*

Country	1987 Births		Infant mortality rate	
	No.	Rate	1988†	1987
Japan	1,346,658	11.1	4.8	5.0
Sweden	105,000	12.5	5.8	5.7†
Finland	59,241	12.0		6.1
Switzerland	76,100	11.6		6.8
Canada	369,441	14.4		7.3
Hong Kong	69,811	12.4	7.4	7.4
Ireland	58,864	16.6		7.4
Singapore	43,889	16.8	7.0	7.4†
France	768,040	13.8	7.7	7.6†
Netherlands	186,651	12.7	7.5	7.6
Denmark	56,300	11.0		8.3
German Federal Republic	640,752	10.5		8.3
Norway	54,501	13.0		8.4
German Democratic Republic	225,959	13.6	8.1	8.5†
Spain	434,490	11.2		8.5†
				(1985)
Australia	244,347	15.0	9.2	8.7
United Kingdom	776,400	13.6	8.8	9.1†
Belgium	117,402	11.8		9.7†
Austria	85,923	11.3	8.1	9.8
New Zealand	55,248	16.8		10.0
Italy	548,116	9.6	9.5	10.1
United States	3,809,394	15.7	9.9	10.1
Israel	99,022	22.7		11.5
Greece	105,899	10.8		12.6†
Czechoslovakia	214,505	13.8	11.9	13.1†
Cuba	179,477	17.4	11.9	13.3†
Portugal	123,218	12.0		14.2
Bulgaria	115,586	13.0		14.7

*Data from United Nations Statistical Office. Countries listed in order of 1987 infant mortality rate. Birth rate per 1000 population. Infant mortality rate per 1000 live births.
†Provisional data.

4. Viral infections
5. Cigarette smoking
6. Alcohol and substance abuse

A lack of prenatal care has been demonstrated to bear a direct relationship to the rate of prematurity and low birth weight. In the United States where a baby is born, what color he or she is and how much money the parents earn affect the infant's chances of surviving the first year of life. Infant mortality rates are highest in rural, nonmetropolitan counties and in inner-city areas of large cities.

It is very apparent when viewing the alarmingly higher rate of infant mortality among blacks and other minorities that something is radically wrong. The people most in need of instruction regarding preconception and conception health actually receive the least amount of education. Although women attending tax-supported prenatal clinics often receive minimal instruction, the opposite is occurring for women obtaining private medical care, since classes in prepared childbirth are proliferating throughout the United States for families who can afford private care.

Studies have demonstrated the effectiveness of preterm birth prevention education, increased visits, and specific interventions to prevent preterm delivery. By providing enhanced prenatal care services, including psychosocial, health education, and nutritional services, preterm births can be reduced in a cost-effective manner.

Although prenatal programs can improve outcomes, formidable financial and cultural barriers to the use of perinatal services exist for many women in the United States. Understanding these barriers is important to solving the problem.

To decrease the U.S. infant mortality rate will require a combination of medical, nursing, and social efforts to change a maternity care system that is fragmented and overly complex, particularly for low-income women, uninsured women, homeless women, teenagers, newly arrived immigrants, and inner-city residents.

Maternal Mortality

Maternal death rates in the United States have declined more than thirtyfold since 1940. Greater use of prenatal care, improved intrapartal care, technical advances in medical care, lower parity, fewer unwanted births, and a decrease in the number of illegal abortions have all contributed to the lower rate of maternal mortality. However, as with infant mortality, the rate of maternal mortality for black women and other minority races is three times higher than that for white women. Increased efforts to provide access to family planning and prenatal services for black women and women of other minority races could probably reduce this differential.

IMPROVING MATERNITY CARE

In view of the overwhelming effects of social influences on infant and maternal mortality rates, it would seem that we should seriously reexamine our priorities. A step in the right direction may be to change our goal from discovering a new substance in the amniotic fluid or developing a new and better electronic monitoring system to alleviating prematurity and low birth weight.

Since 80% of women experience normal childbirth, a new maternity model may be appropriate, designating two levels of care:

1. *Low risk*—a simple, humanistic model for healthy women
2. *High risk*—a more complex but still humanistic model for women with medical complications or complications of pregnancy

In keeping with the concept of levels of care, many states have regionalized maternity and newborn care with the goal of ensuring access to the appropriate level of care. Basically this involves dividing a state into regions according to population distribution and geography and providing levels of care ranging from routine care for uncomplicated births to complex care for complicated births. These levels follow:

Level III ("tertiary" care): A teaching and research hospital providing care for high-risk maternal-fetal and neonatal patients with complications. This regional center has a minimum of 2000 births a year, many of these being normal deliveries.

Level II ("intermediate" care): A hospital providing care for the normal mother and newborn and limited care for the high-risk mother and newborn. This district center has 1000 to 2000 births per year and special care nurseries for stabilization of newborns prior to transfer to the Level III center. This hospital also has 24-hour laboratory, radiology, ultrasound, and in-house anesthesia services.

Level I ("primary" care): A hospital providing primarily routine maternity and newborn care. This is usually a small community hospital with at least 1000 births a year. The goal of such hospitals is to detect high-risk mothers and babies and transfer them early to the regional center.

If regionalization of care is to work, a team approach must be developed with physician referral to appropriate medical facilities for Level III care and referral for "stepped-down" care (that is, referral from intensive to intermediate care) as well.

THE FAMILY

The family is the oldest human institution, and in many ways it is the most important. Families have existed since earliest times and will continue to exist in *some form* as long as human beings live on earth. Families began and survived as the basic unit of society because they serve vital human needs (Fig. 1-8).

There are five models of the family, each with its own definition. The two most frequently considered when hospital maternity policies are written are the legal family model and the family structure model. Three other models are (1) the normative or moral model, (2) the social-psychological model, and (3) the functional model. These five models of the family are explained in Table 1-4.

Each family is defined by its unique history, culture, and set of values. A family functions as a nurturing center for human development (Fig. 1-9). In a contemporary family the following functions are important aspects of family life: (1) affection, (2) personal security and acceptance, (3) satisfaction and a sense of purpose, (4) continuity of companionship and association, (5) socialization, and (6) establishment of limits. These functions of a family can be met by changing family forms of diverse styles and shapes that include the following:

Communal families. Groups of people, not all from the same family, sharing living accommodations and

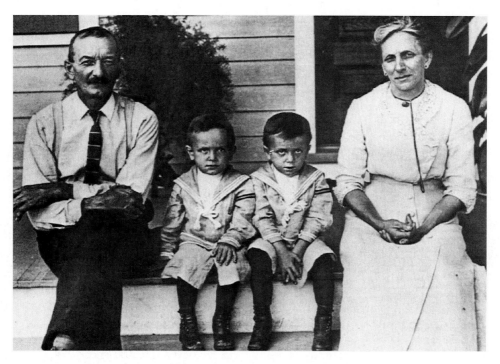

Figure 1-8 Turn-of-the-century American family.

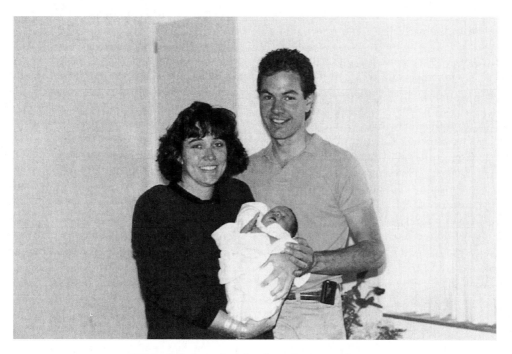

Figure 1-9 A nuclear family today: a new image.

goods and working together to achieve the group's goals.

Social contract marriages. Couples "living together" without a marriage ceremony.

Single parents. One out of every four children in the United States (or 16.2 million children) is in a single-parent family. Single parenting can be the result of separation, divorce, or death of a partner or can simply be a matter of individual choice. Although many single parents worry about being an effective mother or father to their children, they can fill the dual role successfully. An understanding of what forces (other than parental) con-

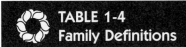

TABLE 1-4
Family Definitions

Model	Definition
Legal family model	Defined by law and varies from one state to another but commonly consists of married heterosexuals and their legitimate children. (There were 2,444,000 marriages reported in 1983.)
Family structure model	Defined by the U.S. Census Bureau for statistical purposes as two or more persons, residing together, who are related by blood, marriage, or adoption.
Normative or moral model	Defined by most religions as the nuclear family for the purpose of determining biological links, legal recognition, and patriarchal hierarchy. Families headed by women are excluded.
Social-psychological model	Defined as a group in which parents and children interact, live in residence, or have significant and frequent contact. The phrase "significant other" identifies them.
Functional model	Defined by linking family and society. The family is viewed as passive, whose purpose is sharing of consumption of material goals.

Modified from Sydner DP: *The family in post-industrial America*, pp. 25-33, Boulder, Colo, 1979, Westview Press.

tribute to childhood development, how these forces interact, and how to find and use them is essential for single parents.

Blended families. Blended families are defined as one adult plus one or more children from one family and one adult plus one or more children from another family. Developmental issues for blended families include commitment to a new marriage and to a newly formed family, and being ready to deal with complexity and ambiguity.

Divorced families. In 1983 there were three times as many divorces as there were in 1955 and twice as many as in 1965. The median duration of marriage before divorce was 7 years. Demographers project that half of all first marriages made today will end in divorce.

Lesbian parents. A review of women's health literature suggests that the lesbian pregnancy experience is characterized by the use of donor insemination. Because of the lack of societal acceptance of the lesbian life-style, the lesbian couple may have to depend on peers rather than family networks for social support.

Skip-generation parents. This nontraditional family is often formed when parents cannot or will not assume responsibility for their children. This phenomenon is often linked to parental drug or alcohol abuse. Grandparents assume responsibility for the rearing of their neglected or abused grandchildren.

Nuclear family. The family of marriage, parenthood, or procreation, consisting of husband, wife, and children, either natural, adopted, or both.

Extended family. The nuclear family plus the relatives of either or both spouses, all living together.

Adolescent parents. The terms *adolescent parent, teenage parent,* and *school-aged parent* all apply to parents at an

age or developmental stage that is considered premature or inappropriate.

Adolescent Parent

It is estimated that one million adolescent girls become pregnant each year. One third of these pregnancies will end in abortion, and the other two thirds will result in adolescent parenthood.

Changing life-styles with an evolution in attitudes toward adolescent sexuality have resulted in an earlier onset of sexual intercourse, although the use of contraception is not generally well accepted among adolescents.

Adolescence can be divided into three stages of growth and development: early, mid, and late (Table 1-5). Regardless of the stage adolescence is a time of turmoil during which many developmental tasks must be achieved. Perhaps the most difficult task an adolescent must accomplish is to develop a personal identity. This can be very difficult for a young woman who has to recognize the growing fetus inside her as a separate person.

Complicating adolescent pregnancy is the fact that this is a high-risk population for medical and social complications. Risk factors (such as late prenatal care; family stress; poor nutrition; use of alcohol, tobacco, and other drugs; and sexually transmitted infections) are not age related but are often correlated with early sexual intercourse and pregnancy. In the general population the rate of perinatal mortality in teenage pregnancies is elevated compared with pregnancies of women in their 20s (30% higher in some studies).

Adolescents experience higher levels of pregnancy

TABLE 1-5
Stages of Adolescence

Area	Early adolescent 11-14	Midadolescent 15-17	Late adolescent 18-20
Body	Rapid changes leading to discomfort and self-consciousness; body image in flux	Growing comfort with body	Acceptance of adult body
Family	Strong but ambivalent ties to family	Struggle for independence and autonomy; constant testing of limits	Reestablishment of ties with family
Peers	Same-sex friends most common	Strong peer influence assists in separation from family	Individual relationships sought and valued
Sexuality	Undifferentiated relationships with same and opposite sex; fantasy common but actual activity infrequent	Sexual experimentation and risk taking; need to feel grown-up; tendency to be easily influenced	Intimate, committed relationships sought
Cognition	Concrete, here-and-now thinking; inability to appreciate long-term consequences of actions; denial as major defense	Impulsive and unpredictable behavior; variable ability to think abstractly	Abstract thinking achieved by most but not all
Identity	Self-concept changing from child to adult; awkward and shy in social situations; authority figures looked to for guidance	Preoccupation with self and own concerns; moodiness; limited social skills; authority figures viewed as threats to autonomy	Ability to appreciate others' needs and feelings; authority figures viewed as equals

From Fuller SA: Care of postpartum adolescent, *MCN* 11:399 Nov/Dec 1986.

complications than older women and a higher incidence of low birth weight infants. The unfavorable outcome of these infants appears to be the major childbearing hazard of adolescent pregnancy. Pregnancy-induced hypertension (PIH) is the most prevalent medical complication in young, pregnant adolescents. Because adequate prenatal care is an important determinant of birth weight and prematurity, the key to reducing complications in adolescent pregnancy is the timing, quality, and quantity of prenatal care.

Although the motivations for pregnancy in adolescence can be as numerous as those for any pregnancy, during adolescence the pregnancy is frequently unwanted and therefore a crisis. With an adequate support system some young mothers are very capable of child care, whereas others have a very difficult time with mothering. The adolescent needs a great deal of help in decision making from a support person who can be trusted for honesty, consistency, and stability. The crisis of adolescent pregnancy can be a time of responsible planning and difficult decision making and ultimately result in the adolescent's becoming mature and assuming increased responsibility.

Both adolescent mothers and fathers are less likely than their peers to graduate from high school. When they do graduate, they are more apt to enter the work force earlier and take low-paying jobs with little opportunity for advancement.

In the process of providing support and counseling for the adolescent mother, the single father is often forgotten. It is wrongly assumed that he is unconcerned about the pregnant girl, her safety, or the well-being of his child. If he wants to be involved, it is important to include the single father in planning alternative solutions regarding the child's future. Many young, single fathers-to-be have difficulty believing that they are about to become fathers. Being involved in the prenatal care, pregnancy outcome planning, and even labor and birth can help them face the reality of the situation and the responsibilities involved.

It is very important to identify referral sources for social, educational, and vocational resources for both adolescent parents. Programs in child development and infant stimulation have proven useful for infants of teenaged mothers. In addition, support and counseling, information on contraception, reproductive physiology, and child development will help give adolescents the skills necessary to improve their parenting.

Family Trends

Because we live in a time of transition and rapid change, we cannot understand families without recognizing the economic factors, life-styles, and values that influence them. Corporate restructuring with numerous layoffs, unemployment, the economy, and the increased costs of raising children often cause family stress.

A smaller proportion of women today fill the traditional full-time housekeeping role. Two thirds of all American mothers are in the labor force, and almost half of all mothers with infants under 1 year of age work outside the home. With these social changes, pregnancy no longer has to end a woman's career. The Pregnancy Discrimination Act mandates that employers can neither force a pregnant woman to quit working nor can they deny a woman a job or pass her over for a promotion because she is pregnant.

There is a definite trend in this country toward delaying the age at which couples have their first child. Many factors influence this trend, including late marriages, career choices, education, control over fertility and infertility, and financial concerns. Most of the women postponing pregnancy until their 30s are post-World War II baby boomers. As this group aged in the 1980s, the total number of women aged 35 to 40 increased by 42%, from 13.0 to 18.5 million. In the early years of the 1990s the tail end of the baby boom generation reached the 30 to 40 age range. For the most part these women have good support systems and economic stability. They have planned their pregnancies and consider their experience to be a "premium pregnancy." These "older" or "mature" women often shop for a facility and a maternity program that offer the benefits they feel are important. Thus in the highly competitive and cost conscious health care environment of the 1990s, the older primigravida is an important consumer.

Although many women are shopping for a place to give birth, a growing population of women have limited access to health care. Thirty-seven million Americans have no insurance. Sixty percent are women of childbearing age or children. One out of every five children lives in poverty; the rate is twice as high among blacks and Hispanics.

These changing economic factors, life-styles, values, and childbirth practices affect children and their families in many ways. How family members see their roles may vary significantly within different cultural groups; nevertheless, in every family the action of one individual affects all other members. A birth in the family affects each family member according to that person's own needs and expectations. A new baby in the family can mean competition for a sibling, more work for the grandparents, financial worry for the parents, loss of privacy for some family members, less physical space in the house, and change in life-styles for all family members. As pregnancy and the idea of a new baby are introduced to the family, the effect of the physical and emotional changes of the mother on her relationship with the family must also be considered.

Cultures

FCMNC is applicable to all racial, socioeconomic, cultural, and ethnic groups. The goal of FCMNC is to treat each family with dignity and each family member as an individual. The trend for the twenty-first century will be toward greater ethnic, racial, and cultural diversity, with minorities maintaining their cultural identities while participating in American life.

Health care providers sometimes make value judgments about the way family members should act during a woman's labor and birth. These judgments are based on their own cultural norms and standards, developed during childhood from their own personal family values. Attitudes are influenced by each person's own culture and professional socialization.

When values differ from our own, we must listen, be nonjudgmental, reach out, be sensitive to the differences, and understand any reluctance the family may have to accepting new and foreign ideas. In working with a culturally diverse population, there is one rule that always holds true: We *never* have the right to impose our own personal convictions on anyone.

To communicate with a childbearing woman in transcultural health care, it is important to first identify her cultural background, determine her level of acculturation, and determine whether and what type of support systems are present, if any. To achieve this basic level of understanding, anthropologist Alan Harwood suggests determining the following characteristics:

1. Level of education, literacy, and English language skill
2. Number of generations in the United States
3. Household composition
4. Presence of family members in vicinity
5. Previous experiences with the U.S. health care system
6. Country of origin
7. Age at immigration (if applicable)
8. Residence (rural or urban) in native land
9. Contact with birthplace after immigration to United States
10. Closeness of coethnics

With this information, some assumptions can be made about the woman's cultural health-related beliefs and attitudes about childbearing. More specific information on the childbirth practices of the woman's individual culture can be obtained through further interviews.

The childbearing experience can focus on four components of a cultural system: (1) the moral and value system, (2) the kinship system, (3) the knowledge and belief system, and (4) the ceremonial and ritual system. In family-centered maternity care, practices are adapted to the individual woman's culture. Resources to meet the needs of diverse populations, such as interpreters and educational materials in different languages, are made available. Community leaders, resources, and traditional health care providers of various cultures are included in provision of family-centered maternity care.

Rights

As providers of care for the childbearing family, we have a responsibility to ask ourselves again and again: Whose birth is this? To whom does the baby belong?

People do not give up rights when they enter a health care institution. They have the same rights as any other human being in our society. Many patients' rights are derived from the necessity to obtain informed consent. Informed consent simply means that patients have a right to participate in the decisions that determine what may or may not be done with their bodies and their minds. They need to be sufficiently aware of what is going to happen so that they can make appropriate decisions.

The American Hospital Association's "Patient's Bill of Rights" is a national policy statement distributed to its member hospitals throughout the country. This statement is intended to help the consumer understand what to expect in effective patient care. For childbearing families, the Committee on Patients' Rights, headed by Doris and John Haire, published the "Pregnant Patient's Bill of Rights." "The Pregnant Patient's Responsibilities" was prepared by members of the International Childbirth Education Association. Both of these papers are reproduced in Appendix B so that you can study and discuss them.

FATHERING: PATERNAL INVOLVEMENT IN LABOR AND BIRTH

In our culture, the father's role in childbearing has changed greatly in the past 100 years. In the nineteenth century childbirth was accepted as a natural part of the life cycle, usually occurring at home with the assistance of a midwife, a woman relative, a family physician, or the father if he was the only one available to assist. But whether the father assisted in the delivery or not, he was close at hand, proudly interested in the labor and birth.

As society became more complex, more women gave birth in hospitals if they could afford it. Then instead of actively participating at the birth, the father waited in a hospital fathers' waiting room designed just for him.

Our culture's stereotyped sex roles also had a great deal to do with moving childbirth to women's wards in hospitals and keeping it there. A man in our culture has had to repress his feelings of tenderness and gentleness, causing him to downplay his role as father and thus making fatherhood a social obligation, whereas motherhood has always meant nurturing and meeting the physical and emotional needs of the family.

A man in our culture was expected to be "manly" and provide financially for his family, whereas a woman was expected to be "motherly" (nurturing).

The irony of all this is that the role of the father is tremendously important for the mental health of the family. Study after study indicates that emotional disturbances in children can be traced to the detachment or lack of involvement of a father with his children.

Men's reactions to fatherhood are many and diverse. Many expectant fathers have a joyful reaction to impending fatherhood, whereas others may react with depression, fear, anger, or jealousy. How a man reacts may depend on his childhood memories of his own father, his mother's pregnancies, his own childhood, his financial status, and number of children he already has.

During pregnancy a man must deal with the change of his partner's role to "mother" while he is becoming a "father." In addition, he may further be confused when his partner begins to evaluate him in terms of what kind of father he will be, as he may be wondering himself. Pregnancy may be a time when the man also needs mothering and feels strongly dependent.

Pregnancy may be a real testing ground for a man-woman relationship as well as a training ground for parenthood. Pregnancy can be a crisis time for men as well as women.

During pregnancy men are often worried about the increasing financial responsibilities they will have. Also, it is not unusual for some men in pregnancy to unintentionally acquire the symptoms presented by the pregnant women, such as nausea and vomiting in the first trimester.

The labor and birth, as the culmination of pregnancy, and the beginning of the relationship between father and child can have a marked influence on the father, both positive and negative (Fig. 1-10).

Stresses in Father Participation

Today in the United States more than 80% of fathers are present at the birth of their child. However, in most instances the father continues to be seen primarily as the maternal support person, rather than as a man about to become a father. The changing roles of men and women in family life are placing increased stress on

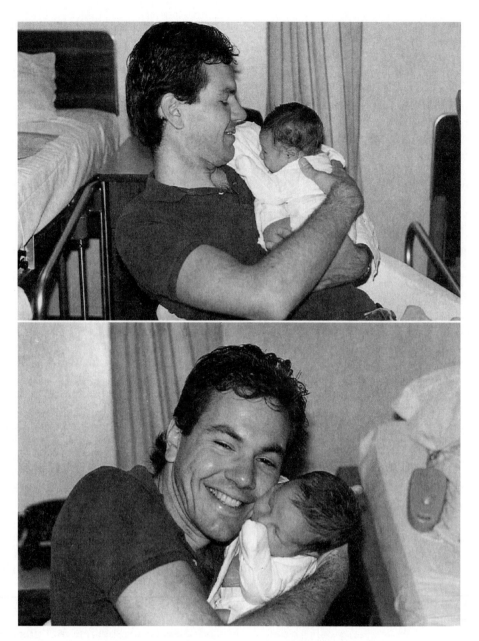

Figure 1-10 Father and newborn son.

both partners. Fathers have increasing pressure because of the growing number of mothers working, shortened hospital stays for birth, lack of supportive extended families, and the expectation that the father *will be* the woman's primary support person for labor and birth.

It is not unusual for fathers to feel very anxious about meeting society's expectations for their performance, first at labor and birth, and then at parenting. It is important to assess each couple individually and to encourage them to discuss their changing roles, wants, and needs early in pregnancy, or better yet, in preconception counseling.

During the birth experience health care providers must be sensitive to the feelings and needs of the expectant father. Expectant fathers may experience a type of "culture shock" when entering a hospital labor and delivery area. An unfamiliar physical environment can be disorienting and cause the father to feel as if he were a visitor instead of a participant. Many fathers begin labor physically tired after weeks of sleep that was interrupted by dreams. Also, their needs for food and for elimination do not stop as their mates labor. The question is: What is meaningful participation for a father in the birth process and what are his needs? Merely being present at birth does not mean that the needs of fathers are being met. It is also important to recognize that some fathers may be perfectly content to wait in a separate room during the labor and birth. When fathers choose *not* to participate, nurses need to respect and support that choice.

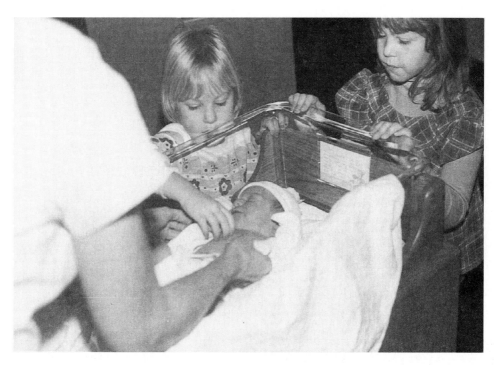

Figure 1-11 Big sisters with baby brother.

PSYCHOLOGICAL ASPECTS

Psychological Aspects for Siblings

Once again, it is important to individualize care. Some parents want their children present at the birth of their new sibling, others do not. There is a diversity of opinions on the issue of sibling presence, as present theories on sibling participation are still quite primitive. Parents have a right to make their own decisions, whereas medicine and nursing provide education, guidance, and sensitive care. If the parents choose sibling participation at birth, preparation for the experience is essential. Issues to cover during preparation include the wetness, smells, and sounds of birth; the basic anatomy and physiology of labor and birth; the hard work, intensity, and pain of labor and birth; plus the procedures involved. It is also essential to have a supportive person, in addition to the father, help the sibling during labor and birth.

Whether siblings participate in the labor and birth, it is very important for them to visit and interact with their mother and their new brother or sister after birth. Our goal should be to *minimize* separation anxiety (from parents) and jealousy toward the new baby. When meeting the new baby, the sibling should be told to examine the baby and discover his or her unique traits, thus bridging the gap between reality and fantasy (Fig. 1-11). Sibling-to-sibling relationships endure beyond parent-child relationships and are longer than husband-wife relationships. In our society sibling relationships are often characterized by life-long struggle, rivalry, and competitiveness. Could this be changed?

Psychological Involvement of Grandparents

Biological links and generational ties are profound. Grandparents who attend the birth of their grandchild provide a special kind of love and support. They want to see and hold the new baby but may feel left out, especially when hospitals limit postpartum visiting time for grandparents.

Many grandparents do not understand the need for childbirth preparation classes because their own birth experiences may have been with liberal use of anesthesia. Often, women who had general anesthesia for their own births may relive their suppressed birth experience when present for their daughters' labor and birth. These women need support so that they may verbalize feelings. Sharing the birth experience between generations can help all family members understand what being a family means.

Psychological Aspects of Postpartum Period

During the postpartum period new parents have to balance their own partner's and infant's needs. They also have to cope with changes in self, relationships, and

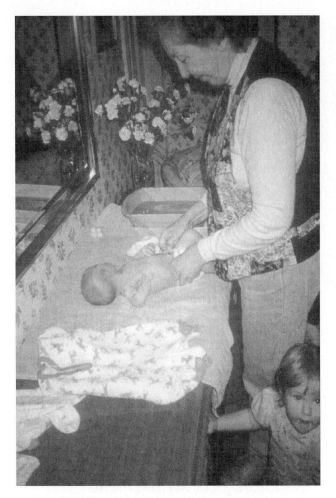

Figure 1-12 Grandma and the new baby.

routines while redefining relationships with parents and friends.

Men become fathers and grandfathers. Women become mothers and grandmothers (Fig. 1-12). Children become brothers and sisters, and numerous other roles change for family members and friends through the birth experience. Although all of these changes began months earlier, the result of 8 to 16 hours of an average labor brings the reality of a new life and all that this means to everyone in the family.

BONDING: PARENT-INFANT ATTACHMENT

Bonding is the early attachment that takes place between parents and infants within the first hours and days after birth. It can be facilitated and reinforced by physical contact and is primarily unidirectional from parent to infant. When there is bonding difficulty, the infant may be at risk of being abused. All health care providers who work with childbearing families should be able to recognize behavior that indicates successful bonding or bonding difficulty or delay.

Attachment is an affectional tie between infants and parents that begins during pregnancy, continues through birth, and flourishes over a lifetime. Attachment is reciprocal between mother and infant and between father and infant. Many variables influence attachment.

Bonding During Pregnancy

Bonding does not occur magically at the time of birth but progresses throughout pregnancy, beginning when the mother confirms the pregnancy. With any pregnancy, whether planned or unplanned, a woman has many new and different feelings, including ambivalence toward the pregnancy. Rubin describes the first trimester for women as the "Who, me? Now?" stage. We will describe the first trimester for men as the "Why me? Why now?" stage. When learning of the woman's pregnancy, the man is often ambivalent, sometimes both pleased that he can "father" biologically but worried about what kind of father he will be. The lack of obvious physical evidence of the pregnancy permeates this stage, and both the mother and the father focus on themselves and their own needs.

As the pregnancy progresses and fetal movement is felt and the woman blossoms out into maternity clothes, Rubin identifies the period as that of "radiant health." Uncertainty about the pregnancy is removed by the positive presence of the fetal movement. If they have accepted the pregnancy and moved through the ambivalence of the first trimester, the couple's focus is now on the baby. During the second trimester many men go through a period of creative, warm feelings. Feeling the baby move for the first time is a profound experience, and they begin thinking seriously about becoming fathers.

Rubin describes the last trimester as a period of "watchful waiting" for women; it is a period of anxious concern and waiting for the father. He is often very concerned about his mate's physical safety as the time for birth approaches. Bonding with their unborn baby begins as both the man and the woman move through these emotional phases of pregnancy on their way to successful role changes (Table 1-6).

All family members of a pregnant woman, as well as the woman herself, should be offered prenatal classes or prenatal counseling and teaching to prepare for the birth and to help them work through the emotional phases and preparatory tasks of pregnancy.

Bonding Behavior

In studying parent-infant behavior immediately after birth, it has been demonstrated that parents want to

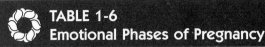

	Women (mother)	Men (father)
First trimester	Who, me? Now?	Why me? Why now?
Second trimester	Radiant health	Creative, warm feelings
Third trimester	Watchful waiting	Anxious concern and waiting

make eye contact with their babies. Very early after delivery mothers have been heard to say, "Open your eyes," "What color are your eyes?," and "Oh, she's looking at me!" The parents and baby need to have eye contact to respond to each other. Since babies can focus on an object 12 to 16 inches away, breast-feeding immediately after birth is an ideal opportunity to have eye contact. The initial position that facilitates eye contact has been given the term "en face." It has been reported that the baby is most alert and can make eye contact with the mother immediately following birth, following her visually for 180 degrees.

Another bonding behavior with infants that has been noted is the manner in which parents first touch their babies. The initial touching is very lightly with the fingertips to the baby's extremities, gradually increasing to touching with the palm and then with the whole hand, encompassing the trunk and head with the hand.

A variety of experiences may interfere with the parent-infant relationship. These happen throughout pregnancy and immediately after birth. Some of the more common experiences follow:

1. Unplanned pregnancy
2. Poor relationship between partners
3. Lack of education about what is happening both physically and emotionally
4. Attitude of health care providers toward parents
5. Separation at time of birth
6. Previous negative experiences in childbirth
7. Disappointment about birth outcome (for example, need for anesthesia, unexpected cesarean, infant with congenital anomalies)

When parents cannot have contact with their infant in the early days of life, they need to be reassured that bonding is an ongoing process and that lack of early contact will not compromise their long-term relationship with their child.

Factors that could be described as bonding difficulty are as follows:

1. Parents not touching infant; holding infant at arm's length
2. Disinterest in infant; perceiving infant to be ugly
3. Anger and noncommunication between parents

4. Expectations for infant; wanting a female or male *only*

Factors that could be described as indicating bonding are as follows:

1. Eye contact (parent-infant-parent)
2. Touching infant and holding infant close to body
3. Talking, cooing, smiling, seeing infant as pretty or cute
4. Undivided attention toward infant
5. Calling infant by name

BONDING PROMOTION STRATEGIES

Klaus and Kennel have developed the following specific recommendations for maternity care to enhance the father-mother-infant bond:

1. Identify specific needs for a mother that would influence the birth and her ability to adapt to mothering (also true for fathers).
2. Encourage all parents to attend prenatal education classes to ensure their role as active participants in childbirth (does not mean natural birth only).
3. Encourage that a significant person be present with the mother during labor and delivery to offer support and reassurance.
4. Enhance attachment by allowing privacy (long periods of father-mother-infant contact and the opportunity for the parents to assume all care for their infant with a nurse available to assist when needed).
5. Avoid putting silver nitrate or erythromycin ointment in the infant's eyes until the parents have been able to have close contact with the baby during the first hour of life.
6. Allow the mother, infant, and father to interact as a new family without interruptions.
7. Encourage rooming-in to assist the parents in recognizing the normal behavior of their infant before going home.
8. Allow families, including children, to make hospital visits to provide emotional support for all the family members and to prevent possible trauma from the separation.

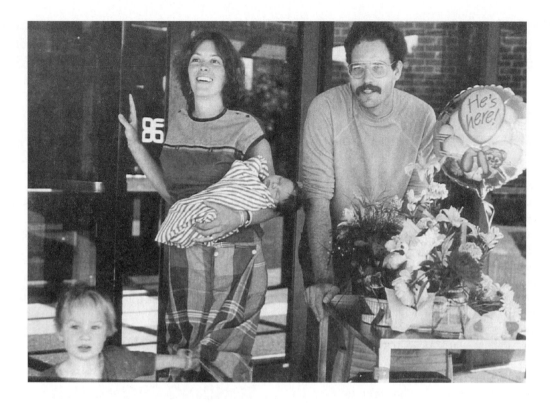

Figure 1-13 The new family leaves the hospital.

BONDING PROMOTION AMONG SPECIFIC POPULATIONS

Economically disadvantaged women may face numerous stressful situations that distract their attention from developing relationships with their infant. They may be worried about lack of money and chaotic home situations. It is important to assess the social networks and resources of these women individually and nonjudgmentally so that they can be enrolled in support programs such as the Special Supplemental Food Program for Women, Infants, and Children (WIC) and Medicaid (if eligible). Ideally, this assessment would be done prenatally. For many low-income mothers, the hospital setting may be more conducive to bonding than the home.

Women and men of diverse cultural groups may not demonstrate the same bonding behaviors as Anglo-Americans. Caution should be used when promoting bonding and interpreting maternal and paternal behavior of women and men of different cultural groups. Female relatives in some cultures provide extensive care of the baby and may almost appear to replace the mother in bonding to the newborn. In some cultures women believe that their colostrum will make their infants sick and do not breast-feed until after their milk comes in.

Always investigate cultural practices before making judgments about the adequacy of bonding.

SUMMARY

Increased participation of women and their families in birth preparation and the birth process creates a history of accomplishment and develops greater self-confidence with regard to child care. Confident and competent parents can be a powerful influence in society because the family (the basic social unit) is responsible for childbearing and child rearing.

The foundation for enduring parent-child relationships begins before pregnancy, extends into the prenatal period, and can be continued through the participation of both parents in the birth and care of their infant.

Support for the family-centered approach stems from the realization that childbearing is not an illness, but rather a time of emotional, social, and physical change and stress. Under these circumstances, it is most appropriate for medical and nursing staffs to make their expertise available to the family rather than controlling the delivery of a service to a passive recipient. The acknowledgement of the birth process as normal leads to a joining of health care providers and family into a functioning team.

Finally, because the family participates to a greater extent, education becomes increasingly important. Armed with knowledge about healthful prenatal practices, childbirth procedures, and postpartum care of the mother and infant, the family is better prepared to assume more responsibility for self-care and thus is more likely to be prepared for early discharge (Fig. 1-13).

The components of family-centered care have proven to be both cost-effective and highly marketable. In this new era in maternity care, the chief beneficiaries will be childbearing families. This time of rapid change is especially exciting for maternity nursing because it offers the opportunity to develop truly comprehensive family-centered maternity care.

The care described in this book is developed from a philosophy of family-centered maternity and newborn care. This first chapter was designed to provide a brief look at obstetric care yesterday and family-centered maternity and newborn care today, with both their problems and their joys. It was also intended to provide a stimulus for you to examine your own feelings and attitudes about pregnancy and birth as you embark on this study of the childbearing family. What you have learned to this point will set the tone and influence the quality of care you provide. As you progress through the other chapters in this text, remember that the major change in maternity care needed to make family-centered care work is *attitudinal*.

BIBLIOGRAPHY

Ahmann E: Family-centered care: shifting orientation, *Pediat Nurs* 20(2):113-117, 1994.

Ahmann E: Family-centered care: the time has come, *Pediatr Nurs* 20(1):52-53, 1994.

Baker TJ: Image of nurse-midwifery: a barrier to practice, *Clin Nurs Spec* 8(1):2-5, 1994.

Berry LM: Realistic expectations of the labor coach, *J Obstet Gynecol Neonatal Nurs* 17(5):354-355, 1988.

Butler J and others: Supportive nurse-midwife care is associated with a reduced incidence of cesarean section, *Am J Obstet Gynecol* 168(5):1407-1413, 1993.

Chow MP: Nurses as primary care providers: an old idea whose time has come, *Calif Hosp* 10-14, 1994.

Committee on Adolescence: Adolescent pregnancy, *Pediatr* 83(1):132-134, 1989.

Committee on Adolescence: Counseling the adolescent about pregnancy options, *Pediatr* 83(1):135-137, 1989.

Committee on Adolescence: Care of adolescent parents and their children, *Pediatr* 83(1):138-139, 1989.

Council on Long Range Planning and Development: The future of obstetrics and gynecology, *JAMA* 258(24):3547-3553, 1987.

Declercq ER: Where babies are born and who attends their births: findings from the revised 1989 United States standard certificate of live births, *Obstet Gynecol* 81(6):997-1003, 1993.

Devitt N: The transition from home to hospital births in the United States, 1930-1960, *Birth Fam J* 4:2, 1977.

Dickason EJ, Silverman BL, Schult MO: *Maternal-infant nursing care*, ed 2, St. Louis, Mosby, 1994.

Eyer DE: *Mother-infant bonding: a scientific fiction*, New Haven, Yale University Press, 1992.

Fonteyn VJ, Isada B: Nongenetic implications of childbearing after age thirty-five, *Obstet Gynecol Surv* 43(12):709-719, 1988.

Footlick JK: What happened to the family, *Newsweek* 14 Winter/Spring, 1990.

Fortier JC and others: Adjustment to a newborn: sibling preparation makes a difference, *J Obstet Gynecol Neonatal Nurs* 20(1):73-79, 1991.

Fullar SA: Care of postpartum adolescents, *MCN* 11(6):398-403, 1986.

Harrison H: The principles for family-centered neonatal care, *Pediatr* 92(5):643-650, 1993.

Harwood A: *Guidelines for culturally appropriate health care*. In Harwood A, editor: *Ethnicity and medical care*, pp 482-507, Cambridge, Mass, 1981, Harvard University Press.

Hobel CJ and others: The west Los Angeles preterm birth prevention project, *Am J Obstet Gynecol* 170(1):54-62, 1994.

Horn M, Manion J: Creative grandparenting: bonding the generations, *J Obstet Gynecol Neonatal Nurs* 3:233-236, 1984.

Interprofessional Task Force on Health Care of Women and Children: *A joint position statement on the development of family-centered maternity/newborn care in hospitals*, June, 1978.

Khazoyan CM, Anderson NLR: Latinos' expectations for their partners during childbirth, *MCN* 19(4):226-229, 1994.

Klaus MH, Kennell JH: Parent-infant bonding, ed 2, St. Louis, 1982, Mosby.

Leavitt JW: Joseph B DeLee and the practice of preventive obstetrics, *Obstet Gynec Survey* 44(9):682-683, 1989.

Lehrman EJ: Findings of the 1990 annual American College of Nurse-Midwives membership survey, *J Nurse Midwifery* 37(1):33-46, 1992.

Lubic RW: Childbearing centers: delivering more for less, *Am J Nurs* 83(7):1053-1056, 1983.

Mattson S, Smith JE, editors: *Core curriculum for maternal-newborn nursing*, Philadelphia, 1993, WB Saunders.

May KA, Mahlmeister LR: *Comprehensive maternity nursing, nursing process and the childbearing family*, ed 2, Philadelphia, 1990, JB Lippincott.

Mitford J: *The American way of birth*, New York, 1992, William Abrahams/Dutton.

Reed J, Schmid M: Nursing implementation of single room maternity care, *J Obstet Gynecol Neonatal Nurs* 15(5):386-389, 1986.

Rooks JP and others: Outcomes of care in birth centers: the national birth center study, *N Engl J Med*, 321:1804-1811, 1989.

Ross MG and others: The west Los Angeles preterm birth prevention project: II. Cost effectiveness analysis of high-risk pregnancy interventions, *Obstet Gynecol* 83(4):506-511, 1994.

Rubin R: Cognitive style in pregnancy, *Am J Nurs* 70:508-520, March 1970.

Sherwen LN: *Psychosocial dimensions of the pregnant family*, New York, 1987, Springer.

Speert H: *Iconographic gynitrica: a pictorial history of gynecology and obstetrics*, Philadelphia, 1973, FA Davis.

Steensma J: A plan for implementing mother-baby nursing, *Birth* 20(3):148-154, 1993.

Stevens KA: Nursing diagnosis in wellness childbearing settings, *J Obstet Gynecol Neonatal Nurs* 17(5):329-336, 1988.

Stevens KA, O'Connell ML: The problem of access: meeting needs of pregnant women, *J Perinat Ed* 1(2):1-11, 1992.

Symanski ME: Maternal-infant bonding: practice issues for the 1990s, *J Nurse Midwifery* 37(suppl):67S-73S, 1992.

Vezeau T, Hallsten D: Making the transition to mother-baby care, *MCN* 12:193-198, 1987.

Waryas F, Luebbers M: A cluster system for maternity care, *MCN* 11:98-100, 1986.

Watters N: Combined mother-infant nursing care, *J Obstet Gynecol Neonatal Nurs* 14:478-483, 1985.

Wegman ME: Annual summary of vital statistics—1988, *Pediatr* 84(6):943-955, 1989.

Wertz R, Wertz D: *Lying-in: a history of childbirth in America*, expanded ed, New Haven, 1989, Yale University Press.

Wismont JM, Reame NE: The lesbian childbearing experience: assessing developmental tasks, *Image* 21(3):137-141, 1989.

DEFINITIONS

Define the following terms:

adolescent
alternative birth center (ABC)
American College of Nurse-Midwives (ACNM)
American College of Obstetricians and Gynecologists (ACOG)
American Society of Psychoprophylaxis in Obstetrics (ASPO)
antepartal
asphyxia
atelectasis
attachment
attitudes
birthing room
bonding
capitated
commune
congenital malformations
culture
ethnic
family-centered maternity and newborn care (FCMNC)
fetal
freestanding birth center
home health aide
infant mortality rate
International Childbirth Education Association (ICEA)
lay midwife
LDR room
LDRP room
low birth weight
maternal-child nurse practitioner
maternal mortality rate
midwife
morbidity
mortality
myths
neonatal mortality rate
nonjudgmental
nuclear family
nurse-midwife
nurse practitioner
obstetrics
obstetric technician
pediatric nurse practitioner
postpartal
prenatal
puerperal sepsis
regionalization
ruptured membranes
Semmelweis
single room maternity care ((SRMC)
urban
values

LEARNING ACTIVITIES

1. Group discussions.
2. Guest speakers: childbearing couples of different ages, races, cultures.
3. Visit a tertiary perinatal center and report on its goals and activities.
4. View audiovisual aids and discuss.
5. Check to see if there is an alternative birth center in your community. What are the ABCs policies? Cost? If possible, visit the center.
6. Are there LDR or LDRP rooms in your community? Evaluate their cost-effectiveness.
7. Guest speakers: certified nurse-midwife, lay midwife, nurse practitioner. Ask these speakers to explain how their educational preparation and daily work differs. What duties would a maternal-child nurse practitioner perform? What duties would a pediatric nurse practitioner perform?
8. Write a paragraph explaining family-centered maternity and newborn care.

ENRICHMENT/IN-DEPTH STUDY

1. Read and report on "A Joint Position Statement on The Development of Family-Centered Maternity/Newborn Care in Hospitals," June 1978, Interprofessional Task Force on Health Care of Women and Children.
2. Design a plan for improving maternity care in your community. Use only current local resources and resources available within a 250-mile radius.
3. Write a paper on the therapeutic use of self in maternity care. Describe how you can best use yourself in a helping way while providing care to childbearing families of a different culture than your own.
4. How many babies are born in your community each year? What are the infant and maternal mortality rates in your community? Do these rates differ by hospital or place of birth? Why? Or why not?
5. Research local resources and support groups for pregnant adolescents in your community. Are there high school education programs for pregnant adolescents?
6. Analyze the clinical facility in which you are studying in terms of the low-income pregnant woman. What practices encourage their attendance in prenatal clinics and what practices discourage them? How would you change the program?

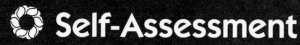

Self-Assessment

For questions 1 through 12, determine if each statement is true or false. Fill in the space to the left of the statement with T for true and F for false.

_____ **1.** The first services provided to women at childbirth really were maternal.

_____ **2.** Milestones in obstetric care occurred in the fifteenth century.

_____ **3.** Obstetric practice was established as part of medicine during the twentieth century.

_____ **4.** During the eighteenth century the physician's role in obstetrics came into vogue.

_____ **5.** In the twentieth century childbirth in the United States was transformed from a normal life event to a medical procedure in a hospital.

_____ **6.** "Childbed fever" (puerperal fever) claimed the lives of many women giving birth before Pasteur discovered the organism causing puerperal fever in 1860.

_____ **7.** In the twentieth century postpartal and antepartal care were recognized as being important in the care of childbearing women.

_____ **8.** The U.S. Congress established a Children's Bureau in 1912 to educate the public in the need for prenatal care.

_____ **9.** The United States ranked second in the world in infant mortality from 1985 to 1989.

_____ **10.** Infant mortality rates are highest in rural nonmetropolitan counties and in inner cities among blacks and other minorities.

_____ **11.** Sometimes people experience childbirth as a warm, giving experience.

_____ **12.** Men in our culture have never been actively involved in the birth process.

For questions 13 through 20, choose the best answers and indicate your choice by circling the answer.

13. A new baby in the family can mean:

    a. competition for a sibling

    b. more work for grandparents

    c. financial worry for the family

    d. no noticeable change in life-style

    e. diminished privacy for all

    Answer (circle one):

      1. a and c

      2. a, b, c, and e

      3. all of the above

14. The pregnant couple during the first trimester often feels that the pregnancy is:

    a. a welcome, wanted responsibility

    b. a threat to their own freedom

    c. both a and b

15. The progression parents use in first touching their baby is:

   a. whole hand to body

   b. fingertip to palm to increased body contact

   c. palm to fingertip

16. The single father may be helped to face the reality of pregnancy by:

   a. involving him in prenatal care

   b. informing him that he has no rights if he does not provide child support

   c. encouraging him to go on "about his business"

   d. involving him in the pregnancy planning

     Answer (circle one):

     1. a and d

     2. b

     3. c

17. According to data gathered from the United Nations Statistical Office, the U.S. ranking for Infant Mortality Rate was tied for:

   a. 21st

   b. 15th

   c. 4th

18. By 1940 the percentage of American babies born in hospitals was:

   a. 50%

   b. 99.2%

   c. 89%

19. Nurse-midwives are certified by a national organization known as:

   a. ACNM

   b. NAACOG

   c. ANA

20. Lay midwives are certified by a national organization known as:

   a. ACNM

   b. they are not certified

   c. ACLM

Supply the correct answer(s) for items 21 through 24.

21. List three factors that could be described as bonding delay.

   a. _____

   b. _____

   c. _____

22. Describe three steps that could be taken by this society to improve maternity care for all people in the United States.

   a. _____

   b. _____

   c. _____

23. List four major causes of infant mortality for premature infants.

   a. _____

   b. _____

   c. _____

   d. _____

24. List three hospital policies that would be considered family-centered.

   a. _____

   b. _____

   c. _____

Fill in the blanks for items 25 through 29.

25. The major change in maternity care needed to make family-centered care work is

_____.

26. Family-centered maternity care includes all family members in

_____ for the birth experience.

27. A goal of family-centered maternity care is to treat each family with

_____ as individuals, no matter what makes them seem

"different."

28. "Rights" always bring with them _____.

29. One million adolescent girls are estimated to become pregnant each year. Of these

pregnancies _____ will end in abortion, and the remainder

will result in adolescent parenthood.

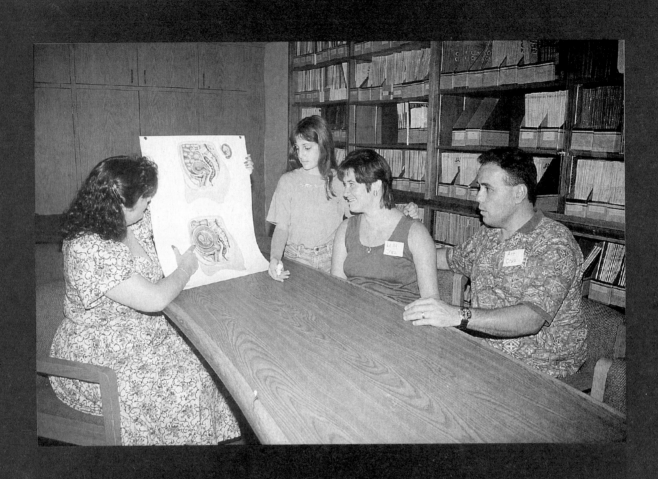

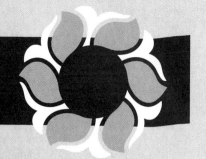

2

BASIC ANATOMY AND PHYSIOLOGY OF THE REPRODUCTIVE SYSTEM

GOALS

This chapter is designed to provide the reader with information that will:
- form a basis for understanding the primary structures and functions of the female and male reproductive systems.

- facilitate explaining basic reproductive system anatomy and physiology to future parents and family members.

STUDENT OBJECTIVES

After studying this chapter, you should be able to:
1. Identify and briefly describe the male and female organs of reproduction.
2. Correctly label diagrams of the male and female internal and external reproductive systems and understand their function.
3. Trace the passage of spermatozoa from their origin until they are ejaculated.
4. Given a diagram of a mammary gland, label the following structures: nipple, areola, milk (lactiferous) duct, alveoli, sinus (ampullae).
5. Demonstrate a basic understanding of the anatomy of the uterus by identifying four distinct areas of uterine demarcation.

6. Demonstrate a basic understanding of the anatomy of the female bony pelvis by:
   a. Listing the four bones of the pelvis
   b. Identifying the three bones that unite to form the innominate bone
   c. Identifying the four joints of the bony pelvis
   d. Identifying the anatomic landmark separating the false from the true pelvis
   e. Identifying the three planes of the pelvis that have obstetric significance
   f. Identifying the axis of the true pelvis
7. Explain the processes of menstruation, ovulation, and fertilization by naming the hormones responsible for these processes and describing their functions.
8. Discuss the menstrual cycle and identify [...] of the cycle and their dominant horm[...]

FUNCTIONS OF THE FEMALE REPRODUCTIVE SYSTEM

Human life begins with the union of two different parent cells: one from the female called the ovum, and one from the male called the sperm. This beginning of life, known as fertilization or conception, begins inside the female, whose body then nurtures the fertilized ovum until it grows and develops into a new and separate human being.

The female reproductive system has three basic functions:

1. To reproduce (to give life)
2. To produce the hormones responsible for female sexual characteristics and reproductive functions
3. To provide sexual gratification

The female reproductive system consists of the external genitals, the internal reproductive organs, the breasts, and the bony pelvis and related pelvic structures.

EXTERNAL FEMALE GENITALIA

The external parts of the female reproductive system are known collectively as the *vulva* (from the Latin word meaning covering) (Fig. 2-1). These include two pair of "small lips," or *labia minora*, which protect the vaginal opening *(introitus)*; the urethral opening *(meatus)*, leading from the bladder; and the *clitoris*, a highly sensitive projection of tissue, nerves, and blood vessels.

The outermost "large lips," called the *labia majora*, are composed of numerous glands and fat and are cov-ered with pigmented skin and pubic hair on the outer surface and are smooth and free from hair on the inner surface. These outer lips are continuous with and extend down from the *mons pubis* (or *mons veneris*), a skin-covered mound of fatty tissue covering the pubic bone.

The two smaller, thinner lips, called the *labia minora*, are folds of hairless skin that lie within the labia majora and meet at the top to form a hood, called the *prepuce*, which covers the clitoris. The triangular or almond-shaped area between the labia minora is called the *vestibule*. Several genital structures are located in the vestibule.

The *clitoris* is a ¼ to 1 inch long, somewhat cylindrical, erectile organ covered with mucous membrane. It is like the male organ, the penis, in that it is the major site of sexual stimulation and *orgasm*. Toward the anus, the labia minora blend together with the labia majora to form a ridge of tissue called the *frenulum of the labia*, or *fourchette*.

The vaginal opening and the urethral orifice through which urine is voided are also found within the vestibule. The vaginal opening is surrounded by a fold of mucous membrane called the *hymen*. Just above and to each side of the vaginal opening are mucus-producing *Bartholin's glands* (also called *greater vestibular glands*). Bartholin's glands secrete a thin mucus that lubricates the vagina and vulva. On each side of the urethral orifice are *Skene's glands* (also called *paraurethral glands*), which discharge lubricating secretions to lubricate the urinary meatus and protect it from bacterial invasion. Both the labia minora and labia majora are responsive to pleasurable and painful tactile sensations.

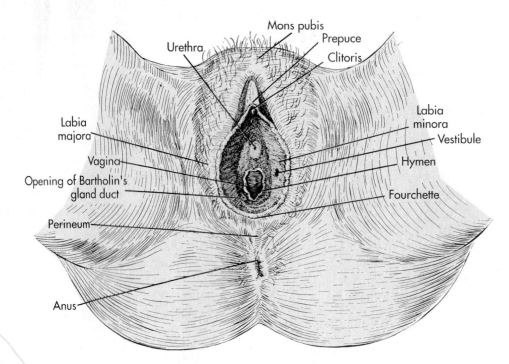

Figure 2-1 External female genitalia.

Not considered to be part of the reproductive system, the *anus* lies below the perineum and serves as an outlet for the rectum. In a woman the area of skin, connective tissue, and muscle between the vulva and the anus is called the *perineum.* The perineum flattens and stretches to accommodate birth of the baby.

FEMALE INTERNAL REPRODUCTIVE ORGANS

The internal reproductive organs are found within the pelvis (Fig. 2-2, *A* and *B*). They consist of the vagina, uterus, fallopian tubes, and ovaries, all of which are target organs for estrogenic hormones.

The two *ovaries,* the female gonads, are the primary sex glands of the female. The female sex cells or ova are produced here. These almond-shaped glands are attached to ligaments and are located on each side of the uterus near the open end of each fallopian tube. Each ovary is about an inch long, half an inch thick, and three quarters of an inch wide. They contain small, secretory sacs, or *follicles,* each of which contains an *ovum* that matures and is discharged from the ovary into the pelvic cavity by the process of *ovulation.* In addition to maturing and discharging ova, the ovaries produce the two major hormones necessary for reproduction to occur: *estrogen* and *progesterone.*

The two *fallopian tubes* (also called *oviducts* or *uterine tubes*) attached to each side of the upper body of the uterus are small, muscular structures about 10 centimeters (4 inches) long with a diameter of about 0.5 centimeters (almost the thickness of a lead pencil or drinking straw). These tubes carry the egg from the ovaries to the uterus by the wavelike action of tiny hairlike structures called *cilia* in the lining of the tubes and by peristaltic activity. There is no direct connection between the ovaries and the fallopian tubes. Extending from the flared, open ends of the tubes are small, finger-like projections called *fimbriae,* which form a cup over the top of each ovary but actually open into the abdominal cavity. Their movements cause a current in the peritoneal fluid, which sweeps the ovum into the tube. It takes about 5 days for the ovum to travel in the tube from the ovary to the uterus.

Fertilization usually occurs in the outer one third of the fallopian tube (farthest from the uterus), and the fertilized egg usually continues down into the uterus where it implants itself. Sometimes a fertilized egg implants itself in the lining of the tube, and this is called a *tubal pregnancy.* Rarely, a fertilized egg does not find its way into the tube at all and attaches itself to the peritoneal cavity, causing an *abdominal pregnancy.* Any pregnancy outside of the uterus is known as *ectopic* or *extrauterine.*

When fertilization does not occur, the egg moves out of the uterus through the cervical canal and is expelled through the vagina. It passes without notice, being no larger than the period at the end of this sentence.

The *vagina* is a muscular, membranous, highly vascular tubular structure about 8 to 10 centimeters (4 to 5 inches) long, which connects the uterus with the vulva. Directly in front of the vagina are the urethra and the urinary bladder, and in back of it is the rectum. Glands in the vaginal lining continuously produce a small amount of thin mucus to keep the area moist. During sexual arousal these lubricating glands increase their output. The walls of the vagina contain many folds, or *rugae,* which allow the vagina to stretch during childbirth and sexual intercourse. The vagina receives the penis and semen during sexual intercourse, discharges menstrual flow in nonpregnant women, and is the passage through which birth occurs.

The *cervix,* or neck, is the lowermost part of the uterus. It dips down into the upper vagina so that a circular space is formed around the cervix and between the walls of the vagina. The areas of this circular space are known as *fornices,* with the deepest of these spaces behind the cervix called the *posterior fornix.* A needle can be introduced into the vaginal canal and then poked through the thin tissue of the posterior fornix and into the abdominal cavity to withdraw samples of any fluid that might have accumulated there. Because this lowermost portion of the abdominal cavity is called the *cul-de-sac,* this procedure is known as *culdocentesis.*

The cervix is divided into three parts (Fig. 2-2, *A*): (1) the *internal os,* which opens into the uterus; (2) the *external os,* which opens into the vagina; and (3) the *cervical canal,* the area located between the internal and external osea. The external os is a round hole before the first childbirth and is often more like a horizontal slit after childbirth. The cervix is composed of fibrous connective tissue. Glands in the cervical canal produce a downward flow of mucus to protect the uterus from bacteria. Also, mucus is produced in response to cyclic hormones: thick, scanty mucus when estrogen levels are low; thin, and slippery, abundant mucus when estrogen levels are high at the time of ovulation. This thick mucus helps sperm penetrate the cervical canal as they make their journey through the uterus to the fallopian tubes to fertilize an ovum.

Commonly known as the "womb," the *uterus* is a hollow, pear-shaped thick-walled, muscular organ, which in the nonpregnant female is about the size of a closed fist. The uterus contains four distinct areas (Fig. 2-3): (1) the uppermost, rounded top portion, above the level where the fallopian tubes enter, called the *fundus,* (2) the middle portion, called the *body* or *corpus,* (3) the *isthmus* (called the lower uterine segment during pregnancy), joining the corpus to the cervix, and (4) th

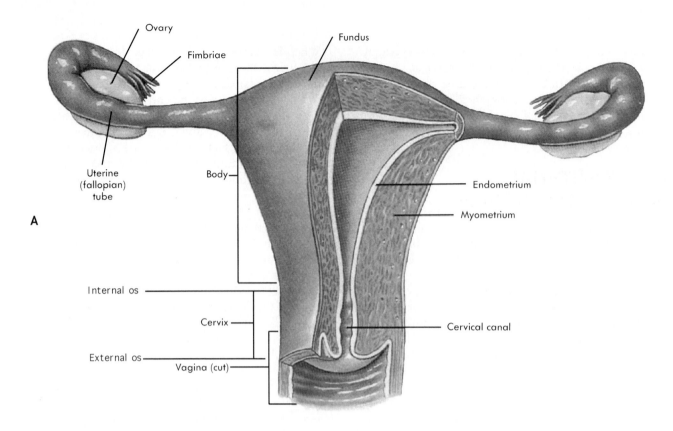

A

Ovary

Fimbriae

Fundus

Body

Uterine
(fallopian)
tube

Internal os

Cervix

External os

Vagina (cut)

Endometrium

Myometrium

Cervical canal

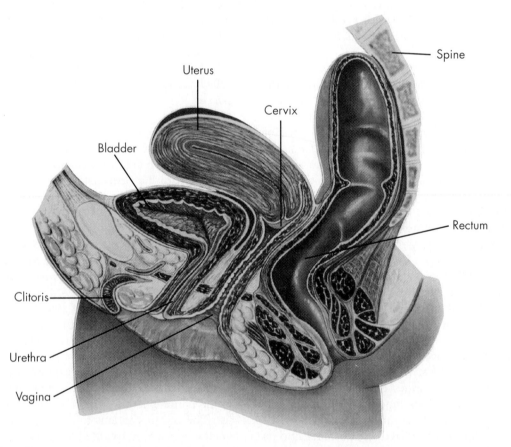

B

Uterus

Cervix

Spine

Bladder

Clitoris

Urethra

Vagina

Rectum

Figure 2-2 A, Internal female reproductive organs: cross section. **B,** Internal female reproductive organs: midsagittal view. *(A, from Thibodeau GA, Patton K:* Structure and function of the body, *ed 9, St. Louis, 1992, Mosby.* **B,** *from Seeley RR, Stephens TP, Tate P:* Anatomy and physiology, *ed 3, St. Louis, 1995, Mosby.)*

lower, smaller portion, called the *cervix,* or *neck.* The prolongations of the uterus into which the fallopian tubes fit are termed the *cornu* (horns). Generally the entire uterus is tipped forward *(anteverted);* the corpus is flexed forward *(anteflexion).*

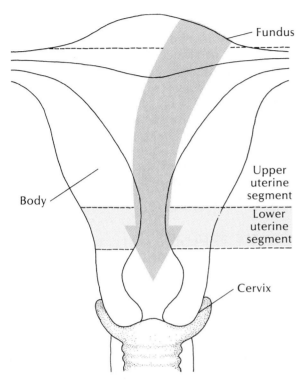

Figure 2-3 Areas of the uterus.

The uterus is located in the middle of the pelvic cavity between the bladder and the rectum. It is held in place by ligaments that stretch to allow the uterus to expand and rise up out of the pelvis into the abdominal cavity during pregnancy.

The interior surface or lining of the uterus, the *endometrium,* is composed of secretive tissue containing blood vessels and glands. This is the layer of the uterus that sloughs away each month during menstruation and is then renewed again each menstrual cycle. The walls of the uterus are made of a smooth muscle called *myometrium.* The outside of the uterus is covered by connective tissue called *perimetrium.* The myometrium is the thickest of the three layers. Its walls contain a network of muscle fibers that can grow and stretch as the uterus grows in pregnancy (Fig. 2-4). The outer layer of the myometrium is made up mainly of lengthwise fibers that extend into various supporting ligaments. The outer layer's longitudinal fibers predominate in the fundus and are needed to push the fetus downward at birth. The fibers of the thick, middle layer form an interlacing network and are arranged in figure eight patterns. Because blood vessels run through these interlacing patterns, when these fibers contract after the birth, the blood vessels are kinked and constricted, thus controlling uterine bleeding. This middle layer is often called a living ligature. The fibers of the inner layer run in a circular direction and provide sphincter action to help keep the cervix closed and hold the contents of the uterus during pregnancy.

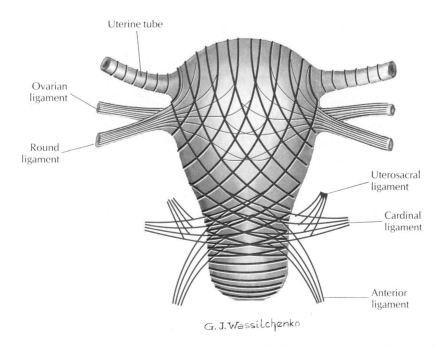

Figure 2-4 Schematic arrangement of directions of muscle fibers. Note that uterine muscle fibers are continuous with supportive ligaments of uterus. *(From Bobak IM and others:* Maternity nursing, *ed 4, St. Louis, 1995, Mosby.)*

Blood Supply

Although the nonpregnant uterus receives only 50 to 60 milliliters of blood per minute, the pregnant uterus at term can receive up to 700 to 800 milliliters per minute. This is equal to 10% of all blood pumped by the maternal heart at term. About 70% of the abundant blood supply of the uterus is provided by the uterine artery and 30% by the ovarian arteries (Fig. 2-5, *A*). To understand where these arteries arise, trace them back to the aorta. As you can see, to get to the uterus, a red blood cell could *either* travel from the aorta through a common iliac artery, through an internal iliac (hypogastric) artery, and then through the uterine artery, *or* the red cell could travel directly off the aorta through an ovarian artery to the uterus. The uterine artery also supplies blood for the cervix, upper vagina, fallopian tubes, and round ligament.

Once the uterine and ovarian arteries reach the uterus, they penetrate the uterine wall to reach the myometrium, the thick middle muscular layer. There they branch into arteries that run parallel to the surface. From these arteries arise the *radial arteries,* which point inward toward the uterine cavity like the spokes of a bicycle wheel. Where the radial arteries terminate, they are very tortuous and convoluted, and thus are called *spiral arteries.* Because the spiral arteries are so coiled and twisted, they can easily stretch out to supply the placenta as it and the uterus change in size and position during pregnancy (Fig. 2-5, *B*).

Blood is supplied to the ovaries by the ovarian artery.

Veins follow essentially the same paths as the arteries. They penetrate all the layers of the uterus and are especially plentiful in the myometrium.

Nerve Supply

The innervation of the female reproductive organs can be divided into efferent (motor) and afferent (sensory) components. Motor fibers to the uterus are primarily sympathetic nervous system fibers, which originate in the lower thoracic and upper lumbar portions of the spinal cord. After leaving the cord and traveling down toward the pelvis, these fibers eventually form large, intertwining tangles called *plexi* (singular: *plexus*). The *hypogastric plexus* is the large plexus formed above the sacral promontory. This plexus sends sympathetic fibers to the uterus, fallopian tubes, vagina, and ovaries. The ovaries and fallopian tubes also receive sympathetic fibers via the *ovarian plexus.* The sympathetic nerves cause muscle contraction and constriction of the veins.

The pelvic organs receive a lesser amount of innervation from the parasympathetic nervous system via the *pelvic splanchnic nerves (nervi erigentes),* which originate from spinal cord segments S2, S3, and possibly S4. The pelvic splanchnics enter the pelvic plexus before reaching the pelvic organs. The parasympathetic nerves inhibit contractions and cause dilatation of the veins.

Sensory fibers from the uterus, as well as pain fibers from the vagina and cervix, are found in the nervi erigentes (S2-S4). However, it is currently thought that sensory fibers also accompany the sympathetic component.

It is currently believed that the sensation of "pain" in labor is transmitted as follows:

1. First stage of labor: dilation and effacement of the cervix sends impulses along with the sympathetic nerves to T11, T12, and L1.
2. Second stage: distention of the vagina and perineum sends impulses along branches of the *pudendal* nerve to S2, S3, and S4.
3. Third stage: dilation of the cervix sends impulses along with the sympathetic nerves to T11, T12, and L1 (Fig. 2-5, *C*).

Uterine Support

The uterus is supported in its position in the pelvic cavity by ligaments (Fig. 2-6). The paired *broad ligaments* attach the uterus to each side of the pelvic cavity. Uterine blood vessels and nerves pass through the broad ligaments. They serve to anchor the ovaries and tubes in place. The *uterosacral ligaments* connect the sacrum to the uterus, one on each side of the rectum. The *cardinal ligament* extends laterally from the vagina and cervix and runs within the lowest part of the broad ligament to the pelvic sidewall. The cardinal ligament is the chief ligament that keeps the uterus from dropping down into the vagina. The *round ligaments* extend from a point on the uterus just below the fallopian tubes through the inguinal canal to the labia majora. Because the uterus is suspended from ligaments (which can be pulled, stretched, and distorted), it can rise up out of the pelvic cavity as it enlarges during pregnancy. The *ovarian ligaments* attach the ovaries to the cornua.

Pelvic Floor

The pelvic floor is a muscular diaphragm composed of three layers of muscles. The two outermost layers are made up mainly of sphincters (Fig. 2-7, *A*). These ringlike muscles, which are relatively weak, close the outer openings of the urinary meatus, rectum, and vagina. The outermost layer contains the ischiocavernosus muscle, the bulbocavernosus muscle, and the superficial transverse perineal muscle. The bulbocavernosus muscle, with the external anal sphincter muscle, forms a figure eight around the vagina and rectum. The middle layer, not visible in the diagram, contains the sphincter

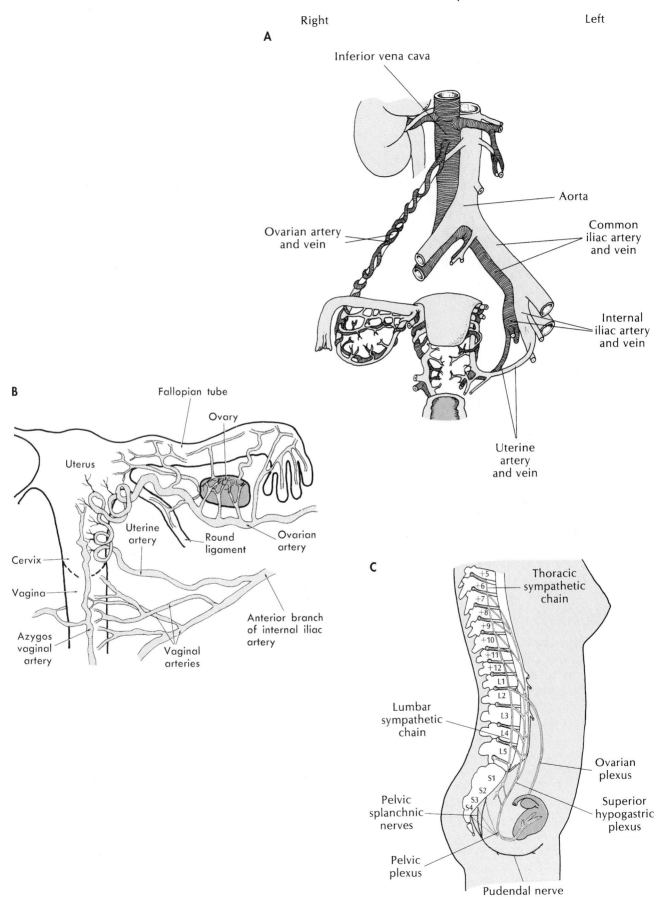

Figure 2-5 A, Blood supply to pelvis. **B,** Blood supply to uterus. **C,** Nerve supply to uterus.

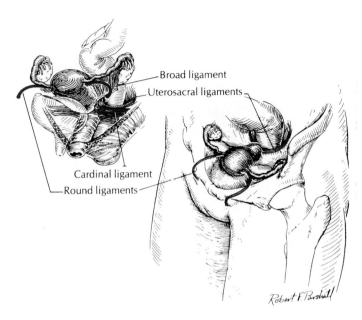

Broad ligament
Uterosacral ligaments
Cardinal ligament
Round ligaments

Figure 2-6 Uterine support. *(From Barkauskas VH, Stoltenberg-Allen K, Baumann LC, Darling-Fisher C:* Health and physical assessment, *St. Louis, 1994, Mosby.)*

urethrae (which surrounds the urethra) and the deep transverse perineal muscle. Lying inside these outer muscle layers are deeper, stronger muscles that run from the pubis to the coccyx and form the base of the abdominal cavity (Fig. 2-7, *B*). These most powerful muscles are the *levator ani* and the *coccygeus*. The levator ani has three portions: (1) pubococcygeal, (2) iliococcygeal, and (3) puborectalis muscles. These muscles form a hammock, or sling, above which the vagina, rectum, bladder, and uterus are suspended by ligaments and fasciae made of connective tissue, strands, bands, and layers. These fascial sheaths surround and embrace each pelvic organ and are subject to tearing during birth.

Breasts

The mammary glands, or breasts, are considered to be accessory reproductive organs (Fig. 2-8). The breasts lie over the pectoralis muscles on the anterior chest and are attached to them by connective tissue ligaments. Each breast is composed of an intricate system of glandular (milk-secreting) tissue containing 15 to 20 divisions or lobes, each lobe containing many lobules. The lobules contain *acini cells,* which begin to secrete colostrum in midpregnancy and milk after birth. The milk-secreting cells are arranged in grapelike clusters called alveoli. Lactiferous ducts connect all lobes and lobules and join under the *areola* (the pigmented area around the nipple) to make sinuses *(ampullae).* These sinuses can enlarge to serve as a reservoir for colostrum and milk. Breast size has no effect on the number of lobes because breast size is determined more by the amount of fat around the glandular tissue. Thus breast

size has little to do with how much milk a woman can produce following childbirth.

In the areola sebaceous glands form *Montgomery's tubercles,* which secrete oil to lubricate and protect the nipples. The tubercles appear as small, white, elevated patches on the pigmented areola. The nipple, located in the center of the areola, is the outlet for the ducts. The nipple is made of sturdy, pigmented erectile tissue. Although the breasts are complex in their structure and function, it is very easy for women to become familiar with how their breasts feel. In fact, women and their partners can become so sensitive to the normal texture of the breasts that breast lumps often are first detected by them.

Female Bony Pelvis

The pelvis is a bony, basket-like structure that carries the weight of the upper part of the body and transfers this weight to the lower extremities. It is a protective bony cage that contains the reproductive organs and through which the baby must pass at the time of birth.

Bones

The *female bony pelvis* is made up of four bones: the coccyx, the sacrum, and the two innominate bones (Fig. 2-9). The sacrum is the wedge-shaped bone at the back of the pelvis. Attached to the bottom of the sacrum is the coccyx. The sacrum and coccyx can be thought of as lowermost extensions of the spinal column. The innominate, or hip, bones make up the sides and front of the pelvis. Each innominate bone is composed of three fused bones: the ilium, the ischium, and the pubis (Fig.

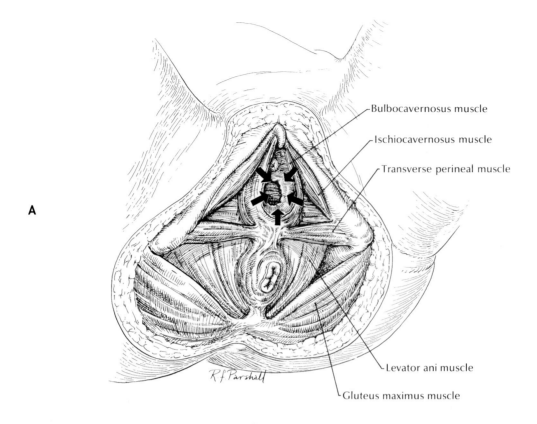

Bulbocavernosus muscle

Ischiocavernosus muscle

Transverse perineal muscle

Levator ani muscle

Gluteus maximus muscle

A

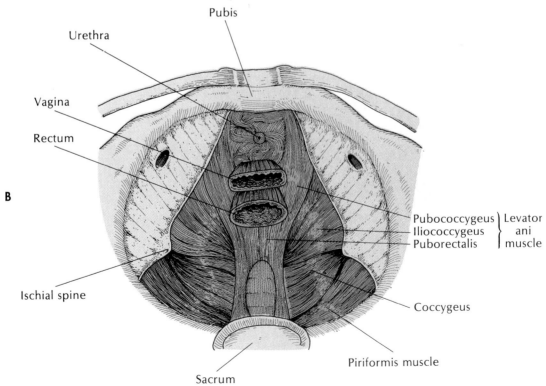

Pubis

Urethra

Vagina

Rectum

Ischial spine

Pubococcygeus ⎱ Levator
Iliococcygeus ⎰ ani
Puborectalis ⎰ muscle

Coccygeus

Piriformis muscle

Sacrum

B

Figure 2-7 A, Muscles of pelvic floor. **B,** Muscles of perineun. *(A, from Barkauskas VH, Stoltenberg-Allen K, Baumann LC, Darling-Fisher C: Health and physical assessment, St. Louis, 1994, Mosby.)*

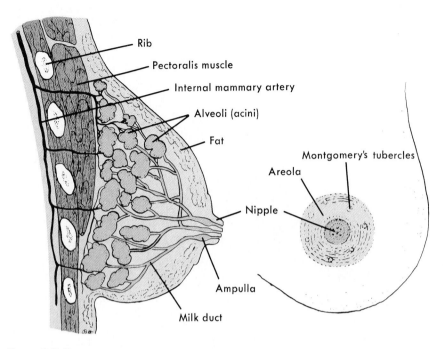

Figure 2-8 Breasts. *(From Hamilton PM:* Basic maternity nursing, *ed 6, St. Louis, 1989, Mosby.)*

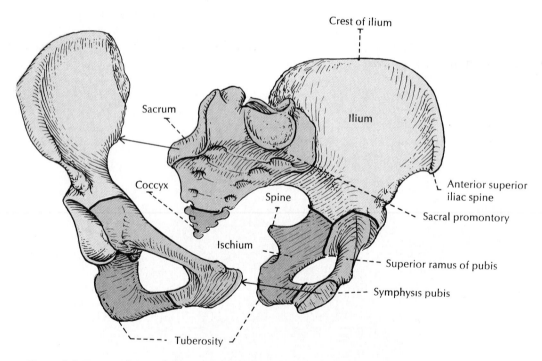

Figure 2-9 Bones of the pelvis. *(From Barkauskas VH, Stoltenberg-Allen K, Baumann LC, Darling-Fisher C:* Health and physical assessment, *St. Louis, 1994, Mosby.)*

2-9). Fusion of these three bones begins at about the twelfth year and is usually complete by the eighteenth. The top anterior portion of the sacrum tilts forward, forming a bony ridge known as the *sacral promontory.* The two pubes join in front to form the *symphysis pubis.* The symphysis forms the top part of the *pubic arch.*

Joints

In the bony pelvis are four joints of importance: the two *sacroiliac* joints, between the sacrum and the ilia on each side; the *symphysis pubis* joint, in the front between the two pubic bones; and the *sacrococcygeal* joint, between the sacrum and the coccyx (Fig. 2-10). These

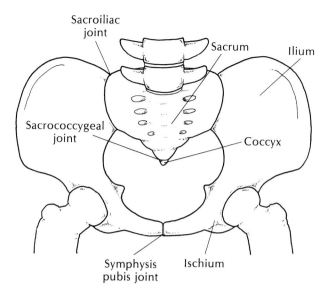

Figure 2-10 Bony pelvis and joints.

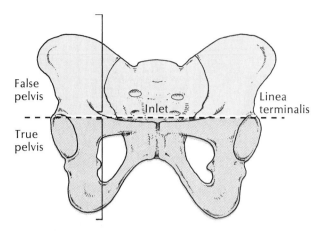

Figure 2-11 False and true pelvis.

joints are lined with fibrocartilage, which becomes thickened and softened by hormones during pregnancy, thus allowing greater mobility of the pelvic bones.

Division

The pelvis is divided by the *linea terminalis* into two parts: the false pelvis (upper flaring part) and the true pelvis (lower part) (Fig. 2-11). The false pelvis forms the lower part of the abdominal cavity and is less important for labor. It can be thought of as a large funnel that supports the uterus during the late pregnancy and directs the fetus into the true pelvis when labor begins.

The pelvic cavity, or true pelvis, is below the abdominal cavity. The true pelvis has three pelvic planes: an inlet, a mid pelvis (tunnel-like cavity), and an outlet (Fig. 2-12, *A*). It forms the bony portion of the birth canal. The *inlet* (the *pelvic brim*) or the entryway to the true pelvis, is the bony ridge that separates the false pelvis from the true pelvis.

The pelvic *outlet* is the space between the ischial tuberosities (the sit-upon bones) on the sides, the coccyx in the back, and the symphysis pubis in the front. Note that the outlet is somewhat diamond shaped (Fig. 2-13). The greatest diameter of the outlet is the anteroposterior (A-P) (from front to back).

Axis

The pelvic cavity, or mid pelvis, is the space between the inlet above and the outlet below and the walls of the pelvis. Note the *axis* of the cavity is curved so that the baby must accommodate itself to the curved path when coming through the canal (Fig. 2-12, *B*). The curve

is similar to that of a slidingboard, and in a favorable position, the baby can slide out head first.

On both sides of the inner part of the ischium are significant bony knobs called the *ischial spines,* which can be palpated during manual pelvic examination (Figs. 2-9 and 2-13). These are landmarks for determining how high the baby is in the pelvis by measuring the height of the baby's presenting part in relationship to the level of these bony ischial spines. The prominence of these ischial spines and the distance between them are important measurements of the adequacy of the pelvis.

The size and shape of the true pelvis is very important because the baby must pass through it to be born.

Pelvic types

There are four basic pelvic types: (1) *gynecoid* (rounded), (2) *android* (wedge or heart shaped), (3) *anthropoid* (oval), and (4) *platypelloid* (flat) (Fig. 2-14). Most women have pelves that do not fit into a single category but incorporate features of several varieties. The preceding classification is based on the shape of the inlet. Although it is generally believed that the gynecoid pelvis is the most favorable for childbearing, the anthropoid pelvis is also suited for vaginal birth. However, a woman's pelvic type is not as important as her individual pelvic measurements compared to the measurements of the head of her baby.

MALE EXTERNAL REPRODUCTIVE ORGANS

The scrotum and penis are the external reproductive organs of the male (Fig. 2-15). The male reproductive system has three basic functions:

1. To reproduce (to give life)

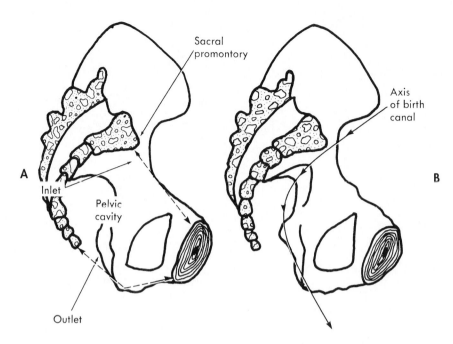

Figure 2-12 Pelvic planes and axis. **A,** Cavity of true pelvis. **B,** Axis of birth canal.

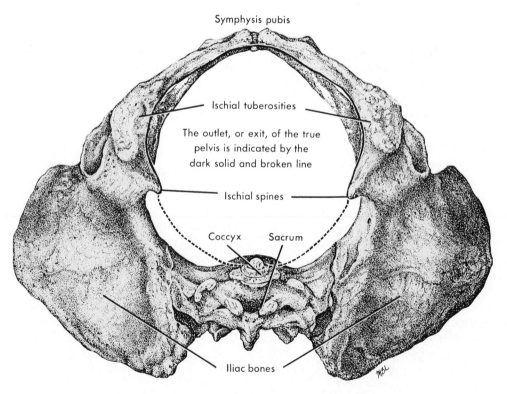

Figure 2-13 Pelvic outlet.

2. To produce the hormones responsible for male sexual characteristics and reproductive functions
3. To provide sexual gratification

The external organs of reproduction in the male are the penis and the scrotum.

The penis is the male organ of copulation.

Penis

The penis is a cylindrical organ made of three chambers of a spongelike tissue containing many blood-filled spaces. These spaces are relatively empty when the penis is in a relaxed state, but fill with blood and distend when sexual excitation occurs, making the penis stiff

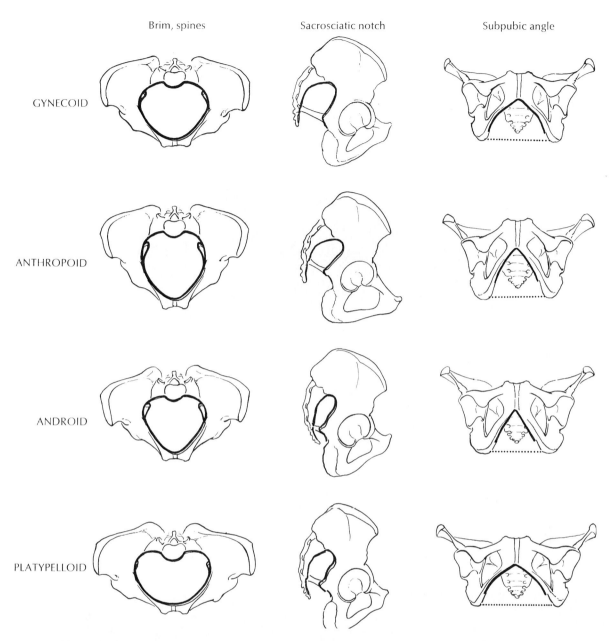

Brim, spines   Sacrosciatic notch   Subpubic angle

GYNECOID

ANTHROPOID

ANDROID

PLATYPELLOID

Figure 2-14 Comparison of various portions of the four basic pelvic types. *(From Barkauskas VH, Stoltenberg-Allen K, Baumann LC, Darling-Fisher C:* Health and physical assessment, *St. Louis, 1994, Mosby.)*

and erect in order to enter and deposit sperm in the woman's vagina during sexual intercourse. The male urethra passes through one of the three chambers. It is through the urethra that the urine empties from the bladder and that the reproductive cells and secretions are carried to the outside.

The head of the penis is composed of an enlarged portion called the glans. Covering the glans is the loosely fitting retractable skin, called the *prepuce* or *foreskin*, unless it is removed by circumcision shortly after birth.

Scrotum

The scrotum is the skin-covered pouch suspended between the thighs that holds the male gonads *(testes)*. The scrotum is divided into two sacs by a septum down the middle. Each sac contains a *testis (testicle)*, an epididymis, and a portion of the spermatic cord. Sperm require a temperature lower than body temperature for their development and maintenance, thus the temperature of the scrotum is a few degrees cooler than that of the body. Muscle fibers in the tissue of the scrotum can move the testes closer to the abdomen when very cold

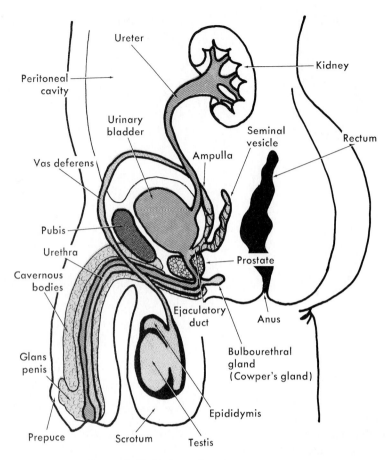

Figure 2-15 Male genitourinary system.

or lower the testes away from the abdomen when very hot.

MALE INTERNAL REPRODUCTIVE ORGANS

The internal organs include two testes (gonads), two epididymides, two seminal ducts and vesicles, two ejaculatory ducts, two spermatic cords, the urethra, the prostate, and the bulbourethral (Cowper's) glands. As these internal reproductive organs are described, refer to Fig. 2-15 to locate each part.

Testes

The testes are paired, oval-shaped glands about 2 inches long and 1 inch wide. Each testis contains specialized tissue arranged in narrow but long and coiled tubules *(seminiferous tubules)* where the sperm are produced. Between the tiny tubes are small specialized cells that produce the male sex hormone *testosterone,* which is responsible for the masculine characteristics of the

male body. Part of the seminal fluid, or *semen,* in which the sperm are transported is also produced in the tubules in the testes.

The tubes for carrying the spermatozoa begin with the tubules inside the testis itself. From these tubes the spermatozoa are collected by a coiled tube, 20 feet long if stretched to its full extent, called the *epididymis,* situated above and behind the testis. The mature spermatozoa enter the epididymis from the testis, become motile there, and pass through it to the *vas deferens* when ejaculated.

Vas Deferens

The vas deferens is a duct about 18 inches long that continues through a small canal in the abdominal wall and then curves back behind the urinary bladder where it joins the duct of the seminal vesicle to form the *ejaculatory duct.* The vas deferens carries the semen to the urethra. Traveling with the vas deferens are the testicular artery, autonomic nerves, veins, lymphatics, and a small muscle. These structures collectively make up the *spermatic cord.*

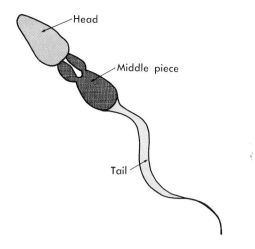

Figure 2-16 Spermatozoon.

Seminal Vesicles

The seminal vesicles are two small muscular glands at the base and rear of the urinary bladder. They are somewhat irregularly shaped and consist of many small sacs, or pockets. Their glandular lining produces a thick, milky secretion that forms much of the ejaculated semen. The ducts of the seminal vesicles join the vas deferens to form the ejaculatory ducts, which empty into the urethra. Semen is alkaline and protects sperm from the acidic environment of the female vagina.

Prostate Gland

The prostate gland is a single, fibromuscular, doughnut-shaped gland completely surrounding the urethra, just below the bladder. The prostate secrets a thin, clear fluid that becomes part of the ejaculate by entering the urethra by way of about 60 tiny *prostatic ductules*. This part of the ejaculate helps to activate the sperm and maintain their motility. The prostate is also composed of muscular tissue that contracts to aid in the ejaculation of semen into the urethra.

Bulbourethral Glands (Cowper's Glands)

The bulbourethral glands are a pair of pea-sized organs located below the prostate gland. These glands secrete mucus into the penile portion of the urethra to serve as a lubricant.

Spermatozoa (Sperm)

Spermatozoa or sperm are very tiny detached cells that look like tadpoles with oval heads, a midsection, and long tails. Chromosomal material is contained in its head and neck, and the tail is responsible for motility. Over 200 million spermatozoa are deposited in the vagina in the average ejaculation. Once ejaculated, spermatozoa have a life expectancy of 24 to 72 hours. Roughly one in a million will actually make the entire journey to the egg. The head of a spermatozoon contains chemicals that help it to penetrate the ovum, and the tail propels it as it swims to meet the ovum (Fig. 2-16).

The spermatozoa are produced in the testes, stored in the epididymis, and travel through the vas deferens to the ejaculatory duct to the urethra and out the penis. In sexual intercourse the spermatozoa are deposited in the vagina by the erect penis through the process of ejaculation.

REPRODUCTION

Puberty is the term given to the period of time (11 to 17 years of age) when the reproductive organs of both the male and female reach maturity. For a female the childbearing years begin when she produces mature ova *(ovulation)*, usually within the year after her first menstrual period *(menarche)*, and end when she experiences a permanent cessation of menses *(menopause)*. For the male the ability to father a child begins when he produces functional spermatozoa, usually during his early teens. Although the female's ovaries contain over 1 million immature ova at birth, males constantly produce new spermatozoa after each ejaculation. Thus the male is capable of remaining fertile until well advanced in years.

Hormones

Hormones are secreted by the gonads, or sex glands. The female gonads are the ovaries; the male gonads are the testes.

The two main female sex hormones are (1) *estrogen*, responsible for the development of female characteristics, and (2) *progesterone*, which prepares the endometrium for pregnancy, maintains the endometrium, and suppresses ovulation during pregnancy.

In the male the primary sex hormone is *testosterone*, which is derived from the interstitial cells of the testes and is secreted directly into the bloodstream. Testosterone contributes to development of secondary sex characteristics; sex urge and behavior; and development, maintenance, and functioning of accessory sex organs.

Ovarian Cycle: Ovulation

Although the ovarian cycle may vary in length from female to female, for purposes of description, a 28-day cycle is generally used, the first day of the menstrual period being day 1. The anterior lobe of the pituitary, a small endocrine gland at the base of the brain, secretes gonadotropic hormones that control the ovarian cycle in women. These hormones are the *follicle stimulating hormone* (FSH) and the *luteinizing hormone* (LH). In turn, release of LH and FSH is controlled by *luteinizing hormone–releasing hormone* (LHRH), a chemical compound secreted by the hypothalamus (a part of the brain) to act on the anterior pituitary gland.

Beginning at puberty one of the ovaries is stimulated about once a month to prepare an egg (ovum) for release and possible fertilization. Each egg, and its surrounding specialized mass of supporting and nutrient-supplying cells, is called a *follicle*. At the onset of each ovarian cycle, FSH released by the anterior pituitary travels through the bloodstream to stimulate the growth and maturation of several follicles (Fig. 2-17). One follicle outgrows the others to form a prominent, mature *graafian follicle*, which becomes large enough to stick out above the surface of the ovary. Thus the first half of the ovarian cycle is termed the *follicular phase*. (Although FSH is generally thought to be the most important anterior pituitary hormone to stimulate follicle growth, *both* FSH and LH are necessary.)

As the graafian follicle matures, some of its cells secrete increasing amounts of estrogen (primarily in the form of estradiol). It has been shown that if estradiol levels in blood are *high enough for long enough* the anterior pituitary will release LH. Thus approximately 14 days into the average ovarian cycle, the anterior pituitary releases a "surge" of LH, which triggers a small area of the graafian follicle to become thin and translucent, resembling a blister. It then bursts, and the ovum, covered by several cell layers, floats out of the follicle into the end of the fallopian tube. This "bursting" is termed ovulation.

After ovulation, the graafian follicle collapses and the mass of tissue forms a new structure termed the *corpus luteum*, or yellow body (see Fig. 2-17). The cells of the corpus luteum (luteal cells) produce both estrogen and progesterone in large amounts for approximately 14 days. Thus the second half of the ovarian cycle is termed the *luteal phase*. About 9 days after ovulation, the corpus luteum begins to wither and die if fertilization does not occur. As the corpus luteum dies, its hormone producing powers die with it, and thus estrogen and progesterone levels in the bloodstream fall to their lowest levels.

One might ask: "If rising estrogen levels cause the anterior pituitary to release the LH 'surge,' why doesn't a second LH 'surge' occur during the luteal phase as estrogen levels rise?" The answer lies in progesterone's ability to inhibit this feedback mechanism. Thus because the corpus luteum secretes large amounts of pro-

gesterone, a second ovulation during the same ovarian cycle is normally prevented.

If the ovum is fertilized by a spermatozoa in the fallopian tube, menstruation does not occur and the corpus luteum continues to secrete progesterone during the first 3 months of pregnancy. The placenta gradually takes over the secretion of progesterone.

Uterine Cycle: Menstruation

The menstrual cycle prepares the endometrium for implantation of the ovum should fertilization occur. We are once again using a 28-day cycle for study. The four phases of the menstrual cycle are described as follows (see Fig. 2-17).

Proliferative phase

This coincides with the last 8 to 12 days of the follicular phase of the ovarian cycle, depending on the duration of an individual woman's menstrual flow. During the proliferative phase, a period of endometrial repair is in progress. Cells from the uterine glands spread over the base of the endometrium as it regenerates and thickens. Endometrial glands become more and more tortuous. This growth is stimulated by the estrogen secreted from the developing ovarian follicle(s).

Ovulatory phase

Ovulation occurs on about the fourteenth or fifteenth day.

Secretory phase

Technically this phase begins at ovulation and includes the ovulatory phase. The secretory phase coincides with the luteal phase of the ovarian cycle. In normal circumstances the secretory phase is a constant 14 days in duration regardless of the length of a woman's menstrual cycle (for example, 28 days, 31 days, 26 days). Progesterone, the hormone responsible for the secretory phase, prepares the already thickened endometrium for possible implantation of the fertilized ovum. The endometrium becomes edematous and highly vascular. By the eighth day of the secretory phase (twenty-second day of the cycle), endometrial activity and gland secretory activity reach their peak, coinciding with maximal corpus luteum activity and highest progesterone levels. From the tenth to fourteenth days, edema subsides and the endometrium regresses. As the endometrium shrinks, the endometrium loses its blood supply and becomes ischemic. Tissue necrosis develops.

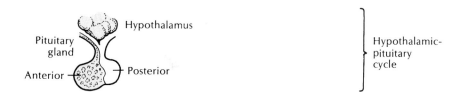

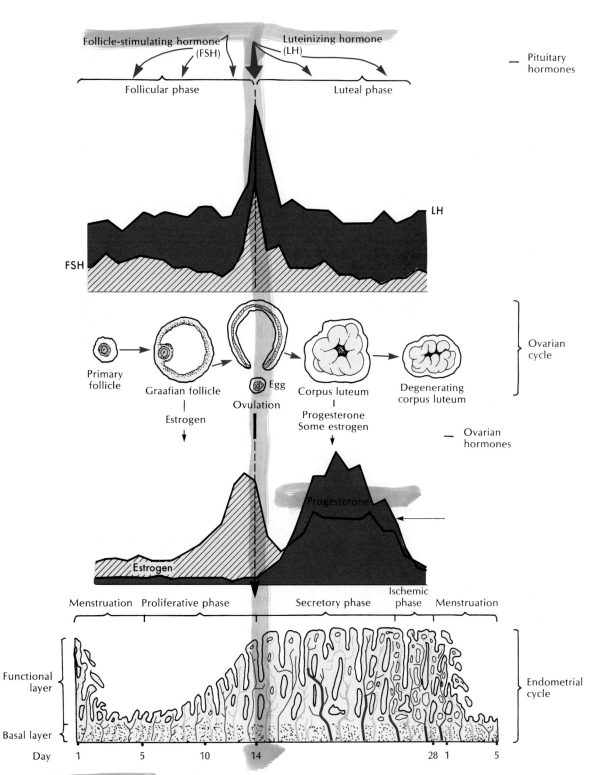

Figure 2-17 Menstrual cycle: Hypothalamic-pituitary, ovarian, and endometrial. *(From Bobak IM and others:* Maternity nursing, *ed 4, St. Louis, 1995, Mosby.)*

Menstrual phase

The tissue necrosis produced during the secretory phase causes blood vessels to open, producing scattered endometrial hemorrhages. These enlarge and form hematomas, which in turn cause shedding of the endometrium. The pattern of this shedding varies considerably in duration and amount of flow and is termed *menstruation*.

Normally the cycle begins again and continues at regular intervals except during pregnancy and after menopause.

SUMMARY

Chapter 2 was designed to provide you with a very basic review of the anatomy and physiology of the male and female reproductive systems, with an emphasis on the female.

BIBLIOGRAPHY

Alexander LL, LaRosa JH: *New dimensions in women's health,* Boston, Mass, 1994, Jones and Bartlett.

Barkauskas VH, Baumann LC, Stoltenberg-Allen K, Darling-Fisher C: *Health and physical assessment,* St. Louis, 1994, Mosby.

Jacob S, Francone CA: *Elements of anatomy and physiology,* ed 2, St. Louis, 1989, Mosby.

Mattson S, Smith JE, editors: *Core curriculum for maternal-newborn nursing,* Philadelphia, 1993, WB Saunders.

McCance KL, Huether SE: *Pathophysiology, the biologic basis for disease in adults and children,* ed 2, St. Louis, 1994, Mosby.

Oxorn H: *Human labor and birth,* ed 5, Norwalk, Conn, 1986, Appleton-Century-Crofts.

Sloane E: *Biology of women,* ed 3, Albany, NY, 1993, Delmar.

Thibodeau GA: *Structure and function of the body,* ed 9, St. Louis, 1992, Mosby.

DEFINITIONS

Define the following terms:

acini cells	cervix
ampulla	cilia
anteflexion	clitoris
anteverted	coccygeus
areola	colostrum
Bartholin's glands	convoluted
bulbourethral gland	copulation

cornu	menarche
corpus luteum	menopause
cul-de-sac	menstruation
culdocentesis	Montgomery's tubercles
ejaculation	myometrium
endometrium	ova
epididymis	ovaries
estrogen	ovulation
fallopian tubes	pelvic floor
fibrocartilage	pelvic splanchnics
fimbriae	perimetrium
follicle	perineum
follicle stimulating hormone (FSH)	peristaltic action
	prepuce
follicular phase	progesterone
fourchette	proliferative phase
fundus	prostate
gamete	rugae
gonad	secretory phase
graafian follicle	semen
gynecoid	Skene's glands
hymen	spermatozoa
hypogastric plexus	spiral arteries
innominate bones	symphysis pubis
ischial spines	testes
ischium	testosterone
labia majora	urethra
labia minora	uterus
levator ani muscle	vagina
linea terminalis	vas deferens
lobes	vestibule
lobules	vulva
luteal phase	

LEARNING ACTIVITIES

1. In an anatomy laboratory inspect a bony female pelvis and a male pelvis. Compare the general shape and curvature of the pubic arch.
2. View and discuss audiovisual aids.

ENRICHMENT/IN-DEPTH STUDY

1. Discover how the pelvic size of your family members who have been pregnant was determined. If you have experienced a pregnancy, how was your pelvic size determined?
2. Prepare a lesson plan to teach basic reproductive system anatomy and physiology to expectant couples in prenatal classes. Determine what information the couple needs in order to understand the physiologic changes that will occur in the pregnant woman. How much information is too much (overload) and how much information is just enough?

✿ Self-Assessment

1. External female reproductive organs. Label the following structures: labia majora, labia minora, vagina, clitoris, anus, perineum.

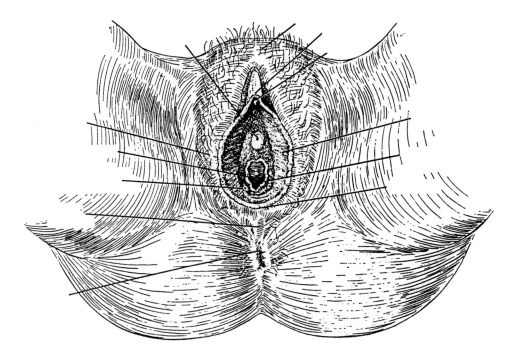

2. Male reproductive system. Label the following structures: bladder, urethra, pelvic bone, penis, scrotum, testis, vas deferens, prostate gland, epididymis, foreskin, glans penis, seminal vesicle.

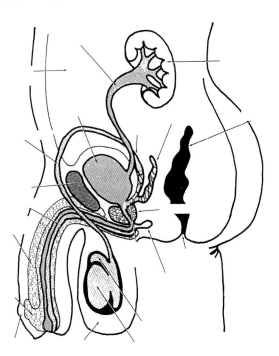

3. Internal female reproductive organs, front view. Label the following structures: fundus, cervix, corpus, fallopian tube, fimbriae, ovum, vagina, endometrium.

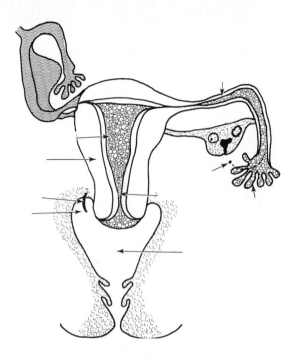

4. Label the following structures of the breast: nipple, areola, Montgomery's tubercles, rib, pectoralis muscle, internal mammary artery, alveoli (acini), fat, milk duct, sinuses (ampullae).

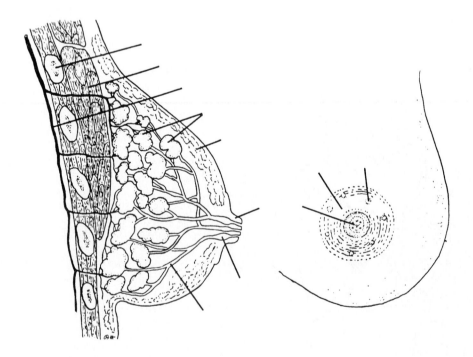

5. Female pelvic bones. Label the following: innominate bones, sacrum, coccyx, sacral promontory, ischial spines, pubis, ischium.

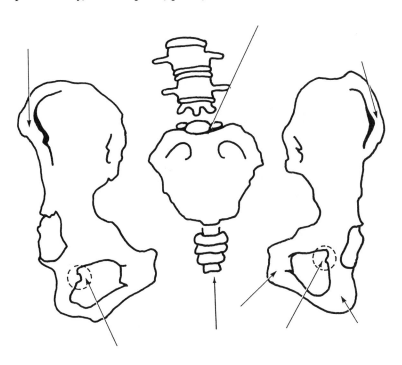

6. Identify the four pelvic types according to their shape:

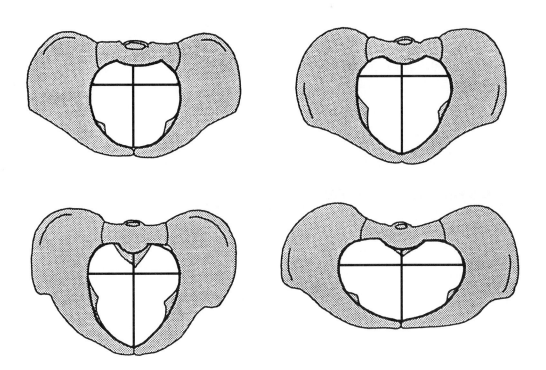

7. Explain two functions of the pelvic floor:

   a. _____

   b. _____

For questions 8 through 15, circle the best answers.

8. The three divisions or parts of the cervix are:

   a. meatus

   b. internal os

   c. corpus

   d. isthmus

   e. external os

9. Three of the bones listed below unite to form the innominate bone. Which one does *not?*

   a. pubis

   b. ilium

   c. coccyx

   d. ischium

10. The lowermost part of the uterus is called the:

    a. clitoris

    b. vagina

    c. endometrium

    d. cervix

11. The uppermost part of the uterus is called the:

    a. cervix

    b. corpus

    c. fundus

    d. myometrium

12. The three layers of tissue comprising the uterus include all of the following except:

    a. embriometrium

    b. endometrium

    c. perimetrium

    d. myometrium

13. The anatomic structure of the breasts that produces milk is:

    a. acini cell

    b. sinus

    c. areola

    d. Montgomery's tubercles

14. In the woman, the area of skin, connective tissue, and muscle between the vulva and the anus is called the:

    a. prepuce

    b. perineum

    c. hymen

    d. mons veneris

15. The male sex hormone responsible for the masculine characteristics of the male body is:

a. testosterone

b. semen

c. progesterone

d. estrogen

Supply the correct answer(s) for items 16 through 20.

16. Which layer of uterine muscle is the thickest and shaped like a figure eight?

17. The three basic functions of the male and female reproductive systems are:

a. _____

b. _____

c. _____

18. List the four bones of the pelvis.

a. _____

b. _____

c. _____

d. _____

19. The four phases of the menstrual cycle are:

a. _____

b. _____

c. _____

d. _____

20. The two phases of the ovulatory cycle are:

a. _____

b. _____

21. On the line to the left of each item in Column A match the appropriate hormones from Column B.

Column A

_____ 1. stimulates development of the follicle

_____ 2. initiates buildup of the lining of the uterus

_____ 3. causes ovulation and develops the corpus luteum

_____ 4. finishes preparation of uterus for pregnancy

_____ 5. a drop in this hormone in particular precedes menstruation

Column B

a. LH (lutenizing hormone)

b. estrogen (estradiol)

c. FSH (follicle stimulating hormone)

d. progesterone

22. Match the structures listed in column B with their proper characteristics in column A.

Column A

_____ 1. a muscular hammock supporting the internal organs

_____ 2. attaches from the uterus to each side of the pelvic cavity

_____ 3. extends from the uterus to the labia majora

_____ 4. connects the sacrum to the uterus

_____ 5. ligament that keeps the uterus from dropping down into the vagina

_____ 6. a superficial muscle that makes a figure eight around the vagina and rectum

Column B

a. uterosacral ligaments

b. broad ligaments

c. levator ani

d. round ligaments

e. cardinal ligament

f. bulbocavernosus muscle

For items 23 through 26, fill in the blanks.

23. Two female sex hormones are _____ and

_____.

24. Ovulation occurs during the _____ phase of the menstrual cycle.

25. The lining of the uterus thickens to prepare for pregnancy during the

_____ phase of the menstrual cycle.

26. The anatomic landmark that separates the false pelvis from the true pelvis is

_____.

27. Name the nerve pathways that transmit uterine pain.

_____

_____

_____

28. Describe in two sentences the function of the corpus luteum.

_____

_____

_____

29. Draw a rough sketch, indicating relative amounts of LH, FSH, estradiol, and progesterone during the menstrual cycle and ovarian cycle. Use a separate sheet for your sketch.

30. Name all of the structures that add fluid to semen.

_____

_____

_____

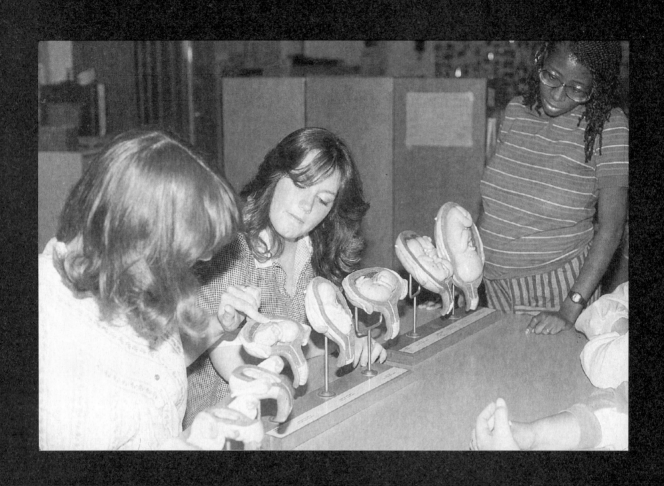

3

CONCEPTION AND PRENATAL DEVELOPMENT

GOALS

This chapter is designed to provide the reader with information that will:
- promote an understanding of conception, implantation, and placental and fetal development.
- develop an awareness of the influence of heredity and environmental factors on reproductive health.
- develop an awareness of the experience of infertility.

STUDENT OBJECTIVES

After studying this chapter, you should be able to:

1. Describe the process of implantation (transition from zygote to blastoderm).
2. Explain the functions of the amniotic fluid.
3. Describe the growth of the embryo from the second to the eighth week after fertilization.
4. Describe the umbilical cord (length and composition) and explain the significance of a single umbilical vein in the cord.
5. Name the functions of the placenta.
6. Characterize the significant changes in growth and development of the fetus in utero at 20 weeks of gestation, 28 weeks of gestation, and 32 weeks of gestation.
7. Trace the flow of blood through fetal circulation and name three unique fetal circulatory structures.
8. Explain how the sex of a person is determined.
9. Explain how common characteristics are inherited in terms of dominant and recessive traits and sex-linked traits.
10. Discuss the relationship between the incidence of Down syndrome and maternal age.
11. Identify a chromosomal abnormality that can be detected by examination of amniotic fluid cells following amniocentesis.
12. Discuss known environmental agents associated with birth defects.
13. List common sexually transmitted diseases and their effect on the newborn.
14. List at least three factors that can cause infertility in the female.
15. Name two tests available for diagnosing infertility.
16. List at least three factors that can cause infertility in the male.
17. Describe the choices available for an infertile couple who desire a child.

FERTILIZATION

During sexual intercourse spermatozoa are ejaculated from the penis into the vagina. At the time of ejaculation over 200 million spermatozoa may be deposited in the vagina. Moving by means of their long, thin tails, they travel up into the cervical canal. Contractions of the uterus and fallopian tubes are primarily responsible for propelling the sperm through these organs to the ovum. Less than 200 sperm actually survive to reach the vicinity of the ovum. The spermatozoa are viable for an average of 24 to 72 hours, swimming about, waiting for an ovum. If the female ovulates during this time, a single spermatozoa can enter the ovum, thereby fertilizing it. A human ovum remains viable for about 12 to 24 hours and is capable of being fertilized for only a short period after ovulation (probably not more than 12 hours). Thus in each woman's menstrual cycle, there is a period called the *fertile period*, during which fertilization can occur. This period occurs approximately 14 days before the next menstrual period begins, regardless of the length of the menstrual cycle.

The spermatozoon releases enzymes that facilitate penetration of the outer covering of the ovum (the *zona pellucida*). When one sperm has penetrated, an immediate cellular change in the zona pellucida makes penetration by other sperm impossible. *Fertilization* usually occurs in the dilated outer one third of the fallopian tube. (See Chapter 2)

Sex is determined by the sperm at the moment of fertilization. If the sperm carries an X chromosome, the baby will be a girl; if the sperm carries a Y chromosome, the baby will be a boy.

The fertilized cell resulting from the union of sperm and ovum is called a *zygote*. The zygote is one cell in which the nucleus of the sperm and the nucleus of the ovum have joined to form a single nucleus containing all of the necessary components for the development of another human being who is different from both parents.

CLEAVAGE

Soon after the zygote has formed, it divides into two daughter cells, called *blastomeres*, then four, eight, sixteen, and so forth by a process of cell division called *cleavage*. This cell division occurs while the fertilized ovum is being moved down the tube by the wavelike action of cilia and the peristaltic action of the tube itself.

Before division each chromosome doubles its hereditary material by a process called *mitosis* (Fig. 3-1, *A*). To divide, the parent cell duplicates each chromosome so that each new cell is an exact replica of the parent cell. The 46 chromosomes in the nucleus of the zygote literally line up in pairs, split lengthwise, and then di-

vide in half. Thus two identical sets of 46 chromosomes are made for the two new cells that are formed from the first. All future cell division proceeds this way. As a result each cell of the developing baby contains an equal number of chromosomes from each of the parents. It is these chromosomes that carry genes.

The trip to the uterus takes approximately 3 to 4 days, during which time the ovum becomes a solid mass of cells called a *morula* because of its resemblance to a mulberry. Although there are more than 16 cells by now, there has been no increase in the size of the developing cell cluster. It is still no larger than the point of a straight pin. As the cells continue to divide, fluid passes into the morula from the uterine cavity, and the cells regroup themselves into a hollow ball filled with fluid. The outer layer of cells, called the *trophoblast*, obtains food for the inner layer (or *embryoblast*) and eventually forms the placenta. The embryo develops from the inner layer of cells. At this stage the fertilized ovum is called a *blastocyst* (Fig. 3-2).

IMPLANTATION

As the blastocyst falls into the uterus, it sheds its outer membrane (the zona pellucida) and prepares to implant in the thick lining of the endometrium by day 6 or 7. By this time the endometrial lining has been prepared by circulating progesterone during the secretory phase and is now thick, edematous, and vascular. (See Chapter 2.) The endometrium is at its "ripest" stage. The blastocyst, by this time consisting of approximately 200 cells, usually implants in the anterior or posterior wall of the upper portion of the uterus (Fig. 3-3). To burrow into the uterine lining the trophoblastic cells secrete an enzyme that dissolves and absorbs some of the endometrium, eating its way into the endometrium and penetrating large maternal sinusoids which have formed. Owing to the increased thickening and enlargement of cells, the endometrium is now called the *decidua,* and the area directly under the trophoblast is called the *decidua basalis* (Fig. 3-4). Enzyme action occasionally opens a maternal vein and artery causing formation of *lacunas* (small blood lakes) in the decidua. The blastocyst now lies in a pool of maternal blood fed by maternal arterioles and drained by maternal veins. As the trophoblastic cells invade, they differentiate into two types: those at the blastocyst-decidua interface blend together to form the *syncytiotrophoblast* in contact with maternal blood, and those trophoblast cells next to the developing embryo remain separate as *cytotrophoblasts*. This proliferation of cells greatly increases the surface area and facilitates fetal-maternal exchanges.

Increased circulation at the site of implantation sometimes causes slight bleeding about 2 weeks after conception. Since this bleeding coincides with the men-

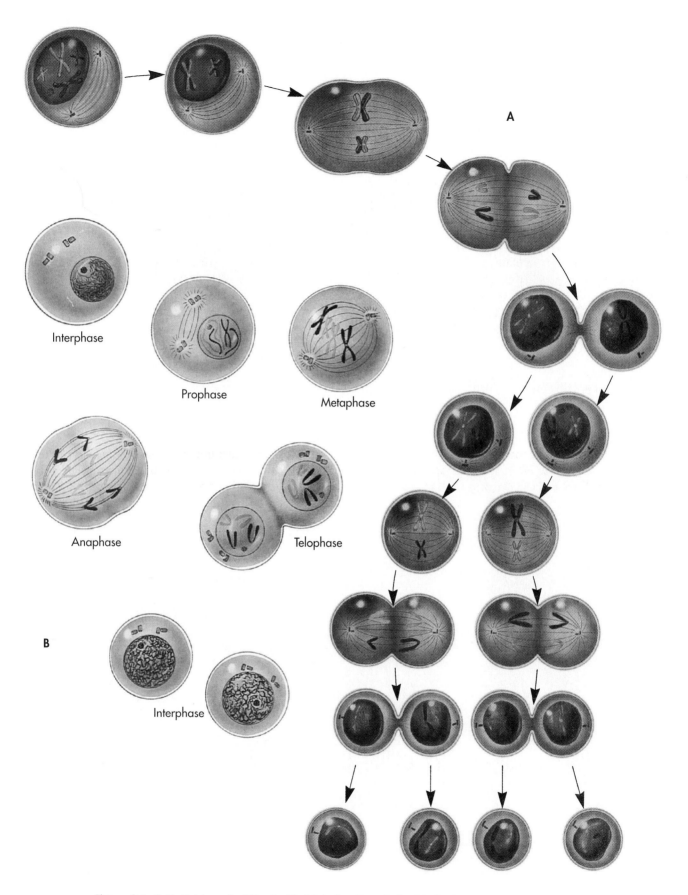

Figure 3-1 Cell division. **A,** Mitosis. **B,** Meiosis. *(From Seeley RR, Stephens TD, Tate P:* Anatomy and physiology, *St. Louis, 1989, Mosby.)*

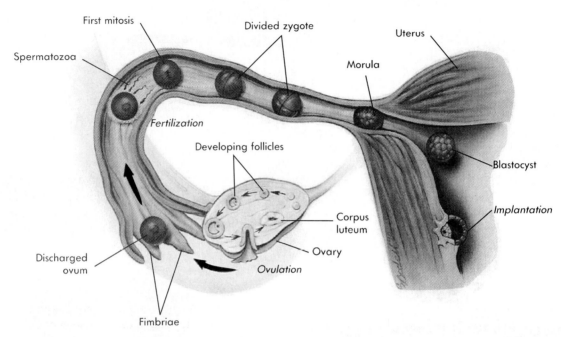

Figure 3-2 Fertilization, cleavage, and implantation. *(From Thibodeau GA, Patton KT:* Structure and function of the body, *ed 9, St. Louis, 1992, Mosby.)*

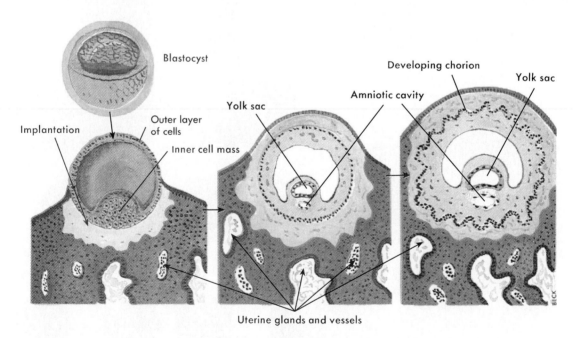

Figure 3-3 Implantation and early development. *(From Thibodeau GA, Patton KT:* Structure and function of the body, *ed 9, St. Louis, 1992, Mosby.)*

strual period in a 28-day cycle, it may lead to miscalculation of the expected date of delivery by approximately 1 month.

TROPHOBLASTIC STAGE

Once implantation has occurred the growing embryo can no longer survive only on nutrients from its own yolk sac; therefore the trophoblastic cells begin to form the *chorion,* or outermost sac. Covering the chorion are thousands of rootlike projections called *villi,* which further dig into the decidua and lay the foundation for the *placenta,* which will nourish the developing fetus.

The yolk sac gradually disappears as the amniotic cavity encloses the embryo. The embryo develops from the body stalk within the amniotic cavity, and as development continues, the chorionic villi that are not attached to the decidua fall off, leaving a transparent sac called the fetal membranes, which are made up of the *amnion (inner)* and *chorion (outer)* membranes. These membranes help to protect the embryo (and later the fetus) by sealing it off from the outside (Fig. 3-4). This

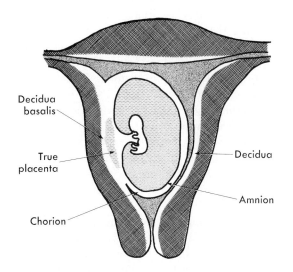

Figure 3-4 Fetal membranes.

amniochorionic sac is more commonly known as the "bag of waters."

The syncytiotrophoblast cells produce the hormone *human chorionic gonadotropin* (hCG), which signals the corpus luteum in the ovary to continue to manufacture levels of progesterone and estrogen high enough to prevent menstruation and ovulation. After the first few weeks of gestation the corpus luteum is no longer essential to maintain pregnancy, and thus hCG's function thereafter is unclear. The hormone hCG is excreted in the woman's urine and blood and is the basis of pregnancy testing, beginning 1 or 2 weeks following a missed menstrual period. Implantation is completed by about day 12 (Fig. 3-5).

AMNIOTIC FLUID

The amnion secretes *amniotic fluid* in which the fetus floats and moves for the duration of the pregnancy. This fluid-filled space contains 500 to 1000 milliliters of clear, slightly alkaline fluid by the end of the pregnancy.

The functions of the amniotic fluid include keeping the fetus at an even temperature, serving as a protective cushion for the fetus, equalizing pressures, and allowing the fetus to move freely without adhering to the amnion. Contributing to the formation of amniotic fluid is fluid from the maternal blood, the fetal lungs, and the fetal kidneys. This fluid is not static but is removed and replaced at a rate of approximately one third its volume every hour. The fetus near term drinks about 500 milliliters of amniotic fluid each day, which is about the same as the daily milk consumption of the newborn. Because the fetus drinks and inhales amniotic fluid, urinates into the amniotic fluid, and constantly sheds cells into it, studies of amniotic fluid obtained by *amniocentesis* (withdrawing some fluid from the amniotic sac for cell study) can reveal fetal maturity, sex, and general well-being (Fig. 3-6). Too much amniotic fluid *(polyhydramnios)* or too little *(oligohydramnios)* often indicates fetal abnormalities. Certain genetic disorders can also be diagnosed by utilizing amniocentesis.

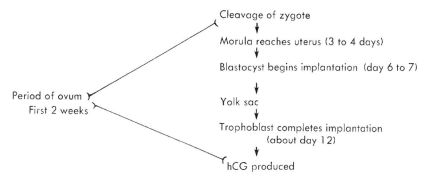

Figure 3-5 Preembryonic period.

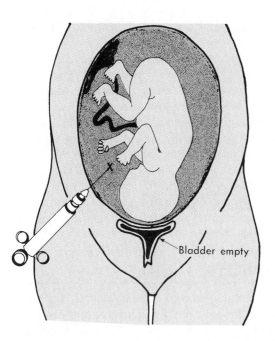

Figure 3-6 Amniocentesis.

EMBRYO

Embryonic Development

The time between fertilization and the first 14 days of development is the *preembryonic* period or stage of the ovum. It is a time of rapid cell division with differentiation of tissues and establishment of the embryonic membranes and primary germ layers—the *ectoderm*, *endoderm*, and *mesoderm*. The spinal cord, the brain, all the nerves, the sensory organs, and the skin will be formed from the ectoderm. The epithelial lining of most of the body systems will develop from the endoderm. The skeleton, muscles, and many internal organs will develop from the mesoderm.

At the third week the mass of growing cells is termed an *embryo*. By this time the groundwork for development of the new human being has been established, and the woman has missed her menstrual period for the first time in the pregnancy.

By the end of the first 28 days following conception (the first lunar month or month by the moon), the heart and brain are beginning to form. There are the beginnings of eyes, ears, nose, and small buds that will eventually become arms and legs. Development of the embryo generally proceeds from the head to the tail *(cephalocaudal)*.

During the next 28 days (second lunar month) the embryo grows to be about 1⅛ inches long. Because of the rapid development of the brain, the head is very large in comparison with other parts of the embryo. External genitalia appear, but sex cannot be differentiated

(Fig. 3-7). By the end of the seventh week, the beginnings of *all* major structures are present.

Development of the growing embryo is most easily affected by harmful environmental agents—including drugs, chemicals, radiation, and certain viruses—during the *organogenetic period*. Because this is the time when the body's basic organ systems are being formed (week 3 through week 8), it is at this time that the embryo is most sensitive to agents known to cause congenital malformations (Fig. 3-8).

Fetal Period

In the ninth week of pregnancy the embryo has developed into a *fetus*. All the major systems and external features are well established or at least begun. During the next 7 months the fetus will continue to grow until birth, when it will become a *newborn* (infant).

PLACENTA

As the developing embryo continues to grow, the chorionic villi (fetal side) embedded in the decidua basalis and the decidua basalis (maternal side) form the *placenta* during the third week. At the end of a full-term pregnancy, about 80% of the normal placenta is of fetal origin. The capillaries unite to form larger and larger veins, until finally they join to form the umbilical vein in the body stalk. Blood is sent back to the placenta from the embryo through two umbilical arteries (Fig. 3-9). The large umbilical vein and two smaller arteries are enclosed in the umbilical cord, which is about 2 feet long at birth and filled with a whitish, gelatinous substance that is called *Wharton's jelly*. Wharton's jelly prevents kinking of the cord and interference with circulation.

The umbilical cord should always be inspected at the time of birth. In 1 out of every 500 deliveries the umbilical cord contains only one artery instead of two. If this is the case the baby should be examined carefully because there is a higher risk of abnormalities in babies with a single umbilical artery.

The embryo is now floating in fluid and is anchored to the uterine wall by the umbilical cord and placenta. The placenta consists of maternal portions (decidua basalis) and fetal portions (chorionic villi) and acts as the organ of transfer between the mother and the fetus. The maternal surface is deep red and divided into sections, or *cotyledons*. The fetal surface (covered with amniotic membrane) is smooth and grayish with prominent blood vessels. The umbilical cord usually arises from the middle of the placenta (Fig. 3-10). At the end of pregnancy the placenta is about 8 inches (20 centimeters) in diameter, 1 inch (2.5 centimeters) thick, and weighs more than 1 pound (2.2 kilograms).

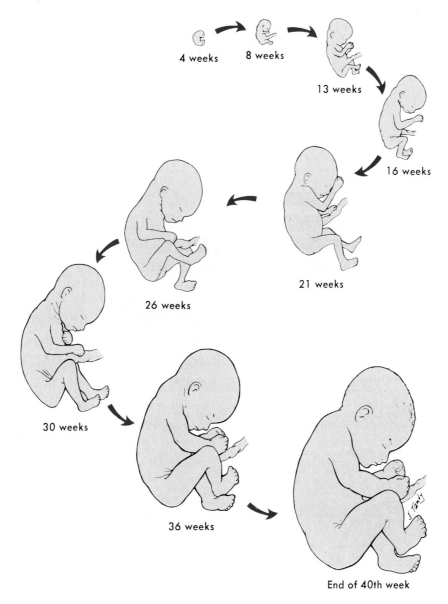

Figure 3-7 Growth and development. *(From Jensen M, Benson RC, Bobak IM:* Maternity care: the nurse and the family, *St. Louis, 1977, Mosby.)*

Placental Transfer

It is important to understand that the maternal and fetal blood are in separate systems and do not mix. There are three tissue layers between maternal and fetal blood in the human placenta. These are (1) fetal trophoblast, (2) the connective tissue core of the fetal villus, and (3) the endothelium of fetal capillaries. Any substance passing between mother and fetus must cross these three permeable tissue layers (often known as the *placental barrier*). Contrary to the old myth that this placental barrier stops all harmful substances and protects the fetus, we know now that the placenta is literally a bloody sieve, allowing almost all substances, if small enough, to cross it in varying degrees. Only substances of high molecular weight such as insulin or heparin and complex structures such as red blood cells cannot cross the placental barrier.

Nourishment passes from the maternal side to the fetal side, and waste products pass from the fetal side to the maternal side as a result of several factors, both static and dynamic. Oxygen from the maternal side passes through the placenta to the fetal side, and CO_2 passes from the fetal side to the maternal side by *diffusion* (the passive passage of gases from an area of high concentration to one of low concentration). On the mother's side of the placental barrier, the uterine arteries bring blood into the intervillous space, and uterine veins drain the blood. On the fetal side, umbilical ar-

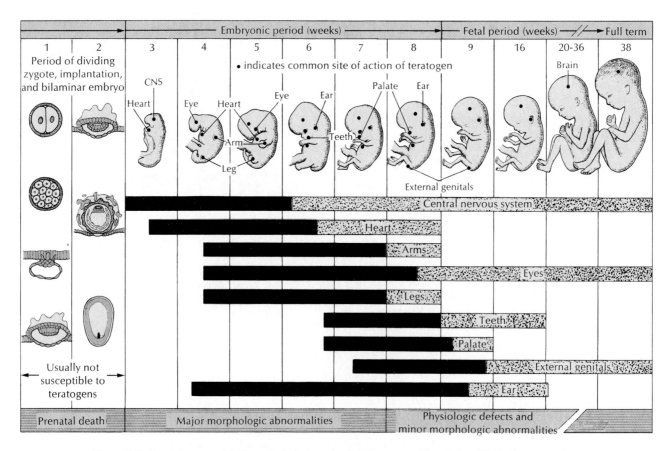

Figure 3-8 Sensitive, or critical, periods in human development. *(From Moore KL:* Before we are born, *Philadelphia, 1989, WB Saunders.)*

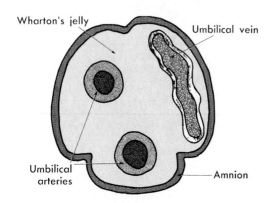

Figure 3-9 Cross-section of the umbilical cord.

teries bring blood into the fetal placental area, and the umbilical veins drain it. To recall this terminology, remember that the term *artery* always refers to a vessel that brings blood *away* from a heart (maternal or fetal), and the term *vein* always refers to a vessel that brings blood *to* a heart. As these two separate blood systems come close at the placental membrane site, the exchange of substances occurs (Fig. 3-11).

The placenta has three major functions: (1) transfer—O_2, CO_2, nutrients, electrolytes, some antibodies,

and waste; (2) metabolism—the placenta manufactures fatty acids, glycogen, and cholesterol; and (3) endocrine secretion—hCG, human chorionic somatomamotropin (hCS), thyrotropin, estrogens, and progesterones. As stated earlier, during the first part of pregnancy the corpus luteum produces the progesterone, but after about 3 months of pregnancy, the placenta takes over the secretion of progesterone, which is essential for the maintenance of pregnancy. At this point the corpus luteum is no longer needed and degenerates.

The placenta also secretes estriol, an estrogen, and human placental lactogen (hPL), a hormone similar to prolactin.

FETAL DEVELOPMENT

Fertilization age is measured from the time the zygote is formed by the union of sperm and ovum. However, because this date is not usually known with certainty, a more useful term is *gestational age*. Gestational age is dated from the time of onset of the last menstrual period. From the first day of the last menstrual period, the length of an average pregnancy is 280 days, 10 lunar months (month by the moon), 9 calendar months,

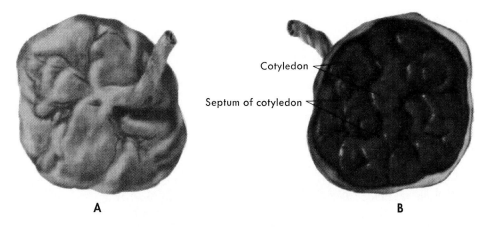

Figure 3-10 **A,** Fetal surface of placenta. **B,** Maternal surface of placenta. *(From Placental circulation, Nursing Education Aid No. 2, Columbus, Ohio, Ross Laboratories.*

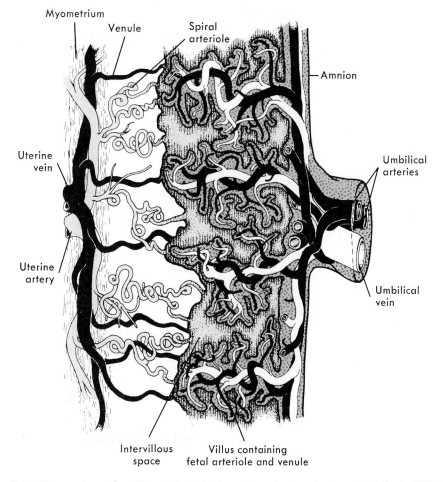

Figure 3-11 Placental transfer. *(From Tucker S:* Pocket guide to fetal monitoring ed 2, *St. Louis, 1992, Mosby.)*

or 40 weeks. As you study fetal development, refer again to Fig. 3-7.

By the *fourth lunar month (16 weeks of gestation)* the fetus usually looks like a miniature baby with pink skin but a rather large head. It is 6 inches (15.2 centime-ters) long, weighs 6 ounces (170 grams), and has formed fingers and toes. The buds for "baby" teeth are present, and the kidneys are developing and secreting small amounts of urine. Brain configuration is nearly complete, and heart muscle is developed. *Meconium* (a thin, dark green to black sterile substance) begins to be present in the intestines.

By the *fifth lunar month (20 weeks of gestation)* the fetus has grown considerably and is approximately 8 inches (19 centimeters) long, weighing 1.0 pound 0.5 ounces (435 to 465 grams). A fine, downy hair called *lanugo* covers the body. The fetus is able to suck and swallow amniotic fluid. Fetal movements are felt by the mother *(quickening),* and the heartbeat can be heard with a fetoscope. (Actually the heartbeat can be heard as early as the sixteenth week with the sensitive electronic instrument called an *ultrasonic fetoscope,* or Doppler.)

By the *sixth lunar month (24 weeks of gestation)* the fetus is 11.2 inches (28 centimeters) long and weighs 1 pound 10 ounces (780 grams). The skin of the fetus is red and wrinkled, and the fetus has a reflex handgrip, and will exhibit a startle reflex. If born, the infant may not survive.

By the *seventh lunar month (28 weeks of gestation)* the fetus is about 14 inches (35.4 centimeters) long, has a head circumference of approximately 26 centimeters, and weighs 2½ pounds (1136 grams). A cheesy, greasy, white substance, called *vernix caseosa,* covers the wrinkled red skin to serve as a protective coating for the fetus floating in the amniotic fluid. Without this lubricating vernix, the fetus might shrivel like a prune. The eyes have lids that open and close, eyebrows, and lashes. Lungs are capable of breathing air. If born, the fetus may survive with life support systems and expert intensive care.

By the *eighth lunar month (32 weeks of gestation)* the fetus is approximately 16 inches (40.6 centimeters) long, has a head circumference of about 30 centimeters, and weighs about 3½ pounds (1590 grams). The fetus now has the appearance of a "little old man" and is gaining weight from an increase in muscle and fat. If born at this time, the fetus has a chance of surviving if given expert care.

By the *ninth lunar month (36 weeks of gestation)* the fetus is approximately 18 inches (45.6 centimeters) long, has a head circumference of about 32 centimeters, and weighs about 6 pounds (2600 grams). The fetus now has fingernails reaching to the fingertips and has a fairly good chance of surviving if it is born at this time.

By the *tenth lunar month (40 weeks of gestation)* the fetus is 20 inches (50.8 centimeters) long, has a head circumference of about 35 centimeters, and weighs about 7 pounds (3200 grams). The body has filled out because of subcutaneous fat deposits. The soft lanugo hair has almost disappeared except on the shoulders and upper back, and vernix caseosa is mainly in the folds and creases of the skin. The fetus is considered full term and ready to be born.

The fetus of a pregnancy that goes past a 42-week gestation period is termed *postmature.* This can be a serious situation for the fetus because as the placenta ages, the mother deposits fibrin in the placenta. Extensive fibrin deposits can cut off the villi and cause a compromised placenta that becomes less and less efficient in supplying O_2 and nutrients. A postmature baby appears to have very dry, parchment-like skin with little subcutaneous fat and no vernix. This postmature baby is at risk of developing major problems such as meconium aspiration and hypoglycemia.

There are biochemical and biophysical tests that can determine both the gestational age and the wellness of the fetoplacental unit. If the tests indicate that the fetus is being compromised, the pregnancy can be terminated and the baby born before life-threatening complications occur.

Fetal Capabilities

The fetus has many varied experiences before birth. Research in prenatal and perinatal psychology indicates that a fetus can see, hear, feel, and perhaps even form a basic level of awareness inside the uterus. There is mounting evidence that by the fourth month after conception the fetus has a well-developed sense of touch and taste and can perceive and respond to light shining on the mother's abdomen. There is evidence that by the sixth month in utero the fetus hears clearly and moves in rhythm to the mother's speech; when the fetus is startled, the legs are first drawn up and then stretched out.

As discussed in Chapter 1, bonding begins during pregnancy and is accelerated at birth and throughout the postpartum period. With information on the sensory capabilities of the fetus, parents can be encouraged to interact with their baby during pregnancy. Parents can be encouraged to sing to their baby and play calming music. Also, light, rhythmic stroking of the mother's abdomen, talking to the fetus, and responding to fetal movements are all communication channels that can be used to promote intrauterine bonding.

Fetal Circulation

Because the source of oxygen for the fetus is the placenta, the fetus does not need its lungs to exchange oxygen; and because the source of nutrients for the fetus is the placenta, it does not need its own liver to serve as a nutrition factory. Consequently, there are three special shunts to route most of the fetal blood past the fetal lungs and liver. These shunts are the *ductus venosus,* which goes straight through the liver, and the *foramen ovale* and *ductus arteriosus,* which bypass the lungs (Fig. 3-12). These will be discussed subsequently.

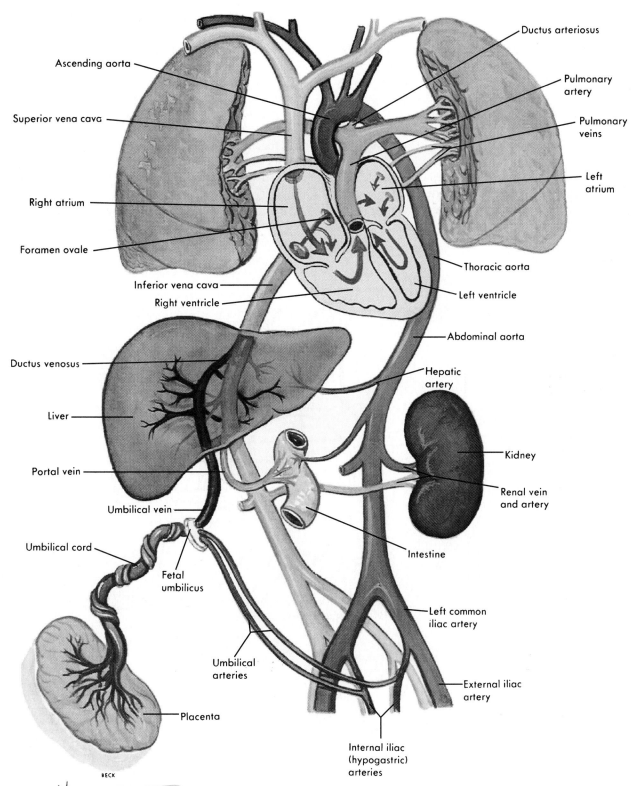

Figure 3-12 Fetal circulation. *(From Thibodeau GA, Patton KT: Structure and function of the body, ed 9, St. Louis, 1992, Mosby.)*

Comparison of Fetal and Adult Circulation

Adult circulation

In an adult the unoxygenated blood returns to the heart via the superior vena cava (SVC) and inferior vena cava (IVC). The blood enters the right atrium, travels next to the right ventricle, then leaves via the pulmonary artery for oxygenation in the lungs. In the capillary beds of the pulmonary circulation, the blood not only picks up O_2 but also gives off CO_2. The blood then returns to the left atrium by way of the pulmonary veins. From the left atrium it travels to the left ventricle and then is pumped out of the aorta, under high pressure, to perfuse the rest of the body. (Trace the path just described in Fig. 3-13.)

Fetal circulation

Because in the fetus the source of O_2 is the placenta and not the fetal lungs, blood rich with O_2 and nutrients flows through the umbilical vein. (Remember: blood returning from an oxygen source always travels through veins.) Blood from the umbilical vein enters the *portal venous system* (which drains all blood from the intestines and other digestive organs), and then 20% to 80% of this mixed blood is shunted quickly through the liver, bypassing the normal liver by way of the special ductus venosus. It is not known what factors determine how much umbilical vein blood goes through the ductus venosus and how much traverses the liver.

Once fetal blood leaves the liver, it enters the IVC and continues its journey toward the heart. One would

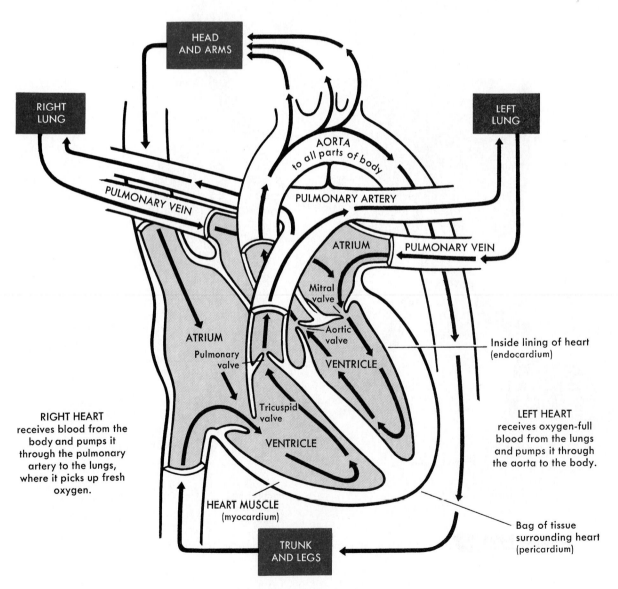

Figure 3-13 Adult circulation.

think that IVC and SVC blood would mix completely in the right atrium; however, this is not the case. Much of the blood from the IVC is directed preferentially through the right atrium to the left side of the heart via the *foramen ovale* (a small hole between the two atria). Thus this relatively oxygen-rich blood (remember: it has just recently returned from the placenta) flows from the left atrium to the left ventricle and out the ascending aorta to the oxygen-hungry fetal brain.

On the other hand, blood returning from the fetal head is relatively oxygen-poor. Thus most SVC blood is efficiently streamlined to pass through the right atrium into the right ventricle and out the pulmonary artery. However, blood traveling through nonbreathing lungs serves little purpose (except to provide the small amount of blood necessary to keep the fetal lungs alive). Thus the third fetal shunt is the *ductus arteriosus,* a short artery between the pulmonary artery and the descending aorta. The ductus arteriosus allows 85% to 90% of pulmonary artery blood to bypass the lungs and thus begin its trip down the descending aorta toward the placenta to be reoxygenated. The fetal heart pumps the blood to the body at a rate of 120 to 160 beats per minute. (Trace the path of fetal circulation in Fig. 3-12.)

Circulation changes at birth

With the first breath the lungs expand and the pulmonary vessels open. This drop in pulmonary vascular resistance lowers the blood pressure on the right side of the heart, thereby reversing the blood flow through the shunts (foramen ovale and ductus arteriosus). The foramen ovale closes by a small flap of tissue sealing over the hole during the first 24 hours. The closure of the fora-

men ovale normalizes the course of blood flow. The ductus venosus and ductus arteriosus shrivel up and are converted to fibrous ligaments within 2 to 3 months. The umbilical arteries wither from disuse and are converted to fibrous cords. The umbilical vein becomes a round ligament of the liver (the ligamentum teres).

SEX DETERMINATION

Except for the spermatozoon and the ovum, each human cell contains 23 paired *chromosomes* (total 46) within its nucleus. There are 22 matching pairs (total 44) of autosomes (nonsex chromosomes) and one pair of chromosomes that determines the individual's sex (*XX* if female, *XY* if male). During *meiosis,* or germ cell division in preparation for fertilization, the *diploid* (double) number of 46 is reduced to the *haploid* (single) number of 23 chromosomes (Fig. 3-1, *B*). However, because each resulting *gamete* (egg cell or sperm cell) receives one chromosome from each of the matching pairs, the gametes still carry all of the genetic information from the parents.

Each ovum carries 23 chromosomes, one of which is the *X* chromosome (sex chromosome). Each spermatozoon carries 23 chromosomes, one of which is the sex chromosome, which can be either *X* or *Y*. If an *X*-carrying spermatozoon fertilizes an ovum, two *X*s are joined, creating a female. However, if a *Y*-carrying spermatozoon fertilizes an ovum, an *X* and *Y* are joined, creating a male. Thus it is the father rather than the mother whose gamete determines the sex of the embryo.

$$X + X = XX = \text{female}$$
$$X + Y = XY = \text{male}$$

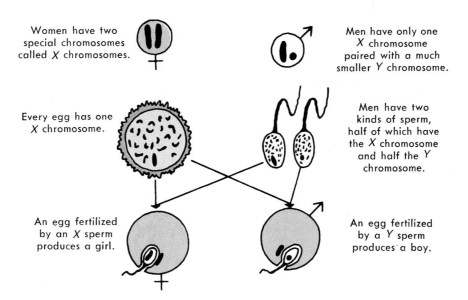

Women have two special chromosomes called X chromosomes.

Men have only one X chromosome paired with a much smaller Y chromosome.

Every egg has one X chromosome.

Men have two kinds of sperm, half of which have the X chromosome and half the Y chromosome.

An egg fertilized by an X sperm produces a girl.

An egg fertilized by a Y sperm produces a boy.

Figure 3-14 Sex determination. *(From Morgan C:* Introduction to psychology, *ed 2, New York, 1961, McGraw-Hill.)*

When the sperm and ovum unite at conception, the resulting zygote contains 46 chromosomes: 23 chromosomes, including a sex chromosome, from each parent (Fig. 3-14).

HEREDITY

Chromosomes are made up chemically of protein and DNA (deoxyribonucleic acid), a complex protein that carries the genetic information.

DNA could be called the master template for cell building. In humans DNA occurs as a double-stranded helix found in the cell nucleus. Two long chemical chains of DNA molecules are wrapped around each other and linked by chemical bonds to form a shape like a spiral staircase. The instructions contained in the DNA are carried to all parts of the body by RNA (ribonucleic acid), another nucleic acid present in the genes.

Each chromosome contains thousands of minute structures called *genes,* which carry the factors responsible for transmitting the characteristics or traits of an individual. Thus each individual inherits characteristics from his or her mother and father by receiving their genes.

Dominant and Recessive Traits

Some physical traits passed on from generation to generation are said to be either *dominant* or *recessive.* If the genes the individual receives from each parent are different *(heterozygous),* the dominant gene will determine the characteristic more likely to appear . If there are like recessive genes present *(homozygous),* a recessive trait will appear. People may carry a recessive trait without showing the trait themselves.

Some dominant traits	Some recessive traits
Dark hair	Blue or grey eyes
Brown eyes	Light hair
Curly hair	Rh negative blood

Example: Gene for eye color

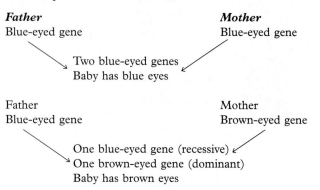

Father
Blue-eyed gene

Mother
Blue-eyed gene

Two blue-eyed genes
Baby has blue eyes

Father
Blue-eyed gene

Mother
Brown-eyed gene

One blue-eyed gene (recessive)
One brown-eyed gene (dominant)
Baby has brown eyes

Sex-linked Characteristics (X-linked)

Still other physical traits are associated with the genes in the *X* and *Y,* or sex, chromosomes and do not affect the two sexes equally. Rare sex-linked (*X*-linked) recessive disorders occur almost exclusively in males, with females being carriers. This occurs because very few genes are present on the *Y* chromosome. Thus a gene present on one *X* chromosome is easily "dominant" in a male who can offer no other *X* genes. More than 50 traits are known to be inherited in this manner, including color blindness and hemophilia.

Example: Hemophilia

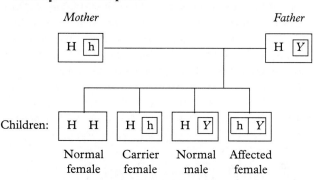

risk: 50% for female carrier
50% for male with hemophilia

H = normal gene

h = hemophilia gene

Y = absence of hemophilia gene on *Y* chromosome

It is possible as early as 12 to 14 weeks of gestation to determine the sex of the fetus in utero by doing an early amniocentesis. If a Barr body (sex chromatin found in female cells) is found in 20% to 40% of the nuclei of the fetal cells collected, the fetus in utero is probably a female. It could be important to predict fetal sex in the event of sex-linked diseases such as described previously. The parents may choose to abort a fetus who could be a carrier or may have a sex-linked disorder; or by simply knowing the probabilities, they may be better prepared to cope with potential problems.

BIRTH DEFECTS

Between 3% and 5% of babies born in the United States have some sort of genetic disease or congenital malformation (birth defect). Although traits and abnormalities can be passed on from generation to generation, as previously discussed, birth defects can result from three other major causes: (1) chromosomal abnormalities, (2) environmental agents, and (3) a combination of genetic and environmental factors.

Chromosomal Abnormalities

As previously discussed, each spermatozoon and ovum has 23 chromosomes, which unite at conception to form 46. Rarely, a sperm or ovum keeps one complete pair, thus giving it 24 chromosomes, or drops a pair, giving it 22 chromosomes. If an ovum with an extra chromosome is fertilized by a normal sperm, the resulting fetus is either aborted or a baby is born with *autosomal trisomy.* The most frequent chromosomal abnormality is trisomy 21 (Down syndrome), associated with an extra chromosome 21. The incidence of Down syndrome increases as the mother's age increases. In women under 20 years of age, the incidence is 1:1500 to 2000. In women over 44 years of age, the incidence is 1:50. In this case it is thought that the ova of the older woman, having been present in her ovaries since birth, may have begun to deteriorate. These women are also candidates for amniocentesis because trisomies can be detected by a study of the amniotic fluid.

If this problem arises in a sex chromosome, it is called a *sex-linked trisomy.* An example of this is Klinefelter's syndrome, in which the male has an *XXY* trisomy and usually has immature sexual organs, may be impotent, and is often mentally retarded.

In *monosomy,* only one of a particular pair of chromosomes is present. An example of this is Turner's syndrome, in which the female has an *XO* monosomy and usually has no ovaries, a webbed neck, and congenital heart disease. Fortunately, these aberrations are usually one-time occurrences and are not passed on to the next generation.

Prenatal diagnosis

When couples are at risk for having a child with an inheritable disease, prenatal testing can be done. *Prenatal diagnosis* is the detection of birth defects prior to delivery. The three most common obstetric screening procedures for identifying genetic problems are family history, alpha-fetoprotein (AFP) screening and ultrasound evaluation. Family history is the primary means for identifying women who need genetic counseling.

Alpha-fetoprotein (AFP) is the major protein in the serum of the embryo and early fetus. It crosses the fetal membranes into maternal circulation and can be measured in maternal serum.

Routine maternal serum screening for alphafetoprotein can uncover a higher than normal level of AFP in maternal blood. This higher level of AFP may indicate that the fetus has major open neural tube defects such as spina bifida or anencephaly, or an open abdominal wall defect such as omphalocele. When there is a positive AFP test, ultrasound evaluation can be done for further screening. Ultrasonography can detect fetal structural abnormalities such as spinal defects, cardiac anomalies, abdominal wall defects, cleft lip and palate, and urinary tract abnormalities. Maternal AFP screening at 15 to 18 weeks of gestation is mandatory in some states.

Traditional amniocentesis is the safest and most widely used prenatal diagnostic technique. It is performed between 15 and 18 weeks of gestation. It is an outpatient procedure with risk for complications of less than 0.5% when the procedure is done by experienced clinicians. Early amniocentesis can be effectively performed at 12 to 14 weeks of gestation, thus decreasing the anxiety of a longer waiting period before receiving results. However, the risk of complications such as miscarriage after early amniocentesis is approximately 1%. Amniocentesis can provide chromosome, DNA, enzyme, and alpha-fetoprotein analysis.

Chorionic villus sampling (CVS) performed in the first trimester of pregnancy can provide chromosome, DNA, and enzyme analysis. CVS can be performed between 10 and 12 weeks of gestation. It involves the removal of a small tissue specimen from the fetal portion of the placenta. CVS carries a higher risk for complications than do traditional or early amniocentesis.

Chromosome analysis can be performed by obtaining any tissue that contains cells capable of dividing. Usually the sample is blood or amniotic fluid fetal cells. This sampling allows rapid *karyotyping.* Abnormalities in the number of chromosomes can be detected by analysis of karyotypes—the chromosomal elements typical of a cell, arranged according to a definite classification (Fig. 3-15). The entire process should take from 7 to 10 days to complete.

A variety of disorders that were not previously detectable can be diagnosed using DNA analysis now. Because this testing is complex and variable, when a DNA analysis is being considered, the family should be referred for an in-depth family history and counseling.

GENETIC COUNSELING

Genetic counseling services are available to couples who suspect that their future children may be at risk for inheriting a disorder or to couples following the delivery of a baby with a birth defect. There are counseling centers throughout the United States where people can go to gather the information necessary to obtain a probability estimate for genetic problems. In addition, these centers provide extensive counseling.

The well-informed nurse can help with genetic counseling by case finding, making referrals, and explaining

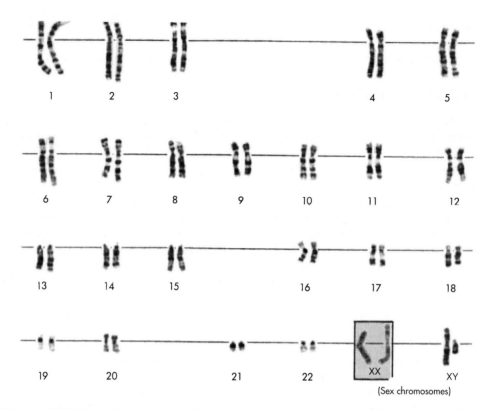

Figure 3-15 High-resolution G-banded human karyotype (male). *(Courtesy Bradshaw C, UCSD Medical Genetics, La Jolla, Calif.)*

the genetic counseling procedure to couples, thereby preventing or alleviating anxiety. Reproductive choices are methods to decrease or eliminate the risk for a particular genetic disorder. Donor insemination is an alternative in some autosomal recessive disorders or if the male has an autosomal dominant disorder. Surrogate mothers provide an alternative when the mother has an autosomal dominant disorder. Adoption can become a choice if the other alternatives are not acceptable.

Scientific knowledge in human and medical genetics is expanding rapidly during the last decade of the twentieth century. Almost every day there is a news release about the discovery of a new gene, the relationship of a gene to illness, the effect of the environment on genetics, or genetic therapy. The ethical implications of this research involve the possibility of genetic science in ways that may go beyond using it for human good and the avoidance of preventable harm.

When reproductive decisions must be made, nurses can help parents to consider their choices and then can support parents in their decisions.

Environmental Agents

Exposure to toxic agents can cause prematurity, birth defects, spontaneous abortions, stillbirths, intrauterine growth retardation, and a decrease in fertility. Agents (such as a drug, chemical, or infection) capable of causing permanent damage to the developing fetus are called *teratogens*. Even before a woman may realize that she is pregnant, the embryo is particularly vulnerable to the teratogenic effects of environmental agents. The third through eighth weeks of gestation (the period of embryogenesis) is a time during which major structural defects can occur after exposure to a hazardous agent. Teratogens may include prescription drugs and over-the-counter medicines, environmental pollutants, tobacco, alcohol, crack/cocaine, radiation, hyperthermia, viral diseases and infections, communicable diseases, and sexually transmissible diseases (STDs). A chart of potentially harmful medicines should be consulted whenever a pregnant (or possibly pregnant) woman gives a history of taking prescription medications or other drugs. Because many teratogens cause birth defects before a woman knows she is pregnant, educational efforts regarding teratogens must begin before pregnancy.

Many environmental agents are currently under investigation after reports of potentially harmful effects. A disproportionate amount of spontaneous abortions and birth defects have been reported in women who work with video display terminals and computers. It is unclear whether this is a true correlation or merely statistical chance. Industrial solvents found at toxic waste dumps have been associated with a variety of birth defects and high rates of infant mortality. Exposure to dioxin, used by the U.S. government on forests, highways, and power lines, has been associated with birth defects and spontaneous abortions. Although environmental agents do not usually cause abnormalities during the fetal period, if exposure to them occurs during the fetal period, they can cause abnormalities of the external genitalia, teeth, brain, and palate because the development of these structures is not completed during the embryonic period. Because the brain is particularly susceptible, adverse environmental conditions may cause mental retardation.

Paternal Causes of Teratogenesis

Although the possible mechanisms of paternally caused birth defects are speculative, recent studies indicate that paternal exposure to lead, anesthetic gases, or caffeine, and possibly smoking, may adversely affect the fetus. Counseling about potential workplace hazards is necessary so that the couple can make informed decisions regarding their work situations.

Behavioral Teratogenesis

Illicit drug use is particularly dangerous. Any pregnancy complicated by substance abuse should be considered high risk. During the first trimester, substance abuse alters organogenesis. Neurologic growth can be adversely affected at any time during the pregnancy because the central nervous system continues to develop throughout pregnancy. During the third trimester substance abuse can alter labor patterns. Cocaine abuse during pregnancy is associated with preterm labor, perinatal complications (miscarriage, prematurity, and stillbirth), low birth weight, and congenital cardiac anomalies, as well as maternal and fetal death. Abuse is further complicated when drugs are taken in combination. The dangers of maternal drug abuse do not end with delivery. Many substances can be passed to babies during breast-feeding, posing long-term threats to infant development.

More commonly encountered is the pregnant woman who smokes cigarettes or drinks alcohol. Heavy cigarette smoking has been correlated with an increased incidence of low-birth-weight babies and preterm birth. Even light smoking (less than 10 cigarettes per day) has been shown to increase the risk of fetal death, damage in utero, abruptio placentae, and placenta previa. There also are reports of an increased risk of sudden infant death syndrome (SIDS) in babies of women who smoke during and after pregnancy. Prenatal use of marijuana seems to have effects similar to those of cigarette smoking.

Heavy and steady alcohol consumption has been correlated not only with a high incidence of newborn mental retardation but also with fetal alcohol syndrome, in which one or more of the following characteristics occur: growth retardation, microcephaly (small head size), central nervous system abnormalities, joint anomalies, kidney abnormalities, and heart defects. Facial characteristics may include increased space between the eyes; depressed, broadened nasal bridge; increased space between nose and upper lip; and thin upper lip. It appears that there is a dose-effect relationship; that is, the more one drinks, the more likely one is to have a baby with the full-blown syndrome. However, no one knows whether drinking even a small amount of alcohol during pregnancy could have harmful effects on the fetus. Thus it is best to avoid exposure to alcohol during pregnancy.

TORCH

The infections that have been convincingly shown to cause serious birth defects are known as the TORCH group:

T for toxoplasmosis
O for "other" (hepatitis B)
R for rubella
C for cytomegalovirus (CMV)
H for herpes simplex virus (HSV)

Women who contract these infections while pregnant have an increased risk of delivering malformed offspring because each of the five diseases crosses the placenta and may adversely affect the developing fetus. The effect of each varies, depending on the developmental stage at the time of exposure.

Toxoplasmosis is caused by the parasite *Toxoplasma gondii*. Infectious organisms are transmitted primarily in the feces of cats who hunt rodents that harbor the parasite. However, the disease can also be spread by eating undercooked or raw meat from sheep, pigs, or cattle that feed from contaminated sources. Associated congenital anomalies include intrauterine growth retardation (IUGR), microcephaly or *hydrocephaly* (large, fluid-filled brain), *microphthalmia* (small eyes), *chorioretinitis* (an inflammation of the eyes), calcifications in skull radiographs, low platelet counts, and jaundice. An infected infant that survives the neonatal period is usually mentally retarded, affected by seizures, and has neuromuscular disease and poor vision. Pregnant women should avoid contact with cat feces or kitty litter boxes and raw meats. Women and newborns infected with toxoplasmosis are not contagious and need not be isolated.

Hepatitis B (HBV) is caused by a virus and is spread by contact with contaminated blood, urine, saliva, feces, vaginal secretions, tears, and other bodily fluids.

Population groups in the United States from areas where the disease is endemic are at high risk for HBV infection. These geographic areas are China, Southeast Asia, sub-Saharan Africa, Pacific Islands, and Haiti.

Major routes of transmission are intravenous drug abuse, tattoos, blood transfusions, dialysis, sexual transmission, and perinatal exposure. Offspring of infected mothers can be infected either transplacentally (in utero) or during delivery. Most infected infants are asymptomatic. However, 90% of infected newborns become chronic carriers of the virus, continually shedding the virus in their bodily fluids. Even when perinatal transmission of the virus does not occur, the chances of HBV transmission from the infected mother to her child are great.

The U.S. Centers for Disease Control and Prevention (CDC) recommend testing all pregnant women for the presence of hepatitis B surface antigen (HBsAg), providing immunoprophylaxis to the newborns of HBsAg-positive women, and providing routine vaccinations to all infants. Universal inoculation with hepatitis B vaccine for all newborns will prevent future HBV infections. Neonatal infection with HBV from HBsAg-positive mothers is prevented in 85% to 95% of cases with one dose of hepatitis B immune globulin (HBIG) and a series of three hepatitis B vaccines. Nurses must educate families about HBV so that parents will give informed consent to hepatitis B vaccination.

Health care workers routinely exposed to blood and bodily secretions should be vaccinated against hepatitis B. Antibody status should be checked every 2 years and boosters given if needed. Of course all health care workers should use meticulous universal precautions at all times.

Rubella (German measles) is caused by a viral organism that can cross the placenta. If the mother becomes infected while pregnant, there is a 20% to 60% chance that the offspring will have major anomalies. These may include low platelet count, hepatitis, microcephaly, congenital heart disease, low birth weight, cataracts, deafness, and mental retardation.

Congenital rubella in infants is contagious, and the virus may be shed for 6 to 12 months after birth. Gown and handwashing precautions and isolation of the infant will help prevent the spread of infection to other babies.

Because there is no treatment, women should be vaccinated against the virus before becoming pregnant. Women who have not been vaccinated are tested for rubella antibodies in the prenatal period, and if no immunity is present, the rubella vaccine may be given after birth. It is advised to wait at least 3 months after vaccination before becoming pregnant again.

Cytomegalovirus (CMV), a member of the herpes virus family, can cause a mononucleosis-type illness in adults or an asymptomatic infection. The general mode of transmission is sexual (either oral or genital contact). Although most neonates infected are asymptomatic, congenital CMV infections vary from mild (jaundice, feeding difficulties, irritability, muscle weakness, spasticity) to severe (IUGR, microcephaly, mental retardation, and involvement of multiple organ systems). Infants may excrete the virus in saliva and urine for years; therefore, infected infants should be isolated while in the hospital and gown and linen precautions should be used. Women with CMV in one pregnancy have increased risk of CMV with subsequent pregnancies. There is no specific treatment.

Herpes simplex virus type II (HSV-2) is the organism thought to be responsible for congenital herpes infection. Although cases of herpes simplex virus type I (HSV-1), which is typically present in the mouth and causes "cold sores," have been reported in the genital mucosa, it is usually HSV-2 that is responsible for genital herpes. HSV-2 lesions are typically fluid-filled vesicles and ulcers on the genitalia. In women they can involve the vagina, cervix, and bladder. There may be extreme pain and tenderness in the infected tissues until the lesions heal. Typically the virus remains latent for a time, only to reappear with recurrent vesicles later.

Congenital herpes is acquired in the birth canal as the fetus descends past active lesions. Infection of the infant can be prevented by cesarean delivery if maternal lesions are present. After membranes rupture, cesarean delivery is effective only if done within 4 hours after the rupture. Prolonged rupture of the membranes may expose the infant to ascending infection. Congenital herpes is associated with skin lesions (which can cover the entire body), psychomotor retardation, microcephaly, seizure disorders, optic atrophy, cataracts, and eye inflammation.

If a woman has an active lesion or a positive cervical culture and her baby is delivered by cesarean section without rupture of the membranes, the infant may be admitted to the newborn nursery and may go out to the mother for care. It is recommended that the mother be in a private room and be taught to use good handwashing technique when handling her infant. Women who deliver by cesarean section or vaginally after rupture of membranes with an active cervical lesion or positive culture should have their babies in their rooms, not in the nursery. The infant should be observed for any clinical signs of infection, and the mother should be taught to use good handwashing technique when handling the infant.

Hospital personnel should wear gloves when touching the lesion or secretions from the lesion and when handling equipment and linen contaminated with lesion secretions. Good handwashing practices should be followed. Routine cleaning of the patient's room should be performed. To prevent nosocomial spread of the virus, hospital personnel with an oral HSV lesion or a skin lesion should not provide care for a mother or infant until the lesion is dried and crusted.

A mother, father, or visitor with an oral HSV lesion should be instructed to refrain from kissing the infant, and on occasion a mask may be appropriate. Good handwashing should be taught.

Treatment of herpes for both mother and baby includes acyclovir; however, data are not clear regarding safety in pregnancy.

Infectious agents other than those of the TORCH group have been linked to harmful effects on the fetus and/or newborn. These may include *chlamydia, syphilis, gonorrhea, human papilloma virus* (HPV), *Group B strep infection (GBS),* and *acquired immunodeficiency syndrome (AIDS)* caused by *human immunodeficiency virus (HIV).*

Sexually transmitted diseases (STDs)

Chlamydia is caused by the intracellular microorganism *Chlamydia trachomatis.* This infection is difficult to diagnose clinically and eludes detection because it produces few or no symptoms and signs are nonspecific. Some women may have a vaginal discharge and pain when urinating; others may have fever and pelvic pain. It is a prevalent, sexually transmissible disease in the United States, with approximately 3 million new cases of genital chlamydia per year. Perhaps 5% of pregnant women are infected. Chlamydia can cause *pelvic inflammatory disease (PID),* an infection in the reproductive organs. When an infection occurs in the fallopian tubes, it can lead to tubal obstruction and ectopic pregnancies. Maternal chlamydia infection has been thought to cause *IUGR* (intrauterine growth retardation), premature delivery, and stillbirths. However, the evidence for this correlation is still incomplete. What is known with certainty is that maternal chlamydia infection can cause newborn infection as the organism is transferred to the fetus during delivery. Newborn infections may include *inclusion conjunctivitis* (eye), *pneumonitis* (lung), and *otitis media* (ear). Treatment is with antibiotics such as erythromycin, doxycycline, bactrim, and tetracycline.

Syphilis is caused by the bacterium *Treponema pallidum* and is spread by direct contact with infectious lesions (usually sexually). The earlier in pregnancy the fetus is exposed to the organism through transplacental infection, the more severe the fetal infection. If an infant is born with symptoms, these are likely to include a bullous rash (syphilitic pemphigus); enlarged liver, spleen, and lymph nodes; anemia; low platelet count; and inflammation of the mouth and respiratory tract (producing the "syphilitic snuffles"). However, newborns with congenital syphilis are often asymptomatic

when born and do not receive potentially curable treatment with antibiotics. They can develop tooth abnormalities ("Hutchinson's teeth" and "mulberry molars"), eye disease, facial anomalies (the "saddle nose"), and bowing of the legs ("saber shins"). These deformities are not reversible.

Gonorrhea is caused by the bacterium *Neisseria gonorrhoeae* and is spread by sexual contact. Although sometimes women with gonorrhea have no symptoms, urinary frequency and pain, purulent vaginal discharge, and pelvic pain may be symptoms of gonorrhea. The infection can be transmitted to the newborn during delivery through the birth canal and can result in *ophthalmia neonatorum,* a congenital eye infection that can result in blindness unless the infant's eyes are treated with an antibiotic ointment or 1% silver nitrate within 1 hour of birth. Treatment of the infected woman is with ceftriaxone, doxycycline, and erythromycin.

Human papilloma virus/(HPV)/genital warts (HPV)/condylomata acuminata. Genital warts are caused by many types of HPV. Said to be one of the most common sexually transmitted diseases, HPV is usually asymptomatic. However, HPV may cause warts anywhere on human epithelial surfaces, including the cervix, vagina, and vulva. Certain types of HPV are associated with the development of cervical dysplasia. Whether the virus can be vertically transmitted from the mother to fetus (transplacentally or intrapartum) is unknown.

Treatment includes topical chemotherapy (podophyllin and trichloroacetic acid), surgery or ablation, and immunologic therapy. Some cases of HPV respond to treatment, others do not. HPV has also been known to regress on its own. With appropriate screening, treatment, and follow-up care, cervical cancer can be prevented in women with HPV.

Group B strep infection (GBS). GBS is a bacterium in the streptococcal family. Although GBS can be transmitted sexually, there is disagreement as to whether GBS is a true sexually transmitted disease. In the United States as many as 12,000 infants and 50,000 pregnant women become ill each year from strep infection. GBS infection in the newborn can be obvious with the infant showing clinical signs of infection-bacteremia (bacteria in the blood), pneumonia or meningitis, within hours or days of life. Late-onset illness can also occur with signs of clinical disease not appearing until after the first week of life and up to three months of age. In contrast to early-onset illness, late-onset GBS often begins with meningitis. Signs may be fever, irritability, poor appetite, conjunctivitis, otitis media, and impetigo.

Treatment of GBS is vigorous with antibiotic treatment during the antepartal period if the mother is a carrier of the infection. Penicillin or ampicillin are the antibiotics of choice. Symptomatic infants and those less than 34 weeks of gestation should be treated with antibiotics.

The *acquired immunodeficiency syndrome (AIDS)* is caused by a retrovirus known as the *human immunodeficiency virus (HIV)*, which damages the body's immune system. There are three primary ways of transmitting HIV: sexual contact, exchange of blood, and perinatal acquisition. Although the disease usually affects intravenous drug abusers, homosexual men, and hemophiliacs, the incidence of the disease among women and men who are in bi-sexual and heterosexual relationships is increasing steadily. Women at high risk for AIDS may include (1) women who have abused intravenous drugs; (2) those who are or have been sexual partners of IV drug-abusing, bisexual, or HIV-infected men; (3) those who have engaged in prostitution; and (4) women who were born in areas where heterosexual transmission of HIV is very prevalent, such as Haiti, Africa, or South East Asia.

The mode of transmission of the virus from mother to infant is not entirely clear. It is possible that the virus may be acquired by the fetus in utero. However, the most frequent mechanism of transmission is through infant contact with infectious maternal blood and body fluids at the time of birth. There is also documentation of transmission of the virus through breast milk, and it is not recommended that HIV-infected women breast-feed. The rate of perinatal transmission is estimated to be 40% to 50%, and most affected infants develop clinical symptoms during the first year of life.

The Centers for Disease Control and Prevention (CDC) have issued recommended guidelines for health care workers and patients to follow to prevent transmission of HIV. These include the following universal blood and body fluid precautions for all patients:

1. Gloves for all contact with moist body substances, nonintact skin, and mucous membranes.
2. Masks and protective eyewear during procedures that are likely to produce splashes to eyes, nose, or mouth.
3. Gowns or plastic aprons during procedures that are likely to generate splashes of body fluids.
4. Handwashing if contamination with body fluids occurs and immediately after gloves are removed.
5. Careful disposal of needles and sharps. Avoid recapping.
6. Use of ventilation devices to avoid mouth-to-mouth resuscitation.
7. Clean up of blood spills immediately with detergent and water. Use of a solution of 5.25% sodium hypochloride (household bleach) diluted from 1:10 to 1:100 parts water for disinfection.

Pregnant health care workers are not known to be at greater risk of contracting HIV infection. Pregnant health care workers should be especially familiar with

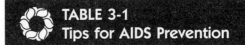

TABLE 3-1
Tips for AIDS Prevention

- AIDS can only be transmitted by an exchange of blood, semen, or vaginal secretions. And such exchange has the same chance of occurring through vaginal intercourse as it does through anal intercourse.
- When engaging in sexual activity always use a latex condom and a foam that includes the ingredient nonoxynol-nine. Nonoxynol is effective in preventing the transmission of many STDs including: herpes, chlamydia, syphilis, hepatitis B, genital warts, yeast infection, and HIV—the virus that causes AIDS. It is also an effective spermicide. Use a lubricant but make sure it is waterbased because oil lubricants like Crisco or Vaseline will weaken the condom.
- If sharing needles make sure to sterilize them after every use so that blood is not transmitted. The same goes for tattoo and earpiercing needles. Bleach is an effective cleanser.
- Store condoms in a cool dry place, and always PREPARE FOR SPONTANEITY!

From *Genesis* 9:3, June/July 1987.

and strictly adhere to precautions designed to minimize the risk of transmission of HIV and other infectious agents.

Treatment of the primary infection of HIV is limited to use of zidovudine (AZT). Although AZT is being used in infants, it is not being used in HIV-seropositive pregnant women. Women and their sexual partners need counseling concerning HIV and ways to practice safe sex. (See tips for AIDS prevention in Table 3-1.)

Table 3-2 (p. 82) summarizes the sexually transmitted diseases and recommended treatments.

Nursery-specific issues
1. Place HIV-infected infant in nursery.
2. Do not use DeeLee Suction.
3. Use Universal Blood Precautions for all infants during delivery and before first bath.
4. Establish policy regarding circumcision for HIV-infected babies.
5. Establish policy regarding breast-feeding for HIV-infected babies.
6. Establish policies and referral support for HIV-infected babies to go to adoption or emergency shelter care.

Nursing Implications

Screening for sexually transmitted diseases should be done during the prepregnancy period so that the disease can be treated appropriately. With all STDs, the only absolute approach to lifetime prevention is sexual abstinence or having one sexual partner, who also has had no other partner, for life, If this is not reality for a couple, the use of latex condoms may afford some protection. However, to be effective latex condoms must be used properly, consistently, and not break. Nurses have an important role in informing people about STDs and the prevention and treatment options available.

INFERTILITY

In the United States one out of every six couples (15%) of childbearing age experiences *infertility*, which is defined as the inability to achieve conception after 1 year of unprotected sexual intercourse. In *primary infertility* there has never been a pregnancy for either the male or female; *secondary infertility* follows one or more pregnancies. An infection, adhesions, or a change in a male factor may all contribute to secondary infertility.

Contrary to public perception, the United States is not experiencing an epidemic of infertility. In the past decade there has not been a rise in the percentage of couples who are infertile. It is the number of people seeking treatment that has steadily climbed as many more baby boomers who postponed child rearing reached the 25-44 age group. With age the odds of being infertile increase from 4.1% at ages 15-24 years to 13.4% at ages 25 to 34 years and 21.4% at ages 35-44 years. As the childbearing population aged new drugs and techniques for treating women with infertility, plus an increased number of physicians specializing in infertility, and extensive media coverage all combined to encourage more people to seek help. However, review of a national sample of women aged 15-44 in the United States disclosed that older, white, married women of higher socioeconomic status were those most likely to obtain specialized infertility services.

Causes of Female Infertility

Factors that cause infertility are almost equally divided between male and female. Today idiopathic or unexplained infertility encompasses only about 10% of infertile couples. Because infertility can be caused by either or both partners, both partners should be evaluated together in an infertility investigation. Evaluation may include a thorough history and physical examination, documentation of ovulation by basal body temperature, endometrial biopsy, examination of cervical mucus, post-coital test (PCT), determination of tubal patency, assessment of hormonal function, and analysis of seminal fluid.

The major causes of female infertility are tubal, hormonal, uterine, and cervical. Causes of blocked tubes include pelvic inflammatory disease (PID), postabortal

sepsis, adhesions, and other pathology. The diagnosis can be made with either a *hysterosalpingogram*, in which an x-ray picture is taken of the uterus and fallopian tubes after contrast material is injected through a catheter into the uterus, or with *laparoscopy*, in which a viewing tube (laparoscope) is inserted through a small abdominal incision for direct inspection of the fallopian tube. Tubes that have been closed can often be opened by tubal insufflations with CO_2 gas, sexual rest, antispasmodics, and tubal surgery *(tuboplasty)*.

Hormonal factors causing infertility usually involve lack of ovulation *(anovulation)* or irregular ovulation *(oligoovulation)* because of low levels of hormones or deficiencies in endocrine organs. Fertility drugs to induce ovulation provide effective treatment for ovulatory dysfunction. Clomiphene-citrate (Clomid) therapy is used to stimulate ovulation in women with these problems. The drug is relatively safe, with few side effects. It stimulates the LH "surge." (See Chapter 2.) For women who become pregnant after treatment with clomiphene, multiple births are possible. The incidence of twins born to such women is 1 in 16 (versus 1 in 89 in the general population), and 1 in 200 will have three or more children born at the same time. Since prematurity often accompanies multiple birth, there is some fetal risk involved.

Women who fail to respond to clomiphene will sometimes respond to human menopausal gonadotropin (hmg). Menotropin (Pergonal) is an injectable form of hmg used to induce ovulation. Pergonal is a combination of two pituitary hormones: FSH and LH. For some women, treatment with Pergonal is the only option to induce ovulation. There is also a higher than normal rate for multiple births with hmg medication.

Cervical and uterine factors causing infertility include cervical "incompetence," which may be corrected by a *cerclage* procedure—placement of a suture around the cervix to hold it closed. The cerclage may be done before conception or during pregnancy. The procedure of choice may be "permanent" (subsequent delivery will have to be by cesarean birth) or "temporary" (the suture can be removed prior to delivery). Congenital abnormalities of the uterus that can predispose to abortion are bicornuate, septate, and double uteri. The treatment for these uterine abnormalities is surgical. Also, DES (diethylstilbestrol) exposure in utero may have caused anatomic abnormalities of the woman's uterus, which could prevent implantation.

Endometriosis is also considered when evaluating infertility because it may be a causative factor. In this condition endometrial tissue, normally found inside the uterus, is present in abnormal locations such as the fallopian tubes, ovaries, and peritoneal cavity. The cause is unknown. Retention of this endometrial tissue causes scarring and adhesions within the tubes and in the peritoneal cavity, preventing passage of the ovum and

TABLE 3-2
A Guide to Sexually Transmitted Diseases

Disease	Agent	Symptoms in mother	Symptoms in child	Treatment
Viruses				
Acquired immunodeficiency syndrome (AIDS)	Human immunodeficiency virus (HIV)	Weight loss, malaise, Kaposi's sarcoma, *pneumocystis carinii*, widespread opportunistic infections	Same as in mother	No recommended treatment
Genital herpes	Herpes simplex virus (HSV)	Burning in pelvic area, itching, sores that heal very slowly	Mental impairment, TORCH syndrome*	Acyclovir
Bacteria				
Chlamydia	*Chlamydia trachomatis*	Vaginal discharge, inflamed cervix endometritis, pelvic inflammatory disease	Conjunctivitis, blindness, pneumonia, otitis media	Erythromycin for pregnant women
Lymphogranuloma venereum	*C. trachomatis*	Swollen lymph glands, genital sores, rectal sores	Same as for chlamydia	Erythromycin
Chancroid	*Haemophilis ducreyi*	Swollen glands, sores on genitals or anus, rash	(Effects seldom seen in U.S.)	Erythromycin
Syphilis	*Treponema pallidum*	Sores in mouth, genitals, anus; swollen glands, rash	TORCH syndrome*	Penicillin
Gonorrhea	*Neisseria gonorrhoeae*	Discharge, malaise, pelvic inflammatory disease	Conjunctivitis, meningitis, premature birth	Penicillin or gentamicin and spectinomycin

Disease	Organism	Symptoms	Fetal Effects	Treatment
Anaerobic vaginosis	*Gardnerella vaginalis*† *Ureaplasma urealyticum Mycoplasma hominis*	Discharge, nongonococcal urethritis, pelvic inflammatory disease, unpleasant odor	Premature birth, low birth weight	Ampicillin
Group B hemolytic streptococcus	*Streptococcus agalactiae*	Rash, fever, spontaneous abortion	Infection, meningitis, premature birth	Penicillin
Donovanosis (granuloma inguinale)	*Calymmatobacterium granulomatis*	Slowly spreading genital sores	No known fetal effects	No recommended treatment
Hepatitis	Hepatitis A virus (HAV) Hepatitis B virus (HBV)	Jaundice, fever, inflamed liver	Premature birth	Vaccine for HBV, gamma globulin
Cytomegalovirus	Cytomegalovirus (CMV)	Symptoms very hard to find in mother; sometimes symptoms of mononucleosis	Mental impairment, TORCHES syndrome*	No recommended treatment
Protozoa				
Trichomoniasis	*Trichomonas vaginalis*	Discharge, bleeding, nongonococcal urethritis, pelvic inflammatory disease, unpleasant odor	No known fetal effects	Clotrimazole in mother, metronidazole in child
Fungi				
Candidiasis (monilia)	*Candida albicans*	Discharge, itching, rash	Thrush, diaper rash	Antifungal agents

*TORCHES syndrome refers to various combinations of encephalitis, hepatitis, skin disease, and widespread blood disorders (intravascular coagulation). The syndrome is found in infants affected by toxoplasmosis, rubella (German measles), cytomegalovirus, herpes, and syphilis.
†Also called *Haemophilus vaginalis* and *Corynebacterium vaginale.*
From *Genesis* 9:3, June/July 1987.

sperm. Surgical treatment or drug therapy may be useful in treating endometriosis. Danazal (Danocrine), a synthetic weak androgen, suppresses gonadotropins FSH and LH so endometriosis is inhibited and the tissue regresses and atrophies. Surgical intervention using a laser with laparoscopy to remove adhesions from endometriosis can also offer promising results for some women.

Causes of Male Infertility

Causes of male infertility include lack or deficiency of sperm, low sperm motility, mechanical obstruction for passage of sperm, and impotence. It has been found that 25% of infertile males have varicose veins of the left testicle *(varicoceles)*, which can reduce sperm production. These may be responsible for up to 40% of male infertility.

Infertility diagnostic studies begin with semen analysis. Seminal fluid is analyzed for volume of fluid, sperm count, sperm shape, and sperm motility. Because of variability, at least two specimens should be examined before a diagnosis of fertile, subfertile, or sterile is made. Normal values are as follows: volume, 3 to 5 cc; count, 20 million per cc; size greater than two thirds normal; and motility greater than 50% at 1 to 2 hours. Excessive use of drugs, alcohol, or tobacco affects sperm production, as do some genitourinary problems, infections, or surgery.

Hormonal, environmental, nutritional, occupational and immunological factors, as well as chronic illness, stress, and fatigue can also contribute to male infertility. In addition, chronic exposure to certain chemicals can have a detrimental effect on sperm production.

If the semen analysis is normal or the male is somewhat subfertile, the infertility evaluation would then continue with the woman while further investigation and possible treatment could be initiated on the man.

Surgical Intervention

Surgery to deal with the problem of varicoceles *(varicocelectomy)* has improved fertility in the majority of cases. The procedure involves entering the scrotum via the abdomen and tying off the main vein from the left testicle. Patients can resume normal activities, including sexual intercourse, within 1 week.

Immunologic Infertility

When a couple is infertile despite normal sperm and hormone levels, immunologic factors may be the cause. In some cases women produce antibodies against the antigens found in their partner's semen. When this happens, the sperm may be unable to move past the cervix and into the uterus. Treatment for immunologic infer-

tility may include the use of condoms until the woman's serum antibody titer is lowered, immunosuppressive medications, and sperm "washing."

In working with infertile couples, it is important to remember that infertility is a stressful situation for people who want to have a child. They should be encouraged to express their feelings and understand that their emotional response is normal.

Adoption, surrogacy, donor insemination, and embryo transplantation are possible alternatives for those couples who remain infertile after evaluation and treatment. Adoption is the legal placement of an infant or child with parents, to whom the state gives full legal responsibility for the child. For adoption to occur, the infant's biologic mother usually gives up her rights to her baby voluntarily. In some instances the court terminates her rights; however, when this happens, it is usually because of abandonment. There are also times when the father is required to renounce parental rights.

An alternative to adoption is donor insemination, in which donor semen or a combination of the husband's and a donor's sperm is deposited in the woman's vagina via syringe during her fertile period. When donor sperm is used, an attempt can be made to match the physical characteristics of the donor to those of the husband.

Additional Choices to Promote Fertility

Infertility care has become a burgeoning business in this country with more than $1 billion spent on infertility treatment each year. There are medical specialists in infertility and a professional organization of fertility care providers, the American Society for Reproductive Medicine. A *reproductive endocrinologist* is an obstetrician/gynecologist who has completed an additional two-year fellowship in reproductive endocrinology. In addition to expertise in menopause and menstrual cycle abnormalities, this specialist is certified to provide all aspects of infertility care.

In vitro fertilization

Choices for the childless couple include *in vitro fertilization and embryo transfer (IVF/Et)*. IVF/Et involves recovery of an ovum from the woman using the laparoscope or ultrasound imaging, with subsequent fertilization and incubation in a laboratory medium and then implantation in her own uterus 48 to 72 hours after insemination of the recovered oocytes. Although pregnancy rates of 20% to 25% have been achieved after two cycles of treatment with this technique, there is wide variation in the rates of success cited by different fertility centers.

Although one third of IVF/Et pregnancies spontaneously abort in the first 3 months, many couples undergo the procedure several times. The financial and emotional costs are high (intense anxiety is followed by grief if a treatment attempt fails). Thus comprehensive information beforehand and emotional support are the primary needs of couples undergoing IVF/Et.

Gamete intrafallopian transfer

The technique with the highest pregnancy rate for previously infertile couples is called *gamete intrafallopian transfer (GIFT)*. It involves removal of eggs through a minilaparotomy, mixture of egg and sperm in a laboratory solution and then return of the ovum and sperm to the fallopian tubes where fertilization occurs. According to the American Society for Reproductive Medicine, GIFT has a success rate of 26.6%. GIFT can be accomplished as a one-step procedure without the need to return for embryo transfer as with IVF/Et.

Zygote intrafallopian transfer (ZIFT, also known as PROST, for pronuclear state transfer)

Some women respond better to a variation called *ZIFT*, in which an egg is fertilized in a petri dish and the preembryo (zygote) is transferred to a fallopian tube via a catheter through an incision in the woman's abdomen. There is reported to be a 19.7% success rate with ZIFT.

IVF/Et, GIFT, and ZIFT require hormone therapy to stimulate ovulation, close monitoring, and emotional support. Success rates, of course, depend on retrieving an egg and often times require four attempts at the procedure chosen. Many couples choose to undergo more than four attempts at a procedure.

There are risks to mother and baby in all of these procedures. For the woman there is the possibility of organ perforation (estimated to be 1 in 1000), and ectopic pregnancy (five times greater than normal). A great deal of information is still not available about the effect of taking massive doses of hormones. A Stanford University study in 1994 linked the use of fertility drugs to a two- to threefold increase in the risk of ovarian cancer. Then there is the risk of prematurity with multiple births and the problems that could cause for the baby.

Embryos not transferred can be *cryopreserved*, a process in which the unused embryos are frozen in liquid nitrogen. The embryos can be thawed and then transferred to the woman's uterus, eliminating the need to repeat egg retrieval and fertilization.

A highly complex experimental technique is being researched for treating failure of the sperm to fertilize the egg. In this procedure a single sperm is injected directly into the egg via a catheter through an incision in the side of the woman's abdomen.

In the case of high-technology treatment for infertility, it is clear that serious emotional stresses can be treated. As with IVF/Et, couples experiencing GIFT or ZIFT may experience emotional upheaval and require intensive counseling and support. In spite of all the high-tech intervention, many women will not become pregnant. One author estimated that 40% to 50% of infertile couples never achieve a pregnancy. Couples will need help to live with each other in a quality relationship whether the procedure results in a pregnancy.

Surrogacy

The most controversial of solutions to infertility involves hiring surrogate mothers to bear children for infertile couples. Surrogates are used in cases in which the man is fertile, but his partner is unable to sustain pregnancy. Usually the surrogate mother is artificially inseminated with the man's sperm and carries the baby to term for the infertile couple. There is a great deal of apprehension about the use of paid surrogates, and there are strict guidelines for screening would-be surrogates and the couples who hire them for both medical and psychological fitness. The legal aspects of surrogacy are complex, with laws varying from state to state.

Nursing implications

Many infertile couples feel isolated from family and friends because of strong social and cultural expectations to have children. Mutual support and education are available to these couples through local support groups and the national self-help organization for infertile couples known as RESOLVE. The nurse's role when dealing with infertile couples is to be nonjudgmental, to support their right to choice of treatment, to be their advocate, and to offer understanding and encouragement as needed.

SUMMARY

Chapter 3 has briefly described the fascinating trip of the fertilized ovum to its bed in the uterus as life begins. We traced the development of both the embryo and the fetus and became aware of some of the hazards along the way to conception and to healthy development when conception occurs. As the chapter concluded we reviewed both the problems of infertility and the advances in infertility care. The next chapter explores ways to assure optimal wellness for the new life.

BIBLIOGRAPHY

American Academy of Pediatrics (AAP) Committee on Infectious Diseases and Committee on Fetus and Newborn: Guidelines for prevention of Group B streptococcal (GBS) infection by chemoprophylaxis, *Pediatr* 90(5):775-778, 1992.

American College of Obstetricians and Gynecologists: Group B streptococcal infections in pregnancy, *ACOG Technical Bulletin*, No. 170, 1992.

Bernhardt J: Sensory capabilities of the fetus, *MCN* 12:44-46, 1987.

Bernhardt JH: Potential workplace hazards to reproductive health: information for primary prevention, *J Obstet Gynecol Neonatal Nurs* 19:53-61, 1990.

Blenner JL: Passage through infertility treatment: a stage theory, *Image* 22(3):153-158, Fall 1990.

Cefalco RC, Moos MK: *Preconceptual health care*, ed 2, St. Louis, 1995, Mosby.

Conover E: Hazardous exposures during pregnancy, *J Obstet Gynecol Neonatal Nurs* 23(6):524-532, 1994.

Crawford NG, Pruss AM: Preventing neonatal hepatitis B infection during the prenatal period, *J Obstet Gynecol Neonatal Nurs* 22(6):491-497, 1993.

Davis DC, Dearman CN: Coping strategies of infertile women, *J Obstet Gynecol Neonatal Nurs* 20(3):221-228, 1990.

Forsman I: Evolution of the nursing role in genetics, *J Obstet Gynecol Neonatal Nurs* 23(6):481-486, 1994.

Gaffney KF: Prenatal maternal attachment, *Image* 20(2):106-109, Summer 1988.

Haggerty L: TORCH: a literature review and implications for practice, *J Obstet Gynecol Neonatal Nurs* 14:124-129, 1985.

Jones LC, Bennett M: Human immunodeficiency virus (HIV) during pregnancy, *ICEA Rev* 14:21-28, 1990.

Kelley KF, Galbraith MA, Vermund SH: Genital human papillomavirus infection in women, *J Obstet Gynecol Neonatal Nurs* 21(6):503-515, 1992.

Mattson S, Smith JE, editors: *Core curriculum for maternal-newborn nursing*, Philadelphia, 1993, WB Saunders.

Milne BJ: Couples' experiences with in vitro fertilization, *J Obstet Gynecol Neonatal Nurs* 17:347-352, 1988.

Moore KL: *The developing human*, ed 4, Philadelphia, 1988, WB Saunders.

Pace-Owens S: Gamete intrafallopian transfer (GIFT), *J Obstet Gynecol Neonatal Nurs* 18:93-97, 1988.

Pritchard JA, MacDonald PD, Gant MF: *Williams obstetrics*, ed 17, New York, 1985, Appleton-Century-Crofts.

Raff BS: Nursing and genetics for the 21st century, *J Obstet Gynecol Neonatal Nurs* 23(6):477-480, 1994.

Sandberg EC: Only an attitude away: the potential of reproductive surrogacy, *Am J Obstet Gynecol* 160:1441-1446, 1989.

Thibodeau GA: *Structure and function of the body*, ed 9, St. Louis, 1992, Mosby.

Verny T: *The secret life of the unborn child*, New York, 1982, Dell.

Wilcox LS, Mosher WD: Use of infertility services in the United States, *Obstet Gynecol* 82:122-127, 1993.

Wright L: Prenatal diagnosis in the 1990s, *J Obstet Gynecol Neonatal Nurs* 23(6):506-515, 1994.

Zacharias JF: The new genetics, *J Obstet Gynecol Neonatal Nurs* 19(2):122-128, 1990.

DEFINITIONS

Define the following terms:

amniocentesis	homozygous
amnion	human chorionic gonadotropin (hCG)
anovulation	
Barr body	"incompetent" cervix
bicornuate	infertility
biochemical	lacunas
biophysical	laparoscopy
blastoderm	meconium
cephalocaudal	meiosis
cerclage	mitosis
chromosomes	morula
chorion	ovulate
cleavage	placenta
cytomegalovirus (CMV)	primary infertility
decidua	pulmonary
decidua basalis	quickening
dominant	recessive
double uteri	retroverted
ductus arteriosus	rubella
ductus venosus	secondary infertility
endometriosis	septate
endothelium	surrogacy
embryo	syphilis
fertilization	toxoplasmosis
fibrin	trisomy
foramen ovale	trophoblast
gamete	tuboplasty
genes	variocele
genetic counseling	vernix caseosa
gestational age	villi
heterozygous	zygote

LEARNING ACTIVITIES

1. Group discussions.
2. Guest speakers: a genetic counselor, a couple who has experienced genetic counseling.
3. View audiovisual aids and discuss.
4. Obtain a placenta from a hospital maternity department and examine it. Check the number of vessels in the cord.
5. Look at a three-dimensional model of placental circulation.
6. Look at three-dimensional models of growth of embryo and fetus.
7. Write for information on services of RESOLVE, Inc., 1310 Broadway, Somerville, MA 02144-1731. This association deals with infertility.

ENRICHMENT/IN-DEPTH STUDY

1. Visit a biology laboratory to examine specimens of embryos. If there are embryos of animals present, compare their development with that of a human embryo. What are the principal differences?

Chapter 3 Conception and Prenatal Development   **87**

2. Survey your community to determine if preconception classes or counseling exist. If yes, what is the focus? What is the average age of people attending class? What are their most commonly asked questions? Why?

3. Determine which reproductive technologies are available in your community. What is the cost? What are the success rates? Will insurance companies cover the cost? What is the average income level of people utilizing these reproductive technologies? Why?

4. Visit local pharmacies and grocery stores to find what over-the-counter drugs are available to pregnant women. Is there potential for teratogenic substances to be present in these drugs? Are there warning labels on the packages?

5. Develop a teaching aid to use in explaining fetal development to families in early pregnancy classes. Keep in mind stages of development and their relationship to maternal diet and life-style. How do a woman's life-style choices influence her fetus in utero at 6 weeks, 20 weeks, and 34 weeks of gestation?

6. Determine if there are smoking intervention programs available for pregnant women in your community. If yes, what is the content of these programs and what is their cost? What is their success rate?

Self-Assessment

For questions 1 through 15, determine if each statement is true or false. Fill in the space to the left of the statement with T for true and F for false.

____ **1.** Human development begins when an ovum is fertilized by a sperm.

____ **2.** Fertilization takes place in the tube at the point where the tube enters the uterus.

____ **3.** The ovum lives 12 to 24 hours if not fertilized.

____ **4.** The genes carry the chromosomes.

____ **5.** The spermatozoon cell determines whether the baby will be a boy or a girl.

____ **6.** The sex of the embryo is determined at conception.

____ **7.** Each ovum and each sperm carries 23 chromosomes, one of which is the sex chromosome.

____ **8.** The fertilized cell resulting from the union of a sperm and ovum is called a gonadotropin.

____ **9.** During pregnancy the endometrium is termed the decidua.

____ **10.** The zygote moving through the fallopian tube is called an embryo.

____ **11.** The cells that provide nourishment for the developing zygote are the trophoblasts.

____ **12.** Implantation usually occurs near the cervix of the uterus.

____ **13.** The period of the ovum lasts 8 weeks.

____ **14.** The transparent sac in which the fetus floats is made up of two membranes: amnion and chorion.

____ **15.** Implantation is completed by the trophoblast.

For questions 16 through 27, circle the best answer.

16. Which of the following functional activities is *not* performed by amniotic fluid?

   a. protection

   b. fluid exchange

   c. temperature regulation

   d. gas exchange

17. The structures in fetal circulation that allow a detour of most blood past the fetal lungs and liver are:

   a. ductus venosus

   b. foramen ovale

   c. ductus arteriosus

   d. mitral valve

   Answer (circle one):

     1. a, b, and c

     2. a, b, and d

     3. all of these

18. Traits are passed on from parents to their offspring by:

    a. genes

    b. chromosomes

    c. hormones

19. The zygote contains the following number of chromosomes:

    a. 46 plus 2 sex chromosomes

    b. 44 plus 2 sex chromosomes

    c. 42 plus 2 sex chromosomes

20. The embryo can be affected by all *except* one of the following:

    a. viruses affecting the mother

    b. drugs taken by the mother

    c. nutritional deficiency of the father

    d. nutritional deficiency of the mother

21. An example of a recessive trait is:

    a. dark hair

    b. brown eyes

    c. diabetes mellitus

    d. curly hair

22. The umbilical cord ordinarily contains:

    a. two arteries and one vein

    b. two veins and one artery

    c. one vein and one artery

23. If a woman's menstrual cycle was 33 days in length, when was her fertile period in that cycle?

    a. Day 14

    b. Day 17

    c. Day 19

    d. Day 12

24. The process of cell division that takes place soon after the zygote is formed is called:

    a. blastomeres

    b. peristalsis

    c. chromosomes

    d. cleavage

25. The embryo becomes a fetus after:

    a. 12 weeks

    b. 14 days

    c. 8 weeks

    d. 20 weeks

26. Oxygen (from the maternal side of the placenta) and CO_2 (from the fetal side of the placenta) pass through the placenta by means of:

    a. diffusion

    b. osmosis

    c. fetal circulation

27. Infertility is defined as the inability to achieve conception after unprotected intercourse for what period of time?

    a. 1 year

    b. 6 months

    c. 2 years

28. On the line to the left of each item in Column A, match the appropriate time periods from Column B. Each item in Column B may be used more than once.

Column A	**Column B**
____ 1. fetus weighs 3½ pounds	a. 28 weeks of gestation
____ 2. lanugo covers fetus	b. 32 weeks of gestation
____ 3. if born, fetus might survive	c. 20 weeks of gestation
____ 4. fetal heartbeat can be heard through stethoscope	
____ 5. vernix caseosa covers fetus	

29. On the line to the left of each item in Column A, match the appropriate time periods from Column B.

Column A	**Column B**
____ 1. rapid development of brain	a. end of first 3 weeks
____ 2. heart and brain formed	b. end of first 4 weeks
____ 3. formation of eyes, ears, and nose	c. end of first 7 weeks

30. Draw a sketch of adult circulation and of fetal circulation, tracing the flow of blood through the adult heart and the fetal heart. Label structures in the fetal heart that differ from adult circulation. Use a separate sheet for your sketch.

For questions 31 through 39, fill in the blanks.

31. The incidence of Down syndrome increases as the mother's _____ increases.

32. There is a higher risk of _____ in babies born with only one umbilical artery in the cord.

33. At the sixth week of pregnancy, the product of conception is termed the _____.

34. The fetal period extends from the eighth week until _____.

35. Development during the fetal period is primarily concerned with _____ and _____ of tissues and organs.

36. Three major functions of the placenta are _____, _____, and _____.

37. Identify the infections known as the **TORCH** group:

    T for _____

    O for _____

    R for _____

    C for _____

    H for _____

38. At birth the closure of the _____ changes the course of blood flow from fetal to that of a normal adult human.

39. Today one in _____ American couples is experiencing infertility.

40. The Centers for Disease Control and Prevention (CDC) have issued recommended guidelines for health care workers and patients to follow to prevent transmission of human immunodeficiency virus (HIV). List six universal blood precautions:

a. _____

b. _____

c. _____

d. _____

e. _____

f. _____

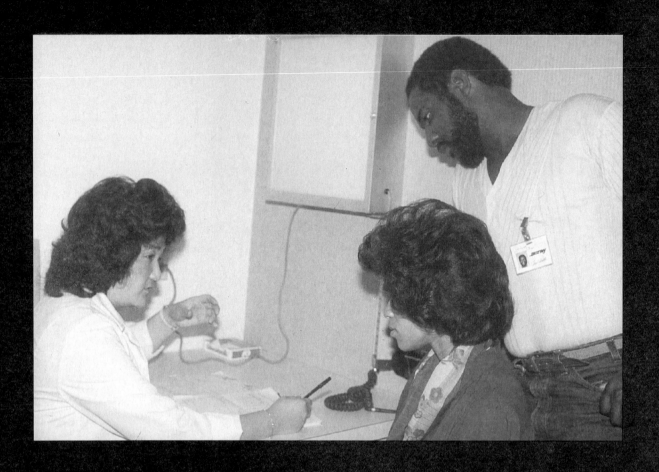

4

THE ANTEPARTUM FAMILY

GOALS

This chapter is designed to provide the reader with information that will:
- develop awareness of the psychological responses to pregnancy.
- promote an understanding of the physiologic changes of pregnancy.
- develop a basis for understanding recommended care during pregnancy.
- explore the nursing role in antepartum care.

STUDENT OBJECTIVES

After studying this chapter, you should be able to:

1. Explain both the basic physiological and psychological factors affecting attitudes and feelings on love, sex, and intimate relations during pregnancy.
2. Describe changes in sexual feelings and behaviors in pregnancy.
3. Indicate the time interval when intercourse can be resumed for most well couples following childbirth.
4. Describe the physiological changes resulting from pregnancy by identifying at least one change in each body system.
5. Differentiate among the presumptive, probable, and positive signs and symptoms of pregnancy and explain when they occur, why they occur, and a possible other cause for each.
6. Describe the care provided during the first prenatal visit.
7. Explain Nägele's rule in determining the estimated date of delivery.

8. Identify the normal values for the following laboratory tests commonly done during the antepartum period: Hct (hematocrit), Hgb (hemoglobin), serology, Rh factor, rubella, urine content of sugar, and albumin.
9. Design a plan to cover a woman's basic nutritional needs during pregnancy and lactation.
10. Identify appropriate weight gain in pregnancy.
11. Explain the cause of the following common discomforts of pregnancy and suggest ways to alleviate them:
    a. frequent urination   g. dyspnea
    b. nausea and vomiting   h. varicose veins
    c. heartburn   i. hemorrhoids
    d. flatulence   j. leg cramps
    e. constipation   k. fatigue
    f. backache   l. vaginal discharge
12. Discuss common breast-feeding problems and nursing interventions.
13. List the danger signs that may indicate complications of pregnancy.

MOTIVATIONS

The decision to become pregnant may be conscious and well thought out or may be buried deep in the subconscious. Many times a couple decides to have a baby because they love each other and want to have a child to share their life. This is the beginning that each human being deserves but may not have if any of the following motives for pregnancy are present:

1. To have a child for a status symbol
2. To have a child to please others
3. To have a family heir
4. To escape a job or new responsibility
5. To prove femininity or masculinity
6. To save a relationship
7. To prove independence
8. To convey hostility toward a parent or "the system"

Being pregnant and alone or deciding to place the baby for adoption does not necessarily mean that the woman or the couple were ignorant of contraception. One or more of the preceding motives may have precipitated the pregnancy, or a complex psychological mechanism revolving around feelings of guilt and punishment if contraceptives are used, may have been involved. If one prepares for intercourse by obtaining contraceptives, then the act is planned. Some may fear that the fantasized "magic" and "hearing violins playing" may not happen if the act is not "spontaneous."

MYTHS

Just as there are numerous reasons why a woman becomes pregnant, there are also many myths or old wives' tales surrounding childbearing and birth. Some of these center around harm to the unborn child, such as: (1) "Don't reach above your head or the cord will strangle the baby," (2) "If you see a monkey, your baby will look like a monkey," and (3) "If you walk in the moonlight, your baby will be a lunatic."

Other myths are concerned with the sex of the baby, such as: (1) "If you carry the baby low, it will be a boy," and (2) "If you stick out in front, the baby will be a girl."

Still other myths involve the physical symptoms a woman may have, such as: (1) "If you have heartburn, your baby will have curly hair," and (2) "If your baby is active, he or she will be a poor sleeper."

We could go on at great length about myths because each culture has its own. It is necessary to explore the attitudes, motivations, and myths each person brings to the childbearing experience; many times what one believes to be true is often as important as what is actually true.

SEXUALITY

Pregnancy, labor, and birth are all aspects of female sexuality, closely related physiologically and psychologically. Consequently, because childbirth is a sexual experience, we need a basic understanding of the attitudes as well as the feelings couples may have on love, sex, and intimate relations during pregnancy.

Sexual arousal and response are highly individualized physical, emotional, and mental processes. Research conducted in laboratories by Masters and Johnson has shown that sex habits vary widely among different couples and these habits may change throughout pregnancy. Therefore it is important to individualize and not compare the needs of one couple with those of another. A couple's sexual interest before and during pregnancy may remain the same or differ, depending on their expectations.

The human sexual response cycle as observed by Masters and Johnson has shown women to be as sexually responsive as men, if not more so. In both men and women, the two principal physiological responses to sexual stimulation are (1) vasocongestion of tissues in the pelvic region and (2) an increase in voluntary and involuntary muscle tension. The phases of sexual arousal and stimulation are excitement, plateau, orgasm, and resolution. The excitement phase develops from sources of physical or psychological stimuli. In the plateau phase sexual tension becomes intensified and may lead to orgasm, the involuntary climax of sexual tension. In orgasm, vasocongestion and muscle tension often intensify, and although the total body is involved, the sensations are concentrated in the pelvic region. During the resolution phase sexual tension subsides, and the person returns to the preexcitement state (Fig. 4-1). Some women have a multiorgasmic potential and, if adequately stimulated, may experience another sexual response cycle before resolution. The male experiences a refractory period following ejaculation during which he cannot be restimulated. This sexual response cycle is both highly individualistic and subjective in regard to what is sexually arousing and what is adequate physical stimulation. The female sexual response is not an isolated phenomenon of the vaginal area. A woman's brain, hormones, and senses are all integrated in her sexual response.

SEXUALITY DURING PREGNANCY

Physiological sexual responses during pregnancy are very similar to those of nonpregnant women. Although the usual wide range of physiological response exists, sexual interest, frequency, and satisfaction often change for both men and women as pregnancy progresses.

To understand what is happening to the couple, we

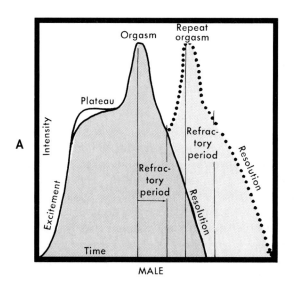
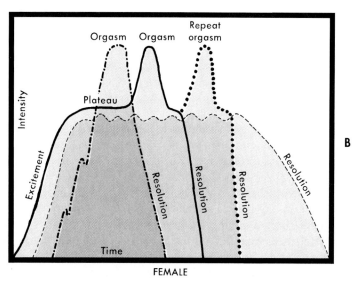

Figure 4-1 A, Male sexual response cycle. **B,** Female sexual response cycle.

must look at the entire couple, not just their pregnancy. How childbearing couples integrate sexual expression into their lives during pregnancy and postpartum depends on many factors. These factors include their sexual value systems, religious beliefs, folklore, general health and specific pregnancy-related health concerns, and the quality of the couple's relationship.

When sexuality is incorporated into counseling sessions or teaching plans, the approach and information shared should vary according to the individuals involved.

First Trimester Changes

For most women during the *first trimester* (first 3 months of pregnancy) there is a decrease in sexual desire and consequently in the frequency of sexual intercourse. Normal physiological alterations of pregnancy that may cause this decrease in sexual desire follow:

1. Nausea and perhaps vomiting
2. Breast tenderness
3. Fatigue
4. Feeling of fullness
5. Pelvic vasocongestion

Psychologically a woman may feel that she is now a "mother" and should behave differently or that she should protect her baby from possible trauma during intercourse.

Fathers often view the newly pregnant woman with awe and worry that they may harm the baby during intercourse, which causes their uncertainty and reluctance to engage in sexual activity. On the other hand,

some men, having impregnated their partners, feel more "manly" and desire sexual contact more often than before. The couple may have decreased sexual desires and responses because of cultural taboos against sexual activity during pregnancy or because of myths about lovemaking in pregnancy.

Second Trimester Changes

In the second 3 months of pregnancy *(second trimester)* most women experience a general feeling of well-being, with the fatigue gone and an increase in pelvic engorgement all contributing to easier and more frequent sexual arousal. If the woman is happy with her pregnancy and things are going well with the couple in other areas of their lives, the woman's desire for sexual encounter may be greatly increased.

Fathers often feel very warm, loving, and protective toward their mates as they bloom in the second trimester. The initial fear of harming the fetus is put aside as physical evidence of the pregnancy in the form of the growing uterus reassures both partners that the pregnancy is a reality and seems to be going well.

The couple may enjoy sexual activity more because there is no fear of pregnancy or need for contraceptives. The second trimester is often a time of loving caresses, expressions of appreciation for each other, and a fulfilling sex life.

Third Trimester Changes

During the last 3 months of pregnancy *(third trimester)* there is often again a decrease in sexual interest and reduced sexual activity.

The mother often loses interest in sex because she is increasing in size, concentrating on her baby, and mentally preparing herself for motherhood. As she "rests," the father's fears of sexual activity injuring the baby often return and he shows less interest in sexual intercourse to support his mate's increased needs and to protect the fetus from any harm.

Until recently it was traditional for physicians to prohibit sexual intercourse for all couples during the last 6 weeks of pregnancy and the first 6 weeks postpartum. This practice was recommended because it was believed that for 6 weeks before birth sexual intercourse could induce premature labor and for 6 weeks after birth it could cause serious infection. Not only were these reasons invalid, but many couples continued to have intercourse in spite of the instructions and then had to deal with guilt feelings associated with what should be an act of love and giving.

Today it is recognized that sexual intercourse is contraindicated in pregnancy when the following complications are present:

1. Vaginal bleeding
2. Ruptured membranes
3. Incompetent cervix
4. Threatened premature labor
5. Prematurely ripe cervix
6. Vaginal infection
7. History of miscarriage (abortion)

All women are no longer instructed to refrain from intercourse during the last 6 weeks of pregnancy and the first 6 weeks postpartum. Advice is based on a realistic appraisal of each couple's individual needs, desires, and circumstances. Following childbirth, sexual intercourse can usually be resumed when vaginal discharge has stopped, when there is no perineal discomfort, and when the couple is psychologically ready. For the first few months the vagina may not lubricate well and a water-soluble gel may be recommended for lubrication. If the woman has had an episiotomy, there may be tenderness and discomfort. Positions for intercourse that can take pressure off the episiotomy site will be necessary.

Pregnancy and the postpartum period need not be a time of sexual frustration for the pregnant couple but can be a time to increase intimacy and strengthen their bonds.

TERMS

The physical and psychological health care a family receives during pregnancy is termed antepartal (*ante*, before; *partal*, birth) care, or prenatal care. In beginning a study of the antepartum, there are several terms you should become familiar with because they will be used frequently. These are:

gravid the state of being pregnant.

gravida the number of pregnancies a woman has had, regardless of outcome. It includes the present pregnancy. It is the pregnancy that is counted and not the number of babies in utero.

nulligravida a woman who has never been pregnant.

primigravida a woman pregnant for the first time.

multigravida a woman who has been pregnant more than once.

para the pregnancy that terminates in the birth (live or dead) of a fetus or fetuses who reached the stage of viability (generally designated at 24 weeks of gestation).

nullipara a woman who has not yet carried a pregnancy to viability.

primipara a woman who has given birth to a fetus or fetuses (live or dead) who reached the stage of viability.

multipara a woman who has given birth to more than one infant (live or dead) at the stage of viability.

A woman who has delivered three children and is in labor now with her fourth pregnancy is gravida IV, para III. A woman who is pregnant for the first time is a primigravida. When she gives birth to her first child, she will be a primipara.

PHYSIOLOGIC CHANGES
Reproductive System

In the healthy, regularly menstruating woman, an absence of the menses beyond 2 weeks of the expected menstrual date is suggestive of pregnancy.

In the first 3 months of pregnancy, the uterus becomes enlarged and more anteflexed than normal. Uterine growth is due to stretching and enlargement of existing cells rather than growth of new cells. By the end of pregnancy each cell is approximately 4 times wider and 10 times longer than before pregnancy. Also, new muscle fibers are developed and there is an increase in fibrous tissue in the body of the uterus. This results initially from the effects of estrogen on the uterus and later from mechanical stretching. The blood supply to the uterus increases, and the blood vessels become larger. (See Chapter 2.)

By the end of pregnancy approximately one fifth of the mother's total blood volume is in the uterine blood vessels because of the circulatory requirements of the uterus. The sound of blood *(uterine souffle)* in the uterine arteries can be heard with a stethoscope. This uterine souffle matches the maternal pulse rate. The nerve supply increases; lymphatics enlarge. By the end of the pregnancy, the size of the uterus will increase to 20 times that of nonpregnant size.

By the fourth month of pregnancy, the uterus has lost its nonpregnant "pear" shape and is more globular. It emerges from the pelvis and can be palpated above the symphysis pubis. Uterine contractility increases, and during the first trimester irregular, infrequent, painless contractions begin (the so-called *Braxton Hicks contractions*). As the pregnancy progresses, these contractions become more regular but are often unnoticed by the pregnant woman. Braxton Hicks contractions exercise the uterine muscle in preparation for the work it will have to do to expel the fetus.

About 4 weeks after conception, the softening of the cervix *(Goodell's sign)* is detectable by pelvic examination. The endocervical glands become more active and secrete large amounts of thick cervical mucus, and a mucous plug forms. The function of this mucous plug is to prevent infections in the uterus that might be caused by organisms from the vagina. At about the sixth or eighth week of pregnancy, the lower segment of the uterus becomes softer, and this softening *(Hegar's sign)* can be felt by the examiner during a bimanual examination (Fig. 4-2). This is one of the most reliable early signs of pregnancy. Also, during a vaginal examination at 8 to 10 weeks of pregnancy, the examiner can see a bluish violet tinge to the cervical and vaginal mucous membranes *(Chadwick's sign)*. This is caused by the increased vascularity of the pelvic organs. The vagina also

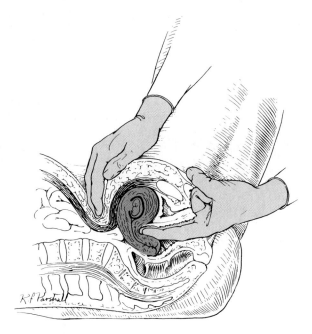

Figure 4-2 Hegar's sign, softening of the lower uterine segment. *(From Barkauskas VH, Stoltenberg-Allen K, Baumann LC, Darling-Fisher C: Health and physical assessment, St. Louis, 1994, Mosby.)*

becomes softer and more congested. Vaginal secretions become more acidic (pH 3.5 to 6.0), which plays a role in preventing infection.

In the first 3 to 4 months of pregnancy, the fetus is small compared with the amount of amniotic fluid; therefore it will rebound against the examiner's fingers *(ballottement)* when the examiner gently pushes against the uterus through either the vagina or the abdomen.

Breasts

High estrogen and progesterone levels cause the areolae to enlarge and become dark, the nipples to become firmer, and the size and weight of the breasts to increase. The breasts also become tender and often sensitive to touch, and light blue veins are visible beneath the skin. Visible striations may develop as the lobules enlarge and stretch the connective tissue and skin of the breasts. After the first few months of pregnancy, a thin, yellowish, clear fluid called pre *colostrum* may sometimes be expressed from the nipples. In the third trimester, colostrum is secreted. This is the substance that precedes the milk from the breasts when milk letdown occurs 3 to 4 days after delivery. Neither the presence of colostrum nor the size of the breasts indicates whether the woman will be able to breast-feed.

The external structures of the perineum enlarge as a result of increased blood supply, hypertrophy (thickening) of skin and muscle, and the fat deposits that occur during pregnancy. Softening of the connective tissue causes some relaxation of the area. All of these changes facilitate stretching as the baby is born.

Skeletal and Muscular Systems

The increase in both hormone supply and blood supply to the pelvis causes relaxation of the pelvic joints during pregnancy, which can cause a "waddling" walk. The pelvic bones actually spread out slightly, thus shifting some of the weight of the heavy uterus to surrounding muscles and ligaments. The normal lumbar curve of the spine becomes more pronounced as the weight of the uterus and its contents tilt the pelvis forward. This extra burden on the muscles and ligaments may cause the backache that many women experience toward the end of pregnancy.

Circulatory System

Because there is an increase in the amount of blood needed for the reproductive system in pregnancy, the blood volume in the body increases by approximately 40% to 50% so that supplies in the rest of the body will not be depleted. This means an increase of 500 to 1000 milliliters of blood added to the circulatory system, with the volume reaching its peak at 30 to 32 weeks of gestation. Palpitation of the heart and shortness of breath may occur at this time. Also, the increase in circulation to the surface areas of the body may cause a woman to feel warmer than usual.

The increase in plasma volume is greater than the increase in red blood cell volume, so there is a slight dilution of the hemoglobin content of the blood. This hemodilution is normal and called physiological anemia of pregnancy. The hemoglobin-hematocrit ratio in pregnancy is often 12.1 g/dl to 36, instead of 13.3 g/dl to 40, as seen in nonpregnant menstruating women. However, a hemoglobin concentration below 11.0 g/dl, and hematocrit lower than 35%, especially late in pregnancy, are indicative of anemia.

The heart is displaced upward and to the left by the enlarging uterus and the displaced abdominal organs. Cardiac output increases by approximately 30% early in pregnancy and remains elevated until delivery. During labor there is a further increase in cardiac output. Uterine contractions can increase output by up to 400 milliliters per minute. There is a marked positional effect: in the supine position the enlarged, heavy uterus frequently lies against the inferior vena cava and obstructs venous return to the heart, reducing cardiac output by as much as 1 liter per minute. (See Chapter 3.) This compression can lead to serious hypotension and even fetal compromise.

Heart rate increases early in gestation by approximately 20% (10 to 15 beats per minute). Although there is no significant change in systolic blood pressure, there is a slight decrease in diastolic blood pressure. A pressure of 90/70 is not unusual in the pregnant woman. The increased blood flow in pregnancy occurs mainly to the breasts, gut, skin, kidneys, and uterus.

As the pregnancy progresses, the pressure on the enlarged veins of the pelvis and lower extremities increases because of the pressure of the growing uterus. This makes the woman a good candidate for varicose veins in the legs, thighs, and vulva, as well as for dependent edema, phlebitis, and hemorrhoids.

Integumentary System

Increases in hormone levels cause many skin changes in pregnancy. Some of these are *linea nigra*, a dark vertical line running from the umbilicus to the mons pubis (veneris), and *melasma* formerly known as *chloasma* ("mask of pregnancy"), irregular mottled brownish pigmentation of the face. The *linea nigra* and *melasma* fade and sometimes disappear after pregnancy. It is thought that these skin changes may be the result of increased levels of melanocyte-stimulating hormone (MSH) during pregnancy, causing increased production of the pigment melanin. Women with darker skins experience these increases in pigmentation more than fair skinned women. *Angiomas* or tiny capillary branches ("vascular spiders") frequently occur on the skin of the shoulders, arms, hands, or face and tend to disappear after birth. They are thought to be caused by estrogen. There are also silvery-blue stretch marks *(striae gravidarum)* on the sides of the abdomen, breasts, and thighs (Fig. 4-3). These are caused by connective tissue fragility and may fade but never entirely disappear.

Itching is a common complaint during pregnancy. It

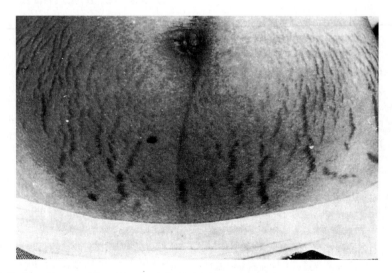

Figure 4-3 Striae. *(Courtesy Mercy Hospital and Medical Center. From Novak JC, Broom BL: Ingalls and Salerno's Maternal and Child Health Nursing, ed 8, St. Louis, 1995, Mosby.)*

often begins on the abdomen and occasionally becomes generalized. In addition, during pregnancy there is increased activity of both sweat and sebaceous glands.

Respiratory System

The pregnant woman breathes more deeply and more frequently than the nonpregnant woman to maintain optimal pressures of O_2 and CO_2 for herself and the fetus. Because respiratory rate is slightly increased and tidal volume increases, the total amount of air exchanged is elevated approximately 40%. However, oxygen consumption increases only 15% to 20% (primarily accounted for by the uterus and its contents). The pregnant woman frequently experiences difficulty breathing *(dyspnea)* in the latter months of pregnancy as the large uterus displaces the diaphragm. Although the lungs are crowded, the ribs flare out so that lung capacity is not decreased.

Gastrointestinal System

Nausea and vomiting ("morning sickness") are common in early pregnancy. The high level of circulating hormones is probably one of the primary causes of nausea. By the third or fourth month of pregnancy, the placenta has assumed major responsibility for progesterone production, and circulating estrogen levels begin to exceed progesterone. At this time nausea stops being a problem for most women.

During pregnancy there is relaxation of the sphincter between the esophagus and stomach causing a reflux of gastric juices into the esophagus. This reflux causes heartburn. Constipation and flatulence are very common, resulting from pressure of the growing fetus on the large intestines and a generalized reduction in gastric tone and motility. Because of uterine enlargement pushing the intestines aside, the pain of appendicitis may actually present in the upper abdomen (near the rib cage) rather than in its traditional position in the right lower abdomen. Gallbladder emptying time is prolonged, which can lead to formation of gallstones.

Urinary System

Frequency of urination is common in both early and late pregnancy because of the pressure of the uterus on the bladder. This frequent urination is alleviated to some degree in the second trimester as the uterus rises out of the pelvis to the level of the symphysis. However, because the edema of pregnancy (swollen feet and ankles) is relieved when the pregnant woman lies down at night, this fluid is often mobilized. Thus it is common for the pregnant woman to have to get up several times at night to urinate. The increased hormone level in pregnancy causes the walls of the ureters to soften and lose much of their muscular tone, thus causing them to dilate. As a result urinary tract infections, such as *cystitis* (bladder infection) and *pyelonephritis* (kidney infection) frequently occur in pregnancy. In order to accommodate a heavier work load, there is also a change in the kidney filtration system in pregnancy, with the glomerular filtration rate (GFR) increasing 50%. This increase in GFR, along with a decrease in kidney threshold for glucose, sometimes results in *glucosuria* (sugar in the urine) after a meal. Even though glucosuria is common in pregnancy, all pregnant women should be screened to determine whether diabetes is present.

Proteinuria does not occur normally during pregnancy, although it may appear occasionally after vigorous activity, in concentrated urine, or in the first voided specimen in the morning.

Endocrine System

The thyroid gland increases in size during pregnancy, and as it does, the basal metabolic rate (BMR) increases. The posterior lobe of the pituitary secretes the oxytoxic hormone, which stimulates uterine muscle to contract. Oxytocin production gradually increases as the fetus matures. The anterior lobe of the pituitary secretes hormones necessary to the normal physiology of pregnancy and also the hormone *prolactin,* which causes breast milk to be secreted after birth.

In response to increased estrogen levels, adrenal cortical secretion increases. The result is increased carbohydrate and protein metabolism. As the placenta matures, there is an increased pancreatic secretion of insulin. However, the increase in human placenta lactogen (hPL) diminishes the effectiveness of the insulin.

Insulin production is increased throughout pregnancy to compensate for decreased tissue sensitivity to insulin that is caused by placental hormones.

WEIGHT GAIN

The recommended weight gain in pregnancy is 25 to 35 pounds. However, there are exceptions. Recommendations for weight gain are based on prepregnancy weight and height. Women who are underweight when first pregnant should gain between 28 to 40 pounds. Women who are overweight when they become pregnant should gain no more than 15 to 25 pounds. Short women (under 62 inches) should have lower weight gain goals of 18 to 30 pounds. Extremely obese women should limit their weight gain to 15 pounds with adequate nutrient intake. The weight gain recommenda-

Presumptive Signs
1. Amenorrhea (cessation of menses)

2. Frequency of urination (micturition)

3. Nausea and vomiting in the morning ("morning sickness")
4. Quickening (first fetal life felt by mother)
5. Enlargement of breasts

6. Pigmentation of the skin
7. Chadwick's sign

Other Causes
Could also result from hormone imbalance, emotional disturbance, disease, environmental changes, or excessive exercise
Could also be caused by a bladder infection, diabetes, a pelvic tumor, or congestive heart failure
Could have emotional causes, or be caused by a "flu" or a variety of intestinal disturbances
Could be intestinal activity ("gas")
Could be caused by hormonal changes other than pregnancy
May be present in all women
Could be present when any pelvic congestion occurs

Probable Signs
1. Enlarged uterus and abdomen
2. Braxton Hicks contractions
3. Hegar's sign
4. Ballottement
5. Positive pregnancy test
6. Uterine souffle (a soft, blowing rhythm the same rate as the mother's pulse, caused by blood passing through large uterine vessels)

Other Causes
Could also be fibroid tumor, ascites, or ovarian cysts
Probable indication
Probable indication
Could also occur with some tumors
Probable indication
Audible after sixteenth week

Positive Signs
1. Fetal heart beat—audible from eighteenth to twentieth week on with stethoscope; by 9 to 11 weeks with Doppler ultrasound
2. Fetal movement—palpable after 20 weeks
3. Sonography–will show fetal outlines as well as movements by 5 to 6 weeks (occasionally at 4 weeks)

tion is individualized for each woman and is based on her prepregnant weight and height.

The average weight gain when plotted on a grid reflects a gradual and progressive increase in weight (Fig. 4-4). Women with healthy prepregnancy weights should gain an average of one pound a week during the second and third trimesters (underweight women, a little more and overweight, a little less). The weight gain of pregnancy is distributed as follows:

Fetus	7.0-8.0 pounds
Placenta	1.5-2.0 pounds
Amniotic fluid	2.0-3.5 pounds
Increased uterine size	2.5-3.0 pounds
Increased blood volume	3.0-4.5 pounds
Increased breast size	1.0-1.5 pounds
Increased extracellular fluid	4.0-6.0 pounds
Fat	4.0-6.5 pounds
TOTAL	25.0-35.0 pounds

SIGNS AND SYMPTOMS

The *presumptive* (presumed but not proved) signs and symptoms of pregnancy are mostly those that occur very early in pregnancy. The *probable* (likely but not definite) signs are those that occur generally after 6 to 8 weeks of pregnancy. The *positive* (no doubt about it) signs and symptoms appear after approximately the twentieth week of pregnancy. (See box above.)

PREGNANCY TESTS

Although pregnancy can usually be easily diagnosed once a women is well along in her pregnancy (simply by observing and palpating her distended abdomen), there are now simple examinations of the blood and urine that make it possible to diagnose pregnancy as early as 8 days after ovulation.

Pregnancy tests differ in their sensitivity, the time they take to complete, and whether urine or blood is used. Obviously the more sensitive and sophisticated the test, the more it costs to do. All currently available tests detect levels of human chorionic gonadotropin (hCG), a hormone produced by the fertilized egg that can be found in the pregnant woman's blood and urine. (See Chapter 2.) The urinary excretion of hCG doubles every 1½ to 2 days, and thus the more sensitive the test, the earlier pregnancy can be detected.

The five main types of pregnancy tests are latex agglutination inhibition (LAI), hemagglutination (HAI),

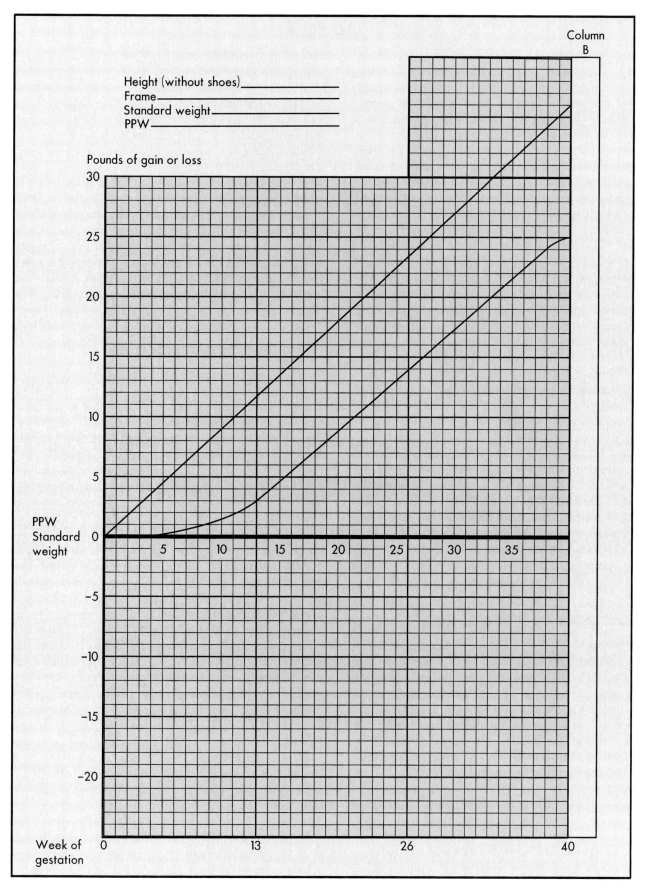

Figure 4-4 Chart for weight gain. *(Dimerio D:* Prenatal nutrition: clinical guidelines for nurses, *White Plains, NY, 1988, March of Dimes Birth Defects Foundation. From Dickason EJ, Silverman BL, Schult MO:* Maternal-Infant Nursing Care, *ed 2, St. Louis, 1994, Mosby.)*

radioreceptor assay (RRA), radioimmunoassay (RIA), and direct agglutination (DA). LAI tests are usually done by mixing a drop of urine onto a slide and agitating for 2 minutes. A clumped solution indicates a negative result (no pregnancy) and a milky-smooth solution indicates a positive result (pregnancy). LAI is cheap but is accurate only 21 to 24 days after conception. HAI tests are similar to LAI but usually require test tubes and take 1 to 2 hours. Most home pregnancy tests are of this type. A mat of debris at the bottom of the tube signals a negative result, and a ring at the tube base indicates a positive result. HAI is accurate from 14 to 18 days after ovulation. RRA tests, done in sophisticated laboratories, take about 1 hour to perform and can detect pregnancy approximately 14 days after ovulation. RIA tests, done on blood or urine, are the most sensitive of the currently available pregnancy tests and can detect pregnancy as early as 8 days after ovulation (actually *before* the missed menstrual period). These are the tests of choice for assessment of ectopic pregnancies, hydatidiform mole, or threatened spontaneous abortions. DA tests are also very sensitive and accurate early in pregnancy.

PRENATAL CARE

The overall objectives of prenatal care are to promote the health and well-being of the pregnant woman, the fetus, the infant, and the family for up to 1 year after the infant's birth. To achieve these objectives requires that prenatal care be available and used. It should include (1) early and continuing risk assessment, (2) health promotion, and (3) a balance of medical and psychosocial interventions and follow-up.

Importance of Prenatal Care

There is no doubt that improved prenatal care in this country has reduced maternal and infant morbidity and mortality. Detecting possible problems early leads to prompt treatment and greatly improved pregnancy outcome. Because so much of the wellness of pregnancy is dependent on the woman assuming responsibility for her own health maintenance with proper exercise, nutrition, and preventive measures, early diagnosis, assessment of the pregnancy, and a planned regimen of care are essential.

However, because health in pregnancy depends a great deal on a woman's general health before the pregnancy, placing more emphasis on preconception and early pregnancy care is needed. When medical and psychosocial risk assessment is performed before conception, treatment may be started early, as well as health promotion and interventions to reduce psychosocial

risks. The pregnancy may occur or be deferred as appropriate. Preconception care can be made part of family planning visits and health care programs for women in their reproductive years.

The National Institutes of Health/Health and Human Services (NIH/HHS) Expert Panel on the Content of Prenatal Care has recommended fewer prenatal visits for pregnant women whose fetuses are at no apparent risk and intensified prenatal care for high-risk women during their pregnancies.

According to the federal panel, the first prenatal visit should take place within 6 to 8 weeks of gestation and not be delayed to a later time. To meet the education and psychosocial needs of pregnant women, the panel also recommended that childbirth education classes be available to all pregnant women as part of standard care during pregnancy.

Nursing Responsibilities

When you first meet the pregnant woman and her family, remember that rapid physical and emotional changes are occurring, causing anxiety for the parents-to-be. A positive pregnancy test may not cause waves of joy for the woman. As mentioned in Chapter 1, both men and women may have ambivalent feelings when pregnancy is confirmed. Frequently your first introduction to the family will be to the woman only, since pregnancy has been considered "woman's business" in our society. If there is a mate, encourage his presence during prenatal visits. Through understanding the physiological and psychological changes the pregnant woman is experiencing, he is better able to offer help and support. Also, the expectant father has needs as he adjusts to his new role. It is not unusual for men to experience morning sickness, weight gain, and fatigue in early pregnancy. Such physiological changes may be cries for help on his part. Last but not least, consider the siblings and other family members. Including siblings in prenatal care by gradually introducing them to the new family member through listening to the fetal heartbeat, watching the uterus grow, and just making them feel part of this family event may help to reduce sibling rivalry. Grandparents often feel left out because they have difficulty understanding today's trends in maternity care. Remember that pregnancy is wellness. This is the family's pregnancy. Birth is the beginning or further growth of a family and you can contribute immeasurably to the experience.

Women living alone may have considerably more need for emotional support and child care during visits than women with family support. Your role as nurse includes assessing the psychosocial needs of the childbearing women who seek your help and then determining how to meet those needs. Consultaion with other members of the health team is necessary. Community resources should be sought out as well.

Medical History

A thorough medical, surgical, obstetric and gynecological as well as psychosocial history is taken during the first examination to determine the present state of the mother's health. Family and genetic history, nutrition, and infection histories are included. A risk assessment to determine possible risks for a problem pregnancy is essential at the time of the first prenatal visit so that appropriate interventions can follow. Cultural, racial, or ethnic background is always included in this assessment process.

The obstetric and gynecological history usually includes a sexual history, including sexually transmitted disease (STDs) and descriptions of each prior pregnancy, including dates of birth, sex, and weight; lengths of labor and pregnancy; and complications. A commonly used form of obstetric history abbreviation is as follows: number of pregnancies = gravida number; number of deliveries (alive or dead) = para number; number of abortions = "Ab" number. For example, a woman who was pregnant three times, delivered twice, had one abortion, and is now pregnant again would be: gravida$_4$ para$_2$ ab$_1$, or $G_4P_2Ab_1$. The history helps the medical and nursing team plan for the pregnancy and delivery and, if at all possible, prevent complications that may have occurred in previous pregnancies.

A careful recording of the woman's menstrual history will be essential in the calculation of the date of delivery.

Calculation of Estimated Date of Delivery

An approximation of the estimated date of delivery (EDD) can be calculated by using *Nägele's rule:* (1) take date of last menstrual period (LMP), (2) subtract three months, (3) add 7 days and 1 year.

$$
\begin{array}{rl}
\textit{Example:} \quad \text{LMP} = \text{August 7, 1995} & \dfrac{8/\ 7/95}{-3} \\[4pt]
& \dfrac{5/\ 7/95}{+\quad 7/1} \\[4pt]
\text{EDD} = \text{May 14, 1996} & \overline{5/14/96}
\end{array}
$$

The typical pregnancy lasts 40 weeks from the first day of LMP, or 280 days. This is also estimated as 9¼ calendar months, or 10 lunar months. The length of pregnancy varies greatly, and 2 weeks in either direction from the EDD is considered normal.

Psychosocial History

The psychosocial history includes risk assessment relative to substance use or abuse: alcohol, tobacco, illicit or prescription drugs; social support; stress; physical abuse; pregnancy readiness; exposure to teratogens; housing and finances; and extremes of physical work, exercise, or other activity.

Because physical abuse often starts during pregnancy, assessing pregnant women for abuse is important. Pregnancy is the ideal time for nurses to intervene with battered women because the women are seen more often by health care providers during that period.

Physical Examination

After the psychosocial assessment and the woman's medical, surgical, and obstetric history are completed, she is ready for a physical examination. The nurse prepares the woman for a physical examination by first collecting a voided urine specimen to check it for sugar and albumin. The woman's temperature, pulse, respiration, blood pressure, height, and weight are also recorded. Vital signs should *not* be measured with the pregnant woman lying on her back because compression of the inferior vena cava by the pregnant uterus may cause misleading values to be recorded. Next the nurse provides privacy for the woman in an examination room, instructs her to remove all clothing, provides a robe or drape for covering, and prepares all necessary equipment. The woman may be very apprehensive. The nurse will stay with the examiner to assist if necessary and to provide emotional support for the woman. If the expectant father is with the woman, encourage him to stay at the head of the examining table so that he can reassure her also. This is a very good time for the couple to learn together about the need for and meaning of the physical examination. It also gives him an opportunity for early involvement in the pregnancy.

The physical examination includes examination of all body systems and abdominal palpation (Fig. 4-5). The obstetric examination includes examination of the external genitalia, the hymenal remnant (if present), the urethral orifice, the vagina, the cervix, the corpus of the uterus, the adnexal structures, and the rectum. It also includes a Papanicolaou smear for a cancer cytology test, measurements of the pelvis, and tests to detect sexually transmissible diseases (STDs) or infections if deemed necessary. Before the obstetric examination, always be sure that the woman has emptied her bladder.

One *pelvic measurement* that is taken is the *diagonal conjugate* (from the inferior margin of the symphysis pubis to the sacral promontory) (Fig. 4-6). This is done on vaginal examination when the tips of the first two fingers of the examiner touch the sacral promontory.

The point where the lower margin of the symphysis pubis rests on the finger is measured. Normally the diagonal conjugate is >12.5 centimeters. (Fig. 4-7). The *true conjugate* is obtained by subtracting 1.5 to 2.0 centimeters from the diagonal conjugate measurement. The normal measurement is 10 centimeters. The true conjugate measures the upper margin of the symphysis pubis to the sacral promontory and can be measured *directly* only by x-ray study (which is not recommended in pregnancy). The *prominence of the ischial spines,* the sloping of the pelvic walls, the curve or prominence of the sacrum, the mobility of the coccyx, and the angle of the pubic arch can be felt and estimated during vaginal examination. The *outlet* is measured by the distance between the ischial tuberosities *(intertuberous diameter),* which is usually 10 to 11 centimeters (Fig. 2-13). This measurement is approximated with a pelvimeter or with estimated length using the closed fist of the examiner's hand. The *posterior sagittal* measurement is made indirectly with a pelvimeter. Normal measurement is 8.0 to 9.5 centimeters. It is the distance between the midpoint of intertuberous diameter and the

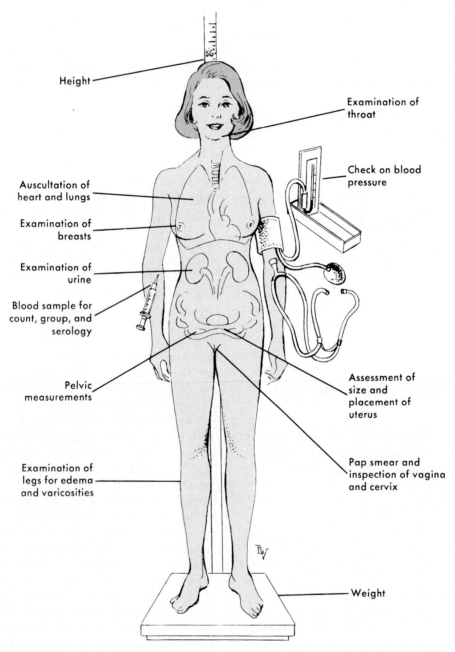

Figure 4-5 Thorough physical examination. *(From Lerch C, Bliss VJ: Maternity nursing, ed 3, St. Louis, 1978, Mosby.)*

tip of the sacrum. If the pelvis is determined to be of adequate size and suitable shape, further assessment of the bony pelvis is usually not necessary.

Laboratory Tests

The following laboratory tests are routinely done:

1. *Serologic testing* should be done. Venereal Disease Research Laboratories *(VDRL)* or rapid plasma reagin (RPR) is done to detect syphilis. If syphilis is present, the test will usually be positive. It is sometimes recommended that testing be repeated before labor begins.

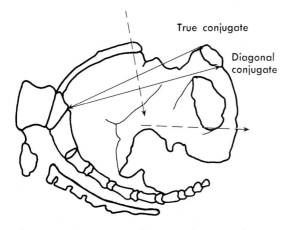

Figure 4-6 Diagonal conjugate and true conjugate.

2. *Rh factor* and *blood type* determinations are done to detect possible maternal-fetal blood incompatibilities. In the United States 85% of the population is Rh positive, which means that they have the Rh antigen in their blood; and 15% is Rh negative, which means that they lack the Rh antigen. A problem can exist if the mother is Rh negative and the father is Rh positive. A potential problem also exists if the mother is type O and the fetus is type A, B, or AB.

3. *Normal hemoglobin and hematocrit levels* are as follows:

	Nonpregnant	Pregnant
Hemoglobin (Hgb)	>13.3 grams/ 100 milliliters	>12.1 grams/ 100 milliliters
Hematocrit (Hct)	>40%	>36%

Note: These values may vary slightly from laboratory to laboratory.

4. *Rubella screening* is usually routine to determine whether the woman is resistant to the rubella virus (German measles). A rubella antibody titer of between 1:8 and 1:20 *or greater* suggests immunity (the exact cutoff point varies from laboratory to laboratory).

5. *Urine tests for sugar* are done to detect maternal diabetes. Urine should be free of sugar, although in the latter part of pregnancy sugar in the urine

A   **B**

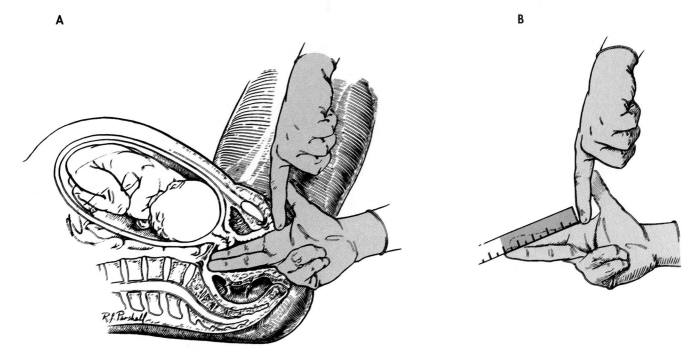

Figure 4-7 Measurement of the diagonal conjugate. **A,** Internal palpation. **B,** Use of a ruler to specify estimation in centimeters. *(From Barkauskas VH, Stoltenberg-Allen K, Baumann LC, Darling-Fisher C:* Health and physical assessment, *St. Louis, 1994, Mosby.)*

may occur as a result of increased amounts of lactose in the blood. Tests for *protein* are done to detect proteinuria, which is indicative of abnormal kidney functioning and pregnancy-induced hypertension (PIH). Urine should be free of protein.

6. *Sickle cell anemia* and *thalassemia* tests are done on women of African or Mediterranean heritage.
7. *Skin testing* for detection of tuberculosis should be done.
8. *Vaginal smears* to detect gonorrhea and chlamydia and laboratory testing for herpesvirus hominis and monilial and trichomonal infections are done if indicated.
9. *Papanicolaou test* (Pap smear) is a screening test to detect cervical cancer. This is usually done on the first prenatal visit.
10. *Hepatitis B antigen* screening is recommended for all women because of the prevalence of these diseases in the general population. Toxoplasmosis and rubeola antibody screens may also be indicated.
11. *HIV screening* should be offered to all women.

Further laboratory tests and repetitions of the preceding tests are done as indicated during the pregnancy.

According to the latest recommendations of the federal panel discussed earlier, families at no apparent risk are encouraged to return for the second pregnancy visit within 4 weeks of the first visit and then again at 24 to 28 weeks, 32 weeks, 36 weeks, and then every week in the last month. Each visit concentrates on risk assessment and health promotion. The visit schedule is adapted and changed as risks are identified for each individual woman. Women determined to be at risk will be followed more closely and have more frequent prenatal checkups than those with low-risk status.

The emphasis in the prenatal care schedule described here is on the preconception period and early pregnancy so that underlying health concerns or problems can be treated before or early in pregnancy.

In addition to risk assessment specific to the needs of each woman at each visit, blood pressure; urine specimens; temperature, pulse, and respiration (TPR); weight gain; height of uterine fundus (Fig. 4-8); fetal well-being; and the mother's general physical and emotional status are assessed. Laboratory examinations are repeated as necessary, and additional laboratory examinations are done as needed.

HEALTH PROMOTION

Counseling to promote and support healthful behavior, general knowledge of pregnancy and parenting, and

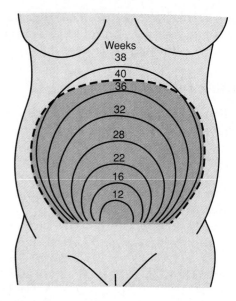

Figure 4-8 Growth of uterus during pregnancy.

information on personal care are all part of the health promotion aspects of prenatal care. When discussing the psychosocial and physiological changes of pregnancy with the woman and her family, the nurse should find out how much they already know, what they believe to be true, and what their cultural background has taught them. Next, the nurse should explain, discuss, clarify, reinforce, and share information, where appropriate, about what they do not know.

Bathing

Because the woman's sebaceous and sweat glands have become more active, she needs a daily bath. Either a tub bath or a shower is all right. There is no danger if bath water enters the vagina. She should not use soap and water on the nipples of her breasts when bathing because soap has a tendency to cause dryness and cracking. The expectant mother, expectant father, or other family member could be encouraged to install safety strips or a nonslip bath mat in the tub or shower to make the area less slippery.

Clothing

Clothing should be nonconstricting. As the breasts enlarge, the bra size may need to increase, and the woman may choose a nursing bra before delivery. It is important to keep the breasts well supported during pregnancy to prevent overstretching of connective tissue, which could lead to sagging of the breasts. Pregnant women should never wear round or rolled garters because they constrict the leg vessels, slow down venous return, and thus cause edema and encourage the formation of varicose veins. Support stockings are helpful for women with varicosities. A girdle is usually not necessary but does offer helpful support to the back and pelvis for some women. Shoes worn by pregnant women should have flat or medium heels because high heels tilt the body forward, upsetting the balance and causing increased curvature of the back to compensate for the forward tilt.

Oral Hygiene

Daily oral hygiene with flossing is essential during pregnancy. A visit to the dentist early in pregnancy will detect any cavities that could make the mother more susceptible to infections. There is no truth in the old adage: "For every child, a tooth is lost."

Sexuality and Feminine Hygiene

As discussed at the beginning of this chapter, unless contraindicated by a medical condition or complication of pregnancy, continuing usual sexual activity is encouraged during pregnancy. A discussion of sexuality can begin by asking the couple what they have heard about sex during pregnancy.

Douching in pregnancy (or at any time) is not necessary unless done specifically under a physician's order to treat a vaginal irritation. It is not unusual to have increased vaginal secretions during pregnancy, and the woman needs to understand this. However, if the secretion is so copious as to require the wearing of a pad, the woman should seek medical attention. This could be indicative of a vaginal infection such as *Trichomonas vaginalis* infection (a profuse, yellowish-green, irritating discharge with an unpleasant odor) or *Monilia* infection (candidiasis, a yeast infection causing a thick, white, cheesy discharge with itching). Both of these infections tend to occur during pregnancy and are treatable.

Bowels

There is a tendency toward constipation (infrequent or hard stools) as a result of decreased peristalsis. Decreased peristalsis causes the feces to remain longer in the bowel, thus increasing the water absorption from the feces. Some iron supplements may make constipation worse. Encourage the addition to the diet of six to eight glasses of liquid per day, roughage, bran, fruits, and fruit juices. Daily exercise also helps to reduce the incidence of constipation. Explain to the woman that if constipation becomes a problem and if changes in her diet and daily exercise do not improve the condition, she may ask the doctor for a mild laxative. However, she should not medicate herself because harsh laxatives can stimulate the uterus to contract.

Exercise, Travel, and Employment

The pregnant woman should remain active during pregnancy, participating in her normal activities but avoiding activity that causes unnecessary fatigue. There are specific exercises that are helpful in maintaining the tone of the abdominal, back, and perineal muscles. Some of these exercises are illustrated in Fig. 4-9.

Today many women continue to be employed outside the home during their entire pregnancy. If the family is dependent on the woman's income, or if she is supporting herself, it is totally unrealistic to encourage this woman to leave her job unless absolutely essential for her health. The nurse can help the family or the single woman decide how to continue working but avoid becoming overtired.

NUTRITION

The nutrition of the mother directly affects the status of the infant; the emphasis needs to be on adequate nutrition in pregnancy, which often leads to a weight gain of 25 to 35 pounds, depending on the prepregnant weight of the woman.

The goals of nutritional management for any prenatal woman should be the optimal growth and development of the fetus and optimal health of the mother.

Well-nourished mothers give birth to healthier children. Poor diet in pregnancy has been associated with decreased infant birth weight, increased stillbirth, spontaneous abortion, and neonatal death. The more poorly nourished a woman is when becoming pregnant, the more important her diet is in pregnancy.

We speak in terms of Recommended Dietary Allowances (RDAs), which are defined as "levels of intake of essential nutrients considered, in the judgment of the Food and Nutrition Board on the basis of available scientific knowledge, to be adequate to meet the known nutritional needs of practically all healthy persons" (Table 4-1).

Generally, pregnant and lactating women have the greatest need for increased nutrient intakes to meet their RDAs. The simplest way to allow for these differences is to adjust the size and number of servings of food. By recommendation of The National Research Council (NRC), a blanket vitamin prescription for all pregnant women is no longer given routinely. Only low-dose iron supplements and folic acid are recommended to be taken as supplements.

The nutrients that must be increased during pregnancy are as follows.

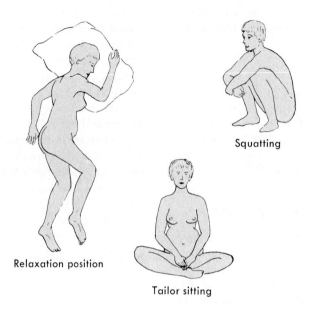

Relaxation position

Squatting

Tailor sitting

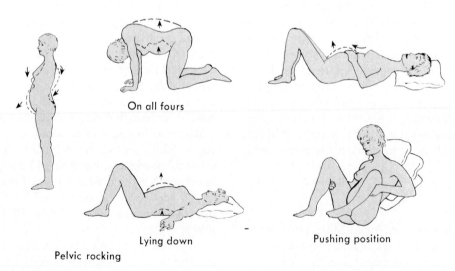

On all fours

Pelvic rocking

Lying down

Pushing position

Figure 4-9 Exercises for prenatal period. *(From Hamilton PM: Basic maternity nursing, ed 6, St. Louis, 1989, Mosby.)*

TABLE 4-1
Food and Nutrition Board, National Academy of Sciences—National Research Council Recommended Dietary Allowances,[a] Revised 1989
Designed for the maintenance of good nutrition of practically all healthy people in the United States

Category	Age (years) or Condition	Weight (kg)	Weight (lb)	Height (cm)	Height (in)	Protein (g)	Vitamin A (μg RE)[c]	Vitamin D (μg)[d]	Vitamin E (mg α-TE)[e]	Vitamin K (μg)	Vitamin C (mg)	Thiamin (mg)	Riboflavin (mg)	Niacin (mg NE)[f]	Vitamin B6 (mg)	Folate (μg)	Vitamin B12 (μg)	Calcium (mg)	Phosphorus (mg)	Magnesium (mg)	Iron (mg)	Zinc (mg)	Iodine (μg)	Selenium (μg)
Infants	0.0-0.5	6	13	60	24	13	375	7.5	3	5	30	0.3	0.4	5	0.3	25	0.3	400	300	40	6	5	40	10
	0.5-1.0	9	20	71	28	14	375	10	4	10	35	0.4	0.5	6	0.6	35	0.5	600	500	60	10	5	50	15
Children	1-3	13	29	90	35	16	400	10	6	15	40	0.7	0.8	9	1.0	50	0.7	800	800	80	10	10	70	20
	4-6	20	44	112	44	24	500	10	7	20	45	0.9	1.1	12	1.1	75	1.0	800	800	120	10	10	90	20
	7-10	28	62	132	52	28	700	10	7	30	45	1.0	1.2	13	1.4	100	1.4	800	800	170	10	10	120	30
Males	11-14	45	99	157	62	45	1,000	10	10	45	50	1.3	1.5	17	1.7	150	2.0	1,200	1,200	270	12	15	150	40
	15-18	66	145	176	69	59	1,000	10	10	65	60	1.5	1.8	20	2.0	200	2.0	1,200	1,200	400	12	15	150	50
	19-24	72	160	177	70	58	1,000	10	10	70	60	1.5	1.7	19	2.0	200	2.0	1,200	1,200	350	10	15	150	70
	25-50	79	174	176	70	63	1,000	5	10	80	60	1.5	1.7	19	2.0	200	2.0	800	800	350	10	15	150	70
	51+	77	170	173	68	63	1,000	5	10	80	60	1.2	1.4	15	2.0	200	2.0	800	800	350	10	15	150	70
Females	11-14	46	101	157	62	46	800	10	8	45	50	1.1	1.3	15	1.4	150	2.0	1,200	1,200	280	15	12	150	45
	15-18	55	120	163	64	44	800	10	8	55	60	1.1	1.3	15	1.5	180	2.0	1,200	1,200	300	15	12	150	50
	19-24	58	128	164	65	46	800	10	8	60	60	1.1	1.3	15	1.6	180	2.0	1,200	1,200	280	15	12	150	55
	25-50	63	138	163	64	50	800	5	8	65	60	1.1	1.3	15	1.6	180	2.0	800	800	280	15	12	150	55
	51+	65	143	160	63	50	800	5	8	65	60	1.0	1.2	13	1.6	180	2.0	800	800	280	10	12	150	55
Pregnant						60	800	10	10	65	70	1.5	1.6	17	2.2	400	2.2	1,200	1,200	300	30	15	175	65
Lactating	1st 6 months					65	1,300	10	12	65	95	1.6	1.8	20	2.1	280	2.6	1,200	1,200	355	15	19	200	75
	2nd 6 months					62	1,200	10	11	65	90	1.6	1.7	20	2.1	260	2.6	1,200	1,200	340	15	16	200	75

[a]The allowances, expressed as average daily intakes over time, are intended to provide for individual variations among most normal persons as they live in the United States under usual environmental stresses. Diets should be based on a variety of common foods in order to provide other nutrients for which human requirements have been less well defined. See text for detailed discussion of allowances and of nutrients not tabulated.

[b]Weights and heights of Reference Adults are actual medians for the U.S. population of the designated age, as reported by NHANES II. The median weights and heights of those under 19 years of age were taken from Hamill et al. (1979) (see pages 16-17). The use of these figures does not imply that the height-to-weight ratios are ideal.

[c]Retinol equivalents. 1 retinol equivalent = 1 μg retinol or 6 μg β-carotene. See text for calculation of vitamin A activity of diets as retinol equivalents.

[d]As cholecalciferol. 10 μg cholecalciferol = 400 IU of vitamin D.

[e]α-Tocopherol equivalents. 1 mg d-α tocopherol = 1 α-TE. See text for variation in allowances and calculation of vitamin E activity of the diet as α-tocopherol equivalents.

[f]1 NE (niacin equivalent) is equal to 1 mg of niacin or 60 mg of dietary tryptophan.

Protein is the building material that forms the structure of every cell. During pregnancy, protein should be increased to 60 grams per day and 70 grams per day during lactation. Special attention to protein intake should be directed at persons on vegetarian diets, women with high-risk pregnancies, and pregnant adolescents.

Excellent sources of protein include poultry, lean meat, fish, and milk. Dried beans, lentils, nuts, eggs, and cheese are other high protein foods.

Calcium and phosphorus are important for maintaining the mother's bones and teeth and for building the infant's bones and teeth. Calcium needs during pregnancy have been determined to be 1200 mg/day. This need for calcium and phosphorus represents increases by 50% over nonpregnant recommendations, both for pregnancy and lactation. Milk, cheese, yogurt, and ice cream are high in calcium. Green leafy vegetables, tofu, and canned salmon are other good sources of calcium.

Iron is an important nutrient during pregnancy for the formation of maternal and fetal hemoglobin, for the increase in maternal blood volume and development of the infant's blood cells, and for the iron reserves the fetus accumulates during the last trimester, which give protection from anemia during the first months of life. The iron requirement doubles during pregnancy from 15 to 30 mg/day. For the general population of pregnant women, daily supplements of 30 milligrams of ferrous iron during the second and third trimesters are recommended. Liver and red meat are particularly rich in iron. Other meats, fish, and poultry are also good sources of iron. Enriched and whole grain breads and cereals, green leafy vegetables, legumes, eggs, and dried fruit also provide iron.

All women capable of becoming pregnant should consume 0.4 milligrams of *folic acid* as a daily supplement, according to the National Research Council (NRC). A deficiency of folic acid has been shown to have a positive correlation with abruptio placentae, late pregnancy bleeding, spontaneous and recurrent abortion, pregnancy-induced hypertension (PIH), prematurity, and neural tube defects. Mothers at risk for folic acid deficiency include those who have had repeated pregnancies, have abused alcohol, use oral contraceptives, have problems with malabsorption, have liver disease, or have restrictive dietary patterns. Food sources of folic acid include legumes, dark leafy green vegetables, fruit and vegetables and their juices, and beef liver.

Intake of *fat-soluble vitamins (A, D, and E)* should be increased in pregnancy and lactation, as should intake of the *water-soluble vitamins* (C, thiamine, riboflavin, niacin, vitamin B_6, and vitamin B_{12}) (Table 4-1). In addition, zinc and iodine requirements also increase . Percent increases over nonpregnant women for recommended dietary allowances can be found in Table 4-2.

The daily calorie (Kcal) increase during pregnancy is 300 Kcal per day during the second and third trimesters and 500 Kcal per day during lactation.

Various food guides have been devised to translate the technical language of nutrients and dietary allowances into the terms of everyday eating. On the basis of their similar nutrient contents, foods can be classified into groups, with recommendations for the amount of food from each group that should be eaten daily. A guide to good eating is a simple plan. The box on p. 114 is based on the Recommended Dietary Allowances (RDAs).

Instead of sodium restriction in pregnancy, the use of iodized salt in moderation is recommended. It has been recognized that women actually need more sodium in pregnancy than during the nonpregnant state. To maintain fluid balance and osmotic integrity when sodium is retained, water must be retained in pregnancy as well. This retained water contributes to the pregnant woman's weight gain. No longer are diuretics prescribed during pregnancy.

Before counseling pregnant families on the changes in approach to nutrition in pregnancy, the nurse needs to determine what their diet is now. A nutrition questionnaire in addition to a diet interview and a counseling session is very helpful. The family can take the questionnaire home, discuss it, and complete it together. This exercise in itself is self-instructional. Also, whenever appropriate, the costs of foods should be discussed and alternatives to high-priced foods found.

LACTATION

Lactating women vary in their nutritional needs according to the volume of their milk production. After feeding is established, a mother produces 500 to 1000 milliliters of milk a day. The composition of each mother's milk may vary. Poor nutrition during the lactating period reduces milk volume before the quality of the milk is lessened.

Caloric Needs

From 0 to 3 months: To make milk, 900 calories per day may be required. This is provided by 200 to 300 calories from mother's fat pad of pregnancy and 500 calories per day extra to manufacture milk.

From 3 to 6 months: The pregnancy fat store is depleted and approximately 1000 calories a day may be required to make milk in addition to her regular diet.

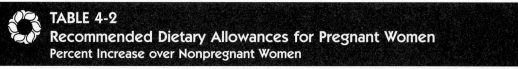

TABLE 4-2
Recommended Dietary Allowances for Pregnant Women
Percent Increase over Nonpregnant Women

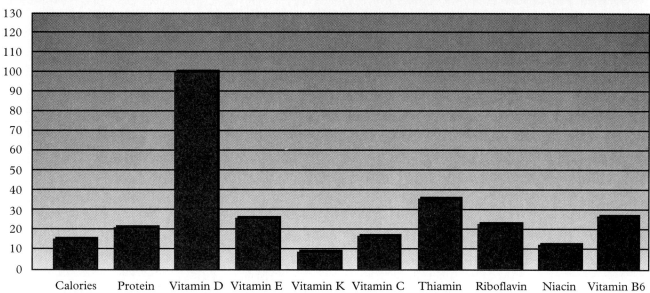

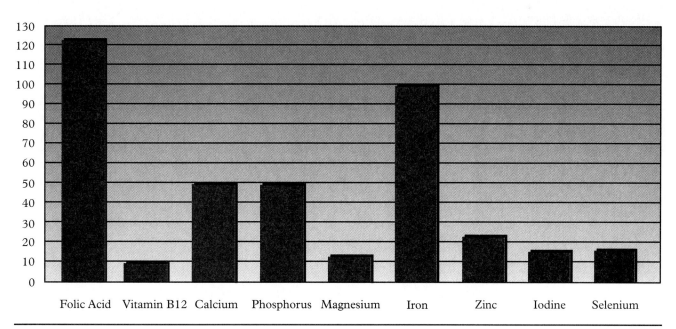

From: *Recommended Dietary Allowances,* ed 10, 1989, National Research Council, National Academy of Sciences.

Guide to Good Eating—A Recommended Daily Pattern

The recommended daily pattern provides the foundation for a nutritious, healthful diet.

Milk Group
Major source of: calcium
riboflavin (B_2)
protein
vitamin B_{12}
magnesium

3 Servings/Child
4 Servings/Teenager
2 Servings/Adult

4 Servings/Pregnant Woman
5 Servings/Lactating Woman
5 Servings/Pregnant/Lactating Woman

Foods made from milk contribute part of the nutrients supplied by a serving of milk.
□ nonfat milk, buttermilk, lowfat milk, plain yogurt
□ whole milk, cheese, fruit-flavored yogurt, cottage cheese
□ custard, milkshake, pudding, ice cream

Meat Group
Major source of: protein
niacin
iron
thiamin (B_1)

2 Servings

3 Servings/Pregnant Woman
3 Servings/Lactating Woman

Dry beans and peas, soy extenders, and nuts combined with animal protein (meat, fish, poultry, eggs, milk, cheese) or grain protein can be substituted for a serving of meat.
□ poultry, fish, lean meat (beef, lamb, pork), dried peas and beans, eggs
□ beef, lamb, pork, luncheon meats, refried beans
□ hot dogs, peanut butter, nuts

Fruit-vegetable Group
Major source of: vitamin A
vitamin C
folic acid

4 Servings

4 Servings/Pregnant Woman
4 Servings/Lactating Woman

Dark green, leafy, or orange vegetables and fruits are recommended three or four times weekly for vitamin A. Citrus fruit is recommended daily for vitamin C.
□ apricot, bean sprouts, broccoli, brussels sprouts, cabbage, cantaloupe, carrots, cauliflower, cucumber, grapefruit, green beans, green peas, leafy greens (spinach, mustard, and collard greens), lettuce, mushrooms, orange, orange juice, peach, strawberries, tomato, winter squash
□ apple, banana, canned fruit, corn, pear, potato
□ avocado, dried fruit, sweet potato

Grain Group
Major source of: carbohydrate
thiamin (B_1)
iron
niacin

4 Servings

4 Servings/Pregnant Woman
4 Servings/Lactating Woman

Whole grain, fortified, or enriched grain products are recommended.
□ whole grain and enriched breads, rolls, tortillas
□ rice, cereals, pastas (macaroni, spaghetti), bagel
□ pancake, muffin, cornbread, biscuit, presweetened cereals

Guide to Good Eating—A Recommended Daily Pattern—*cont'd*

Others
Major source of: carbohydrate
                 fat
   Fats, sweets, and condiments complement but do not replace foods from the four groups. Amounts should be determined by individual caloric needs.
   □ sugar: cake, pie, cookies, doughnuts, sweet rolls, candy, soft drinks, fruit drinks, jelly, syrup, gelatin desserts, sugar, honey
   □ fat: margarine, salad dressing, oils, mayonnaise, cream, cream cheese, butter, gravy sauces
   □ salt (sodium): potato chips, corn chips, pretzels, pickles, olives, bouillon, mustard, soy sauce, steak sauce, salt, seasoned salt
   □ other: spices, herbs

The best way to monitor caloric needs is to monitor maternal weight since there will be some variation of caloric need depending upon volume of milk made and maternal activity.

The increased need for calories, protein, calcium, and vitamins A and D can be met by consumption of extra servings of the food groups identified on p. 114.

Early pregnancy classes are an excellent way to discuss nutrition in pregnancy as well as common discomforts, sexuality, and ways to cope. (See Chapter 5.) When counseling any pregnant family, the nurse must keep in mind the family's attitudes; past experiences with foods; cultural influences on diet; and social, religious, and ethnic influences.

Many people do not consume adequate supplies of milk, which leads to an inadequate calcium and vitamin D (and possibly riboflavin) intake. One quart of milk supplies 100% of the daily requirements of calcium and vitamin D and almost 50% of the protein needed in one day. However, in the United States over two thirds of blacks, Latinos, Native Americans, Ashkenazic Jews, and Asians are lactose intolerant. Lactose is a constituent of milk, and lactose intolerance is the inability to digest and absorb lactose (a sugar) because of low level activity of the enzyme lactase. Symptoms of lactose intolerance are abdominal distention, discomfort, cramps and pain, loose stools, flatulence, and watery, fermentive, acid diarrhea.

Persons who are lactose intolerant should avoid milk and other dairy products except for hard or more aged cheese, such as Swiss and cheddar. These have less lactose than other types and can sometimes be tolerated in small amounts. Very cold milk may be tolerated; also cultured forms of milk, such as acidophilus milk and yogurt, are often tolerated by persons who are lactose intolerant. Calcium and vitamin D supplements can be used. Phosphorus must always be present in the diet to balance calcium intake. Protein foods should also be increased.

Two cups or 8 ounces of tofu or 1½ cups of cooked, dark green leafy vegetables provide approximately the same amount of calcium as 1 cup of milk.

It is beyond the scope of this book to present detailed diets for all ethnic and religious groups; however, the California State Department of Public Health has published an excellent pamphlet on this subject.

COMMON DISCOMFORTS

Many of the symptoms that cause discomfort and concern can be alleviated, and most will disappear as the months pass.

These changes are fairly specific to each of the three trimesters:

First Trimester (0 to 14 Weeks)

Nausea and vomiting, fatigue, breast tenderness, urinary frequency, constipation, flatulence, nasal congestion, dizziness, mood swings, and skin changes are common. Most are related to hormonal changes.

Second Trimester (15 to 26 Weeks)

Unless there is a preexisting condition that can be aggravated by the enlarged uterus (for example, hemorrhoids or varicose veins), the second trimester is relatively comfortable for many women. However, the woman will experience skin changes (increased pigmentation and sometimes acne), striae gravidarium, leg cramps, heartburn, and groin pain from round ligament stretching.

Third Trimester (27 to 40 Weeks)

Changes such as backache, ankle swelling, varicose veins, hemorrhoids, leg cramps, heartburn, constipation, and faintness may begin late in the second trimes-

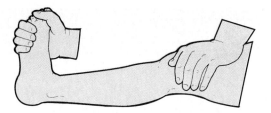

Figure 4-10 Relieving leg cramps.

ter or at this time. These changes are related to mechanical pressure from the enlarging uterus on major blood vessels and internal organs.

For most women and their families, a simple explanation of the cause of the discomfort and ways to possibly prevent or cope with it help tremendously in the acceptance and subsequent solution of the problem. Just knowing that the symptoms are not all psychological and that they will go away is very reassuring. The box on pp. 117 summarizes these common discomforts and suggests prevention and coping methods.

The pregnant woman can be counseled in proper body mechanics to increase her comfort and reduce strain on muscles and ligaments (Fig. 4-11).

BREAST-FEEDING

The World Health Organization (WHO), The American Academy of Pediatrics (AAP), and The American College of Obstetricians and Gynecologists (ACOG) have endorsed breast-feeding as the preferred method of infant feeding in the first year of life. In 1991 the Baby Friendly Hospital Initiative was developed as part of a worldwide program by the United Nations Children's Fund (UNICEF) and the World Health Organization (WHO). Its long-term aim is to contribute to the achievement of global breast-feeding for all. Transformation of maternity and pediatric hospitals into baby-friendly institutions is being encouraged thru implementation of the Initiative's 10 Steps to Successful Breast-Feeding. (See box on p. 120.)

Many women who enter the hospital to give birth are ambivalent about whether or not to breast-feed. Research has shown that nurses and physicians can greatly influence a woman's decision. Unfortunately, health care professionals have often inadvertently discouraged mothers from breast-feeding by supplementing breast-feeding with formula and separating mothers and babies during the first days of life.

The prenatal period is the time to discuss the pros and cons of breast-feeding and to assist the family in making a decision. Once again, early pregnancy classes (Chapter 5) are an excellent place to start encouraging the woman and her family to think about how they will feed the baby (Fig. 4-12). Women need to know that they can breast-feed and that breast size, possible nipple inversion and returning to work are not contraindications. Try to find out what breast-feeding means to the woman and her mate. Breasts are considered a sex symbol in our culture, and frequently modesty dictates, "Keep them covered." For women and men who have a high degree of sexual anxiety, it may be more socially acceptable to bottle-feed. In addition, personal beliefs, cultural attitudes, and the infant's behavior can have major impacts on breast-feeding success (Table 4-3). It may be possible to explore innovative combinations of breast-feeding and bottle-feeding for some families as a compromise to total breast-feeding (Table 4-4). Whatever the family's choice, efforts should be directed at helping them achieve a physically and psychologically healthy start with the method of infant feeding that works best for them. Although breast-feeding is recommended for mothers and infants, the mother should want to breast-feed and should have support from her mate and family, a support group such as the La Leche League, or lactation consultants. In helping the family, the information contained in the box on p. 122 may be useful. It is important to provide this information objectively so that the parents' decision can be made on an informed and factual basis.

Preparation for Breast-Feeding

In most cases the pregnant woman needs to do nothing to prepare her breasts. The average woman can simply open the flaps in the front of her brassiere, exposing the nipple and areola to the soft abrasion of the surface for days and weeks in preparation for breast-feeding. The woman should be counseled to avoid soap on her nipples or rubbing them with alcohol because these practices dry up the natural oils that keep the nipples soft.

If there are anatomic variations such as flat or inverted nipples, the problem can be identified, and recommendations can be made for correction before birth. Inverted nipples can be diagnosed by pressing the areola between the thumb and forefinger. A flat or normal nipple will protrude. An inverted nipple will retract.

Breast Shields

Inverted or flat nipples can be treated with a passive method using breast shields inside the brassiere (Figs. 4-13 and 4-14) over the nipple and areola for 6 to 8 weeks before delivery. These plastic shields put even, gentle pressure over the areola, causing the nipple to evert through the small hole in the center of the shield. *Text continued on p. 123.*

Discomfort	Prevention and Coping
Nausea and vomiting	1. Eat six small meals a day. Avoid any food that might normally make you ill. Stay away from greasy, spicy food or foods that are hard to digest.
	2. Drink a glass of milk before going to bed to have a source of some protein in the body before arising.
	3. Leave crackers or juice at bedside to consume before getting out of bed. Have someone fix tea with honey or prepare food to be brought to you in bed.
	4. Carry snacks in purse to anticipate times of nausea.
	5. Try substituting crushed ice or sherbert for liquids.
	6. Try separating intake of solids and liquids.
	7. Avoid strong odors, especially when cooking.
	Try these measures, and if you are still unable to cope with the situation, consult your physician. *Do not* take home remedies or drugs without your physician's advice.)
Heartburn	1. Eat small amounts of food frequently.
	2. Avoid fatty foods and foods that produce gas.
	3. Eat slowly.
	4. Avoid eating just before bedtime.
Constipation	1. Increase fluid intake
	2. Increase roughage intake (coarse cereal, whole wheat bread, leafy vegetables, salads, bran) to promote regular, unhurried bowel movements.
	3. Increase physical activity.
	4. Take a laxative or use a stool-softener (suppository), if prescribed.
Flatulence	1. Avoid gas-forming foods
	2. Increase roughage intake (coarse cereal, whole wheat bread, leafy vegetables, salads, bran) to promote regular, unhurried bowel movements.
	3. Increase physical activity
Fatigue	1. Treat the symptom, and rest when possible.
	2. Take an afternoon nap, if convenient.
	3. Lay your head down on your desk at work, or elevate your feet when possible.
	4. Go to bed early.
Backache	1. Maintain correct posture, and exercise.
	2. Use bedboards under mattress.
	3. Use massage and hot or cold packs.
	4. Avoid fatigue; get adequate rest.
Leg cramps	1. Increase consumption of foods high in calcium.
	2. Straighten leg and force toes upward; push knee down (Fig 4-10).
Varicose veins	1. Stay off feet as much as possible.
	2. Elevate legs higher than hips.
	3. Avoid tight garments such as girdles or supporters.
	4. Avoid crossing legs, knees, or ankles.
	5. Notify physician immediately if any redness, local soreness, or warmth develops in the veins.
	6. Wear elastic stockings, if indicated.
Vaginal discharge	1. Liberally cleanse external genitalia with mild soap and water.
	2. Seek medical help if irritation and itching are severe.
Itching and dry skin	1. Bathe with mild soap.
	2. Use lotions.
	3. Increase fluid intake.
Swelling of feet	1. Elevate legs and feet for short periods during day.
Excessive salivation	1. Suck hard candy.
	2. Chew gum.
	3. Avoid starches.
	(Treatment is limited.)
Dyspnea (shortness of breath)	1. Sleep with head of bed elevated.
	2. Stand and sit tall, head erect, shoulders slightly back.
Increased perspiration	1. Bathe frequently.
Hemorrhoids	1. Elevate hips on pillows.
	2. Take sitz baths.
	3. Apply cold witch hazel compresses.
	4. Gently push hemorrhoids back into rectum.
	5. Practice pelvic floor contraction and relaxation.

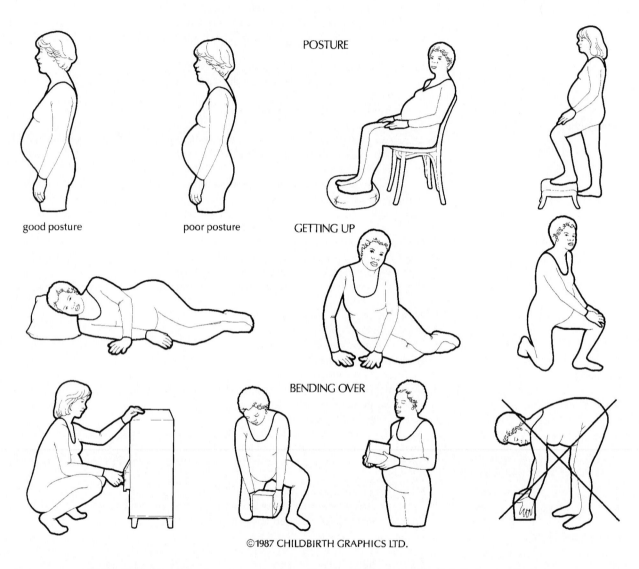

good posture   poor posture

POSTURE

GETTING UP

BENDING OVER

©1987 CHILDBIRTH GRAPHICS LTD.

Figure 4-11 Comforts for your pregnancy. *(Courtesy Childbirth Graphics, Ltd, Rochester, NY, 1987.)*

RELIEF OF BACK PAIN

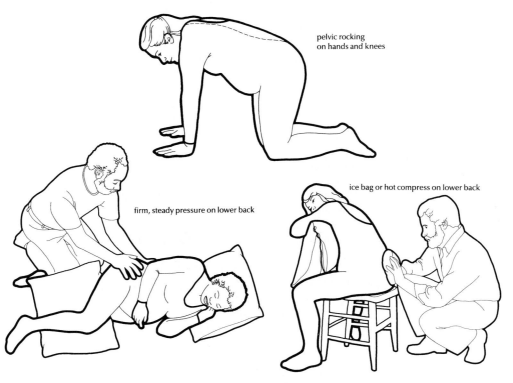

pelvic rocking
on hands and knees

firm, steady pressure on lower back

ice bag or hot compress on lower back

©1987 CHILDBIRTH GRAPHICS LTD.

MASSAGE TECHNIQUES

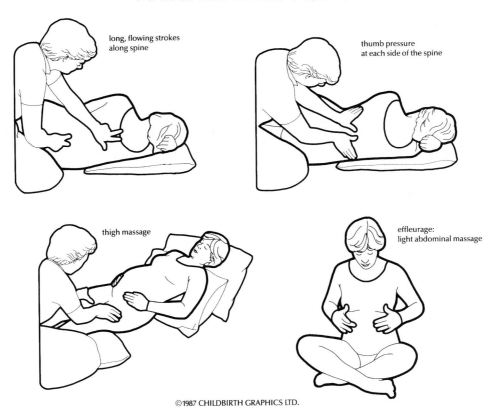

long, flowing strokes
along spine

thumb pressure
at each side of the spine

thigh massage

effleurage:
light abdominal massage

©1987 CHILDBIRTH GRAPHICS LTD.

Figure 4-11, cont'd Comforts for your pregnancy. *(Courtesy Childbirth Graphics, Ltd, Rochester, NY, 1987.)*

Ten Steps to Successful Breast-Feeding

A Joint WHO/UNICEF Statement (1989)

Every facility providing maternity services and care for newborn infants should:

1. Have a written breast-feeding policy that is routinely communicated to all health-care staff.
2. Train all health-care staff in the skills necessary to implement this policy.
3. Inform all pregnant women about the benefits and management of breast-feeding.
4. Help mothers initiate breast-feeding within a half hour of birth.
5. Show mothers how to breast-feed and how to maintain lactation even if they are separated from their infants.
6. Give newborn infants no food or drink other than breast milk unless medically indicated.
7. Practice rooming-in—allow mothers and infants to stay together 24 hours a day.
8. Encourage breast-feeding on demand.
9. Give no artificial teats or pacifiers (also called dummies and soothers) to breast-feeding infants.
10. Foster the establishment of breast-feeding support groups and refer mothers to them on discharge from hospital or clinic.

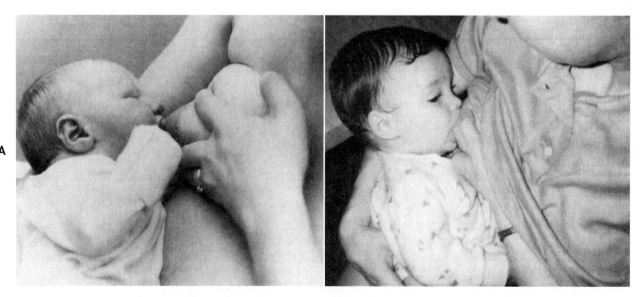

Figure 4-12 Breast-feeding. **A,** Scissor grasp. **B,** Palmar grasp. *(From Lawrence RA:* Breastfeeding: a guide for the medical profession, *ed 4, St. Louis, 1994, Mosby.)*

TABLE 4-3
Risk Factors for Psychosocial Difficulty with Total Breast-Feeding

Personality
Immaturity
Dependency
Displeasure at bodily functions
Rigidity; need for predictability
Insensitivity to infant's needs
Anxiety
Low self-esteem

Family setting
Lack of breast-feeding in family of origin
Partner's dislike or jealousy of breast-feeding
Marital instability
Lack of extended family support where valued

Personal attitudes
Beliefs that breast-feeding is inconvenient, embarrassing, unattractive, overly demanding, in conflict with other responsibilities, and physically or emotionally uncomfortable
Beliefs that bottle-feeding is convenient, more satisfying to infant, less restrictive to mother, and conducive to father-infant attachment

Social environment
Lack of friends who have breast-fed
Bottle-feeding as norm in community
Ambivalence of health professionals
Life-style requiring frequent separation from infant

Emotional state
Depression
Fatigue
Discomfort
Decreased self-esteem
Anxiety
Anger
Frustration with infant

Infant behavior
Excessive crying
Irritability
Early feeding difficulties
Passivity or lack of interest
Weak or ineffective sucking

From Kearney MH: Identifying psychosocial obstacles to breast-feeding success, *Obstet Gynecol Neonatal Nurs* 17:98-105, 1988.

TABLE 4-4
Infant-Feeding Methods

Method	Description	Advantages
Total breast-feeding	Infant nursed on demand; no bottles used	Frequent close physical interaction of mother and infant; immunologic and hypoallergenic benefits; no bottles needed
Breast-feeding/pumping	Breast milk fed by bottle when breast-feeding is inconvenient; breast milk collected by pumping	Infant receives only breast milk; mother can be away from infant at feeding times; feeding responsibility can be shared somewhat, although mother retains responsibility for pumping
Breast-feeding with limited formula	Breast-feeding during some periods of the day; formula-feeding by bottle at other times	Mother can be relieved of both feeding and pumping at selected times; milk supply will continue although quantity may decrease
Comfort nursing	Breast-feeding occurs once or twice daily; formula or other foods are primary sources of infant nutrition	Allows emotional satisfaction of breast-feeding interaction; feeding responsibilities can be shared; reduced milk production may reduce leaking and/or need to pump to relieve engorgement
Formula-feeding	Infant fed formula by bottle	No breast stimulation; feeding responsibility can be shared

From Kearney MH: Identifying psychosocial obstacles to breast-feeding success, *Obstet Gynecol Neonatal Nurs* 17:98-105, 1988.

Breast   **Formula**

Nutritional aspects

1. Easily and completely digested.   1. Formulas today simulate human milk.
2. Uniquely suited to baby.   2. Provides adequate nutrition.
3. Colostrum = laxative.
4. Lower solute load.
5. More unsaturated fatty acids.

Allergies

May reduce allergic responses in infants.

Immunological aspects

Immunoglobulins supply antiviral and antibacterial antibodies to protect baby from certain diseases.

Psychological aspects

1. Prolactin (nature's own tranquilizer) is active in breast-feeding.
2. Creates closeness (skin-to-skin) between mother and baby.

1. Will not have to expose breasts.
2. Can hold baby close.
3. May be a tendency to overfeed, thus causing obesity problems in later life.

Economy

1. Requires no buying of formula.   1. Will cost money.
2. Convenient and economic.   2. Need bottles and supplies as well as formulas.

Safety

1. Clean.   1. Can be contaminated.
2. Not easily contaminated

Convenience

1. No bottles to prepare.   1. Premixed formulas and disposable bottles are available.

Family

1. Instant and natural sex education for older children.
2. Woman should not take oral contraceptives while breast-feeding.

1. Other family members can feed baby.
2. Mother can take oral contraceptives.

Physiological aspects

1. Facilitates mother's physiological return to the prepregnant state (positive effect of oxytocin on uterine involution).
2. Suppresses ovulation and delays immediate return to fertility.

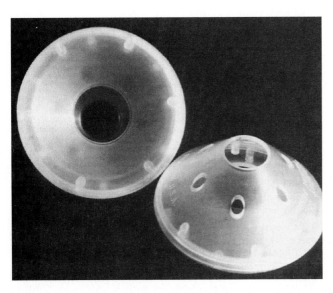

Figure 4-13 Breast shells: vented domes worn over ring that allow nipple to evert. Shell is slipped into cup of well-fitting brassiere. Available in several styles and designs. *(From Lawrence RA: Breastfeeding: a guide for the medical profession, ed 4, St. Louis, 1994, Mosby.)*

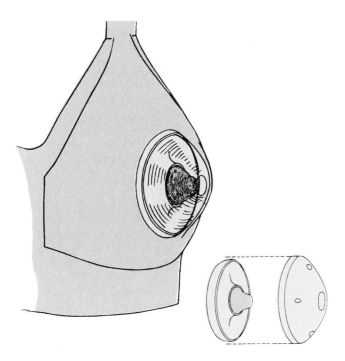

Figure 4-14 Breast shell in place inside brassiere to evert nipple. *(From Lawrence RA: Breastfeeding: a guide for the medical profession, ed 4, St. Louis, 1994, Mosby.)*

Nipple Stretching

Exercises to evert the nipples are rarely successful and may be dangerous. Nipple stimulation can cause uterine contractions and, in some women, labor.

DANGER SIGNS IN PREGNANCY

If a problem arises in pregnancy, it is important that it be taken care of immediately. Alert the mother to report immediately any of the following signs:

1. Signs of pregnancy-induced hypertension (PIH, preeclampsia)
   a. persistent severe headache
   b. blurred vision or visual disturbances
   c. sudden swelling of hands and face
   d. sudden weight gain
2. Signs of problems with the placenta
   a. bleeding from the vagina
   b. abdominal pain
3. Signs of premature labor (before 37 weeks of gestation)
   a. leaking or gushing of fluid from the vagina
   b. sudden increase in mucous discharge
   c. five or more contractions in 1 hour, which may be experienced as:
      • menstrual-like cramps in the lower abdomen, which may come and go or be constant
      • low, dull backache felt below the waistline, which may come and go or be constant
      • pressure in the pelvis, which feels as though the baby is pushing down; pressure comes and goes and may be felt in the abdomen, back, or thighs
      • abdominal cramps with or without diarrhea
   d. vaginal spotting or bleeding
4. Symptoms of urinary tract infection
   a. fever
   b. burning, change in frequency of urination
5. Symptoms of vaginal infection
   a. increased discharge of mucus that causes itching or irritation
   b. any discharge that has a foul odor
6. Any nausea or vomiting that persists
7. Any noticeable change in fetal activity (either much more active or no movement for 12 hours)
8. Any persistent pain anywhere in the body and any fever (temperature over 100° F)

SUMMARY

Chapter 4 has concentrated on providing safe care for the pregnant family. Such care identifies psychosocial and physiologic problems early so that they may be managed by the health care team and the family. An environment in which the family feels free to discuss any and all concerns is essential. To this point, only the low-risk antepartum family has been considered. The high-risk antepartum family is discussed in Chapter 5.

BIBLIOGRAPHY

Alexander LL, LaRosa JH: *New dimensions in women's health,* Boston, 1994, Jones and Bartlett.

American Academy of Pediatrics: The promotion of breast feeding, *Pediatr* 69(5):654-661, 1982.

Auvenshine MA, Enriquez MG: *Comprehensive maternity nursing, perinatal and women's health,* ed 2, Boston, 1990, Jones and Bartlett.

Barkauskas VH, Baumann LC, Stoltenberg-Allen K, Darling-Fisher C: *Health and physical assessment,* St. Louis, 1994, Mosby.

Bing E, Coleman L: *Making love during pregnancy,* New York, 1980, Bantam Books.

Cefalo RC, Moos MK: *Preconceptual health care,* ed 2, St. Louis, 1995, Mosby.

Dickason EJ, Silverman BL, Schult MO: *Maternal-infant nursing care,* ed 2, 1994, Mosby.

Dohrmann KR, Lederman SA: Weight gain in pregnancy, *J Obstet Gynecol Neonatal Nurs* 15:446-453, Nov/Dec 1986.

Howard FM, Howard CR, Weitzman M: The physician as advertiser: the unintentional discouragement of breast feeding, *Obstet Gynecol* 81(6):1048-1051, 1993.

Institute of Medicine: *Nutrition during pregnancy, summary,* Washington, DC, 1990, National Academy Press.

Jarnfelt-Samsioe A: Nausea and vomiting in pregnancy: a review, *Obstet Gynecol Surv* 41(7):422-427, 1987.

Kearney MH: Identifying psychosocial obstacles to breast feeding success, *Obstet Gynecol Neonatal Nurs* 17(2):98-105, 1988.

Lawrence RA: *Breastfeeding: a guide for the medical profession,* ed 4, St. Louis, 1994, Mosby.

Masters WH, Johnson VE: *Human sexual response,* Boston, 1966, Little, Brown & Co.

Mattson S, Smith JE, editors: *Core curriculum for maternal-newborn nursing,* Philadelphia, 1993, WB Saunders.

National Dairy Council: *Nutrition source book,* 1988, Rosemont, IL, The Council.

National Research Council: *Recommended dietary allowances,* ed 10, Washington, DC, 1989, National Academy Press.

Pritchard JA, MacDonald PD, Gant MF: *Williams obstetrics,* ed 17, New York, 1985, Appleton-Century-Crofts.

Public Health Service Department of Health and Human Services: *Caring for our future: the content of prenatal care, a report of the public health service expert panel on the content of prenatal care,* Washington, DC, 1989, U.S. Government Printing Office.

Sharts-Hopko NC: Folic acid in the prevention of neural tube defects, *MCN* 18:232, 1993.

Sloane E: *Biology of women,* ed 3, Albany, NY, 1993, Delmar.

Thibodeau GA, Patton KT: *Structure and function of the body,* ed 9, St. Louis, 1992, Mosby.

U.S. Department of Health and Human Services: *The Surgeon General's report on nutrition and health,* Washington, DC, 1988, U.S. Government Printing Office.

Worthington BS, Williams SR: *Nutrition in pregnancy and lactation,* ed 5, St. Louis, 1993, Mosby.

DEFINITIONS

Define the following terms:

antepartum	micturition
ballottement	Monilia
Braxton Hicks contractions	Nägele's rule
candidiasis	Papanicolaou test
Chadwick's sign	para
chloasma	plasma
colostrum	prolactin
diagonal conjugate	proteinuria
dyspnea	psychosocial
Goodell's sign	reflux
gravida	striae gravidarium
Hegar's sign	*Trichomonas vaginalis*
intertuberous diameter	trimester
lactose	true conjugate
linea nigra	uterine souffle

LEARNING ACTIVITIES

1. Plan a diet for a normal pregnant woman. Use a food value chart to analyze the diet for nutritive value. Such a chart is available from the Superintendent of Documents, U.S. Government Printing Office, Washington, DC 20402.
2. View audiovisual aids and discuss.
3. Design a visual aid to explain to a pregnant woman why the recommended weight gain in pregnancy is 25 to 35 pounds.
4. Compare diagrams of the four phases of the human sexual response cycle for men and women.

ENRICHMENT IN-DEPTH STUDY

1. Work in a pair with another student and practice taking a history with your fellow student playing the role of a pregnant woman. How does your classmate feel about being pregnant; i.e., happy, sad, frightened, etc. Are there preferences for a boy or a girl? What is the gravida and para? EDD?
2. Determine what agencies or persons are available for pregnancy testing in your community. What are the costs? At what time in gestation can the tests be done? Are they accurate?
3. Make a written 1-day food intake record on yourself, then calculate what changes would be needed if you were pregnant. Complete the 1-day food intake record with the necessary nutrient and calorie changes identified.
4. Interview an expectant father in a prenatal clinic. What are his plans for his new role? Do you believe that he is being realistic? How could you help him prepare for the transition to parenthood?

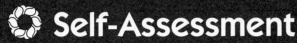
For questions 1 through 4, determine if the statements are true or false. Fill in the space to the left of the statement with T for true and F for false.

_____ 1. During the first trimester there is frequently an increase in sexual desire and frequency of sexual intercourse.

_____ 2. Sexual relations (intercourse) during pregnancy are alright unless the woman is uncomfortable.

_____ 3. It is easy for couples to forego sexual activity for 6 weeks before birth and 6 weeks after birth.

_____ 4. During the second trimester there is frequently an increase in sexual desire.

For questions 5 through 20, circle the best answer.

5. Constipation is best relieved by:
   a. regular use of laxatives
   b. maintenance of good posture
   c. increased roughage and fluid in the diet

6. Frequency of urination during early and late pregnancy is often caused by:
   a. decreased activity
   b. increased weight gain
   c. pressure exerted on bladder by uterus

7. Varicosities on the lower extremities in pregnancy are the result of:
   a. increased cardiac load
   b. pressure of the uterus impeding venous return
   c. increased blood volume

8. The recommended weight gain during pregnancy is:
   a. 25-35 pounds
   b. 10-20 pounds
   c. 20-25 pounds
   d. 15-20 pounds

9. A positive sign of pregnancy is:
   a. Chadwick's sign
   b. nausea and vomiting
   c. fetal heart sounds
   d. linea nigra

10. Which one of these common signs and symptoms associated with pregnancy is a probable sign of pregnancy?
   a. cessation of menses (amenorrhea)
   b. frequent urination
   c. enlarged and tender breasts
   d. Hegar's sign

11. A positive sign of pregnancy is:

    a. a positive pregnancy test

    b. increase in abdominal size

    c. ballottement

    d. hearing fetal heartbeat

12. A presumptive sign of pregnancy is:

    a. enlargement of the uterus

    b. Braxton Hicks contractions

    c. fetal heartbeat

    d. cessation of menses

13. Positive motivations for pregnancy include to:

    a. save a relationship

    b. share lives together

    c. please others

14. The RIA tests (radioimmunoassay) of pregnancy are the most sensitive of the currently available tests and can detect pregnancy as early as how many days after ovulation?

    a. 8 days

    b. 14 days

    c. 21 to 24 days

15. Which of the following lunches would be the best for a pregnant woman?

    a. bologna sandwich, potato chips, cola

    b. cottage cheese, tossed salad and cracker, orange, glass of milk

    c. cold chicken, french fries, French roll, milk

    d. bowl of bean soup, crackers, glass of ice tea

16. Using Nägele's rule, if a pregnant woman's last menstrual period began on August 4, 1995, her estimated due date would be nearest:

    a. May 6, 1996

    b. May 11, 1996

    c. June 11, 1996

    d. May 17, 1996

17. A pregnant woman may develop constipation because of:

    a. diminished motility of the gastrointestinal tract

    b. pressure on the intestines from the enlarging uterus

    c. lack of adequate exercise

    d. lack of adequate fluid intake

    Answer (circle one):

    1. a, b, and d

    2. c, b, and d

    3. a, b, and c

    4. all of these

18. Improved prenatal care in the United States is responsible for:

    a. the population explosion

    b. the increase in pregnancies

    c. reduced maternal mortality

19. A typical pregnancy lasts:

    a. 200 days

    b. 240 days

    c. 280 days

20. A pregnant woman must increase her daily calories by:

    a. 150 Kcal

    b. 300 Kcal

    c. 0 Kcal

Supply the correct answer(s) for items 21 through 33.

21. Prenatal care should include:

    a. _____

    b. _____

    c. _____

22. Advantages of breast-feeding include:

    a. _____

    b. _____

    c. _____

23. Define gravida._____

24. Define para._____

25. Identify the normal findings for the following three laboratory tests in pregnancy:

    a. Hct (hematocrit) and Hgb (hemoglobin)_____

    b. urinalysis

       (1) sugar_____

       (2) protein_____

26. What are four myths you have heard associated with childbearing and birth?

    a. _____

    b. _____

    c. _____

    d. _____

27. Explain how a nurse can help to reduce a woman's anxiety on her first visit to the physician to confirm pregnancy.

    _____

    _____

    _____

28. What would you suggest for relief of varicose veins?

    _____

    _____

29. How many servings of each group of food listed below should be included in the pregnant woman's diet daily?

a. milk group_____

b. grain group_____

c. fruit and vegetable group_____

d. others_____

e. meat group_____

30. What can be done to cope with leg cramps in pregnancy?

_____

_____

_____

31. Preparation of the nipples for breast-feeding includes:

a. _____

b. _____

32. Advantages of formula-feeding include:

a. _____

b. _____

c. _____

33. List eight danger signs during pregnancy:

a. _____

b. _____

c. _____

d. _____

e. _____

f. _____

g. _____

h. _____

34. On the line to the left of each item in Column A, match the physiological change occurring in pregnancy with the body system in which that change occurs.

Column A

_____ 1. respiratory system

_____ 2. integumentary system

_____ 3. circulatory system

_____ 4. GI system

_____ 5. skeletal system

_____ 6. urinary system

_____ 7. endocrine system

_____ 8. reproductive system

Column B

a. linea nigra

b. relaxation of pelvic joints

c. depends on prepregnant state

d. blood volume increase

e. constipation

f. enlarging uterus

g. urinary frequency

h. difficulty breathing

i. increase in basal metabolic rate

35. On the line to the left of each item in Column A, match the correct definition from Column B.

Column A

_____ 1. uterine souffle

_____ 2. colostrum

_____ 3. chloasma

_____ 4. striae gravidarium

Column B

a. mask of pregnancy

b. the substance that precedes the milk from the breasts

c. silvery-blue stretch marks

d. the sound of blood in the uterine arteries

For questions 36 through 38, fill in the blanks.

36. Wearing high-heeled shoes in pregnancy may cause _____.

37. When a pregnant woman's feet swell at the end of the day, the edema is probably the result of _____.

38. If a pregnant woman's hands and face are swollen in addition to her feet, you would _____.

39. When washing her breasts, a pregnant woman should not use _____ on her nipples, since it has a tendency to dry them.

40. The blood volume _____, but the hemoglobin _____ during pregnancy.

41. A woman is $G_5P_4Ab_1$; this means she has been pregnant _____ times, has delivered _____ children, and has had _____ abortions.

42. Late in pregnancy, a hemoglobin concentration below _____ is indicative of true anemia.

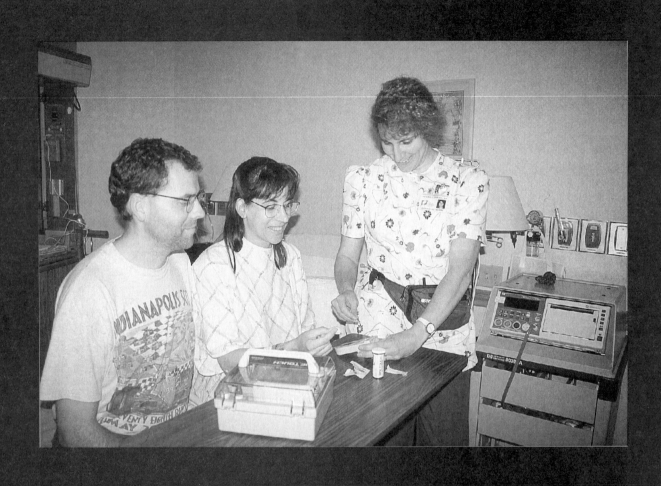

5

THE ANTEPARTUM FAMILY WITH COMPLICATIONS

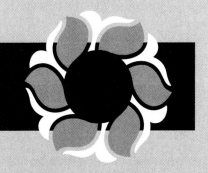

GOALS

This chapter is designed to provide the reader with information that will:
- promote awareness of deviations from normal in the antepartum period.
- explore the nursing role in common complications in the antepartum period.
- promote an understanding of the importance of family-centered care to families with complications in the antepartum period.

STUDENT OBJECTIVES

After studying this chapter, you should be able to:

1. Indicate at least two factors in each of the following categories that classify a woman as high risk in pregnancy: (1) general physical, social, and demographic factors, (2) past complications associated with pregnancy, (3) complications of current pregnancy, and (4) coexistent medical-surgical-psychiatric disorders.
2. Design a plan to illustrate how the nurse can help the high-risk family adapt to the tasks necessary during illness in pregnancy.
3. Briefly describe signs and symptoms of hypertensive states in pregnancy and describe nursing responsibilities.
4. Explain the causes of Rh incompatibility, types of treatment available (before and after birth), and nursing responsibilities with families who have Rh incompatibilities.
5. Distinguish between the meaning of the term *abortion* to the layperson and to professional health personnel.
6. Plan supportive nursing care for women experiencing the three common causes of bleeding problems in early pregnancy.
7. Discuss the significance of diabetes to pregnancy.
8. Describe five common tests of fetal well-being used in high-risk maternity care and the nursing responsibilities in preparing the family for these tests:
   a. ultrasonography
   b. amniocentesis
   c. breast stimulation test
   d. contraction stress test (CST)
   e. nonstress test (NST)

Chapter 1 discussed a two-tiered maternity model, designating two levels of care: (1) normal (a simple, humanistic model for healthy women and their families) and (2) high risk (a more complex but still humanistic model for women with medical complications and/or complications of pregnancy and their families). Also mentioned was the concept of regionalization of nursing care, which provides levels of care appropriate for each level of the childbearing population.

This chapter will introduce you to the high-risk population for whom, ideally, the regional center would provide care.

IDENTIFICATION OF THE HIGH-RISK MOTHER

A high-risk or at-risk pregnancy is one in which the prospects for optimal outcome for either the mother or the fetus are reduced. High-risk mothers and infants have a greater incidence of morbidity and mortality than the general population of mothers and infants. A pregnancy is classified as high risk if certain conditions are present that have been identified as dangerous to the health and life of the mother and infant. These conditions include the following:

1. General physical, social, and demographic factors
2. Coexistent medical-surgical-psychiatric disorders
3. Past complications associated with pregnancy
4. Complications of current pregnancy

The following factors contribute to reproductive risk. The presence of any one or more of these factors merits further assessment and evaluation.

1. *General physical, social, and demographic factors:*
   a. Maternal age of 15 years or younger
   b. Maternal age of 35 years or older
   c. Markedly underweight or overweight
   d. High parity
   e. Small maternal size (under 5 feet)
   f. Poor socioeconomic status
   g. Lack of prenatal care
   h. Inadequate human support resources
   i. Continual presence of stressful situations
   j. Teratogen exposure (radiation, drugs, chemicals, viral infections, and bacterial infections)
   k. Emotional and/or psychological disorders
   l. Maternal social habits (drug ingestion, alcohol consumption, cigarette smoking)
   m. Family history of hereditary disease or congenital anomaly
   n. Some cultural and ethnic practices
2. *Coexistent medical-surgical-psychiatric disorders:*
   a. Infertility of more than 2 years' duration
   b. Genital tract abnormalities

c. Chronic medical disease that adversely affects general health of mother:
   i. cardiac
   ii. vascular
   iii. respiratory
   iv. neurologic
   v. chronic hypertension
   vi. chronic renal problems
   vii. diabetes
   viii. thyroid disease
   ix. hematologic disorders
   x. malignancy
d. Psychiatric disturbances
e. Drug addiction or alcoholism
f. Infection (maternal and neonatal)
g. Parental rejection of pregnancy, particularly maternal
h. Major family upheaval or stress

3. *Past complications associated with pregnancy*
   MATERNAL
   a. Previous premature labor
   b. Previous cesarean or midforceps delivery
   c. Borderline or contracted pelvis
   d. Premature delivery with incompetent cervix
   e. Previous preeclampsia or eclampsia
   f. Prior fetal malpresentation
   g. Medical indication for termination of prior pregnancy
   INFANT
   h. Previous stillbirth or neonatal loss
   i. Two or more spontaneous abortions
   j. Previous infants who were excessively large (over 4000 grams) or excessively small (under 2500 grams)
   k. Known congenital or familial problems
   l. Previous infant requiring special neonatal intensive care

4. *Complications of current pregnancy:*
   a. Suspected ectopic pregnancy
   b. Suspected abortion
   c. Suspected trophoblastic disease
   d. Anemia
   e. Hyperemesis gravidarum
   f. Infections (maternal or fetal)
   g. Gestational diabetes
   h. Pregnancy-induced hypertension (PIH)
   i. Inappropriate fetal growth
   j. Hemorrhage (maternal or fetal)
   k. Hydramnios
   l. Abruptio placentae
   m. Placenta previa
   n. Rh isoimmunization
   o. Multiple pregnancy
   p. Malpresentation of fetus
   q. Premature rupture of membranes

r. Premature labor
s. Postdate pregnancy (gestation of longer than 42 weeks)
t. Dysfunctional labor
u. Intrauterine fetal demise

Risk Scoring

Risk scoring in pregnancy helps to identify those pregnancies that have a significantly greater statistical risk of perinatal morbidity and mortality. As a result those women identified may receive appropriate management. Numerous attempts have been made to quantify obstetrical risk. The usual approach uses scoring systems that range from 100 factors to 5 or 10 factors that identify pregnancies of low, high, or extreme risk. An example of a risk scoring system is integrated into Hollister's maternal and newborn Record System.

Reasons for Avoiding Prenatal Care

Adequate prenatal care effectively prevents numerous maternal and infant health problems, yet many women fail to receive that care. Why? Many simply cannot afford it. Some do not feel that prenatal care is important. There are definite barriers to prenatal care in this country, such as lack of transportation, inconvenient clinic hours, waiting time to obtain an appointment and waiting time at the clinic, child care needs during physician or clinic visits, and language barriers. In addition, a lack of understanding of the value of prenatal care and negative attitudes toward health care providers are other reasons that many women do not seek prenatal care.

Frequently clinics serving the poor offer fragmented, depersonalized care with long waiting periods (often all day) in crowded, unattractive, depressing surroundings. Prenatal clinics are usually open during the same hours that women and their families must work; to complicate the issue even further, these clinics are often geographically distant from the women's homes. It is also important to remember that acceptance of preventive prenatal health care may be incompatible with some people's cultural beliefs and practices.

According to recent studies, preventive health programs that provide prenatal care have been found to be cost-effective. Because these programs reduce the incidence of infant mortality and low birth weight babies, the additional costs of providing comprehensive care are more than recovered. It is possible to change the grim statistics. Comprehensive prenatal care that includes preconceptual health assessment, on-going risk assessment throughout pregnancy, prenatal education, increased evaluation and assistance to meet the psychosocial needs of the pregnant woman, and supplemental nutrition programs for low-income pregnant women can significantly improve pregnancy outcome.

Preparatory Tasks

As stated in Chapter 1, the following preparatory tasks should be completed by the parents-to-be in preparing for the birth: (1) acceptance of the pregnancy; (2) establishment of a bond with the fetus; and (3) adjustment to the change in role from woman (daughter) and man (son) to mother and father.

The high-risk mother and family must work through all these normal preparatory tasks of pregnancy and also those tasks necessary during conditions deviating from normal. Because pregnancy represents a major life change, it is a period of crisis even for the normal family. When the high-risk condition is added, there is a serious crisis for this family because they must also cope with an uncertain outcome.

Nursing Care

The nurse can be extremely helpful to the high-risk family by actively listening to their concerns, by being sure they understand the reasons for all the tests, treatments, and medicines used, and by being open and honest, giving no false assurances or promises. During hospitalization, the nurse can help by giving the woman and her family a chance to control their environment and by helping them prepare for the baby with feeding plans and care instructions for the high-risk infant. It is often difficult for high-risk families to establish a bond with the fetus because the outcome of the pregnancy is so uncertain. It is not unusual for such families to come to the hospital without any baby clothes or articles to care for the baby. They may not even choose a name for the baby until they are certain the baby will live.

Although the family is at risk, it is important to keep in mind all the ordinary concerns of the family, such as breast-feeding, sibling and grandparent adjustment, returning to work, and so on. This family needs plenty of "high-touch" to balance the "high-tech" of high-risk care. Family-centered care has never been more important than in the case of at-risk families.

MAJOR COMPLICATIONS OF PREGNANCY

The danger signals during pregnancy are listed in Chapter 4. Take a few minutes to review the list.

Hypertensive states of pregnancy can be classified as follows:

1. Preeclampsia/eclampsia (pregnancy-induced hypertension—PIH)

2. Chronic hypertension
3. Chronic hypertension with superimposed pre-eclampsia/eclampsia—(PIH)

PIH occurs in approximately 7% of pregnancies. It is one of the three leading causes of maternal death in the United States and is a major cause of intrauterine death and intrauterine growth retardation. Maternal complications of PIH include cerebral vascular accident, pulmonary edema, renal failure, grand mal seizures, disseminating intravascular coagulation (DIC), placental abruption, HELLP syndrome, and death.

Preeclampsia

Preeclampsia is a condition occurring after the twentieth week of pregnancy in 5% to 7% of all pregnancies. Preeclampsia is characterized by a triad of signs: edema, hypertension, and proteinuria. The term *toxemia* has been used to describe preeclampsia and eclampsia but is now considered obsolete because no toxin has yet been found to cause this syndrome.

Pathophysiology

Although the most current theory suggests a disorder of prostaglandin synthesis, the etiology of preeclampsia remains obscure. Preeclampsia occurs primarily during first pregnancies in women under 20 or over 35 years of age. Factors associated with risk include multiple fetuses; vascular disease; diabetes; gestational trophoblastic disease (GTO); severe malnutrition; inadequate prenatal care; poor health care; and family history of preeclampsia, eclampsia, or chronic hypertension.

In PIH, a generalized spasm of the arteries causes a gradual rise in blood pressure and results in decreased blood flow to the kidneys, uterus, liver, and eventually the brain. There is also decreased plasma volume with most of the fluid in the extracellular spaces, resulting in an increased hematocrit. As a result the preeclamptic woman is sensitive to blood loss and to vigorous fluid therapy (overload). A further complicating factor is central nervous system (CNS) irritability evident as jitteriness, hyperactive reflexes, and visual disturbances. CNS irritability can eventually lead to seizures.

Prenatal detection and management

Prevention of maternal and fetal consequences of hypertension is a goal of prenatal care. Visits are scheduled to enhance the probability of detecting PIH early. However, the disease process occurs before signs and symptoms appear, and symptoms may not coincide with prenatal visits. The woman's ability to detect symptoms will facilitate identification and monitoring of PIH. Appropriate education includes advising women verbally or in writing about signs of preeclampsia (headache, visual disturbances, puffiness of hands, face).

Identifying risk factors, determining a reliable estimated date of delivery (EDD), and assessment of baseline blood pressure values are essential in the detection, diagnosis, and management of PIH.

Mild preeclampsia

In mild preeclampsia there is an elevation in blood pressure of 30 mm Hg systolic and/or 15 mm Hg diastolic over the woman's usual blood pressure observed on two or more occasions 6 hours apart with the woman at rest. (A blood pressure of 140/90 usually arouses concern and indicates the need for further evaluation.) In addition, there is abnormal fluid retention, generalized edema, and weight gain of more than 2 pounds per week. Proteinuria of 1+ or greater may be found on a clean-catch urine specimen. The woman may also experience headache and blurred vision.

The primary objectives of treatment are (1) prevention of convulsions, (2) control of blood pressure, and (3) safe delivery of a viable infant.

Nursing care. Care is planned to maximize tissue perfusion, prevent complications, and optimize fetal growth and outcome. Treatment usually includes bed rest in the left lateral recumbent position; close observation and recording of baseline reflexes; urine protein; fluid intake and output; and monitoring of blood pressure, daily weight, and fetal status. Close medical supervision and perhaps sedation, along with education of the woman and her family about a high-protein, high-vitamin diet and treatment regimens are essential. The nurse can be of great help in counseling the woman on the importance of strict adherence to the prescribed treatment by making sure she understands the treatment.

A weight gain of over 2 pounds per week when the woman is on bed rest is significant. Salt restriction, diuretics, or antihypertensives are *not* part of the management of mild preeclampsia.

Intravenous fluid administration may require central monitoring of the intravascular volume and adjustment of rate of main line accordingly.

Severe preeclampsia

If mild preeclampsia is not checked, the woman's blood pressure may be recorded at 160/110 or above on two or more observations taken 6 hours apart. Proteinuria will equal or exceed 3+ or 4+ on routine urinalysis (dipstick), and the edema will worsen. At this point there may be cerebral or visual disturbances, possible epigastric pain, and oliguria of 400 milliliters or less every 24 hours. Treatment for severe preeclampsia includes hospitalization with strict bed rest, sedation, a high-protein diet without added salt, and close monitoring of fetal well-being.

Nursing care. Nursing care becomes extremely important for cases of severe preeclampsia and includes the following: (1) placing the woman in a quiet room, padding the bedrails, and keeping the environment quiet to reduce CNS stimulation; (2) weighing the woman daily; (3) monitoring fluid intake and output hourly (Foley catheter to urimeter); (4) administering medications according to the physician's orders; (5) having eclamptic seizure precautions ready (for example, padded tongue blade, seizure medicines, O_2); (6) frequently checking urine for protein and urine specific gravity; (7) collecting any other necessary laboratory specimens; (8) checking patellar reflexes and clonus at least four times per day and inquiring about other symptoms such as epigastric pain, headache, and visual disturbance; (9) frequently checking blood pressure; (10) monitoring fetal well-being; (11) assessing for pulmonary edema; and (12) accurately recording and immediately reporting any sudden deviations from the baseline in any of these areas. Because fluid overload would worsen hypertension, all intravenous fluids should be regulated with electronic infusers.

This family will be anxious and probably very worried about the pregnancy outcome. There may be problems such as financial and child care needs that must be addressed as the nurse helps to alleviate the woman's anxiety. The fantasy of an uncomplicated, beautiful birth has been replaced by a high-tech atmosphere and possible surgery and preterm delivery. The woman and her family may be angry as well as afraid. The contributions of the social service member of the health care team may be vital in helping this woman and her family to cope with the crisis of hospitalization, which may last for days or even weeks.

Eclampsia

If the symptoms of preeclampsia continue until the woman experiences convulsions, coma, or both, the woman is said to be *eclamptic*. Eclampsia will develop in 5% of treated preeclamptic women. Symptoms and signs that suggest impending eclampsia include intense epigastric pain; severe headache; confusion and disorientation; visual symptoms such as bright spots, flashes, or blurring; increasing activity of reflexes; accelerating hypertension and tremulousness; and urinary output under 30 ml per hour.

Nursing care

The care of an eclamptic woman requires (1) intensive nursing care in a quiet room; (2) hourly recording of vital signs; (3) hourly notation of urine volume (an indwelling catheter) and specific gravity; (4) protective care during convulsions; (5) constant fetal monitoring; (6) frequent checking of reflexes; (7) administration of medications as ordered; (8) lung assessment every 6 to 12 hours; (9) supportive care of the family; (10) explanations of treatment and management to the family and to the woman if she is responsive; and (11) accurate recording and reporting of any sudden deviations from the baseline in any of the areas observed.

Medical treatment

Medications prescribed to treat preeclampsia or eclampsia include the following:
1. Magnesium sulfate ($MgSO_4$), intravenously or intramuscularly, to prevent or control seizures by decreasing central nervous system irritability.
2. Calcium gluconate to reverse magnesium toxicity should it occur.
3. Hydralazine (Apresoline) to lower diastolic pressures greater than 110 mm Hg.

Because $MgSO_4$ is excreted exclusively in the urine, an output of less than 30 ml per hour may lead to magnesium toxicity. Serum magnesium levels are assessed to be sure $MgSO_4$ is in the therapeutic range. Blood levels of $MgSO_4$ should be maintained between 4.6-8.0 mg/dL. Excessive blood levels should be avoided because at 10 mg/dL deep tendon reflexes fade and at 15 mg/dL respiratory paralysis and/or cardiac arrest occurs. Respiratory rates are closely observed while the woman's level of consciousness and orientation to person, place, and time are checked. Calcium gluconate is given if magnesium toxicity occurs.

When $MgSO_4$ is given during labor, the frequency of uterine contractions and progress of labor must be carefully monitored. Slowing of uterine activity can occur with use of $MgSO_4$ because of its smooth muscle relaxation effect. Oxytocin augmentation may be necessary if this happens.

The specific therapy for eclampsia is delivery, which is often accomplished by induction or cesarean birth when the physicians have determined that the infant is better off out of the uterus than in. In eclampsia the rate of maternal mortality may be 5% to 10%.

An acute psychosis may develop in the eclamptic woman 2 to 3 days following delivery. Eclamptic precautions and treatment should be continued after delivery for 24 to 48 hours because there is still a danger of convulsions as long as CNS irritability exists.

In most women, signs and symptoms of pregnancy-induced hypertension disappear within the first week following delivery. In counseling on future pregnancies the family should be informed that if a woman has been eclamptic, she may develop eclampsia in subsequent pregnancies. Of course, the real solution to the problem of eclampsia is prevention. The nurse can be very helpful in counseling on the importance of prenatal care and a high-protein (>80 grams per day) diet during pregnancy to help prevent preeclampsia.

HELLP Syndrome

HELLP syndrome is an extension of severe preeclampsia. It describes, through laboratory values, the organ damage from the vasospasm of severe preeclampsia:

> H = Hemolysis
>
> EL = Elevated liver enzymes
>
> LP = Low platelet count

The HELLP syndrome usually presents during the early third trimester, and its hematologic and hepatic findings are often mistaken for symptoms of other conditions. Women with HELLP syndrome may not meet the standard blood pressure levels for severe preeclampsia. Their symptoms may be related to the impact of the vasospasm on the maternal liver. The woman with HELLP syndrome may complain of malaise, epigastric pain, right upper quadrant tenderness, nausea (with or without vomiting), headache, and edema.

Maternal prognosis is dependent on timely, aggressive intervention. The only definitive treatment for women with HELLP syndrome is delivery, regardless of gestational age. Future pregnancies are dependent on whether permanent organ damage has occurred. Fetal and neonatal outcomes include intrauterine hypoxia leading to fetal distress or fetal demise and intrauterine growth retardation (IUGR) and accompanying complications.

Chronic Hypertensive Vascular Disease

Chronic hypertensive vascular disease includes (1) hypertension known to exist before pregnancy, (2) hypertension discovered before the twentieth week of pregnancy, and (3) hypertension secondary to maternal medical disease (hypertension discovered after the twentieth week of pregnancy). This form of hypertension will also persist for more than 6 weeks postpartum.

Nursing care

The woman with chronic hypertension may have been advised against pregnancy and may have many guilt feelings to work through in addition to carefully

following a treatment regimen. In fact how well the woman and her family accept the antihypertensive treatment regimen may be directly connected to their feelings about the pregnancy. The nurse's support, attentive listening, and teaching can be very helpful in this situation. In hypertensive pregnancies, management of the fetus is of prime importance because it frequently suffers from distress in utero and/or intrauterine growth retardation.

Hypertension with superimposed preeclampsia or eclampsia is development of symptoms and findings of preeclampsia or eclampsia in a woman with chronic hypertension.

Rh Factor

An Rh-negative woman lacks the D antigen on her red blood cells. When an Rh-negative woman is carrying an Rh-positive baby (the baby's father is Rh positive), a few fetal red blood cells may enter the mother's circulation during labor or delivery, causing the mother's immune system to produce antibodies against the fetal D antigens. If a few fetal cells of an Rh-positive baby enter the bloodstream of an Rh-negative mother during the birth of the first baby, the mother will be sensitized (formation of serum antibodies). If this sensitized Rh-negative mother subsequently becomes pregnant with an Rh-positive fetus, the antibodies she has formed cross the placenta, coat the red blood cells of the fetus, and cause their destruction *(erythroblastosis fetalis)*. As the red blood cells are destroyed, the fetus becomes anemic and may go into heart failure. In the most severe form of Rh sensitization, the fetus becomes severely edematous, develops pleural effusion and ascites *(hydrops fetalis)*, and may die in utero or, if born alive, may die in a few days.

Treatment

If the fetus is too immature to survive outside the uterus, it may be given intrauterine transfusions of group O, Rh-negative erythrocytes. The blood type is compatible with that of the mother. The transfusion, which can be repeated often, is given into the peritoneal cavity of the fetus or by percutaneous umbilical blood sampling (PUBS), a new technique that allows direct access to the fetal circulation.

Sometimes transfusions are not necessary in erythroblastic infants until 24 hours after birth. When this happens, exchange transfusion of the infant may be done using Rh-negative blood. If Rh-positive blood were used, the anti-Rh-positive antibodies already circulating in the infant's blood would destroy the new red cells. Exchanging one set of positive cells for another set of positive cells is not the answer.

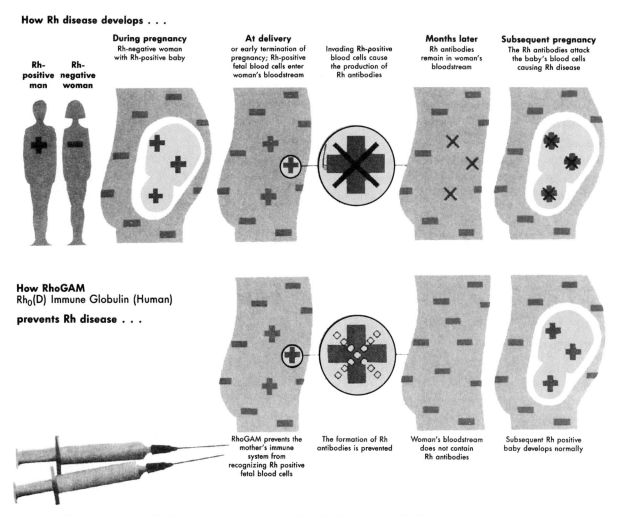

Figure 5-1 How Rh disease develops and how RhoGAM prevents Rh disease. *(Courtesy Ortho Diagnostics, Inc, Raritan, NJ)*

Tests

It is possible to determine whether a pregnant woman has anti-Rh-positive antibodies (anti-D antibodies) in her blood by tests on her serum during pregnancy. Antibody-titer or anti-Rh titers can be used, as well as the enzyme-linked antiglobulin assay and the acid elution test.

Antenatal prophylaxis

Researchers have shown that prenatal administration of anti-Rh-positive globulin (RhoGAM) to Rh-negative pregnant women can reduce the incidence of women sensitized during pregnancy from between 1% and 2% to 0.1%. Established protocols for prenatal prophylaxis recommend administering Rho (D) immune globulin at 28 to 32 weeks of gestation and again within 72 hours after delivery to an Rh-negative mother with no evidence of anti-D antibodies in her bloodstream.

Postpartum treatment

An injection of RhoGAM into Rh-negative mothers within 72 hours after delivery of an Rh-positive infant suppresses the formation of Rh antibodies. To receive RhoGAM, the mother must be Rh negative and have no Rh antibodies in her serum, and the baby must be Rh positive and have a negative direct Coombs' test. The Coombs' test is a technical procedure used to determine the presence of hemolytic disease and/or Rh immunization. Once the mother has been sensitized to factor D, RhoGAM is of no value (Fig. 5-1).

Nursing care

The nurse has a very important role in making sure that each woman who should get RhoGAM is treated. Nursing care for the Rh-negative woman and her family also includes recognition of their concerns, realistic support, and teaching. The woman or man may suffer guilt feelings for having the "wrong" blood type. The couple needs a chance to work through these feelings if they exist, and the nurse is in an excellent position to afford the childbearing couple the help they need.

ABO Incompatibility

A much more common type of blood incompatibility is *ABO incompatibility*, in which the father is blood type A, B, or AB and the mother is type O. If the fetus inherits the blood type from the father and fetal blood crosses the placenta, it can cause the mother to be sensitized to antigens of the foreign blood type. The complications of this type of incompatibility are usually not severe because the anti-A and anti-B immune bodies are not passed easily from mother to fetus. Only 10% of pregnancies identified as ABO incompatible actually develop hemolytic disease of the newborn.

Bleeding in Early Pregnancy

Any bleeding during pregnancy is abnormal. When bleeding occurs early in pregnancy, the most common causes are abortion, ectopic pregnancy, and hydatidiform mole.

Abortion

To the layperson the term *abortion* frequently means inducing the end of pregnancy, and the term *miscarriage* means spontaneous termination of pregnancy. The obstetric definition of abortion is the termination of pregnancy before the fetus has become viable, which generally occurs at 20 weeks of gestation and 500 grams of weight. The great majority of these abortions occur in the first trimester. Abortion may be *spontaneous* (through natural causes) or *induced* (by mechanical or medical agents).

The types of spontaneous abortion follow:

1. *Complete*—spontaneous expulsion of all products of conception.
2. *Incomplete*—partial expulsion of products of conception.
3. *Threatened*—signs and symptoms of abortion present but no passage of tissue from the vagina; this abortion could be reversed.
4. *Inevitable*—vaginal bleeding, usually with cramps and dilation of the internal os; cannot be reversed.
5. *Habitual*—abortion of three successive pregnancies.
6. *Missed*—fetal death occurred, but products of conception still in uterus for over 8 weeks.

An induced abortion is the voluntary ending of a pregnancy. An induced abortion may be therapeutic (for medical reasons) or elective (for social reasons).

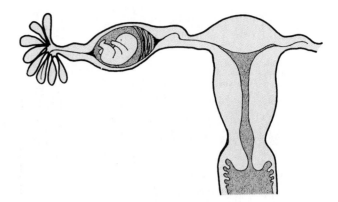

Figure 5-2 Ectopic pregnancy.

A *septic abortion* is any abortion complicated by intrauterine infection and fever.

Ectopic pregnancy

Ruptured ectopic pregnancy is the leading cause of maternal mortality in the first trimester, and its incidence is increasing. On average, 14 in 1000 pregnancies are ectopic pregnancies. An *ectopic pregnancy* is any pregnancy occurring outside the uterine cavity. The most common cause is pelvic inflammatory disease (PID). Also, past or current use of intrauterine devices (IUDs) appears to increase a woman's risk of ectopic pregnancy. Of all pregnancies that occur outside the uterus, 95% occur in a fallopian tube (Fig. 5-2). The fallopian tube stretches to accommodate the growing embryo, but because it is not elastic enough, the tube cannot stretch much. If the tubal pregnancy is not diagnosed and removed surgically, the distended tube will rupture. Ectopic pregnancies frequently are confused with other conditions such as ovarian cyst, PID, and spontaneous abortion.

Symptoms begin usually 6 to 12 weeks after conception. The woman will complain of abdominal pain on one side and usually will have vaginal bleeding that is scant and dark brown, although it is possible to show no outward signs of bleeding. With a ruptured ectopic pregnancy, severe pain is the predominant symptom. The woman may be nauseated or feel faint and may feel rectal or urinary pressure and also referred shoulder pain from diaphragmatic irritation. The woman may exhibit signs and symptoms of shock (cold, moist skin; fall in blood pressure; rapid, weak pulse; thirst; apprehension; pallor; weakness; and "air hunger"). These signs of shock will not be proportional to blood loss because of the enormous pain.

The acute rupture of a fallopian tube constitutes a surgical emergency. After bleeding is controlled, the ectopic gestation is surgically removed and, if the woman so desires, as much of the tube as possible is left for reconstructive surgery.

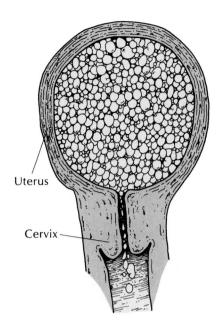

Figure 5-3 Gestational trophoblastic neoplasm (GTN).

Gestational trophoblastic neoplasm (GTN)

Formerly known as *"hydatidiform mole,"* GTN is a developmental anomaly of the placenta causing vaginal bleeding in the first trimester. In 1 of every 2000 pregnancies in the United States, abnormal trophoblastic growth causes higher than normal human chorionic gonadotropin (hCG) levels. The uterus enlarges rapidly, although there is no fetal heart tone, fetal movement, or palpable fetus (Fig. 5-3). Signs and symptoms of preeclampsia may be present as well as vaginal bleeding, often brownish in color. When a GTN is present, no fetal skeleton is seen.

Treatment consists of immediate evacuation of the uterus and follow-up for possible malignancy (approximately 20% of cases progress to invasive *choriocarcinoma*). If there is a metastasis, treatment with chemotherapy is effective. Another pregnancy is contraindicated for 1 year, over which time the chest radiograph and radioimmune assay for the beta-subunit of hCG should have returned to normal.

Nursing care

Abortion, ectopic pregnancy, and gestational trophoblastic neoplasm—the three common causes of bleeding in early pregnancy—require supportive nursing care from nurses knowledgeable about these conditions and their potential complications. The woman and her family had expected a healthy baby and instead are experiencing loss of that baby and loss of a healthy body image. The resolution of grief can begin in the hospital as the nurse helps the mother and family to work through the grief process of denial, anger, bargaining, depression, and acceptance.

Bleeding in Late Pregnancy
Placenta previa

Placenta previa is the most common cause of bleeding during the second half of pregnancy. The bleeding is painless, bright red vaginal bleeding occurring without warning in the absence of trauma. Instead of being implanted in the upper portion of the uterus, the placenta develops in the lower uterine segment, either partially or completely covering the cervix, in approximately 8 of 1000 pregnancies.

There are three types of placenta previa classified according to the degree to which the placenta covers the cervix: (1) partial, (2) marginal, and (3) complete (Fig. 5-4). With placenta previa there is painless vaginal bleeding in the second or third trimester of pregnancy. The dangers to the mother from placenta previa may include hemorrhage, infection (because the area of placental implantation is close to the cervix and susceptible to infection from the outside), and lowered resistance secondary to hemorrhage. With placenta previa, an initial episode is rarely total; however, each succeeding hemorrhage is greater than the last. Profuse hemorrhaging can occur in the third trimester as the os gradually dilates, pulling away from the placenta and causing severe bleeding. The dangers to the baby may include premature birth and hypoxia and/or asphyxiation from the oxygen supply being reduced or cut off.

Nursing care. It is important for the nurse to alert the woman and her family to the significance of *painless bleeding*, which is an early sign of placenta previa and to stress the importance of reporting this to the physician. The mother may be hospitalized or managed as an outpatient on bed rest if she is considered to be a good candidate for outpatient treatment. The nurse should not administer an enema or do a rectal or vaginal examination because it is possible to put an examining finger right through a placenta previa or dislodge it, thus causing life-threatening hemorrhage.

Abruptio placentae

Abruptio placentae is premature separation of the normally implanted placenta after the 20th week of pregnancy or during labor. Premature placental separation occurs in approximately 1% of deliveries and accounts for 15% of all perinatal deaths. The infant mortality rate is 33%, with 50% of these due to prematurity and uterine hypoxia. With abruptio placentae there may be (1) partial separation with concealed bleeding, (2) complete separation with concealed bleeding, or (3) partial

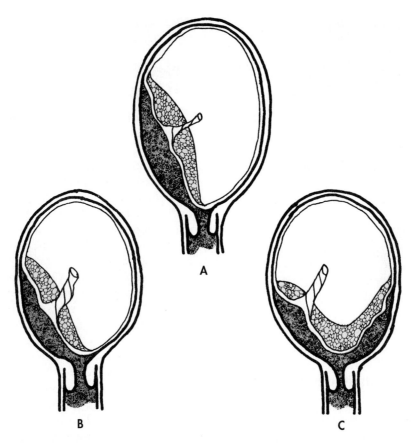

Figure 5-4 Placenta previa. **A,** Marginal implantation: the outer edge of the placenta lies on or near the cervical os. **B,** Partial placenta previa: a portion of the placenta covers the cervical os. **C,** Complete placenta previa: the center of the placenta lies directly over the cervical os.

separation with apparent hemorrhage (Fig. 5-5). The severity of separation may range from being so mild that there are no clinical symptoms to severe separation with maternal shock. In the case of a mild abruption of the placenta the only evidence may be a scar on the maternal side of the placenta found after delivery. In the more severe instances of abruptio placentae the woman complains of uterine tenderness and pain and the uterus becomes rigid. The woman may experience nausea and vomiting. The fetal heart rate may indicate distress or may be absent. For severe abruptio placentae there is no delayed treatment as in placenta previa because delay can result in severe hemorrhage with anemia, fetal death, and the serious coagulation disorder of disseminated intravascular coagulation (DIC). Cesarean birth is usually the method of delivery in severe abruptio placentae.

Nursing care. A family experiencing severe abruptio placentae is usually very aware of the acute emergency situation they are facing. As the nurse prepares the woman for emergency surgery (blood for type and cross-match, Foley catheter in place, recording vital signs, shaving abdomen in preparation for surgery, fetal

heart monitoring, signature of surgery consent forms), it is important to be aware of the fear and shock the woman and her family are experiencing. The woman should not be left alone and should have all procedures explained before or as they are being done.

Incompetent cervix

Cervical incompetence is the premature dilatation of the cervix. The dilatation usually occurs in the fourth or fifth month of pregnancy and results in recurrent, painless spontaneous abortion early in the third trimester or in premature labor. It may be associated with cervical trauma as a result of previous surgery or difficult birth.

Cervical incompetence is treated surgically with a Shirodkar or McDonald procedure, in which an encircling suture is placed around the cervical os. The suture can be removed close to term in order to allow labor to begin spontaneously.

The term *incompetent* can connote to the woman that her body is defective or imperfect. As a result she may feel guilty, hurt, and inadequate. A supportive, sensitive environment and a thorough explanation of the term

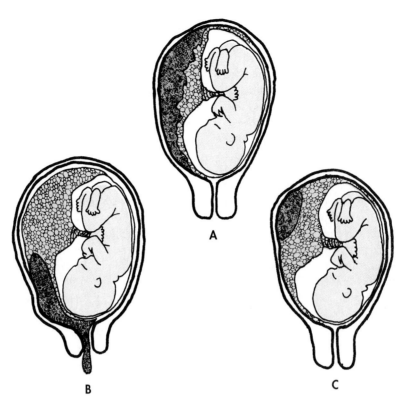

Figure 5-5 Abruptio placentae. **A,** Bleeding concealed. **B,** External bleeding. **C,** Mild concealed bleeding.

can help the woman and her family work through their feelings.

Hyperemesis gravidarum

Hyperemesis gravidarum is frequent, uncontrollable vomiting in early pregnancy. In Chapter 4, it was stated that nausea and vomiting of moderate intensity ("morning sickness") in pregnancy are common complaints during early pregnancy. However, if the nausea and vomiting become severe or continue beyond the first few months of pregnancy, the woman may become severely dehydrated and have electrolyte imbalances. Also, she may become malnourished and experience weight loss.

Hyperemesis gravidarum is estimated to occur in about 1 per 1000 pregnant women. Although the cause of severe nausea and vomiting during pregnancy is unknown, theories include an endocrine (elevated hormone levels, or thyroid dysfunction), psychologic, or allergic origin.

If the condition is severe the treatment consists of hospitalization, with additional treatment ranging from oral supplementation to intravenous supplementation to parenteral nutrition.

No drugs are approved by the Food and Drug Administration for morning sickness, and no consensus exists on the best antinauseant medications for use in morning sickness. However, some antihistamines and phenothiazines are reportedly used in some cases. Women with significant vomiting usually require intravenous fluid replacement and intravenous vitamins, selected minerals, and electrolytes. A few women may require parenteral nutrition (PN). After fluid and electrolyte stabilization and parenteral therapy are initiated in the hospital, the therapy can be maintained at home on an outpatient basis.

Nursing care. Realizing that one cause of hyperemesis may be psychological, the nurse should provide an understanding environment, giving the woman a chance to verbalize her problems and feelings. Communication with the entire family is essential because family problems or attitudes about the pregnancy may contribute to severe nausea and vomiting.

Patient education regarding nutrition and life-style will be important as the nurse helps the woman and her family through this difficult time.

Diabetes

Diabetes is a condition in which insulin production by the pancreas is insufficient or absent so that the body cannot utilize glucose. Approximately 0.3% of all pregnancies in the United States occur among women with established diabetes. Although this number is low, the morbidity associated with these pregnancies may be substantial. Infants born to women with established diabetes are at a high risk for prematurity, congenital defects, macrosomia, respiratory distress syndrome, neonatal hypoglycemia, hyperbilirubinemia, and death—especially when maternal glucose levels are not tightly controlled during pregnancy.

A condition known as *gestational diabetes* occurs in approximately 2% to 3% of pregnancies in the United States. This is a diabetes that develops during pregnancy—usually during the second trimester when the placenta produces increased amounts of hormones.

Pregnancy is characterized by an exaggerated rate and amount of insulin release but with insulin resistance at the cellular level so that the actions of insulin are restricted. As pregnancy progresses, more and more antiinsulin factors are produced by the placenta, and there is more and more stress on the maternal pancreas. Normally the mother meets this stress with increased insulin production. If a woman's pancreatic reserve is low, her insulin production may be inadequate for the first time in her life. This woman is classified as a *gestational diabetic.*

Babies born to mothers with gestational diabetes are at risk for becoming large (macrosomia), birth trauma due to difficult delivery, shoulder dystocia, hypoglyce-mia, hypocalcemia, hyperbilirubinemia, and increased probability of fetal neonatal mortality.

The adverse effects of diabetes on the mother during pregnancy may include increased incidence of preeclampsia; eclampsia; difficult delivery; premature labor; hydramnios; urinary tract and vaginal infections; ketoacidosis; and exacerbated microvascular, renal, ocular, and neural complications (in established diabetes). Women with gestational diabetes are at increased risk for developing diabetes after the pregnancy is over.

There are two methods of classifying diabetes mellitus. White's classification is the oldest method (Table 5-1). In 1979 a new classification (Table 5-2) was developed and is currently used by most health care providers. The old classification was proposed by Dr. Priscilla White at the Joslin Clinic in Boston, Massachusetts. Its purpose was to correlate duration of diabetes and presence of vascular lesions with pregnancy outcome.

Blood glucose screening and diagnostic activities to identify gestational diabetes should be done at 24 to 28 weeks if no risk factors are present, or at first visit for prenatal care and again at 26 weeks if risk factors are present.

For women with established diabetes, prepregnancy counseling is important so that normalization of maternal glucose levels can occur before pregnancy, and strict control of glucose throughout pregnancy can be

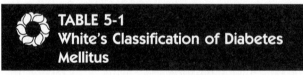

TABLE 5-1
White's Classification of Diabetes Mellitus

Class	Characteristics
Gestational diabetes	Abnormal glucose tolerance during pregnancy; postprandial hyperglycemia during pregnancy
A	Chemical diabetes, diagnosed before pregnancy; managed by diet alone; any age at onset
B	Insulin treatment necessary before pregnancy; onset < age 20; duration < 10 years
C	Onset age 10-20 or duration 10-20 years
D	Onset < age 10 or duration > 20 years, or chronic hypertension (not preeclampsia) or background retinopathy (tiny hemorrhages)
F	Diabetic nephropathy with proteinuria
H	Coronary artery disease
R	Proliferative retinopathy

TABLE 5-2
New Classification of Diabetes Mellitus

Class	Characteristics
Type I insulin-dependent diabetes mellitus (IDDM)	Ketosis prone; insulin deficient owing to islet cell loss; occurs at any age, common in youth
Type II non–insulin-dependent diabetes mellitus (NDDM) Nonobese Obese	Ketosis resistant; more frequent in adults but occurs at any age; majority of affected individuals are overweight; may require insulin for hyperglycemia during stress; requires insulin during pregnancy
Gestational diabetes	This classification is retained for women whose diabetes begins (or is recognized) during pregnancy

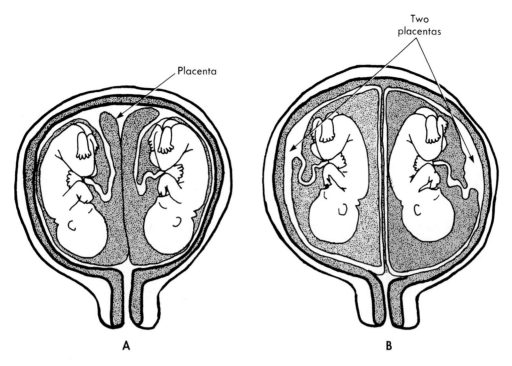

Figure 5-6 Multiple pregnancy. **A,** Identical (monozygotic) twins: two sacs, one placenta. **B,** Fraternal (dizygotic) twins: two sacs, two placentas.

achieved. For these women the goal is to attain eugly-cemia before conception and maintain it throughout gestation.

Complicated diabetic pregnancies may be terminated before term because of the large size of the fetus or because of maternal complications. Tests of placental function and fetal maturity are done to choose the appropriate date for delivery.

The baby of a diabetic mother is placed in neonatal intensive care and treated according to current practice until stable. The infant is at risk for developing rebound hypoglycemia and, if untreated, brain damage and even death.

Nursing care

Comprehensive antepartum education plays a major role in the management of a pregnancy complicated by diabetes. The most successful programs start pre-conceptually and involve the family as active members of the health care team to promote optimal outcomes for mother and baby. Overall objectives may include (1) keeping maternal blood glucose levels as close to normal as possible, (2) providing adequate nutrition for normal development of the fetus, (3) preventing progression of maternal vascular disease, and (4) preventing premature delivery and fetal or neonatal complications.

Multiple Pregnancy

Identical twins *(monozygotic)* result from the union of one sperm and one ovum; fraternal twins *(dizygotic)* result when two ova are fertilized by two sperm (Fig. 5-6). With fraternal twins there are two amniotic sacs and two placentas. With identical twins there are two amniotic sacs and one placenta. Approximately 1 in 90 births in the United States is a twin birth. Because of overdistention of the uterus, twins are usually delivered before term and have extended hospital stays. Twins may be double joy, but they are also double responsibility and more expensive than one baby. The parents need a great deal of support both before and after the twins arrive. It is possible to breast-feed twins. However, the woman who plans to do this needs help with her other responsibilities because breast-feeding will consume a lot of her time.

Heart Disease

Heart disease complicates pregnancy because the diseased or damaged heart may not be able to meet the demands of the increased cardiac work load of pregnancy. Approximately 1% of all pregnant women have some form of heart disease. The majority of these women have either a congenital lesion or heart disease caused by rheumatic fever. Like women with diabetes, women with heart disease should be under close medical supervision during pregnancy. The hemodynamic changes of normal pregnancy may cause significant disability or death in women with heart disease. Early antepartum care and frequent and regular visits to an obstetrician and a cardiologist should be stressed for these women.

Management of the pregnant woman with a cardiac condition is guided by classification based on the presenting symptomatology.

Classification of cardiac disease by functional incapacity is as follows:

1. Class I—Asymptomatic at all degrees of activity. No limitations on physical activity.
2. Class II—Symptomatic with increased activity. Minor limitation of physical activity.
3. Class III—Symptomatic with ordinary activity. Marked limitations of physical activity.
4. Class IV—Symptomatic at rest. Discomfort increased with any physical activity.

Adequate rest and avoidance of activities that cause shortness of breath and fatigue are essential for the pregnant woman with heart disease. Also, excessive weight gain, which could put more strain on the heart, must be avoided. Women with heart disease may experience heart failure at any time during pregnancy. Symptoms of heart failure are difficulty in breathing *(dyspnea), paraoxysmal nocturnal dyspnea* (awakening at night with shortness of breath), *orthopnea* (sleeping on two to four pillows because of shortness of breath), *nocturia* (awakening at night to void), and peripheral edema. Women with heart disease are also at risk for contracting respiratory infections and therefore should seek prompt treatment for a cold or sore throat.

Nursing care

The nurse can be very helpful by encouraging the woman with heart disease to follow the physician's orders. The nurse can also work with the woman and her family in restructuring family chores and activities to reduce the woman's work load and help the family plan their food intake to reduce salt in the woman's diet. Also, continuous psychological support is essential.

Anemia

Anemia is a condition in which there is a reduction in the oxygen-carrying capacity of the blood because of a reduction in red cells and/or hemoglobin.

If the pregnant woman's hemoglobin level falls below 10 in the second trimester, *iron deficiency anemia* is suspected. In iron deficiency anemia inadequate hemoglobin production is the result of decreased heme synthesis. Iron supplementation of 320 milligrams of ferrous sulfate, orally, three times per day, and vitamin C, 500 milligrams, orally, once per day should be recommended when iron deficiency is the cause of anemia.

Folic acid deficiency anemia may result from malabsorption of folate from the intestine, poor intake of folate, liver damage, or frequent pregnancies in which the woman cannot replenish body folate stores. Iron deficiency anemia can be associated with folate deficiency. Folate supplementation of 400 micrograms of folic acid per day in pregnancy should prevent folate deficiency.

Thalassemia primarily affects people of Mediterranean and Southeast Asian origin. In this form of anemia there is inadequate hemoglobin production plus an excessive breakdown of the defective red cells that are produced. The stress of pregnancy frequently worsens the anemia in thalassemia. Iron therapy is *not* recommended.

Sickle cell trait is a sickling of red blood cells found in approximately 8% of black childbearing women. Of the pregnant women who have sickle cell trait, less than 1% have *sickle cell anemia*. In pregnancy complicated by sickle cell anemia, the maternal mortality rate can be as high as 70% and the perinatal mortality rate as high as 50%. These women are susceptible to urinary tract infections, and the fetus may be at risk for hypoxic stress. Iron and folic acid supplementation should be prescribed, and the sources of both should be increased in the diet.

Prenatal Substance Abuse

Abuse of drugs can cause severe problems for both the mother and baby. Approximately 11% of babies in the United States are born to mothers who have used illicit drugs—especially crack cocaine—during their pregnancy. This is a threefold to fourfold increase over 1985 figures. Other abused drugs are phencyclidine (PCP), marijuana, alcohol, amphetamines, nicotine, barbiturates, codeine, diazepam, and narcotics. Frequently women who abuse drugs take more than one drug. Of the infants born to heroin-addicted women, 60% to 90% show signs of withdrawal. Infants born to women on methadone at the time of delivery also experience withdrawal symptoms. The severity of symptoms and time of their onset are related to the duration and type of maternal addiction, as well as to the mother's drug level before giving birth.

The recreational use of cocaine is a major public health issue in the United States, with women of reproductive age making up a growing percentage of all users. Illegal drugs are found in pregnancies and births across the country and are no longer confined to those in hospitals with high percentages of low-income or public-aid patients.

Cocaine can affect a pregnant woman and her unborn baby in many ways. Use of cocaine during pregnancy may lead to premature births, small-for-gestational-age (SGA) babies, abruptio placentae, fetal death, and neonatal addiction through transplacental effects of the drug.

At birth cocaine-exposed infants tend to be irritable and jittery. However, unlike the babies of heroin-addicted mothers, these babies do not go through true withdrawal. Because they cry and startle easily, these babies are difficult to comfort and often are unable to interact with others or respond to their mothers. The mother's continued dependency on cocaine and the baby's reaction to the drug make bonding between mother and baby difficult. Problems faced by these babies may include increased risk for child abuse, neglect, and developmental and learning disabilities.

Nursing care

The nurse must first identify his or her own values and judgments concerning substance abuse during pregnancy. It is not unusual to feel anger, sadness, and disappointment when caring for a withdrawing infant who cannot be comforted, but anger and a judgmental attitude impede therapeutic relationships. Team support among co-workers, identifying and acknowledging one's feelings, and a nonjudgmental approach are necessary.

Denial is an important coping mechanism for the substance-abusing woman. Also, the woman may experience chronic anxiety and depression, and she may lack confidence and hope for the future.

The nurse should be knowledgeable about community inpatient and outpatient treatment programs that accept pregnant women and newborns. Communication and coordination with treatment programs are essential. Educating women of childbearing age about the dangers of drug use in pregnancy is an important function of nurses.

Hydramnios

Hydramnios is the accumulation of excessive amounts (2000 milliliters or more) of amniotic fluid. The reported incidence of hydramnios is approximately 0.4% of pregnancies. The condition is often suspected by the seventh month of pregnancy and can be confirmed by ultrasound screening. Hydramnios is associated with a high incidence of fetal abnormalities; when the diagnosis is made, therefore, further testing is done to see if the fetus has a major abnormality.

Fetal anomalies associated with hydramnios include

anomalies of the CNS (45%), gastrointestinal system (30%), and cardiovascular system (7%), among others. Early detection of anomalies by ultrasonography gives the parents and health care providers warning and adequate time for counseling.

An amount of 100 to 200 milliliters of amniotic fluid is called *oligohydramnios* and is associated with renal anomalies.

DIAGNOSTIC TECHNIQUES

Numerous diagnostic and monitoring procedures are in use today for determining fetal well-being, growth, and maturity. There are advantages, disadvantages, indications, and contraindications for each. The tests are usually confined to the management of high-risk pregnancies. The following are indications for fetal evaluation:

Insulin-dependent diabetes
Preeclampsia or eclampsia
Chronic hypertension
Maternal anemia
Isoimmunization
Previous stillbirth
Intrauterine growth retardation
Post dates
Maternal cyanotic heart disease
Lupus nephritis
Hyperthyroidism
Premature rupture of membranes
Vaginal bleeding
Decreased fetal movement

As the use of technology in high-risk pregnancy increases, it is important that the issues of the safety and the cost-effectiveness of the tests be resolved. New technologies are frequently integrated into systems of care before a long-term analysis of their safety and cost is completed. Professional reluctance to criticize a "revolutionary tool," especially when it represents a major technological advance, may make it difficult to collect objective scientific data once the intervention has been generally accepted.

Ultrasonography

Approximately half the pregnant women in the United States routinely receive ultrasound scans to determine the age of the fetus and location of the placenta. In recent years the benefit-to-risk ratio for use of routine ultrasound in pregnancy has been questioned. This concern led to a 6-year study supported by the National Institutes of Health (NIH).

According to the results of this large randomized study, routine screening with ultrasound offers no benefits and has little effect on the final outcome of low-risk pregnancies. The researchers conclude that ultra-

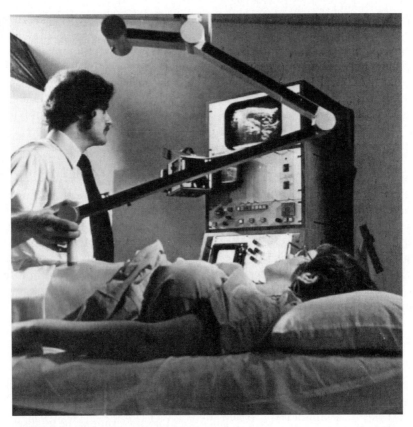

Figure 5-7 Ultrasonography. *(Permission to reproduce this photo has been granted by the National Foundation—March of Dimes as the copyright holder of the original publication.)*

sound exams should be done when the physician believes there is a medical need, but that sonograms should not be done routinely for all pregnancies.

The position paper on ultrasound by the International Childbirth Education Association (ICEA) is reproduced in Appendix H.

Ultrasonography (sonography, sonogram, scan) is a painless technique in which ultra high frequency soundwaves (too high to be heard) are beamed into the body (Fig. 5-7). These soundwaves bounce off soft tissue in different ways, sending out echos, which can be recorded on an oscilloscope and photographed for permanent records in Polaroid photographs. One scanning technique can measure the size of the fetal head to determine whether the fetus is growing normally. Another technique can monitor continuous fetal activity, watch the fetal heart beating, measure fetal breathing and even observe the fetus sucking its thumb. Other uses for ultrasound are to localize the placenta in suspected placenta previa or before amniocentesis so that the operator will not place the needle into the placenta. Sonography can also pick up some fetal anomalies and multiple gestations, tumors in the uterus, and gestational trophoblastic neoplasms.

Nursing care

Pelvic ultrasonography is one test in which the success of the technique is heavily dependent on the woman having a full bladder. For 1½ hours before the test, the nurse encourages the woman to drink a full glass of water every 15 minutes. The full bladder both helps to push the uterus upward and serves as an amplifier for sound. Because a full bladder can make the pregnant woman very uncomfortable, she needs a thorough explanation of the reasons involved.

Endovaginal Ultrasound

Transvaginal sonography with a high frequency probe is more comfortable than conventional ultrasound techniques because it does not require a full bladder. In fact, the woman is encouraged to urinate as completely as possible before the procedure.

Images obtained endovaginally are almost always more detailed than conventional ones and can disclose an embryo at an earlier stage of gestation than through a full bladder. Other uses of transvaginal sonography include diagnosis and treatment in gynecology, ectopic pregnancies, and infertility.

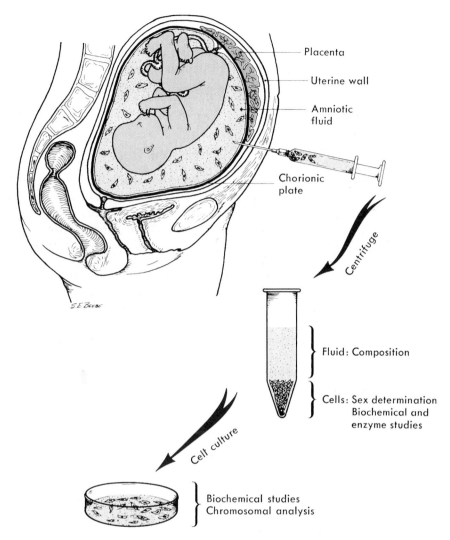

Figure 5-8 Amniocentesis. *(From Tucker SM: Fetal monitoring and fetal assessment in high-risk pregnancy, St. Louis, 1978, Mosby.)*

Nursing care

Women are concerned about the safety, procedure, and comfort of transvaginal sonography. To minimize the danger of spreading infection, the transducer is covered with a sterile glove or sheath before insertion and is carefully cleansed with antiseptic solution once the test is completed. There is no evidence that the endovaginal approach carries any more risk than the older method, even in pregnancy.

In the area of transvaginal sonography, education and support of the woman about to undergo the procedure are the chief nursing functions.

Amniocentesis

Amniocentesis is the removal of amniotic fluid from the amniotic cavity by needle puncture (Fig. 5-8). The risks involved with amniocentesis are abortion in approximately 1% of the pregnancies and trauma to the fetus or placenta resulting in bleeding, infection, and Rh sensitization from fetal bleeding into the maternal circulation. Even though these risks are slight, the fact that they are possible rules out amniocentesis as a routine screening procedure. It is the physician's responsibility to inform the woman and her family of the risks of amniocentesis and to obtain a signed consent form if a decision is made that the benefits from the procedure outweigh the risks. (The need to obtain amniotic fluid to accurately determine fetal maturity or to determine the presence of Down syndrome or other suspected genetic defects in the population at risk are accepted reasons for amniocentesis.)

Nursing care

For amniocentesis, the placenta is localized by ultrasound and fetal position determined. The nurse records the fetal heart rate and prepares the woman's abdomen as for a minor surgical procedure. From 20 to 30 milliliters of amniotic fluid are withdrawn by the physician and placed in taped or amber test tubes to protect the specimen from light. On conclusion of the procedure, the nurse places an adhesive bandage over the puncture site and again listens to the fetal heart tones and watches for any outward symptoms. Before the procedure the nurse explains what will happen to the woman and her family, clarifying anything they do not understand. During the procedure the nurse has the key role in supporting the woman. The Rh− woman with an Rh+ partner receives 300 micrograms of anti-Rh immunoglobulin (RhoGAM) after the test.

Amniotic Fluid Studies

Chromosomal abnormalities such as Down syndrome, the sex of the fetus, and certain genetic defects can be detected by culturing the cells from amniotic fluid and studying them.

Alpha-fetoprotein (AFP) studies early in the second trimester can detect neural tube malformations such as hydrocephalus, spina bifida, and microcephaly. AFP can also be detected in the maternal serum at 12 to 14 weeks of gestation.

Lecithin-sphingomyelin ratios (L/S ratios) can be done on amniotic fluid to determine maturity of the fetal lungs. Lecithin and sphingomyelin are the predominant phospholipids making up *surfactant,* which is the complex detergent-like substance lining the alveoli of the lungs. This surfactant lowers the surface tension in the alveoli and keeps the alveolar walls from collapsing on themselves. L/S are present as a ratio, changing predictably as the pregnancy progresses (Fig. 5-9). When the ratio of lecithin to sphingomyelin is 2.0 or greater, the fetal lung is considered mature. Phosphatidylglycerol is another phospholipid in surfactant. Absence indicates pulmonary immaturity.

Creatinine levels, bilirubin levels, and *the percentage of fat cells* present in the amniotic fluid can also indicate fetal maturity.

Estriol Test

Estriol is a major metabolite of estrogen and is found in relatively large quantities in maternal urine in the last half of pregnancy. The fetus contributes, through its adrenals, to the maternal urinary estriol to the placenta and then into the maternal blood. The synthesis of estriol requires a normal placenta and fetal adrenal cortex. Estriol levels excreted in maternal urine should rise predictably throughout pregnancy (Fig. 5-10). A fall in estriol levels usually signals trouble in the fetal-placental unit and possible impending fetal death. A single estriol level alone is of limited value, but a falling estriol along with other tests indicating a compromised fetal-placental unit is a diagnostic tool. Estriol tests done on the mother's plasma are much faster than the 24-hour urine collection. Because serial estriol determinations alone are not always an accurate indicator of fetal well-being, they should be used in conjunction with other tests.

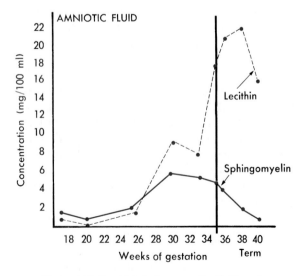

Figure 5-9 Lecithin/spingomyelin (L/S) ratio.

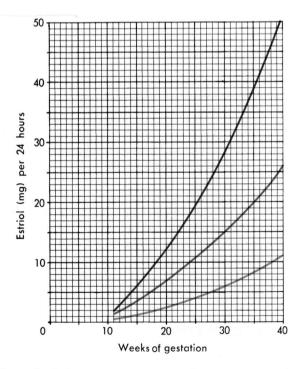

Figure 5-10 Average excretion of urine estriol throughout pregnancy is depicted by the middle line.

Nursing care

In addition to collecting the specimens (whether 24-hour urine or maternal blood), the nurse once again plays the role of explaining to the woman and her family the need for the estriol test and the significance of the test results.

Contraction Stress Test

In a *contraction stress test (CST)*, continuous fetal monitoring is used to test placental respiratory function and reserve. Oxytocin is given intravenously using an infusion pump until the woman experiences three uterine contractions within a 10-minute period. The fetal heart rate is observed in relation to the contractions. If the heart rate remains stable during contractions, the test is negative; however, if late decelerations in the fetal heart rate appear, the test is positive. A negative test means that the present status of the fetus is satisfactory and the pregnancy can continue for another week, when the test should be repeated. If other tests of fetal status are positive, a positive CST may indicate the need for prompt termination of the pregnancy.

Breast or Nipple Stimulation Tests

Many perinatal centers are now using breast stimulation instead of oxytocin for inducing uterine activity. Manual or breast pump stimulation of the nipple and breast releases oxytocin from the pituitary, thus stimulating contractions of the uterine musculature. Because breast stimulation is a potent stimulator of uterine contractions, it should be performed only unilaterally and for short periods.

Nonstress Test

During the last part of pregnancy women may also be monitored using a *nonstress test,* (NST). It is a sign of fetal well-being if the fetal heart accelerates in response to fetal movement. The fetus may move spontaneously or with a Braxton-Hicks contraction or by external manipulation such as rubbing the woman's abdomen.

A reactive NST pattern is fetal movement associated with two accelerations of the fetal heart that last 15 seconds or more and achieve a zenith of 15 beats per minute in one of two 20-minute periods.

The reactive NST and negative CST are highly predictive of fetal well-being but are valid only for the period of the testing. If the maternal condition is stable, most physicians accept a 1 week's predictive value indicating presence of fetal health. However, controversy exists as to which test should be used as the primary screening tool. Many practitioners use a CST after an abnormal NST.

Nursing care

The CST, the NST, and breast stimulation require thorough explanations for the woman and her family both before and during the procedures. Following the tests, the nurse makes sure that the woman and her family understand the results of the tests and their implications for further care.

Vibroacoustic Stimulation (VST)

Fetal acoustic stimulation by sending a loud, vibrating, buzzing signal into the uterus is being used as a test of fetal well-being in some centers. The artificial larynx (placed firmly to the maternal abdomen over the area of the fetal head) is used to produce a loud, vibrating, buzzing sound.

Stimulation is also produced by sound or audio tones, but this is described as sound stimulation or fetal acoustic stimulation (FAS-TEST). VSTs can be useful during NSTs or labor to stimulate an inactive fetus with a flat tracing.

Fetal Movements

Monitoring fetal motion is worthwhile in predicting fetal distress in high-risk pregnancies. It is an inexpensive, noninvasive method and relies on the pregnant woman to observe her own baby.

Since the beginning of time, pregnant women have been known to experience decreased fetal activity before fetal death. Because there is a wide variation in the number of fetal movements daily, each mother needs to determine what is normal for her baby. After 24 weeks of gestation, pregnant women can be instructed to concentrate on fetal movements for specific periods of time daily (according to their risk potential). If the woman notices fewer than three movements in 8 hours or movements that change from strong to weak, this should be communicated to the health care team immediately. Cessation of fetal movement places the fetus in a high-risk category and should alert the care providers to the need for an NST.

Biophysical Profile Scoring (BPS)

Fetal biophysical profile scoring begins with detailed dynamic ultrasound scanning of a pregnant woman (more than 26 weeks of gestation) who has had high-risk factors identified. Five fetal biophysical variables—fetal breathing movements, fetal body movements, fetal muscular tone, qualitative amniotic fluid volume, and the NST—are measured and scored according to fixed criteria. Each variable is assigned an arbitrary score of 2 (if normal) or 0 (if abnormal). When all variables are normal (BPS = 10) or when the amniotic fluid volume

TABLE 5-3
How to Interpret Fetal Well-Being from BPS Scores

Biophysical variable	Normal (BPS = 2)	Abnormal (BPS = 0)
Fetal breathing movements	At least one episode of FBM of at least 30 seconds duration in 30 minutes observation	Absent FBM or no episode of ≥30 seconds in 30 minutes
Gross body movement	At least three discrete body-limb movements in 30 minutes (episodes of active, continuous movement considered a single movement)	Two or fewer episodes of body-limb movements in 30 minutes
Fetal tone	At least one episode of active extension with return to flexion of fetal limb(s) or trunk (opening and closing of hand considered normal tone)	Either slow extension with return to partial flexion or movement of limb in full extension or absent fetal movement
Reactive FHR	At least two episodes of FHR acceleration of ≥15 bpm and of at lest 15 seconds duration associated with fetal movement in 30 minutes.	Fewer than two episodes of acceleration of FHR or acceleration of <15 bmp in 30 minutes
Qualitative AFV	At least one pocket of AF that measures at least 1 centimeter in two perpendicular planes	Either no AF pockets or one pocket <1 centimeter in two perpendicular planes

FBM, fetal breathing movement; *FHR*, fetal heart rate; *bpm*, beats per minute; *AFV*, amniotic fluid volume; *AF*, amniotic fluid.
From Manning FA: Fetal biophysical profile scoring predicts trouble—when it counts, *Contemp Obstet Gynecol* 20:126-137, Jan 1985.

and at least three other variables are normal (BPS = 8), the fetus is considered equivocal and repeat testing is indicated. A score of 4 or less is usually considered abnormal and immediate delivery is indicated. See Table 5-3 for criteria used to interpret fetal well-being from BPS.

Percutaneous Umbilical Blood Sampling (PUBS)

An experimental procedure that is not without risk, PUBS allows direct visualization of the fetus and sampling of fetal tissues, including blood and skin, for antenatal detection of birth defects. At 16 to 20 weeks of gestation, through a spinal needle guided to the exact location by sonography, the physician can withdraw blood and tissue specimens for study.

Because of the substantial risk involved, at present PUBS has a limited but definite application in antenatal diagnosis.

Chorionic Villus Sampling (CVS)

Chorionic villus sampling can diagnose fetal genetic defects during the first trimester, usually at 8 to 10

weeks. Unlike amniocentesis, which relies on fetal cells found in samples of amniotic fluid taken by needle through the abdominal wall, CVS requires no penetration of the walls of the abdomen or uterus or invasion of the amniotic cavity. The findings are ready within 24 hours, and confirming tissue cultures are complete in 5 to 7 days. The procedure, if perfected, may revolutionize prenatal diagnosis of birth defects.

Major indications for genetic amniocentesis and CVS include advanced parental age; a previous child with chromosomal abnormalities; a parent with translocation or other chromosomal abnormality; a fetus at risk for a potentially detectable Mendelian disorder, an X-linked disease, or an inborn error of metabolism; and recurring loss of pregnancy in the first trimester.

Short-term problems may include spontaneous abortion, maternal bleeding, cramping, infection, and amniotic fluid leakage. Long-term complications are yet to be identified.

SUMMARY

Because this is a basic text, this chapter has represented only an introduction to the care of the high-risk woman and her family. Although the major complications of pregnancy were introduced, some of the less common high-risk conditions were not included. As pregnancy screening for identification of high-risk pregnancies becomes more refined and diagnostic techniques are more sophisticated, the need for nurses with special education in the care of high-risk families will increase. In regionalized high-risk centers, continuous in-service education will be needed to update the nursing care provided.

The nurse's role is to provide careful explanations of the procedures and accurate, compassionate, and expeditious counseling. The nurse assists with procedures, supports, teaches, and clarifies information whenever possible. As we continue to expand both knowledge and skills, we must not lose sight of the goal of the high-risk level of the new maternity model—that is, to provide a more complex but still humanistic model for women with medical complications or complications of pregnancy.

BIBLIOGRAPHY

Aaronson LS, Macnee CL: Tobacco, alcohol, and caffeine use during pregnancy, *J Obstet Gynecol Neonatal Nurs* 18:279-287, July/Aug 1989.

American College of Obstetricians and Gynecologists: *Substance abuse in pregnancy*, Technical Bulletin, No. 195, July 1994.

Anderson GD: A systematic approach to eclamptic convulsion, *Contemp Obstet Gynecol* 18:65-70, March 1987.

Bobak IM, Jensen MD, Lowdermilk DL: *Maternity and gynecologic care: the nurse and the family*, ed 5, St. Louis, 1993, Mosby.

Bowman JM: Controversies in Rh prophylaxis, *Am J Obstet Gynecol* 151(3):289-294, 1985.

Brengman SL, Burno MK: Hypertensive crisis in L & D: drugs to get the mother's BP out of the danger zone, *Am J Nurs* 88(3):325-328, 1988.

Capeless EL, Mann LI: Use of breast stimulation for antepartum stress testing, *Obstet Gynecol* 64(5):641-645, 1984.

Centers for Disease Control: Leads from the MMWR; morbidity and mortality weekly report, 35/13, 1986, *JAMA* 255:2544-2564, 1986.

Cnattingius S, and others: Delayed childbearing and risk of adverse perinatal outcome: a population-based study, *JAMA* 268:886, 1992.

Culverwell M: Perinatal effects of cocaine, *Childbirth Instr* 1(1):10-17, 1994.

Dickason EJ, Schultz MO, Silverman BL: *Maternal-infant nursing care*, ed 2, St. Louis, 1994, Mosby.

Droste S, Keil K: Expectant management of placenta previa: cost-benefit analysis of outpatient treatment, *Am J Obstet Gynecol* 170(5):1254-1257, 1994.

Dunn PA, Weiner S, Ludomirski A: Percutaneous umbilical blood sampling, *J Obstet Gynecol Neonatal Nurs* 17:308-313, Sept/Oct 1988.

Enkin MW: Risk in pregnancy: the reality, the perception, and the concept, *Birth* 21(3):131-134, 1994.

Ferguson HW: Biophysical profile scoring: the fetal Apgar, *Am J Nurs* 88(5):662-663, 1988.

Free T, and others: A descriptive study of infants and toddlers exposed prenatally to substance abuse, *MCN* 15:245-249, July/Aug 1990.

Goldenberg RL, and others: Bed rest in pregnancy, *Obstet Gynecol* 84(1):131-135, 1994.

Graham K, and others: Determination of gestational cocaine exposure by hair analysis, *JAMA* 262:3328-3331, Dec 1989.

Hammer RM, Bower EJ, Messina LJ: The prenatal use of Rho(D) immunoglobulin, *MCN* 9:29-31, Jan/Feb 1984.

ICEA Position Paper: Diagnostic ultrasound in obstetrics, *ICEA News* 22:2, March 1983.

Kuczynski HJ: Support for the woman with an ectopic pregnancy, *J Obstet Gynecol Neonatal Nurs* 15(4):306-310, 1986.

Lloyd T: Rh-factor incompatibility: a primer for prevention, *J Nurse Midwifery* 32(5):297-307, 1987.

Manning FA: Fetal biophysical profile scoring predicts trouble—when it counts, *Contemp Obstet Gynecol* 20:126-137, Jan 1985.

Marshall C: The nipple stimulation contraction stress test, *J Obstet Gynecol Neonatal Nurs* 15(6):459-462, 1986.

Mattson S, Smith JE, editors: *Core curriculum for maternal-newborn nursing*, Philadelphia, 1993, WB Saunders.

McCain GC, Deatrick JA: The experience of high-risk pregnancy, *J Obstet Gynecol Neonatal Nurs* 23(5):421-427, 1994.

Modica MM, Timor-Tritsch IE: Transvaginal sonography provides a sharper view into the pelvis, *J Obstet Gynecol Neonatal Nurs* 17:89-95, March/April 1988.

Nagey DA, Bailey-Jones C, Herman AA: Randomized comparison of home uterine activity monitoring and routine care in patients discharged after treatment for preterm labor, *Obstet Gynecol* 82(3):319-323, 1993.

National Institutes of Health: The use of diagnostic ultrasound imaging in pregnancy: Consensus Development Conference, *Cons Statement*, Bethesda, Md, Feb 6-8, 1984.

Newman V, Fullerton JT, Anderson PO: Clinical advances in the management of severe nausea and vomiting during pregnancy, *J Obstet Gynecol Neonatal Nurs* 22(6):483-490, 1993.

Osguthorpe NC: Ectopic pregnancy, *J Obstet Gynecol Neonatal Nurs* 16(1):36-41, 1987.

Peters H, Theorell CJ: Fetal and neonatal effects of maternal cocaine use, *J Obstet Gynecol Neonatal Nurs* 20(2):121-126, 1991.

Portale AM: *Diabetes in pregnancy*, NAACOG update series, vol 3, lesson 5, Princeton, NJ, 1985, CPEC.

Roberts J: Current perspectives on preeclampsia, *J Nurse Midwifery* 39(2):70-79, 1994.

Sleutel MR: An overview of vibroacoustic stimulation, *J Obstet Gynecol Neonatal Nurs* 18:447-452, 1988.

Stain J, and others: Can we encourage pregnant substance abusers to seek prenatal care?, *MCN* 18:148-152, May/June 1993.

Stringer MR: Chorionic villi sampling: a nursing perspective, *J Obstet Gynecol Neonatal Nurs* 17:19-22, March/April 1988.

Sullivan J, Boudreaux M, Keller P: Can we help the substance abusing mother and infant?, *MCN* 18:153-157, May/June 1993.

Surratt N: Severe preeclampsia: Implications for critical-care obstetric nursing, *J Obstet Gynecol Neonatal Nurs* 22(6):500-507, 1993.

Wagner M: Ultrasound evolution, *Mod Health Care*, 26-30, April 1992.

Weinstein L: The HELLP syndrome: a severe consequence of hypertension in pregnancy, *J Perinatol* 6(4):316-320, 1986.

Weiss J, Hansell MJ: Substance abuse during pregnancy, *Nurs Health Care* 13(9):472-479, 1992.

Wenzel L, and others: The psychological, social, and sexual consequences of gestational trophoblastic disease, *Gynecol Oncol* 46:74-80, 1992.

Zacharian R: Maternal-fetal attachment: Influence of mother-daughter and husband-wife relationships, *Res Nurs Health* 17:37-44, 1994.

DEFINITIONS

Define the following terms:

abortion
abruptio placentae
alpha-fetoprotein
antibodies
bilirubin
clonus
Coombs' test
demographic
diabetogenic state
diastolic
diuretics
dizygotic
eclampsia
ectopic pregnancy
electrolyte
estriol
gestational diabetes
gestational trophoblastic neoplasm (GTN)
HELLP syndrome
hyperemesis gravidarum
immunoglobulin
incompatibility
incompetent cervix
induction
isoimmunization
ketoacidosis
macrosomia
monozygotic
oscilloscope
oxytocin
percutaneous umbilical blood sampling (PUBS)
placenta previa
pregnancy-induced hypertension (PIH)
proteinuria
regimen
RhoGAM
sensitization
systolic
titer
transducer
ultrasonography
vibroacoustic stimulation (VST)

LEARNING ACTIVITIES

1. Group discussions.
2. Guest speakers: a nurse from a high-risk maternity clinic.
3. View audiovisual aids, listen to tapes, and discuss.

ENRICHMENT/IN-DEPTH STUDY

1. Discuss the pros and cons of a two-tiered maternity model.
2. Discover community resources for high-risk prenatal care in your community.
3. Investigate resources in your community that provide financial aid to pregnant families in need of such aid.
4. Determine the average cost of prenatal care in your community.
5. Determine the average cost of the hospital stay for delivery and post-delivery care in your community.
6. Investigate community resources for continued schooling, prenatal education, and preparation for birth available in your community for teenaged mothers and fathers.
7. Discuss the emotional reactions a family may experience when receiving results of amniocentesis indicating that the fetus has Down syndrome or neural tube malformations.
8. Attend open meetings of Alcoholics Anonymous, Cocaine Anonymous, and Narcotics Anonymous.

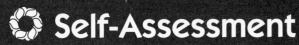

Self-Assessment

For questions 1 through 4, circle the best answer.

1. In which of the following situations is Rh isoimmunization possible?

    a. mother is Rh negative; father is Rh(D) positive

    b. mother is Rh(D) positive; father is Rh negative

    c. both parents are Rh(D) positive

    d. both parents are Rh negative

2. Careful follow-up of the woman who has had a gestational trophoblastic neoplasm (GTN) is important because she:

    a. will probably have twins next pregnancy

    b. will become infertile

    c. may develop choriocarcinoma

3. After delivery from the diabetic mother, the baby is usually placed in the neonatal intensive care unit for close observation because the baby often develops:

    a. hyperglycemia

    b. hypoglycemia

    c. Rh problems

    d. anemia

4. The ratio of lecithin to sphingomyelin indicates the maturity of the:

    a. fetal lungs

    b. fetal kidneys

    c. placenta

For questions 5 through 21, fill in the blanks.

5. The nonstress test uses fetal heart acceleration in response to _____ as a point of reference.

6. A pregnant woman about to undergo pelvic ultrasonography needs a(n) _____ bladder.

7. For amniocentesis, the placenta is localized by _____.

8. A fall in estriol levels during pregnancy could mean _____.

9. The procedure by which a specimen of amniotic fluid is collected for laboratory tests is called _____.

10. When fetal blood cell damage is occurring in utero, the fetus may be given _____ _____.

11. One test that can indicate the severity of fetal blood cell damage during the pregnancy of a sensitized woman is known as the _____.

12. If the Rh-positive infant shows signs of erythroblastosis after birth, the treatment of choice will probably be _____ _____.

13. The anti-Rh-positive globulin that suppresses the formation of Rh antibodies is

    _____ _____.

14. To a layperson the term *abortion* may mean _____.

15. The obstetrical definition of *abortion* is _____.

16. For a woman whose pregnancy is complicated by heart disease,

    _____ is essential.

17. Twins usually deliver before term because _____.

18. Under the category of age and parity, the major high-risk groups are women

    under the age of _____ or over the age of _____,

    as well as women who have given birth to more than _____

    babies.

19. Indicate two previous pregnancy problems that would classify a woman as high risk.

    a. _____

    b. _____

20. Medical conditions that would classify a pregnant woman as high risk include

    _____ and _____.

21. In the eclampsias an elevated blood pressure is detected

    _____ the twentieth week of pregnancy. In the chronic

    hypertensive states of pregnancy an elevated blood pressure is detected

    _____ the twentieth week of pregnancy.

Supply the correct answer(s) for items 22 through 33.

22. Women experiencing abortion, ectopic pregnancy, or gestational trophoblastic
    neoplasm (GTN) are also experiencing loss of their expected baby. Explain
    supportive nursing care for these women.

    _____

    _____

    _____

23. Why is close medical supervision necessary for the pregnant diabetic woman?

    _____

    _____

    _____

24. Which is the most common variety of diabetes in pregnancy?

    _____

    _____

    _____

25. Nursing responsibilities with families who have Rh incompatibilities include:

    a. _____

    b. _____

    c. _____

26. List three common causes of bleeding in early pregnancy:

    a. _____

b. _____

c. _____

27. List two common causes of bleeding in late pregnancy:

    a. _____

    b. _____

28. What are some reasons why women may *not* seek prenatal care?

    a. _____

    b. _____

    c. _____

29. The high-risk pregnant woman has to accomplish specific tasks to achieve stability in a complicated pregnancy. How can the nurse help this woman and her family adapt? Propose a plan of care for a woman and her family when the woman has been hospitalized in the eighth month of pregnancy for treatment of severe preeclampsia. Use a separate sheet for your plan.

_____

_____

_____

30. What would the nurse advise a woman who wants to breast-feed twins?

_____

_____

_____

31. What are three signs of early preeclampsia?

    a. _____

    b. _____

    c. _____

32. When a woman with severe preeclampsia has been admitted to the hospital, the nursing care should include:

    a. _____

    b. _____

    c. _____

    d. _____

    e. _____

    f. _____

    g. _____

    h. _____

    i. _____

33. The classifications of placenta previa are:

    a. _____

    b. _____

    c. _____

34. Match Column A with Column B. Each item in Column B may be used more than once or not at all.

Column A

_____ 1. eclampsia

_____ 2. severe preeclampsia

_____ 3. mild preeclampsia

Column B

a. blood pressure 160/110

b. 3+ to 4+ proteinuria

c. elevation of blood pressure

d. generalized edema

e. convulsions

35. Match Column A with Column B. Each item in Column B may be used once or more than once.

Column A

_____ 1. "morning sickness"

_____ 2. hyperemesis gravidarum

_____ 3. ectopic pregnancy

_____ 4. placenta previa

_____ 5. abruptio placentae

Column B

a. uterine tenderness and rigidity

b. nausea and vomiting

c. abdominal pain on one side and vaginal bleeding

d. dehydration and electrolyte imbalance

e. painless bleeding

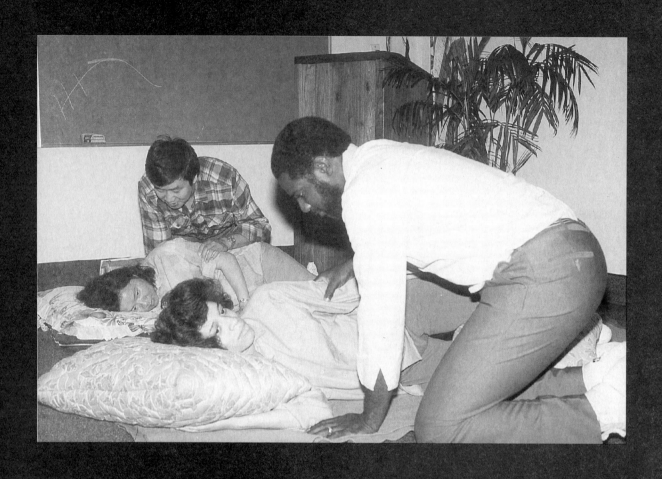

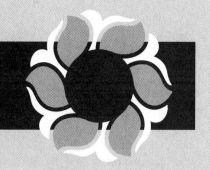

6

PREPARATION FOR CHILDBIRTH

GOALS

This chapter is designed to provide the reader with information that will:
- promote awareness of common factors inherent in all methods of childbirth preparation.
- increase appreciation of the need for physical and psychological support for the laboring family.
- develop an understanding of the role of the support team with both prepared and unprepared childbearing families.

STUDENT OBJECTIVES

After studying this chapter, you should be able to:
1. List the major components that most instructors include in their preparation for childbirth classes.
2. Describe at least five helpful actions the nurse may use when offering verbal or "hands on" support to a couple who have prepared for labor.
3. Demonstrate the following specific breathing techniques widely used in preparation for childbirth classes:
   a. active progressive relaxation
   b. concentration-relaxation
   c. slow-paced breathing
   d. modified-paced breathing
   e. patterned-paced breathing
   f. expulsion breathing
4. Describe types of classes offered in preparation for parenting programs.
5. Identify four benefits of continuous emotional and physical support during labor and explain the role of a doula in providing this support.

HISTORICAL OVERVIEW

Since colonial times in America, women have shared their information on childbirth with other women. In the nineteenth century male physicians gradually came to be recognized as experts to whom women went for information about birth. By 1900 physicians finally usurped women's age-old skills concerning childbirth and became, for many, the sole authorities.

However, as early as 1908 the American Red Cross recognized the need to teach mothers about hygiene and good health practices. In the United States the first formal classes in childbirth education were offered nationally in 1913 by the American Red Cross. Maternity Center Association in New York City followed with classes for expectant parents as early as 1919. Literature on these early attempts at childbirth education revealed that the first classes for childbirth education were developed out of a public health need to teach mothers basic hygiene.

An English physician, Dr. Grantly Dick-Read, published two books in which he theorized that pain in childbirth is caused by a fear-tension-pain syndrome. His first book, *Natural Childbirth*, was published in 1933. Dick-Read's second book, *Childbirth Without Fear*, was published in the United States in 1944. Dick-Read's work became the foundation for the first organized programs of preparation for childbirth and teacher training. The first of such groups to organize was the International Childbirth Education Association (ICEA) founded in 1960.

At about the same time, the Lamaze method, also known as psychoprophylaxis (PPM), was gaining popularity in the United States. PPM opened new perspectives into preparation for childbirth by emphasizing mind control. Marjorie Karmel introduced PPM to the United States in her book, *Thank You, Dr. Lamaze*, which was published in the United States in 1959. Others have written extensively on PPM. This system grew out of Pavlov's work on the higher nervous activity of humans and animals in which he proposed that every vital activity of an organism is a complex reflex process capable of conditioning. In 1960 the American Society for Psychoprophylaxis in Obstetrics (ASPO) was formed in New York as a national organization to promote use of the Lamaze method and prepare teachers of the method.

A Denver obstetrician, Dr. Robert Bradley, published *Husband-Coached Childbirth* in 1965. In this book he advocates what he proposes is the true natural childbirth, without any form of anesthesia or analgesia and with a "husband-coach" and breathing techniques for labor. The American Academy of Husband-Coached Childbirth (AAHCC) was founded to make the Bradley method available and to prepare teachers.

Of the other techniques developed, the most widely known include the work of Kitzinger and Wright, developed in England. Wright's work is based on PPM, described as "levels of breathing." Kitzinger's work is designed around a psychosexual approach, which proposes that birth is a sexual experience. As such, birth is perceived as a normal physiologic process in which the woman works in harmony with her body.

Inevitably, components of one method have been combined with those of others until there are now numerous methods of childbirth preparation. Hypnosis, autogenic training, yogi childbirth, the Gamper method, the Swiss method, and Russian hydrotherapy are examples of the proliferation in techniques to prepare for birth. Although the techniques are more alike than different, explanations of their effectiveness can vary dramatically. (Refer to Appendix H for a list of organizations involved in preparation for childbirth.)

EFFECTIVENESS OF METHODS

Childbirth pain indicates physical effort caused by the uterus contracting and labor progressing. A brief review of the gate control theory of pain provides an explanation for how childbirth preparation is presumed to work. According to this theory, the pain impulses that are transmitted from nerve receptors in the spinal cord to the brain can be modified or altered. Only a limited number of sensations or messages can travel through nerve pathways at one time. Stimulating sensory nerve pathways with distractors such as touch, rubbing, scratching, and vibration can close the gate to pain signals. In addition to blocking the sensory nerve pathways as described, it is also theorized that there are descending control systems so that signals from the brain can close the gate and block pain signals. Utilizing this theory, focusing strategies such as breathing techniques, music, utilizing focal points, and imagery would be effective in decreasing pain perception.

Various studies have been undertaken to determine the physiologic effectiveness of prepared childbirth methods in terms of amount of pain experienced during labor and birth, maternal and fetal complications, and length of labor. When reviewing these studies, contradictory findings can be found concerning physiologic effects of prepared childbirth techniques. Some theorists claim that childbirth preparation can alter the primary pain stimulus arising from the contracting uterus. Others believe that childbirth preparation can only modify the interpretation and perception of pain signals. In the past, few studies were sufficiently well controlled to allow conclusive findings.

Recently childbirth education researchers have started to address these experimental problems. In studies conducted in the past decade, relaxation, presence of a support person, and sensory transformation (the use of imagination to transform painful sensations into pleasant feelings) have been found to be the most helpful in dealing with the pain of labor and birth. Evidence from these studies does suggest that childbirth preparation can decrease the use of analgesic medication and perception of pain. However, there is no clear evidence for the effect of prenatal classes on the duration of labor.

Diminishing fear and learning to cope with the experiences of labor and birth are two important contributions of preparation for childbirth. Women can be taught to experience and to accept the pain of labor as a useful message. Women can also be taught to use constructive ways to relieve the pain so that they emerge from the birth experience with a new sense of strength and self-esteem.

Most childbirth preparation techniques taught today have three components: (1) psychophysical techniques, (2) psychological components, and (3) intellectual components.

METHODS OF CHILDBIRTH PREPARATION

Dick-Read Method: Childbirth Without Fear
Psychophysical techniques

Relaxation and controlled breathing are taught as a way to cope with contractions. Dr. Dick-Read basically recommended three techniques: deep breathing in both abdominal respirations and thoracic respiration, shallow breathing, and breath-holding for the second stage of labor.

Psychological component

According to Dick-Read: "Fear, tension, and pain are three veils opposed to the natural design which have been concerned with preparation for and attendance at childbirth. If fear, tension, and pain go hand in hand, then it must be necessary to relieve tension and to overcome fear in order to eliminate pain. The implementation of my theory demonstrates the methods by which fear can be overcome, tension may be eliminated and replaced by physical and mental relaxation" (Dick-Read, 1959).

Intellectual component

Dick-Read's program educates women to exchange understanding and confidence for fear of the unknown. Adequate prenatal education includes information on

nutrition, basic hygiene, and labor and birth. The approach is holistic, and recognizes that the pregnant woman has been influenced in a complex way by her biology and by her social and cultural environment.

Lamaze (PPM) Method
Psychophysical techniques

Controlled muscular relaxation, breathing techniques, exercises, and expulsion techniques compose the Lamaze method. PPM emphasizes conditioning and repetition.

Psychological component

According to this method, pain in labor is a conditioned response and women can be conditioned not to experience this pain. The essential elements of Lamaze include an external focus of attention and a series of relaxation and breathing exercises with a supportive coach. The presence of a "labor coach" is integral to the Lamaze method.

Intellectual component

The Lamaze method emphasizes understanding the body and how it works so that the woman can learn neuromuscular control techniques to cope with labor.

Bradley Method

The basic foundation of the Bradley method is the use of relaxation as the primary tool for labor.

Psychophysical techniques

Breath control, slow diaphragmatic breathing, and general body relaxation are used in the Bradley method. Working in harmony with the body is emphasized.

Psychological component

The importance of the husband's support is foremost in this method, and the Bradley method has been labeled "husband-coached childbirth." Women are helped to find their own ways to relax and give birth in their own fashion. Sequenced breathing techniques are not taught by Bradley teachers.

Intellectual component

Preparation for birth teaching concentrates on minimizing the need for analgesics or anesthetics. Bradley techniques stress mind-body integration.

Most methods include one or all of the following:
1. Relaxation and breathing techniques
2. Pushing techniques and second-stage coping techniques
3. Good posture and body mechanics
4. Genital and pelvic floor awareness and exercises
5. Physical exercises (squatting, tailor sits, pelvic rock, etc.)
6. Teaching about physical happenings and emotional responses of pregnancy

Finally, an umbrella covering all methods of preparation for birth is the philosophy that knowledge can liberate people from the chains of fear of the unknown. Therefore all childbearing people need knowledge of pregnancy, birth, and parenting, and positive information to replace myths and superstitions. When people are informed of all the options and choices open to them, they should be able to make informed decisions, thus becoming intelligent consumers of maternity care. The coping strategies that are learned for labor and birth can also help people to deal with the challenges of early parenting.

NURSING ACTIONS

Even if the laboring woman and her partner (or family or support persons) are well prepared, the nurse is still an important member of the childbirth team. Labor is a crisis time, and all people, no matter how well prepared, enter labor with some level of anxiety. Women respond differently to labor depending on the pain associated with their labor, fears, coping styles, and goals and expectations. Remember that labor is stress even if the couple is prepared. They need you. Do not leave them totally alone. Provide support when they need it—and privacy when they need it.

The following are some helpful actions the nurse may use to offer both verbal and "hands on" support during labor:

1. Encourage moving around during labor. If labor is progressing slowly, walking may accelerate it. Changing positions frequently (from sitting to standing to hands and knees to lying down to walking or rocking) will help relieve pain.
2. Talk of contractions, not pains.
3. Relax and get as near to the woman's level as possible. If she is lying down, sit by the bedside. Do not tower over her. Touch! Make eye contact.
4. The labor bed can provide for comfortable positions. She should never be flat on her back because the weight of the uterine contents puts too much pressure on major blood vessels, thus reducing the blood flow back to the brain. Use pillows to support all dependent body parts.

5. Use comfort measures such as cold cloths, backrubs, warm showers, baths, and massages. Suggest ice chips, water, and fruit juices for hydration. Keep the room warm, with bright lights dimmed but still providing enough light in the room for her to see the "focal point" if she is using one. Play relaxing music.
6. Carry on a conversation only between contractions if necessary.
7. Talk with the father or other support person. Give reassurance and remember that the father has needs for nourishment, rest, and elimination as well as the mother. Let him know where the bathroom is and where he may purchase food. Reassure him that you will stay with the laboring woman if he needs to leave for a while to tend to his own needs.
8. Do not ask irrelevant questions. Keep talk to a minimum. It uses energy needed to cope. Be aware of attitudinal changes as labor progresses.
9. Keep your voice well modulated at all times. Remain calm and encouraging.
10. Remind the mother to urinate frequently. A full bladder can slow the descent of the baby.
11. Encourage the mother to rest between contractions.
12. Keep the couple and family members informed of what is happening: how many centimeters dilated, station, effacement, and fetal position.
13. Assure the mother that she is doing well, offer encouragement, agree with her if she says it hurts but offer positive comments too.
14. To conserve the mother's energy, encourage her to use the lowest pattern of breathing that is effective.
15. Breathe with the woman if she is faltering. Encourage her to follow your breathing. Guide her in her breathing: "Breathe with me—that's the way—good—stay with it—it's going away—rest—good."
16. Use words and touch to help her relax. Use a soothing voice and phrases such as "Release," "Let go," and "Loosen."
17. Look for signs of relaxation: soft, heavy muscles; loose joints; curved fingers; and an expression of peace.
18. Do not distract her during contractions. Wait until a contraction is over to do a nursing procedure.
19. Remember that the time period just before complete dilatation may be the most intense time in labor. Because the woman may fall asleep between contractions, they may overpower her. She may become very irritable.

20. During the actual birth stage, trust her and work with her body. This is not an athletic contest; the goal is pelvic floor release and relaxation. Encourage a series of quick breaths, holding each one for 5 to 6 seconds while pushing and then again. Take a new breath while maintaining abdominal pressure. Give verbal support such as: "Beautiful," "Go with it," "Let it flow," "Open up below," "Soft and loose," "Open the door," "Relax your bottom!" Avoid shouting "push, push, push" at the mother. You might even give the woman a mirror so that she can watch her own progress as she pushes the baby out.

21. As you encourage relaxation, encourage release toward your hand on her body. This will help the woman to increase her body awareness and to release tension by utilizing touch relaxation.

22. Always encourage the breathing that feels right for each woman. She may have practiced one type of breathing before labor only to find that it is not helpful during a certain part of labor. If this happens, be flexible. Encourage her to find what is working for her and to stick with it.

23. There is no failure. Some people who have prepared faithfully for a "natural" childbirth will not be able to achieve that goal because of circumstances beyond their control. They may need analgesia, anesthesia, or a cesarean birth. If they are disappointed, encourage them to talk about their disappointment and then help them to work through it by emphasizing that there is no failure. When they have achieved a meaningful and safe birth, they have achieved their goal.

24. And last, but maybe most important, be constantly and consistently aware of the needs of the fetus throughout the entire labor process. When the couple have prepared diligently for labor and are extremely intent on what they are doing, it is often easy for the support person to get caught up in that intensity and feel reluctant to do any procedure that might "spoil" their experience. Continually think of yourself as a fetal advocate, and use your knowledge and skills to make sound judgments that will lead to a safe birth experience for all family members, especially the baby.

CHILDBIRTH EXERCISES

The nurse who has a basic understanding of the exercises and breathing techniques widely used in preparation for childbirth classes will be able to work effectively with laboring people. Therefore you should practice each of the prepared childbirth techniques that follow. You may find it easier and more fun to practice by working with a fellow student. One of you pretends to be the woman in labor and the other assumes the role of support person. Find a quiet, comfortable place where you will not be disturbed for about an hour. Because the best way to practice is on the floor, you will probably be most comfortable on a carpeted floor or on a mat.

Exercises for the Pelvic Floor (Kegel Exercise)

Many women are not aware of the muscles of the pelvic floor until it is pointed out that these are the muscles used during urination and sexual intercourse and are therefore consciously controlled. Because pelvic floor muscles ring the outlet through which the baby must pass, it is important that they be exercised because an exercised muscle can stretch and contract readily at the time of birth. To locate these muscles, a woman can practice stopping the flow and starting it again while urinating.

Once the muscles are located, this exercise needs to be practiced many times a day to be effective. A good time to practice is during trips to the bathroom, but additional practice at other times is also beneficial. Because it is not obvious when a woman is practicing, she might practice anytime and anywhere.

The procedure is to tighten the pelvic floor muscles as in holding back urine, hold for 10 seconds, and then release. Or think of the vagina as an elevator and practice ascending and descending slowly. This exercise can be done 10 times in a row, 5 to 10 times or more per day. Although some people recommend doing this exercise as many as 100 times in a row, this only fatigues the pelvic floor muscles. After delivery, this exercise helps the pelvic floor muscles return to normal and should be begun immediately after delivery.

Active Progressive Relaxation

Relaxation is the foundation for all other techniques in labor. The first step in learning how to relax is knowing the difference between relaxation and tension in order to recognize tension during labor (Fig. 6-1).

1. Find a position that can support your body completely. Do not have a part of you resting on any other part, and do not have any of your joints straight. Support all your dependent parts by placing a pillow under head, knees, and arms if necessary. (See Fig. 6-1.) Allow your eyes to close.

2. Begin with a cleansing breath of deep inhalation followed by slow exhalation by sighing or blowing. Breathe slowly and naturally. Focus on re-

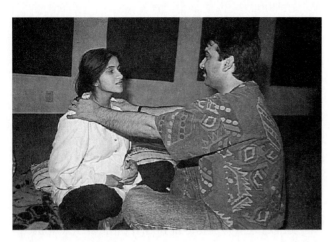

Figure 6-1 Practicing relaxation. *(Courtesy Lifecircle, Marjorie M. Pyle, Costa Mesa, Calif.)*

leasing and allowing yourself to become more comfortable each time you exhale. When you first begin to learn relaxation, it is important that you relax systematically by tightening muscles in a structured order and then letting them go slowly so that you can feel the contrast.

a. Starting with your left foot, tighten it and then relax it. Tighten your left leg next, keeping your left foot relaxed. Now relax your left foot and leg.

b. Next tighten your left hand and then relax it. Tighten your left arm, keeping your left hand relaxed. Now relax your left arm and hand.

c. At this point, your left foot, left leg, left hand, and left arm should be relaxed. They should feel warm and loose.

d. Now work on the right side of your body in the same order: right foot to right leg and right hand to right arm, as you exhale slowly and deeply.

e. When both feet, legs, hands, and arms are relaxed, gently and firmly pull in on the abdomen; draw the buttocks tightly together; and then release gradually. Allow the tension to melt away.

f. Continue to breathe slowly and easily, trying to make your mind a blank slate. Don't permit thoughts to enter in. If you find this difficult, concentrate completely on one simple, pleasant thought, excluding all others. Count sheep, if that helps.

g. Now draw your shoulders and back firmly upward and release slowly, allowing warmth to replace the tightness.

h. Last, make a face by tightening your face and neck muscles, pinching your mouth and eyes closed. Release your mouth, neck, and eyelids,

letting the lower jaw fall loosely. Now work on the upper half of your body. Draw your shoulders and back firmly upward, clench fists and tighten arms. Release slowly. Finally, tighten your face and neck muscles by frowning, clenching your eyes closed, wrinkling your nose upward, clenching your jaws, drawing your lips back over your teeth, and pressing neck muscles together. Release your jaws, lips, neck, cheeks, and nose, letting your lower jaw fall slack and your tongue hang loose. Let your eyelids and brow fall smooth so that your eyes remain gently closed. Feel the tension flow away from your face.

When you have loosened and released all the muscles in your body, concentrate on sights, sounds, or sensations especially appealing to you.

Let your support person's touch or massage be your signal to loosen and release the area touched. Imagine that the tension is being drawn out of your body by this person's hands. Release the muscle tension to your partner's hands. Accept this touch as a nonverbal message saying "Relax" and "I care."

Once fully relaxed, take a minute to enjoy the good feeling, experiencing warmth and well-being throughout your body. Conclude this relaxation exercise by taking in a deep, relaxing breath and feeling energized as you exhale.

To return to a normal state of wakefulness, gradually move your legs and feet, then your hands and arms, as you open your eyes. When you are ready, stand up. You will retain a relaxed feeling as you continue with the practice of the following childbirth exercises.

When entirely relaxed, your bones, muscles, and joints feel heavy at first; later there is little or no feeling. It is as though you had "melted away" or sunk into the floor. When a woman uses this controlled-relaxation technique during contractions, much energy is conserved, and the working uterus is enabled to do a more efficient job (Fig. 6-2).

Different positions will be necessary for comfort as the baby moves through the birth canal. Relaxation should be practiced in many positions, including standing, sitting, semisitting, getting on hands and knees, squatting, and lying on your side.

Music can establish an inviting environment and serve as a pleasing distraction from the stress or pain of labor (especially early labor). Familiar and well-loved music increases endorphin production, which relieves pain by acting on specific receptors in the brain.

Concentration-Relaxation Exercise

Lie on the floor; put a pillow under your head and another under your knees so you are completely sup-

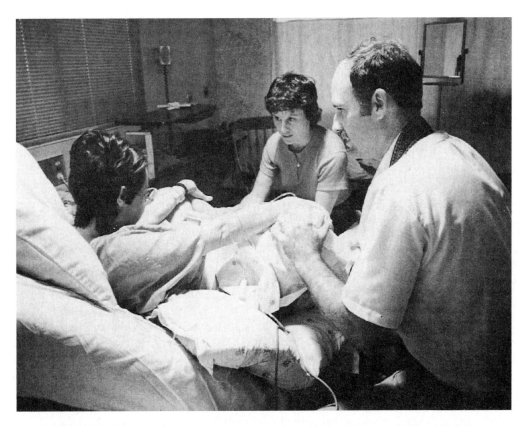

Figure 6-2 Team work. *(Photo by Paul O'Mara, Courtesy Vance Simpson and Sharon Baker.)*

ported. Relax your body using the relaxation techniques just practiced. With the rest of your body as completely relaxed as possible, contract your right arm: tighten your shoulder, elbow, fist, and raise your arm. Release it; let your entire arm go limp and let it fall to the floor. Contract your left arm in the same way; release. Contract your right leg, tighten your entire leg; release. Contract your left leg; release. Contract your right arm and left leg; release. Do not tighten the other limbs. *Continue to keep the rest of your body relaxed.*

If you are practicing with a partner, the support person should check to see if the opposite limbs are relaxed when they should be; for example, if the right arm and left leg are contracted, the left arm and right leg should be totally relaxed. (Practice by alternately contracting and relaxing opposite limbs.)

Slow-Paced Breathing

Slow-paced breathing is the easiest and most relaxing of the techniques and is used in early labor. Slow-paced breathing provides good oxygenation and aids relaxation.

Sit comfortably on the floor with legs relaxed and pillows supporting all dependent parts. Assume a contraction is beginning. Take a deep *cleansing breath* (inhale through your nose and exhale through your mouth). This serves as a signal to relax and focus and gives both the mother and baby an extra boost of oxygen. Following the cleansing breath, breathe deliberately and slowly with your chest, inhaling through your nose and exhaling through your mouth. The rate is approximately half the number of the resting breathing rate (six to nine breaths per minute, excluding cleansing breaths). Relax completely and focus on an object in the room or your support person as you breathe. This will be your focal point. Keep your breathing quiet and abdominal muscles relaxed. When the contraction is over, take another cleansing breath and rest. (To begin a "practice" contraction, simply look at the second hand on a clock or watch and choose a starting time. Allow the contraction to last 60 seconds.)

After you can breathe comfortably with slow-paced breathing, use a light circular stroke *(effleurage)* to massage the abdomen to the rhythm of your breathing. Hold your hands just above your pubic bone and stroke with your fingertips upward over your abdomen while breathing in and down again to the starting point while blowing out (Fig. 6-3).

(The support person could give definite directions at the beginning and end of the contraction by signaling "contraction begins" and "contraction ends" and should check for relaxation of all muscles during the contrac-

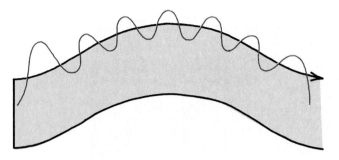

Figure 6-3 Slow-paced breathing.

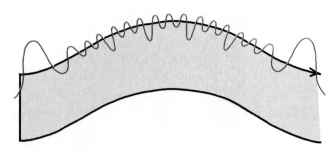

Figure 6-5 Patterned-paced breathing.

Patterned-Paced Breathing

Patterned-paced breathing is for the transition stage of labor, which is often the most stressful time. It is performed at the same rate as modified-paced breathing but with blowing out softly at intervals (Fig. 6-5).

Begin by taking a cleansing breath. Then take four light, shallow breaths, counting as you exhale—"1-2-3-4." Now breathe in another shallow breath and as you exhale, blow out with a small puff of air. Return to light, shallow breaths and blow out according to the 1-2-3-4 pattern established. The rhythmic sound has a calming effect.

Transition contractions may last 60 to 90 seconds, with only short intervals between them. The support person may find it necessary to encourage two or three forceful BLOWS to block an early urge to push.

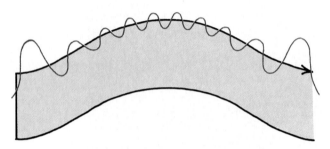

Figure 6-4 Modified-paced breathing.

tion, while offering encouragement and a concerned touch.)

Modified-Paced Breathing

Modified-paced breathing occurs at a rate faster than the mother's normal rate. It should not exceed twice the resting rate (Fig. 6-4).

Take a cleansing breath and relax. Breathe faster than your normal rate with shallow inhalation followed by shallow exhalation. Breathe quietly. Listen to your breath move in and out.

Shift back to slow-paced breathing as the practice contraction ends. Take a cleansing breath and rest.

After you have mastered this breathing, adjust your timing to the "wavelike" flow of contractions. Start breathing slowly as the contraction begins, then speed up your breathing as the contraction increases in strength, and slow down again as it goes away. Remember to keep your eyes open and focus on an object in the room while you practice and keep your body relaxed. If you should feel lightheaded, you may be hyperventilating. Simply rebreathe your own air by breathing into a paper bag or into your hands.

The support person could continue to signal "contraction begins" and "contraction ends," timing the contraction to last 60 seconds.

In addition to being the timer, the support person should continue to check for complete relaxation and offer verbal and "hands on" support.

Expulsion Breathing

To push the baby down through the vagina, when the contraction begins, assume a comfortable position. Because of the detrimental effects of the supine position, semisitting, kneeling, squatting, lying on one's side, standing, and semistanding are all positions women choose. Remember that to push effectively along the axis of the curved birth canal, you must be in a position complementing this curve. The baby moves down, forward, and out as though descending on a sliding board. Breathe in and out very slowly (so as not to waste your energy by pushing too soon). Again, breathe in slowly and hold your breath, fixing your diaphragm downward, and push downward using your abdominal muscles. Again, remember to keep the muscles of your pelvic floor relaxed. Continue to push for the count of 5 or 6, then take another breath. Repeat this effort until the contraction is gone. When the contraction has ended, breathe in and out several times, assume a comfortable position, and rest (Fig. 6-6).

Sometimes you will hear people helping women push by saying, "Push as though you were going to have a bowel movement." Remember this woman is pushing a baby out through the vagina and needs to relax the vagina and pelvic floor to do this. Talking to her about

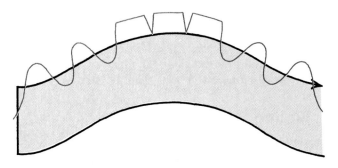

Figure 6-6 Expulsion breathing.

having a bowel movement may only serve to confuse her pushing efforts.

Also, sometimes you will hear helping people ask a woman to "hold her breath" and push as long as she can before coming up for air. When a woman holds her breath, there is greatly reduced exchange of gases across the placenta to the fetus. This reduction in perfusion could be dangerous to the fetus by causing a reduced oxygen supply. So when you push or help women to push, encourage them to push as *they* feel like pushing, without holding their breath more than 5 to 6 seconds at a time, if at all possible.

After you have practiced each of these six specific breathing techniques, exchange roles so that the support person becomes the laboring woman and vice versa.

Because these techniques may not be exactly like those being taught in your community, attend a series of preparation for birth classes so that you can become acquainted with what expectant parents are being taught.

Now that you have experienced breathing patterns for birth, you are probably thinking that preparation for childbirth is a lot of work—and you are right. Breathing techniques are only a part of the birth preparation and should be practiced daily in the last weeks of pregnancy. In addition to the breathing and relaxation skills, childbirth preparation classes usually include information on the anatomy and physiology of labor, the mechanisms of labor, pain relief methods available, ways of coping with the stress of labor, characteristics and care of the newborn, and of course, emotional preparation for parenting.

Childbirth preparation classes further emphasize self-responsibility. A benefits versus risks teaching approach is utilized, presenting current, research-based, accurate information. People are presented with options and choices available for labor and birth and encouraged to choose those that they believe are right for them. Assisting in preparing a birth plan is an important function of the childbirth educator. Also, key factors in selecting health care providers (physicians and mid-

wives) and a place for birth are discussed. There is also opportunity to practice communication skills and support their use. As a result people are empowered and helped to have the kind of birth experience they choose.

PREPARATION FOR PARENTING PROGRAMS

Classes in preparation for the birth itself are only a small part of an extensive preparation for parenthood program that should be available to all childbearing people, whether single or in couples. Such a program recognizes that pregnancy is not a disease state but is a state of wellness, during which individuals move from the role of expectant parents to the role and responsibilities of parents of a new baby. Pregnancy and parenting education programs are part of a continuum that begins before conception and extends through early parenting.

A typical preparation for parenthood program recognizes that childbearing people have different interests and information needs as the pregnancy progresses; consequently, the program is designed to meet the concerns of those involved before pregnancy, at the three major stages of pregnancy, and after birth.

The National Institutes of Health/Health and Human Services (NIH/HHS) Expert Panel on the Content of Prenatal Care has recommended that prenatal care begin before conception, preferably within 1 year of a planned pregnancy. We have known for a long time that pregnancy may be too late for the expectant mother and father to correct poor health habits or avoid teratogens. Many risks to women and their developing infants can be reduced or eliminated if identified before pregnancy.

Preconception Classes

Preconception classes, risk assessment, and counseling offer a positive, preventive approach to women's health care. One of the prime objectives of these classes is to help women and couples decide whether to reproduce.

Classes include discussion of behavior and health considerations that may affect conception and pregnancy (importance of good nutrition and avoidance of alcohol, nontherapeutic drugs, and cigarettes), personal and family medical and genetic factors, reproductive anatomy and physiology, early signs of pregnancy, the importance and benefits of prenatal care, timing and readiness for pregnancy, and choosing a health care professional and working within the system.

Early Pregnancy ("Early Bird") Classes

Early pregnancy classes provide fundamental information about early fetal growth, development, physiologic and emotional changes of pregnancy, human sexuality, and the nutritional needs of the mother and fetus. In addition, appropriate exercise, environmental hazards, and birthing options are discussed.

Midpregnancy Classes

Midpregnancy classes provide information on preparation for breast- and bottle-feeding, basic hygiene, self-help for discomforts, health maintenance (rest, exercise, nutrition), infant health, and parenting. Infant stimulation concepts can be taught in midpregnancy to help facilitate the development of prenatal bonding and parenting skills.

Late Pregnancy Classes

Late pregnancy classes include the preparation for childbirth classes already discussed.

Throughout the series of classes there is discussion of the support systems that people can use during pregnancy and after birth so that they can function independently and effectively by developing their own health awareness and health maintenance behavior. During all the classes the open expression of feelings and concerns about any aspect of pregnancy, birth, and parenting is welcomed.

After Birth Classes ("What Do We Do Now?")

After birth classes include coping mechanisms for the reality of parenting, support systems, infant care and growth and development, family planning, human sexuality, community resources, adapting to new roles (wife/lover⇄mother and husband/lover⇄father), parent-infant interaction, and health promotion.

Preparation for parenthood programs are multiplying throughout the country as new parents tell friends, neighbors, and families about their prepared births, and health care reform emphasizes a wellness and prevention approach to childbirth and parenting. It is exciting to watch well-informed, interested people become active, intelligent consumers of health care. Table 6-1 presents a prenatal teaching guide.

Prenatal Classes for Repeat Parents

Prenatal classes for repeat parents are especially for expectant parents who already have children. The fo-

cus is on preparing the older child for the arrival of the new baby as well as reviewing previously used childbirth preparation techniques. In addition, the classes deal with the physical, social, and emotional changes unique to the growing family (Fig. 6-7).

Sibling Preparation Classes

Sibling preparation classes are designed to ease the anxiety children face when mother goes to the hospital or birth center to give birth. Children are prepared for the role of big brother or big sister, thereby enhancing the experience for the entire family (Fig. 6-8). A hospital or birth center tour is part of the class, children are shown what a newborn really looks like, and basic ways to help are explained.

Grandparenting Classes

The content of grandparenting classes includes looking at the changing role of being a grandparent. The role of grandparent is compared with and contrasted to the role of parent. The content includes an update on childbirth choices, the role of the father as active participant, and "new" infant care trends. The rights of grandparents are explored as well as changes in infant care philosophies and techniques.

Other Classes

Other classes in a comprehensive program might be on cesarean preparation, adolescent pregnancy and family classes, prenatal and postpartum exercise, pregnancy after 30, preparation for vaginal birth after cesarean (VBAC), blended families, breast-feeding, infant massage, and parenting and adult living. There are also orientation classes to specific hospital programs, tours of the birth facility, and opportunities to meet the facility's staff. Involving families in mother and baby care programs can be an effective educational approach.

Although the emphasis in this chapter has been on labor support for the prepared couple, not all couples come to labor prepared and not all laboring women have partners for support. The helpful actions for labor support presented are still very useful for all laboring people. However, if there is no family or friend to support the laboring woman, then the nurse's role becomes even more crucial. A woman should never have to labor alone. If the realities of staffing shortages on busy days prevent your constant attendance to women laboring alone, you could seek labor support persons from community volunteers.

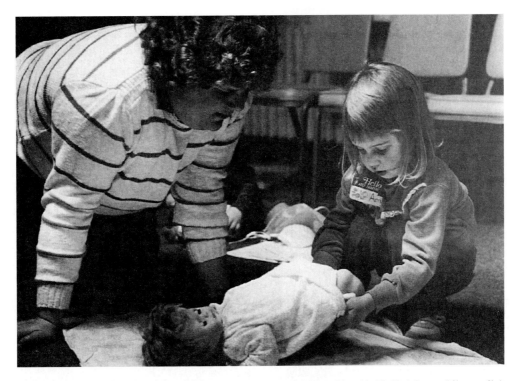

Figure 6-7 Preparing the older child. *(Courtesy The Birthplace at Riverside Medical Center, Minneapolis.)*

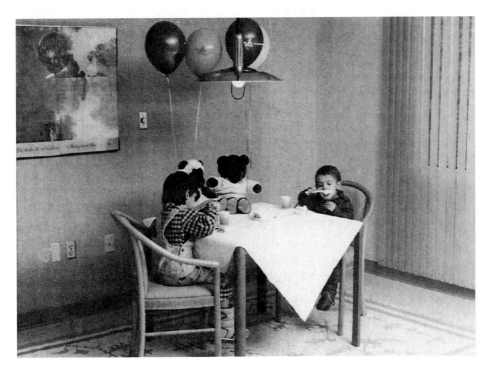

Figure 6-8 Sibling party. *(Courtesy Valley Hospital and Medical Center, Spokane, Wash.)*

TABLE 6-1
Prenatal Teaching Guide

1st-12th Weeks	12th-24th Weeks	24th-32nd Weeks	32nd-36th Weeks	36th week to term
Woman more concerned with herself, physical changes with pregnancy, and her feelings about the pregnancy	Woman has usually resolved the issue of the pregnancy and becomes more aware of the fetus as a person	Woman becomes more interested in baby's needs as a corollary to her own needs now and after birth	Woman anticipates approaching labor and caring for baby after birth	Woman should feel "ready" for labor and for the assumption of care-taking responsibilities for baby, even though she may feel anxious about both of these as well
Changes that are normal for pregnancy	Growth of fetus	Fetal growth and status	Fetal growth and activity	Review signs of labor (or teach)
Breast fullness	Movement	Presentation and position	Personal hygiene	Review or continue
Urinary frequency	FHT	Well-being—FHT	Positions of comfort	instruction regarding
Nausea and vomiting	Personal hygiene	Personal hygiene	Rest and activity	relaxation and breathing
Fatigue	Comfortable clothing	Comfortable clothing	Vaginal discharge	techniques
Emotional adjustments	Breast care and	Body mechanics and	Sexual activity	Finalize home preparations
EDC—calculate and explain	supportive bra	posture	Alleviation of discomfort	Anticipation of
Compare with uterine size	Recreation, travel	Positions of comfort	Backache	hospitalization
Expectation for care	Vaginal discharge	Physical and emotional	Round ligament pain	Admission
Initial visit	Employment or school plans	changes	Constipation or	Labor and birth plans
Subsequent visits	Method of feeding baby	Sexual needs and changes	hemorrhoids	Care in labor
Clinic appointments	Breast or bottle	Intercourse	Leg ache or edema	Medication and
Need for iron and folic acid	Give literature re methods	Alleviation of backache	Dyspnea	anesthesia available
Resources available	Avoidance or alleviation of	Braxton Hicks contractions	Recognition of "false	Postpartum care
Education	Backache	Dyspnea	labor"—Braxton Hicks	Supplies needed: bra,
	Constipation	Round ligament pain	contractions	

Dental evaluation
Medical service
Social service
Emergency room
Danger signs
Drugs, self-medication
Spotting, bleeding
Cramping, pain
Evaluate life style
Stop smoking, drinking
Safe sex STDs
Seat belt usage

Hemorrhoids
Leg ache, varicosities, edema, cramping
Round ligament pain
Nutritional guidance
Weight gain
Balanced diet
Special nutritional needs
Danger signs
Physiological changes
Birthing options LDR
LDRP,
Birthing centers
Infant stimulation
Bonding
Attachment

Leg ache or edema
Confirm infant's feeding plans
Prepare for breast- or bottle-feeding
Nipple preparation
Massage and expression of breast
Preparation for baby
Supplies
Household assistance
Danger signs
Pre-eclampsia
Headache, excessive swelling, blurred vision
Tubal ligations (papers prepared ahead)
Selection of infant's care provider
Pediatrician
Family Practice Provider
Nurse Practitioner

How to cope and "practice" with these
Nature of "true labor" signs—Difference between "bloody show" and bleeding
What happens during labor
Labor contractions and progress
What she will experience
Relaxation techniques
Breathing techniques
Abdominal
Accelerated pattern
Panting and pushing
Involvement of husband or significant other
Provision for needs of other children
Anticipation of baby
Care for children at home while mother is in hospital

personal items, money
Family visitation
Tour of maternity unit
Confirm plans to get to hospital; care of other children
When to go and where
Consider family planning needs
Emergency arrangements
Precipitate delivery
Premature rupture of membranes with or without contractions
Care away from home
Vaginal bleeding
Newborn screening procedures
Infant care
Feeding
Car seats

Modified from Roberts J: Prenatal teaching guide, *J Obstet Gynecol Neonatal Nurs* 5:17-20, May/June 1976.

Childbirth Companions

Randomized trials of continuous emotional and physical support during labor have demonstrated a significant effect on reducing the stress of labor. Findings from these studies included the following benefits: shorter labor; significantly less pain medication; and fewer medical interventions, including cesarean section, forceps delivery, and epidural anesthesia. Many HMOs and health insurance plans are beginning to understand the medical and financial benefits of doula support and are funding doula services.

This continuous emotional and physical support can be provided by two types of women who are filling this role: The *doula* (from the Greek, meaning "in service of") provides physical and emotional support during birth but does not assess the mother's or fetus's well-being. The *monitrice* (from the French, meaning "to watch over attentively") combines nurturing skills with clinical assessment skills.

All childbirth companions have a minimum of 2 to 3 weeks of intensive training to be able to function as a support person to the mother before, during, and just after childbirth.

The childbirth companion can offer support to the laboring woman alone or to the couple. In many instances a woman needs not only the father or chosen partner but also a nurturing, experienced person such as a doula to help her through labor and birth.

It is recommended that the doula visit with the childbearing couple in the antepartum period in order to establish a rapport and discuss the labor expectations of the couple-to-be. The childbirth companion can provide support at home for early labor so that women do not have to go to the birth facility until in active labor. Once in the birth facility the childbirth companion can serve as the woman's advocate while providing support.

Women alone or couples who have not attended preparation for birth classes can learn relaxation and slow chest breathing techniques with your help during labor. Inform them that there are ways to cope with labor and that you can help them to learn these techniques right then and there. A motivated learner is the best learner, and most laboring women are highly motivated for relief of discomfort.

There are times when no matter how much support you offer and no matter what you do, the woman or couple will choose to request analgesia and/or anesthesia (total or partial). Each person has a right to labor and give birth in whatever way she chooses, provided the way is safe for both mother and baby. Success and failure should not be part of the vocabulary relating to participation in labor. Chapter 7 discusses analgesia and anesthesia used for labor and delivery and responsibilities of the helping person.

SUMMARY

This chapter has given you an opportunity to become familiar with some of the breathing techniques widely used in preparation for childbirth classes and support techniques for labor so that you will be able to work effectively with childbearing couples. Preparation for childbirth has been presented before the discussion of intrapartum care, which contains the mechanisms of birth, so that you can begin to get the feeling of the birth experience before you learn the mechanics of it. To become a skilled maternity nurse, you will need to develop feelings and sensitivity for this profound experience in addition to many skills.

BIBLIOGRAPHY

Association of Women's Health, Obstetric, and Neonatal Nurses: *Competencies and program guidelines for nurse providers of perinatal education,* Washington, DC, 1993, The Association.

Bing E: *Six practical lessons for an easier childbirth,* New York, 1982, Bantam Books.

Bradley R: *Husband-coached childbirth,* ed 3, New York, 1981, Harper & Row.

Broussard AB, Rich SK: Incorporating infant stimulation concepts into prenatal classes, *J Obstet Gynecol Neonatal Nurs* 19(5):381-187, 1990.

Chabon I: *Awake and aware,* New York, 1966, Dell.

Chertok L: Psychosomatic methods of preparation for birth, *Am J Obstet Gynecol* 98(5):698-707, 1967.

Copstick S, and others: A test of a common assumption regarding the use of antenatal training during labor, *J Psychosom Res* 29(2):215-218, 1985.

Davis-Floyd R E: *Birth as an American rite of passage,* Berkeley, 1992, University of California Press.

Dick-Read G: *Childbirth without fear,* ed 2, New York, 1959, Harper & Row.

Dick-Read G: *Childbirth without fear,* ed 5, New York, 1987, Harper & Row.

Hassid P: Textbook for childbirth educators, ed 2, Philadelphia, 1984, J B Lippincott.

Hathaway T, Hathaway M, editors: *The Bradley method,* Sherman Oaks, Calif, 1985, American Association of Husband Coached Childbirth.

Henderson JS: Effects of a prenatal teaching program on postpartum regeneration of the pubococcygeal muscle, *J Obstet Gynecol Neonatal Nurs* 12(6):403-408, 1983.

Herzfeld J: *Sense and sensibility in childbirth,* New York, 1985, WW Norton & Co.

Hetherington SE: A controlled study of the effect of prepared childbirth classes on obstetric outcomes, *Birth* 17(2):86, 1990.

Karmel M: *Thank you, Dr. Lamaze,* New York, 1983, Harper & Row.

Kitzinger S: *The experience of childbirth,* Middlesex, England, 1970, Pelican.

Klaus MH, Kennell JH, Klaus PH: *Mothering the mother,* New York, 1993, Addison-Wesley.

Lamaze F: *Painless childbirth: the Lamaze method,* Chicago, 1970, Henry Regnery.

Lindell SG: Education for childbirth: a time for change, *J Obstet Gynecol Neonatal Nurs* 18(2):108-112, 1988.

MacMahon AT: *All about childbirth,* ed 4, Maitland, Fla, 1994, Family Publications.

Mattson S, Smith JE, editors: *Core curriculum for maternal-newborn nursing,* Philadelphia, 1993, WB Saunders.

McKay S, Roberts J: Second stage labor: what is normal? *J Obstet Gynecol Neonatal Nurs* 14(2):101-106, 1985.

McKay S: Squatting: an alternative position for the second stage of labor, *MCN* 9:181-183, 1984.

Melzack R: The myth of painless childbirth (the John J Bonica Lecture), Obstet Gynecol Surv 40(5)297-298, 1985.

National Institutes of Health/Health and Human Services: *Caring for our future: the content of prenatal care—A report of the expert panel on the content of prenatal care,* 1989, Washington, DC, US Government Printing Office.

Nichols F, Humenick S: *Childbirth education: practice, research, theory,* Philadelphia, 1988, WB Saunders.

Noble E: *Childbirth with insight,* Boston, 1983, Houghton Mifflin.

O'Neill M Leclaire: *Creative childbirth: the Leclaire method of easy birthing through hypnosis and rational-intuitive thought,* Pacific Palisades, Calif, 1993, Papyrus.

Perez P, Snedeker C: *Special Women: the role of the professional labor assistant,* Seattle, 1990, Pennypress.

Redman BK: *The process of patient education,* ed 7, St. Louis, 1993, Mosby.

Schorn MN, and others: Water immersion and the effect on labor, *J Nurse Midwifery* 38(6):336-342, 1993.

Sloane E: *Biology of women,* ed 3, Albany, NY, 1993, Delmar.

Velvovsky I, and others: *Painless childbirth through psychoprophylaxis,* Moscow, 1960, Foreign Languages.

Wertz RW, Wertz DC: *Lying in: a history of childbirth in America,* rev ed, New Haven, Conn, 1989, Yale University Press.

Wright E: *The new childbirth,* New York, 1966, Hart.

DEFINITIONS

Define the following terms:

analgesia	focal point
anesthesia	Kegel exercise
Bradley method	Lamaze (PPM) method
cleansing breath	monitrice
disassociation	natural childbirth
doula	perfusion
effleurage	psychoprophylaxis
fetal advocate	Dick-Read method
fetus	transition

LEARNING ACTIVITIES

1. Group practice sessions.
2. Guest speakers: Bradley instructor, Dick-Read instructor, Lamaze instructor, a couple who experienced a prepared childbirth.
3. View and discuss audiovisual aids, and read the following:
4. Chabon L: *Awake and aware,* New York, 1966, Dell.
5. Dick-Read G: *Childbirth without fear,* ed 2 (rev), New York, 1959, Harper & Row.
6. Karmel M: *Thank you, Dr. Lamaze,* Philadelphia, 1959, JB Lippincott.
7. Lamaze F: *Painless childbirth: the Lamaze method,* New York, 1972, Pocket Books.

ENRICHMENT/IN-DEPTH STUDY

1. Write a short, thoughtful paper on: "Should everyone try natural childbirth?"
2. Determine the types of classes on prepared childbirth that are available in your community. Compare the philosophies of the different programs. Do they discuss options in childbirth or only describe hospital policies and procedures?
3. Are fees charged for attendance in the prepared childbirth programs? If someone cannot afford the fee, are there scholarships available?

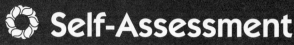
1. List the six broad categories that most preparation for childbirth methods include in their teaching:

    a. _____

    b. _____

    c. _____

    d. _____

    e. _____

    f. _____

Situation: A laboring couple, Catherine and Duncan, have attended preparation for childbirth classes at the local YWCA and are now in the early stages of labor. Catherine is relaxing well and using the slow-paced breathing pattern. Questions 2 through 7 relate to this situation. Circle the best answer.

2. As a member of this team, you would be sure Catherine is in the best position for early labor, by:

    a. rolling her bed down flat so that she is flat on her back

    b. encouraging Catherine to assume a position of comfort

    c. placing pillows to support Catherine's head

3. Between uterine contractions, you would:

    a. carry on a polite conversation

    b. encourage rest

    c. explain to Catherine and Duncan the activities going on in the maternity department

4. During a long, intense contraction, Catherine says, "Oh, that one really hurt!" Your best response would be:

    a. "No, it doesn't hurt. You must be losing control."

    b. "Would you like an anesthetic now?"

    c. "Would you like medicine to relieve your pain?"

    d. "That was really a good contraction that probably helped your progress very much, even though it did hurt a bit."

5. You would encourage Catherine to urinate every half hour during labor because a full bladder can:

    a. cause urine to leak on the bed during a contraction

    b. cause painful uterine contractions

    c. slow down the descent of the baby

6. As labor progresses, it is necessary for you to have Catherine sign a hospital form. You would do this:

    a. quickly at the peak of a contraction

b. between contractions

c. just as the contraction is ending

7. During the labor process, Duncan needs your support, too. Recognizing this, you would:

a. ask him to sit down, rest, and conserve his strength because he is not needed now

b. encourage him to go to the visitors' waiting room to rest

c. offer him nourishment, inform him of the rest and bathroom areas, and offer him encouragement

For questions 8 and 9, circle the best answer.

8. The overall philosophy of preparation for childbirth education includes:

a. developing muscle strength by calisthenics to prepare for labor as an athlete would for a race

b. preparing for labor so one never has to take drugs for pain relief

c. sharing information with people about pregnancy, birth, and parenting so that they can make informed choices

9. The procedure to use when doing the Kegel exercise is:

a. to breathe in slowly through the nose and out the mouth six to nine times a minute

b. to breathe out, abdominally, holding the abdominal wall up off the uterus for 30 seconds

c. to tighten the pelvic floor muscles as in holding back urine, hold for 10 seconds, and then release

10. Before completing this chapter of study, demonstrate the following to your instructor during a group meeting held for return demonstration purposes:

a. active progressive relaxation

b. concentration-relaxation

c. slow-paced breathing

d. modified-paced breathing

e. patterned-paced breathing

f. expulsion breathing

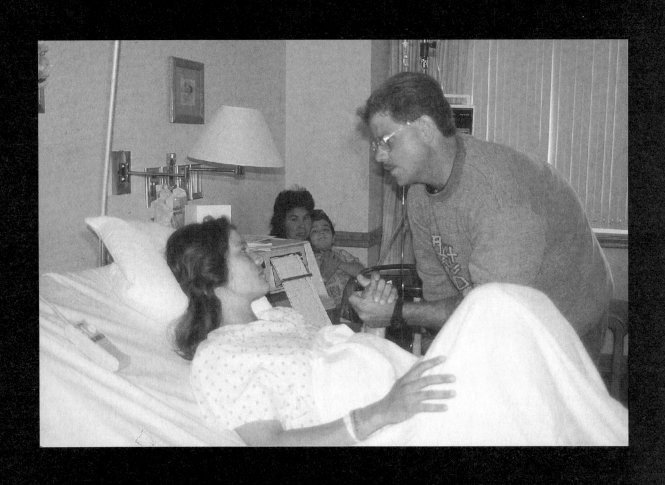

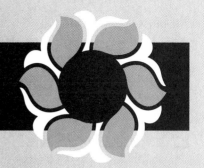

7

THE INTRAPARTUM FAMILY

GOALS

This chapter is designed to provide the reader with information that will:
- promote an understanding of the labor and birth process.
- increase awareness of the psychological stress of labor.

STUDENT OBJECTIVES

After studying this chapter, you should be able to:

1. Recognize circles representing dilation from 1 to 10 centimeters.
2. Identify six possible causes of the onset of labor.
3. Distinguish among the four stages of labor and briefly describe what occurs in each stage. (Include usual duration for a nullipara and a multipara.)
4. Name the two main phases of cervical dilation during stage one of labor and indicate their average duration for a nullipara and a multipara.
5. Describe a uterine contraction in terms of (1) increment, (2) acme, (3) decrement, (4) duration, and (5) time interval between contractions.
6. Recognize the average blood loss during the third stage of labor.

7. Demonstrate a basic understanding of fetopelvic relationships by:
   a. defining lie and presentation
   b. identifying the following bones composing the fetal head: (1) occipital, (2) parietal, (3) temporal, (4) frontal
   c. identifying the anterior and posterior fontanels
   d. recognizing fetal position according to the four quadrants of the mother's pelvis
8. Distinguish among six types of fetal position and identify the letters of the alphabet used to designate each.
9. Describe the seven movements in the mechanisms of labor.
10. Demonstrate an understanding of the stress of labor by:
    a. identifying the psychologic stressors in labor
    b. discussing coping behaviors of women in labor

The physiological and psychological care a family receives during labor and birth is termed intrapartum care (*intra*, during; *partum*, birth).

ONSET OF LABOR

Labor is the process by which a baby is born. An interplay of physiological and emotional forces influences the process of labor. However, exactly what causes labor to begin is not known. It is probably caused by one or more of the following factors: (1) Near term the placental production of progesterone drops. It is thought that progesterone is essential for the maintenance of the pregnancy. (2) Any hollow organ distended to an extreme extent will attempt to empty itself. At term (or before in the case of twins or polyhydramnios) the uterus is certainly distended. The stretching of the muscle fibers seems to increase their irritability and then the uterine muscles contract. (3) Laboring women have increased levels of oxytocin and estrogen, which stimulate the uterus to contract. (4) Prostaglandins, found in amniotic fluid during labor and in the plasma of pregnant women in labor, may play a role in causing labor to begin. (5) The pressure of the fetal presenting part on the cervix and the nerves around the cervix may stimulate labor. (6) The fetus itself may decide the time to be born. It has been proposed that at the proper time the fetal adrenal glands release a pair of substances that trigger the release of other chemicals in the mother's uterus to begin labor. The human fetus may indeed be in control of its own destiny with respect to the onset of labor.

Although labor technically begins when the cervix dilates, it is difficult to identify the exact moment when that happens. Often when women are examined in the last weeks of pregnancy, their cervixes are found to be partially dilated. In fact few women enter effective labor without some cervical dilatation. Therefore because the actual time this dilatation occurred is not likely to be known, the onset of labor is considered to be the same as the onset of regular uterine contractions. Because labor is unique, careful questioning of the woman about when and how she felt that labor had begun usually gives a fairly accurate estimation of the onset time.

Prelabor

Throughout pregnancy the uterus contracts at slightly irregular intervals. These contractions may be felt as tightening of the abdomen, but they are not painful. They were described by Braxton Hicks many years ago and have become known as *Braxton Hicks contractions*. Sometimes women will be aware of Braxton Hicks contractions occurring on and off for hours, days, or even weeks before true labor begins. Most of the time they are felt only in the front of the abdomen and do not increase in intensity. These contractions usually are not regular or rhythmical and can often be relieved or even stopped by walking or by taking a warm shower or bath.

True Labor

As labor begins the woman will usually feel uterine contractions different from the Braxton Hicks contractions she has experienced during much of the pregnancy. The contractions of labor are more uncomfortable and rhythmical and recur at regular intervals (every 5 to 15 minutes, lasting 30 seconds or more). As these regular contractions continue, the interval between them gradually grows shorter. True labor contractions usually become stronger when a woman walks around.

There are other signs that may be present when labor begins. (1) "Show," a small amount of blood-tinged, thick, stringy mucus escaping from the vagina. This mucous plug filled the cervix during pregnancy. (2) Rupture of the membranes ("bag of waters") with a trickle or gush of clear or slightly cloudy, colorless fluid from the vagina. This bag of waters is the transparent sac (amnion and chorion) in which the fetus floated during the pregnancy. Although the bag may rupture before labor, it frequently remains intact and ruptures sometime during the course of active labor. (3) Diarrhea with no apparent cause. (4) Low backache that often starts in the lower back and encircles the abdomen like a tight band. However, for labor to have begun, the preceding signs must be associated with contractions of the uterus and dilation of the cervix.

Proof that labor has begun may have to be a vaginal examination to check for dilation of the cervix. If the cervix has begun to dilate, true labor has begun. However, even though dilation has started, true labor may stop for a few hours or even days.

To differentiate between true labor and prelabor, review their characteristics in Table 7-1.

PROCESS OF LABOR

Pregnant and Nonpregnant Uterus and Cervix

Both the uterus and cervix undergo remarkable changes during pregnancy. Briefly review the divisions of the cervix. (See Fig. 2-2 A, p. 38.) Note that the cervix is composed of a canal, with an internal os at the upper position, separating the cervix from the uterine cavity, and an external os below, which closes the cervix from the vagina. The cervix is about 2.5 centimeters long. The area between the internal and external ossa is the cervical canal.

The cervix is composed mostly of connective tissue interspersed with muscle fibers. In the nonpregnant state it feels firm, somewhat like the tip of one's nose. During pregnancy the cervix softens and feels somewhat like the lower lip. (Feel your lips and your nose. Note the difference?) This softening is caused by increased vascularity, edema, and hyperplasia of the cervical glands. *Ripening* is the softening of the cervix that takes place in late pregnancy.

Cervical Dilation

Dilation (or dilatation) of the cervix means the enlargement of the external os from an orifice of 0.5 centimeters to an opening large enough to permit passage of the fetus—that is, to a diameter of about 10 centimeters. At this stage cervical dilatation is termed *complete* or *full*.

Figure 7-1 is an exact reproduction of a ruler showing centimeters on one side and inches on the other.

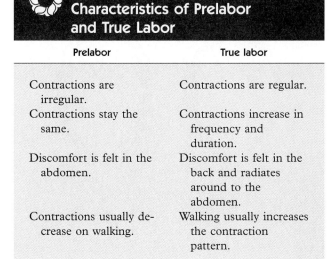

TABLE 7-1	
Characteristics of Prelabor and True Labor	

Prelabor	True labor
Contractions are irregular.	Contractions are regular.
Contractions stay the same.	Contractions increase in frequency and duration.
Discomfort is felt in the abdomen.	Discomfort is felt in the back and radiates around to the abdomen.
Contractions usually decrease on walking.	Walking usually increases the contraction pattern.

Put the tip of your index finger on a centimeter. Does the tip of your finger cover the centimeter? Note that:

4 inches = approximately 10 cm

1 inch = approximately 2 ½ cm

½ inch = approximately 1 ¼ cm

At the beginning of dilation, the cervix usually admits one finger easily (the tip of the index finger is approximately 1 centimeter wide). At the end of the first stage of labor, the cervix is dilated to 10 centimeters.

Cervical Effacement

Effacement is the thinning and shortening of the cervical canal from a structure of 2.5 centimeters in length to one in which no canal at all exists but merely a circular orifice with almost paper-thin edges. Effacement is usually completed in the early part of labor. In a multigravida, both effacement and dilation can occur at the same time. However, a primagravida's cervix usually effaces before dilation begins (Fig. 7-2).

Figure 7-2 shows the length of the area between the internal os and external os before labor. This is the area that thins out and shortens (or effaces). Note the edges of the internal os drawn several centimeters upward, drawn up even more, and finally, the completely effaced cervix.

Effacement is determined during a vaginal examination and is measured in percentages from 0% to 100%—the higher the percentage, the thinner and shorter the cervix. "Zero percent effacement" means the cervix is long and has not begun to thin; "80% effacement" means that the cervix has shortened and is almost completely thinned.

Effacement can be compared with a funneling process in which the whole length of a moldable tube (the cervical canal) is converted into a very large, flaring funnel with only a small circular orifice for an outlet.

Figure 7-3 is a schematic drawing illustrating the change in the uterus during effacement. It is as if a gallon bottle has been converted into a gallon jar.

Both cervical effacement and dilatation are measured by vaginal examination.

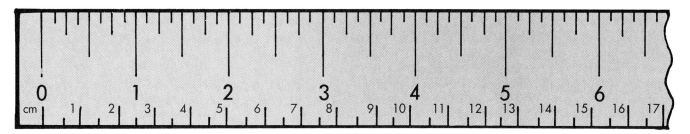

Figure 7-1 Exact reproduction of a ruler.

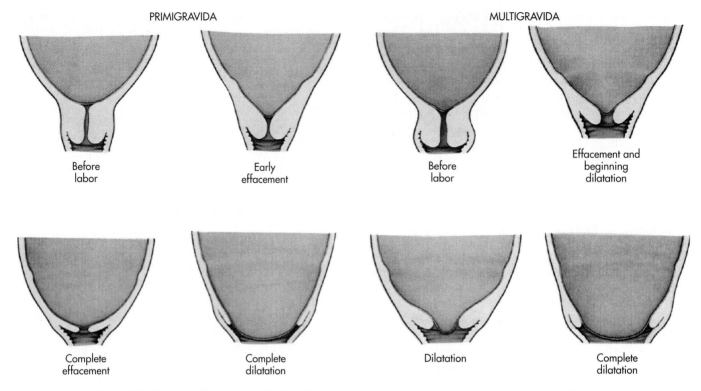

PRIMIGRAVIDA

Before labor

Early effacement

Complete effacement

Complete dilatation

MULTIGRAVIDA

Before labor

Effacement and beginning dilatation

Dilatation

Complete dilatation

Figure 7-2 Cervical effacement and dilatation. *(From* Mechanisms of normal labor, *Ross Laboratories Clinical Education Aid, No 13, Columbus, Ohio, Ross Laboratories.)*

THE FOUR STAGES OF LABOR

Labor progresses in four stages. The first stage begins with true labor contractions and ends with complete effacement and dilation of the cervix. The second stage begins with complete cervical dilation and ends with the birth of the baby. The third stage begins with the birth of the baby and ends with delivery of the placenta. The fourth stage is the period of recovery, from delivery of the placenta to 1 to 2 hours after birth.

Labor is work. It may be the hardest physical work a woman ever does, and when it is over, she may be more tired and yet happier than she has ever been in her life.

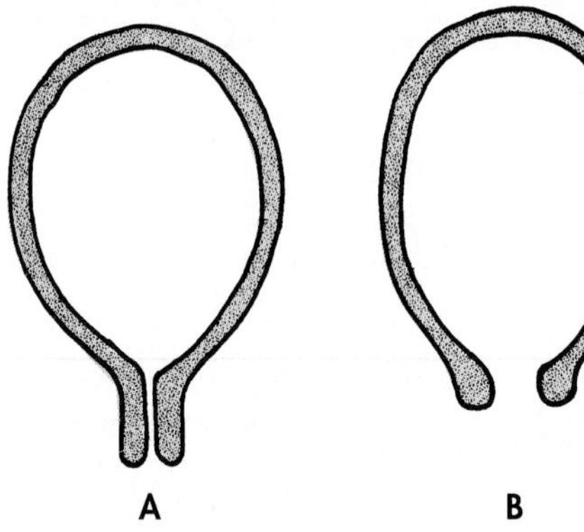

Stage One

The first stage of labor is the stage of dilation and effacement of the cervix. It begins with true labor contractions and ends with complete dilation of the cervix (average 10 centimeters) (Fig. 7-4). This is the longest and most tedious stage for everyone concerned. The entire first stage of labor is not under voluntary control, and the only thing the woman can do is relax and work with labor at the same time. Although as labor begins, contractions can be 15 to 20 minutes apart (lasting 30 seconds); toward end of the first stage they are usu-

A   B

Figure 7-3 Schematic illustration of effacement. **A,** Uneffaced cervix. **B,** Effaced cervix.

ally coming every 2 to 3 minutes and lasting 60 to 90 seconds.

Phases

The first stage of labor can be divided into two main phases of cervical dilation: the latent phase and the active phase. The *latent phase* is the long, slow climb during which the cervix dilates to 3 to 4 centimeters. The *active phase* describes active dilation of the cervix from

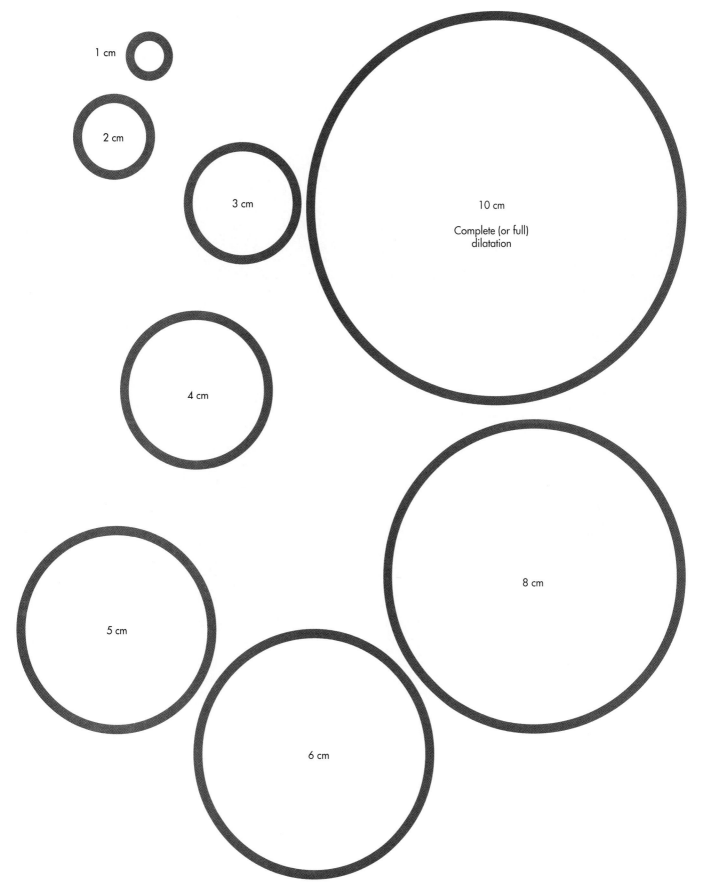

Figure 7-4 Dilation of 1 to 10 centimeters.

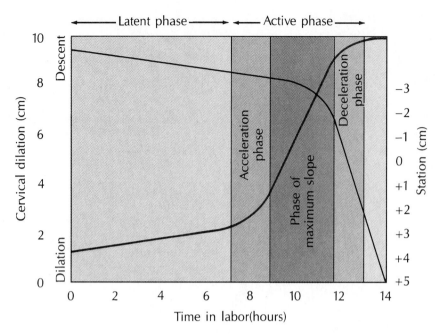

Figure 7-5 Normal labor curve, with functional divisions.

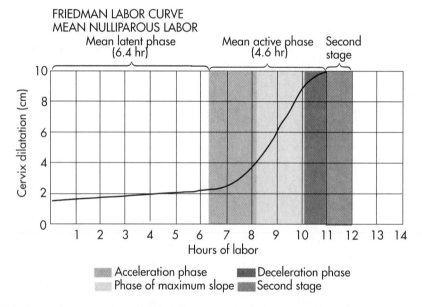

Figure 7-6 The Friedman labor curve formed by plotting the rate of cervical dilatation of the mean nulliparous (primiparous) labor (*mean* indicates average). (*Modified from revised mean labor statistics in Friedman EA: Labor; clinical evaluation and management, ed 2, New York, 1978, Appleton-Century-Crofts; and personal correspondence.*)

4 to 7 centimeters and has been further subdivided into an acceleration phase, a phase of maximum slope, and a deceleration phase (Fig. 7-5).

The deceleration phase, also known as *transition,* is the period from 8 centimeters to full dilation. This transition phase represents the last 2 centimeters of cervical dilation and is often the peak of intensity, pain, and difficulty. The woman's body is still in the first stage of labor but is showing signs of moving into the second stage of labor.

Graphic analysis of labor for the average nullipara is illustrated in Fig. 7-6.

Normal labor curve

The normal labor dilation curve depicted in Fig. 7-5 is drawn from the work of Dr. Emanuel Friedman. Based on an analysis of the labor patterns of a large number of women, Friedman found that the pattern of normal labor takes on the shape of a sigmoid curve

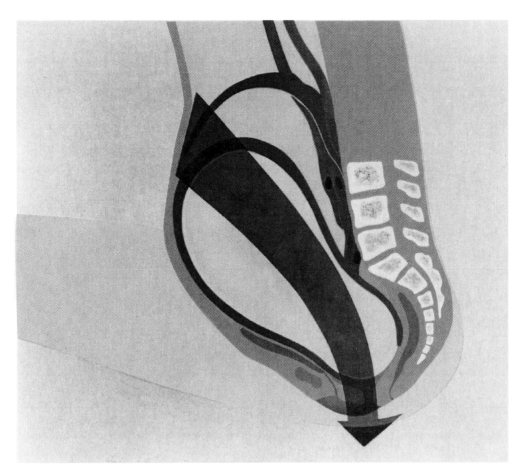

Figure 7-7 The uterus contracts from top to bottom.

(S-shaped) with functional divisions. His analysis led to predictive times for all the stages of labor when normal. (See Fig. 7-6.)

Current active labor management is based on the premise that any variation in the curve can reflect an abnormal labor pattern. The following are averages accepted as the norm: the latent phase for a nullipara—8 to 10 hours but not more than 20 hours; the latent phase for a multipara—3 to 5 hours but not more than 14 hours.

The use of centimeters per hour can allow for early recognition of labor problems. During active cervical dilation, the nullipara averages 3.0 centimeters per hour and at least 1.2 centimeters per hour. During active dilation, the multipara averages 5.7 centimeters per hour and not less than 1.5 centimeters per hour.

Placing strict time limits on the stages and phases of labor according to the normal labor curve has contributed to a lot of anxiety for both laboring women and their health care providers. Lengths of labor will vary according to whether or not the woman is rested, well hydrated and nourished, well prepared, healthy, and approaching labor with minimal fear and tension. The la-

bor environment, ability to move around and assume positions of comfort, and presence of a support person or persons also influence the length of labor.

It is important to remember that Friedman's statistics represent an average length of labor. Although this work has become the standard against which all labors are measured, it is entirely possible that a woman who does not follow the Friedman labor curve will still experience a normal labor for that particular woman.

The cervix dilates as the uterus contracts from top to bottom (Fig. 7-7). A contraction moves down the uterus in a descending gradient (strongest at the top, intermediate strength in the middle, and weakest at the bottom). As labor progresses the uterus is divided into two distinct portions: (1) an active upper portion or segment (fundus and body of the uterus) and (2) a passive lower portion or segment (isthmus and cervix).

As the muscles of the upper uterine segment contract and become thicker, reducing the size of the upper uterine cavity, the muscle fibers of the lower uterine segment become thinner and longer, increasing the area of

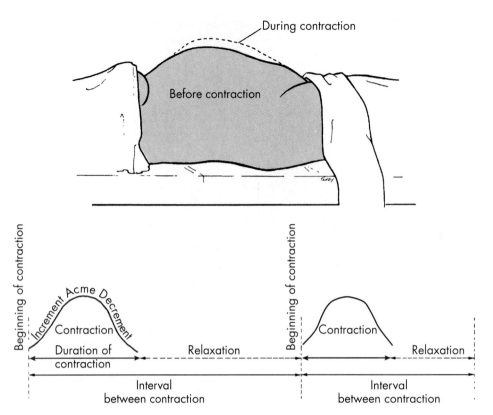

Figure 7-8 Uterine contraction. *(From Bobak IM, Jensen MD: Maternity and gynecologic care: the nurse and the family, ed 5, St. Louis, 1993, Mosby.)*

the lower uterine cavity. When the uterus contracts, it rises up by a pull of the ligaments that support it; consequently, during a contraction the long axis of the uterus is in line with the axis of the birth canal. This change in the shape and angle of the uterus causes the fetus to be forced farther down into the mother's pelvis. At the same time the cervix dilates and effaces as the muscle fibers of the uterus are pulled tight and up. The pressure of the presenting part against the cervix stimulates the release of oxytocin, which stimulates the uterus to contract even more.

Uterine contractions come and go like ocean waves and have great force just like waves in the ocean. Each uterine contraction has three phases: (1) the *increment* phase, during which the intensity of the contraction builds, (2) the *acme*, or peak, during which the contraction is at its height, and (3) the *decrement* phase, during which the intensity decreases (Fig. 7-8). The duration of a contraction is from the beginning of the increment to the end of the decrement and is measured in seconds. The frequency, or interval between contractions, is defined as being from the beginning of one contraction to the beginning of the next contraction. The frequency is measured in minutes and increases as labor progresses.

Intensity, or strength, is the force of the contraction and is described and recorded as mild, moderate, or strong. When an examiner's hands cannot indent the uterine fundus during a uterine contraction, the contraction is said to be strong. When a contraction is mild the fundus is easy to indent with the examiner's hands; moderate contractions are firm but dentable. Contractions can be assessed by palpation of the fundus to determine the firmness, electronic monitoring with an intrauterine catheter, or visually noting the change in abdominal contour as the uterus rises up or falls forward when a contraction occurs.

The degree of relaxation of uterine musculature between contractions is very important because it allows the fetus and the mother to recover from the stress of a contraction. Using an internal electronic monitor to measure the strength of a contraction by recording the amniotic fluid pressure, during normal relaxation the normal tone or *tonus* is approximately 10 mm Hg. At 20 mm Hg, a contraction can be felt as mild by abdominal palpation. A tonus of 10 mm Hg is below the pain threshold and should allow the woman rest between contractions. Electronic fetal monitoring is explained in Chapter 8.

Stage Two

The second stage of labor is the stage of *expulsion*. It begins with complete dilation of the cervix and ends

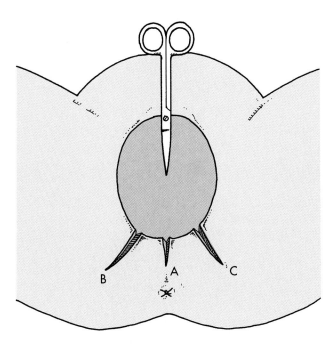

Figure 7-9 Episiotomy. **A**, Median or midline. **B**, Left mediolateral. **C**, Right mediolateral. Fetal head is crowning.

with the birth of the baby. It usually takes 30 minutes to 2 hours in a primigravida and 5 to 30 minutes in a multipara. The uterine contractions change in character and become very strong but slightly farther apart. The woman can actively participate in this stage by pushing the baby out, using her abdominal muscles.

As the second stage begins, the fetus leaves the uterus and begins its descent into the birth canal, pushed forward by the contractions of the thickened upper uterine segment and the voluntary pushing of the woman. The vaginal tissue bulges *(bulging)*, the rectum dilates, the pelvic floor muscles stretch, and a small part of the head of the fetus will appear at the vaginal opening. When the widest diameter of the fetus's head is visible at the vaginal opening, it is said to be *crowning*. With additional effort, a baby is born.

Episiotomy

When the head crowns, an episiotomy may be done. An *episiotomy* is an incision into the perineum and may be made (1) midline (ML), (2) right mediolateral (RML), or (3) left mediolateral (LML) (Fig. 7-9). Episiotomies are also done to facilitate delivery when fetal distress occurs.

Since the early part of this century routine episiotomy has been based on the following rationales: (1) that episiotomy reduces perineal trauma and infection, (2) that episiotomy prevents subsequent pelvic relaxation, (3) that a clean cut is easier to repair and heals better than a laceration, and (4) that the baby's head is not sub-

jected to lengthy pushing and subsequent pressure against the perineum.

There is much debate on the necessity for episiotomy and little evidence to support its routine use. As with any surgical intervention, episiotomy carries its own risks, including excessive blood loss, hematoma formation, and possibility of infection. Recent studies have documented that midline episiotomy is associated with an increased risk of third- and fourth-degree perineal lacerations. In addition, these studies indicate that mediolateral episiotomy does not protect the rectum in spontaneous vaginal deliveries. Other studies have concluded that routine episiotomy results in more need for surgical repair after delivery without a decrease in serious perineal tears. Episiotomies also cause more pain after birth.

Many times massaging the perineum with warm oils, applying warm compresses, and stretching the perineum with the attendant's fingers before delivery will prevent tearing. In addition, stretching, perineal massage, and Kegel exercises performed during pregnancy often permit the mother to relax her perineal muscles at birth, thus allowing the fetal head to emerge over an intact perineum.

Pushing in the correct position (see Chapter 6) with each contraction and relaxing the perineal muscles will help the woman control pressure on her perineum in the second stage. Switching from pushing to panting as the baby's head crowns will also prevent excessive trauma to the perineum. In addition, intelligent use of positioning (sitting, standing, or squatting) so that the perineum is not unduly stretched may help to eliminate the necessity of an episiotomy.

Stage Three

The third stage of labor is the *placental stage*, consisting of two phases: (1) placental separation and (2) placental expulsion. It begins with the birth of the baby and terminates with the delivery of the placenta. During this stage the membranes are separated and expelled from the body. This may require from 5 to 30 minutes.

Placental separation

With the fetus gone the uterus is now smaller and the fundus lies at or just below the umbilicus. Because the uterus is smaller, the placenta will no longer fit in it without buckling on itself. The spongy layer of the lining of the uterus gives way, and the placenta separates from the uterine wall. The signs that indicate the placenta is separating are bleeding from the vagina, a lengthening of the umbilical cord protruding from the vagina, and a globular shape to the uterus, which may rise up in the abdomen (Fig. 7-10).

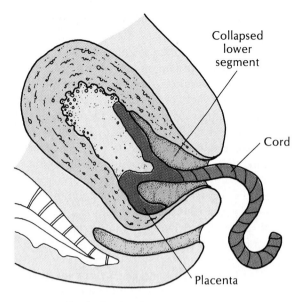

Figure 7-10 Placental separation.

Placental expulsion

Uterine contractions plus voluntary pushing by the mother will expel the placenta from the lower uterine segment and then the vagina. When the uterus is empty, it becomes firm and hard and the fundus can be felt at the umbilicus.

The average blood loss accompanying the third stage is 200 to 500 milliliters. If the placenta is not expelled within an hour after delivery and uterine massage and downward pressure on the fundus do not cause the placenta to be expelled, manual removal is necessary.

Stage Four

The fourth stage of labor is the period following delivery of the placenta until the mother's condition is stabilized. This usually requires 1 to 2 hours for both primiparas and multiparas. If anesthesia was used or if labor was complicated, this fourth stage may last longer. This is a very important stage for close observation because if the uterine muscles do not contract, the blood vessels running through them will not constrict, causing hemorrhage.

FETOPELVIC RELATIONSHIPS

Lie

The lie refers to the relationship of the fetus to the long axis of the mother. In most cases the long axis of the fetus is parallel to the long axis of the mother and is called a *longitudinal* lie. Rarely, the long axis of the

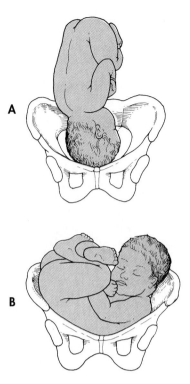

Figure 7-11 A, Longitudinal lie. **B,** Transverse lie.

fetus lies across the mother's pelvis and is termed a *transverse* lie. (Fig. 7-11).

Presentation

Fetal presentation is determined by the part of the baby that is lowest in the mother's pelvis. In approximately 95% of all births the fetal head is the part that enters the birth canal first. Thus the head is most often the *presenting part*. When the head presents, the presentation is termed *cephalic*. Cephalic presentation is referred to as a *vertex* presentation if the fetal head is flexed. If the frontal area of the fetal head is presenting, it is a *brow* presentation. If chin, it is a *face* presentation. When the buttocks present, the presentation is termed *breech* (this occurs in approximately 4% of all births). The rarest (approximately 1% of all births) type of presentation is *shoulder* (or transverse lie) (Fig. 7-12).

Fetal Skull

The fetal head is composed of the bony skull and the face. The bones making up the fetal skull are two *frontal* bones, two *parietal* bones, two *temporal* bones, and one *occipital* bone (Fig. 7-13). Joining these bones are membranous attachments known as *sutures*: the *sagittal* suture joins the two parietal bones; the *lambdoidal* suture joins the parietal and occipital bones; and the *co-*

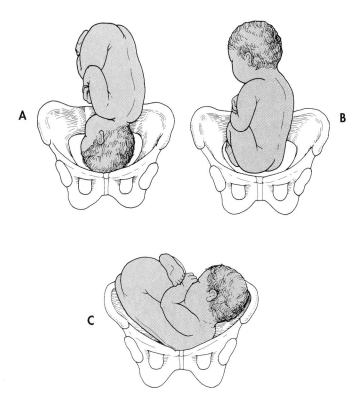

Figure 7-12 Fetal presentation: **A,** Cephalic. **B,** Breech. **C,** Shoulder.

I. **Cephalic Presentations**
1. LOA Left occiput anterior
2. LOT Left occiput transverse
3. LOP Left occiput posterior
4. ROA Right occiput anterior
5. ROT Right occiput transverse
6. ROP Right occiput posterior

II. **Face Presentations**
1. LMA Left mentum anterior
2. LMT Left mentum transverse
3. LMP Left mentum posterior
4. RMA Right mentum anterior
5. RMT Right mentum transverse
6. RMP Right mentum posterior

III. **Breech Presentations**
1. LSA Left sacrum anterior
2. LST Left sacrum transverse
3. LSP Left sacrum posterior
4. RSA Right sacrum anterior
5. RST Right scarum transverse
6. RSP Right acrum posterior

IV. **Transverse Presentations**
1. LScA Left scapula anterior
2. LScT Left scapula transverse
3. LScP Left scapula posterior
4. RScA Right scapula anterior
5. RScT Right scapula transverse
6. RScP Right scapula posterior

ronal suture joins the parietal and frontal bones. The *fontanels* are the areas where several sutures meet: the anterior fontanel ("soft spot") is diamond shaped, and the posterior fontanel is triangular. Because the relatively thin bones of the skull are joined together by these membranous attachments, they can override and mold to fit through the birth canal.

The three distinct sections of the fetal skull are (1) the *vertex,* the area between the anterior and posterior fontanels; (2) the *occiput,* the occipital bone; and (3) the *brow,* the area between the anterior fontanel and the eyes. The widest transverse diameter of the fetal skull is the *biparietal diameter.* The smallest diameter of the head is the *suboccipitobregmatic.* When the fetus flexes its head onto its chest, it presents the smallest diameter of its head to the birth canal.

✓ Position

Position refers to the relation of the presenting part of the fetus to the four quadrants of the mother's pelvis, right or left, front (anterior) or rear (posterior). There are six positions for each presentation. The six positions for the cephalic presentation, three for the face, and three for the breech can be seen in Fig. 7-14. When the head (occiput) is presenting, it is designated by the letter O for occiput. Its position in relation to

the quadrants of the mother's pelvis may be left occiput anterior (LOA), left occiput posterior (LOP), or left occiput transverse (LOT). On the right it may be right occiput anterior (ROA), right occiput posterior (ROP), or right occiput transverse (ROT). The LOA position is the most common (Fig. 7-14). A buttocks presentation is designated by the letter S for sacrum; a face presentation by the letter M for mentum; and a shoulder presentation by the letters SC for scapula.

The six positions for each presentation are identified in the box above.

Presentation and position can be determined by abdominal palpation, vaginal examination, and auscultation.

Lightening

In nulliparas, the fetus usually drops into the pelvis 2 weeks before labor begins. When this happens it is called *lightening.* The mother truly feels lighter since there is more room in the abdominal cavity. Although she can breathe deeply again, walking and moving about may be more difficult and she may experience more frequent

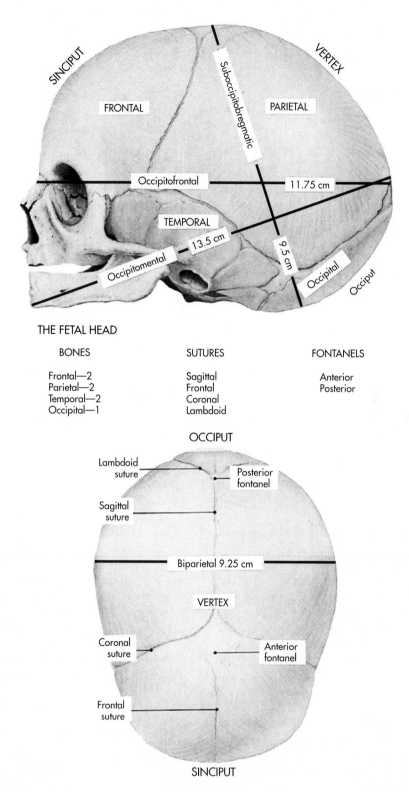

THE FETAL HEAD

BONES	SUTURES	FONTANELS
Frontal—2	Sagittal	Anterior
Parietal—2	Frontal	Posterior
Temporal—2	Coronal	
Occipital—1	Lambdoid	

Figure 7-13 The fetal head. *(From* Mechanisms of normal labor, *Ross Laboratories Clinical Education Aid, No 13, Columbus, Ohio, Ross Laboratories.)*

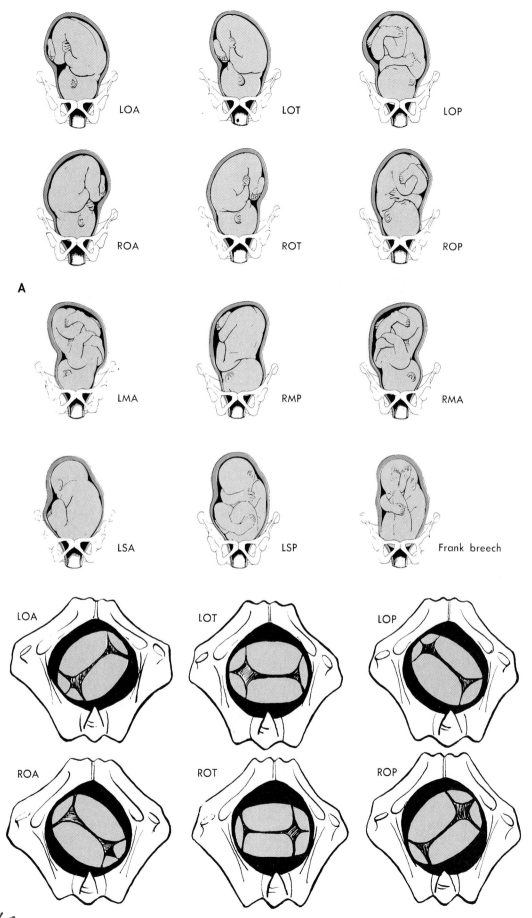

Figure 7-14 A, Categories of presentations. **B,** Positions of occipital presentation as seen looking upward from the outlet. *(A from* Obstetrical presentation and position, *Ross Laboratories Clinical Education Aid, No 18, Columbus, Ohio, Ross Laboratories; **B** from Lerch C:* Maternity nursing, *St. Louis, 1978, Mosby.)*

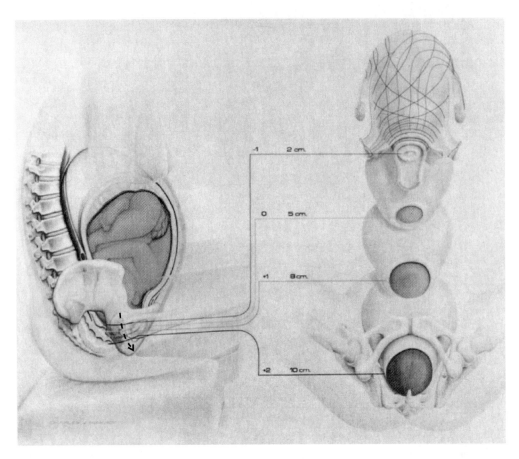

Figure 7-15 Fetal descent. *(Drawing by Charles Pomeroy.)*

urination because of the increased pelvic pressure. However, in multiparas lightening may not happen until after labor begins.

Descent

To be born the baby must be moved down and out by force of the contractions and, in the second stage, by the additional force of the mother's voluntary pushing. The normal curve of descent was illustrated in Fig. 7-5. As for the curve of dilatation, norms for the timing of fetal descent have also been established and can serve as a guide to recognition of early problems. For the primigravida the fetus usually descends at 3.0 centimeters per hour (with 1.5 centimeters per hour being the least amount acceptable). In multiparas the fetus usually descends at between 2.1 centimeters to 5.0 centimeters per hour.

Descent is a dynamic and constant process that is measured by identifying station. Fetal descent is presented diagrammatically in Fig. 7-15.

Engagement and Station

When the largest diameter of the presenting part of the fetus descends into the true pelvis, passing the pel-

vic inlet, engagement has occurred. At this point in time the presenting part is level with the mother's ischial spines.

Station is the relationship of the presenting part to an imaginary line drawn between the ischial spines and is used to indicate the degree of advancement (descent) of the presenting part through the pelvis.

Stations are expressed in centimeters above (minus) and below (plus) the level of the ischial spines (zero).

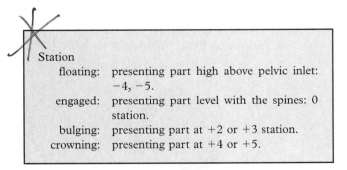

Station	
floating:	presenting part high above pelvic inlet: −4, −5.
engaged:	presenting part level with the spines: 0 station.
bulging:	presenting part at +2 or +3 station.
crowning:	presenting part at +4 or +5.

In Fig. 7-16 note that the fetal head is at zero station and is referred to as engaged. Observe the minus and plus stations in relation to the ischial spines. Women who start labor with the fetal head high above the inlet

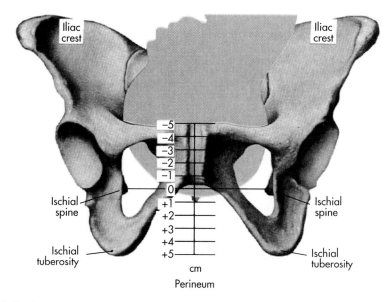

Figure 7-16 Station zero. *(From* Mechanisms of normal labor, *Ross Laboratories Clinical Education Aid, No 13, Columbus, Ohio, Ross Laboratories.)*

usually have lesser degrees of cervical dilation. A low station may be associated with a cervix that is more effaced and dilated, both at the onset of labor and in the beginning of the active phase.

The station is determined by vaginal examination.

MECHANISMS OF LABOR

The largest diameter of the inlet to the pelvis is transverse (side to side) while the largest diameter of the outlet is anterior-posterior (front to back) (Fig. 7-17). The fetal head enters the pelvis in a transverse position and during labor turns its head to emerge from the outlet in an anterior-posterior position with the occiput up and the face looking at the floor. The series of passive, adaptive movements that the fetal head and shoulders make through the birth canal are called the *mechanisms of labor* (Fig. 7-18). By means of these mechanisms the fetus adjusts itself so that its smallest diameter is presented to the irregular shape of the mother's pelvis, thus encountering as little resistance as possible.

Although these seven cardinal movements do not occur in separate steps, but rather overlap or occur in combination, they can be listed in their most frequent order of happening:

1. *Engagement:* With a vertex presenting, the head is engaged when the biparietal diameter (largest diameter) has cleared the pelvic inlet.
2. *Descent:* Occurs intermittently with contractions.
3. *Flexion:* The fetal head tips forward so that the chin rests on the chest to present the smallest diameter, which is caused by the head meeting re-

sistance of the pelvic inlet and soft tissues of the pelvic floor and being flexed.
4. *Internal rotation:* The occiput usually rotates 45 to 90 degrees anteriorly to the midline under the symphysis, which is brought about by twisting of the neck, *not* by any movement of the shoulders.
5. *Extension:* The head sweeps upward and forward under the symphysis.
6. *Restitution:* (external rotation) The head untwists, returns to its original right or left position, and resumes its normal relationship with the shoulders.
7. *Expulsion:* Usually the anterior shoulder presents and delivers first, with the posterior next, and then the rest of the body is born.

PSYCHE

To this point in this chapter, the discussion has centered on the physical, physiologic, and mechanical aspects of labor; or we could say on the *passage* (the pelvis), the *passenger* (the fetus), and the *powers* (the contractions). However, our discussion is not complete until we also consider the factors that contribute to the psychological stress of labor and the ways in which women cope.

Maternal stress has been identified as an important contributor to maternal and fetal complications of labor. Excessive maternal stress can cause an increase in the woman's cortisol and catecholamine levels (epinephrine and norepinephrine), leading to vasoconstriction and decreased uterine perfusion with resulting pain for the woman. In addition, this decreased uterine per-

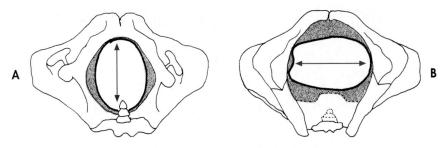

Figure 7-17 A, Anterior-posterior (front to back) diameter of outlet. **B,** Transverse (side to side) diameter of inlet.

fusion can reduce the oxygen and nutrient supply to the fetus. Prolonged or dysfunctional labor may also result, along with increased maternal discomfort and fatigue. The type of childbirth environment can play an important role in moderating maternal stress response.

When a woman and her partner and/or family enter a hospital to give birth, they are confronted with many strange faces, sounds, and smells in an unfamiliar environment. Glaring lights, hospital routines, and equipment can be extremely disconcerting. The woman may be asked to give up her own clothing and to put on a small, unattractive hospital gown that exposes most of her body. She may have to relate to numerous nurses and hospital personnel. There may be a definite lack of privacy as the hospital personnel go in and out of the labor area. If the woman has been in early labor during her normal sleeping hours, she may be very tired and feel irritable. All of these factors are environmental stressors over which the woman usually has very little control. The father or other people with the woman experience similar environmental stressors. The sights, sounds, and smells are new to the woman's partner and family as well, and they may feel anxious and fearful as efficient hospital personnel come and go, sometimes without speaking to them.

Some hospital labor rooms are still narrow, dark, windowless, cell-like rooms designed for the "twilight sleep" era of 30 to 40 years ago. A woman may have to labor in such a room without a bathroom. The other extreme is laboring in a large ward with other laboring women and only curtains between the labor beds. Such an environment for labor does not offer privacy or adequate space to walk around or have family members present.

In other birth settings the environment may be highly technological with a focus on the monitoring equipment and devices and little emphasis on meeting the woman's psychological needs. Women may still be moved from labor bed to stretcher and transported down a hall to a delivery room for birth. They must move or be lifted from stretcher to delivery table to give birth. This is a painful and often frightening and humiliating experience for women. Is it any wonder that women in labor

often find it difficult to use the techniques they have learned in prenatal classes?

If the couple have prepared for the birth, as discussed in Chapter 6, they will begin to cope with the stress of the environment and the discomfort by using the techniques they have practiced. Whether the couple is prepared, the stimulus of pain can bring unresolved feelings, fears, and attitudes about labor to the surface. Remembering previous experiences with hospitals can stir up old fears. A woman's unresolved feelings may threaten her self-confidence as the reality of labor and fast-approaching motherhood crowd in on her. If the relationship of the couple is unstable, many negative feelings may come between them, and their communication system may literally break down.

The ideal childbirth environment does not stress technology but provides a private, homelike, supportive setting in which present technology is available if and when it is needed. In this setting the laboring woman can experience her labor and birth without interference in normal processes.

Adapting

In spite of the stress on the psyche and no matter what their environmental stressors are, women do cope with labor and have done so since the beginning of time.

During the latent phase (0 to 3-4 centimeters of dilation) the uterine contractions are usually mild. The woman usually seems happy that labor has finally begun and smiles, talks, and answers questions freely. She may be anxious but can verbalize her anxiety.

As labor progresses and the cervix is about 4 centimeters dilated (beginning part of active phase), the contractions get closer together (every 5 minutes) and last longer (35 to 40 seconds). The woman's face may flush, her respiration may deepen, and her anxiety may increase. She may start to feel that there is a force outside of her body that is controlling her, and thus she may start to feel helpless. She may use aggressive and hostile behavior to maintain control at this point.

At 6 centimeters of dilation the woman usually becomes serious, talks less, and focuses on herself. Her

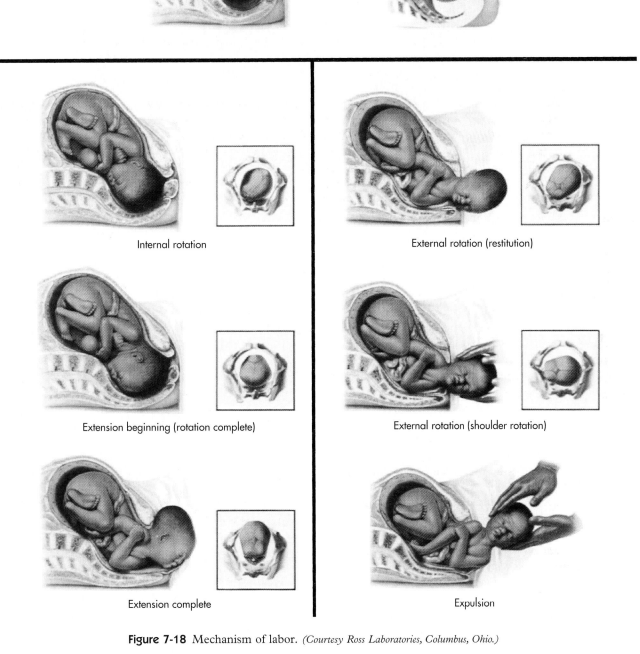

Engagement, descent, flexion

Internal rotation

Extension beginning (rotation complete)

Extension complete

External rotation (restitution)

External rotation (shoulder rotation)

Expulsion

Figure 7-18 Mechanism of labor. *(Courtesy Ross Laboratories, Columbus, Ohio.)*

breathing may become labored, and she may become restless, exhibiting moderate to severe anxiety. She may verbalize a fear of abandonment. At this point the contractions are coming every 3 to 5 minutes and are lasting 40 to 50 seconds.

At 8 to 10 centimeters *(transition)* the mother may feel that labor is never going to end and she simply wants to stop the whole process and go home. She may perspire heavily, shake, have chills, hiccups, and nausea and vomiting. She will become more withdrawn, focus-

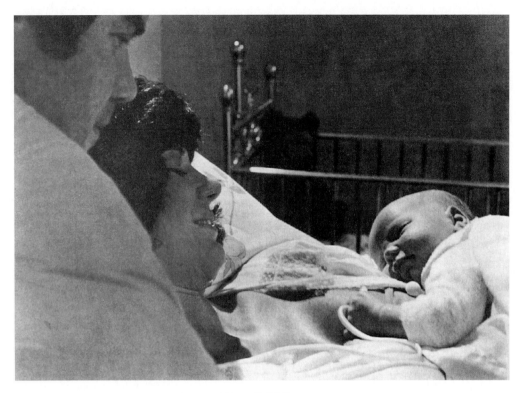

Figure 7-19 Joy.

ing on herself, and become very restless. At the same time, she may be amnesic and actually sleep between contractions. The contractions may be coming every 1 to 3 minutes and last 60 to 90 seconds.

As the second stage begins the woman may feel she has to move her bowels. She may verbalize the urgent need to bear down and become very anxious if she is restrained from pushing. As she bears down her face becomes flushed, the veins in her neck protrude, and she may grunt and groan, making guttural noises with each expulsive effort. This is hard work, and everyone around her knows it. Some women say that they felt like they were experiencing a prolonged and intense sexual orgasm as the baby's head crowned. Other women say that they felt like they were splitting apart as the head was born. The father or other support person may become very worried by the noises the woman makes as she pushes, especially if not prepared for them.

Immediately after the baby is born, most women and their partners experience a moment of pure joy—unlike anything they have ever experienced before (Fig. 7-19).

SUMMARY

In this chapter you have been introduced to the dynamic events of the intrapartum experience—perhaps the most exciting and rewarding experience of a lifetime, although certainly not without dangers. Chapter 8 will help you to learn the meaning of individualized care for the intrapartum family and the nursing care of women during labor and birth.

BIBLIOGRAPHY

Anderson BG, Shapiro PJ: *Obstetrics for the nurse,* ed 6, Albany, NY, 1994, Delmar.

Argentine Episiotomy Trial Collaborative Group: Routine vs selective episiotomy: a randomised clinical trial, *Lancet,* 342:1517-1518, Dec 1993.

Davis-Floyd RE: *Birth as an American rite of passage,* Berkeley, 1992, University of California Press.

Dickason EJ, Schult MA, Silverman BL: *Maternal-infant nursing care,* ed 2, St. Louis, 1994, Mosby.

Friedman EA: *Labor: clinical evaluation and management,* ed 2, New York, 1978, Appleton-Century-Crofts.

Helwig JT, Thorp JM, Bowes WA: Does midline episiotomy increase the risk of third- and fourth-degree lacerations in operative vaginal deliveries? *Obstet Gynecol* 82:276-279, 1993.

Mattson S, Smith JE, editors: *Core curriculum for maternal newborn nursing,* Philadelphia, 1993, WB Saunders.

Nathanielsz PW: A time to be born: implications of animal studies in maternal-fetal medicine, *Birth,* 21(3):163-169, Sept 1994.

Novak JC, Broom BL: *Ingalls and Salerno's maternal and child health nursing,* ed 8, St. Louis, 1995, Mosby.

O'Driscoll K, Meagher D, Boyean P: *Active management of labor,* ed 3, Great Britain, 1993, Mosby–Year Book Europe Limited.

Oxorn H: *Human labor and birth,* ed 5, East Norwalk, Conn, 1986, Appleton-Century-Crofts.

Pritchard JA, MacDonald PC, Gant NF: *Williams obstetrics,* ed 17, Norwalk, Conn, 1985, Appleton-Century-Crofts.

Thorp JM, Bowes WA Jr: Episiotomy: can its routine use be defended? *Am J Obstet Gynecol* 160:1027-1030, 1989.

Zlatnick F: *Normal labor and delivery and its conduct,* in Scott, James and others, editors: *Danforth's obstetrics and gynecology,* ed 6, Philadelphia, 1990, JB Lippencott.

DEFINITIONS

Define the following terms:

acme
active phase
axis
biparietal diameter
Braxton Hicks contractions
bulging
cephalic
crowning
decrement
descent
dilation (dilatation)
effacement
engagement
episiotomy
flexion
floating
fontanels
hyperplasia
increment
intensity
latent phase
lie
lightening
occiput
position
presentation
prostaglandins
restitution
ripening
"show"
station
sutures
tonus
transition
vertex

LEARNING ACTIVITIES

1. Group discussions.
2. Guest speakers: a midwife or obstetrician to discuss experiences with normal labor; a new mother and father to relate their experience.
3. View audiovisual aids and discuss.

ENRICHMENT/IN-DEPTH STUDY

1. Demonstrate the mechanisms of the passage of the fetus down the birth canal by twisting, turning, and thus manipulating a pliable rubber doll through an imaginary delivery. You might sketch the uterus and birth canal in chalk on the board or on the floor and move the doll through it.
2. Study Ross Laboratories' charts on the mechanisms of labor.
3. Prepare a teaching guide to explain the difference between prelabor and true labor to a pregnant woman.
4. Tour all of the facilities for birth in your community and compare and contrast the settings.

Self-Assessment

1. The percentage of births that occur with a cephalic presentation is
   a. 20%
   b. 8%
   c. 95%
   d. 5%

2. Painless, intermittent uterine contractions are known as
   a. Braxton Hicks contractions
   b. colostrum
   c. true labor
   d. "show"

3. The only sure sign of true labor is
   a. pain
   b. bleeding
   c. cervical dilation
   d. Braxton Hicks contractions

4. The first stage of labor covers the time period from the first true labor contraction until _____ of the cervix.

5. What is the average length of time of the latent phase of labor in a nullipara? _____ to _____; in a multipara? _____ to _____

6. The second stage of labor covers the time from complete dilation of the cervix until _____.

7. What is the average length of the second stage of labor in a primigravida? _____; in a multipara? _____

8. The third stage of labor is the _____ stage.

9. What is the average length of time of the third stage of labor?
   _____

10. The fourth stage of labor is the period following _____.

11. What is the average length of time of the fourth stage of labor?
    _____

12. The distance of the presenting part above or below the level of the ischial spines is known as _____.

13. A woman's ways of coping with stresses of labor include all of the following behaviors: _____, _____, _____, _____, and _____.

14. Give a brief description of true prelabor contractions.

_____

_____

_____

15. Identify the cervix that is completely effaced. A or B? _____

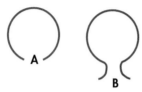

16. A completely dilated cervix is open to the diameter of how many centimeters?

_____

17. Approximately how many centimeters does the circle A below measure?

_____

18. Approximately how many centimeters does the circle B below measure?

_____

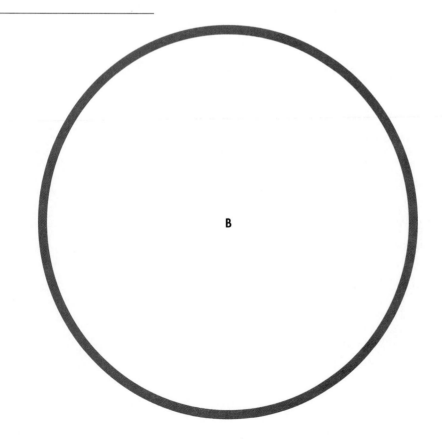

19. The nurse can identify the transition period of labor by signs the woman presents. Four of these signs are:

a. _____

b. _____

c. _____

d. _____

20. A woman has confided in you that she experienced sexual orgasm during the birth of her child and is concerned that she is "weird." How would you respond?

_____

_____

_____

21. Explain why the head of the fetus must rotate in the birth canal to be born.

_____

_____

_____

22. List the seven cardinal movements of the fetus through the birth process to delivery.

a. _____

b. _____

c. _____

d. _____

e. _____

f. _____

g. _____

23. The fetus can present to the birth canal in five different ways. What are they?

a. _____

b. _____

c. _____

d. _____

e. _____

24. What is the average blood loss during the third stage of labor? _____

25. What are four rationales given for routine episiotomy in the United States?

a. _____

b. _____

c. _____

d. _____

26. During what stage of labor may the woman be an active participant? _____

27. After the placenta is expelled, in what condition should the uterus be? _____

28. The widest transverse diameter of the fetal skull is:

a. biparietal

b. bitemporal

29. When the long axis of the fetus is parallel to the long axis of the mother, the lie is called _____.

30. The presenting part is usually the _____.

31. On the line to the left of each item in Column A match the appropriate positions of the fetal occiput from Column B. (See Fig. below columns.)

Column A	Column B
____ A	ROA
____ B	ROP
____ C	LOA
____ D	LOP
____ E	ROT
____ F	LOT

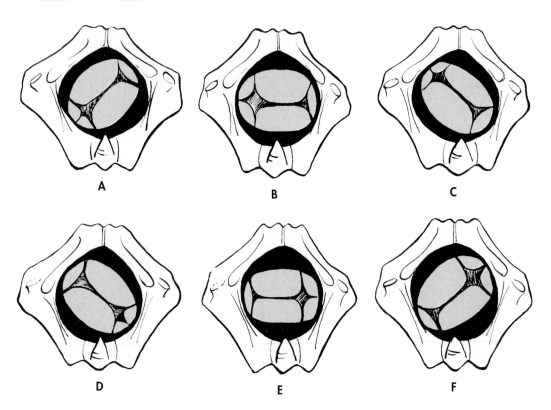

32. On the line to the left of each item in Column A match the appropriate designation from Column B.

Column A	Column B

Designation of the presenting part:

____ 1. head	a. shoulder (Sc)
____ 2. breech	b. sacrum (S)
____ 3. face	c. mentum (M)
	d. occiput (O)

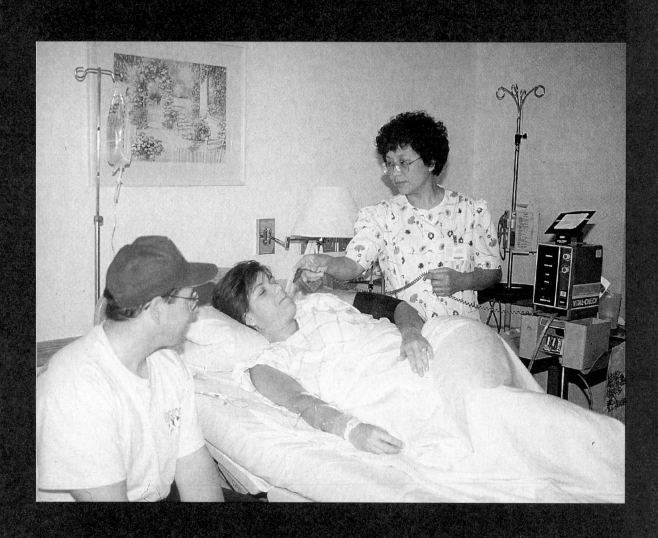

8

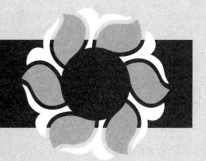

THE INTRAPARTUM FAMILY AND THE NURSE

GOALS

This chapter is designed to provide the reader with information that will:
- promote awareness of nursing care responsibilities for intrapartum families.

- provide the basis for understanding individualized care for the intrapartum family.

STUDENT OBJECTIVES

After studying this chapter, you should be able to:

1. Identify information about the progress of labor that can be assessed by a nursing history.
2. Demonstrate Leopold's maneuvers for determining fetal position.
3. Identify (a) the normal fetal heart rate range during labor, and (b) nursing responsibilities for regular and periodic checking.
4. Differentiate among four types of periodic changes (accelerations, and early, late, and variable decelerations) in the fetal heart rate during labor and state nursing care for each.
5. Give one advantage and one disadvantage for both external and internal fetal heart rate monitoring.

6. Describe the normal appearance of amniotic fluid and two common variations from normal appearance, explaining the significance of these variations.
7. Differentiate among the characteristics of the four degrees of perineal lacerations.
8. List three common drugs used to cause uterine contractions in the third and fourth stages of labor. Include dosages and methods of administration.
9. Discuss the most frequent causes of excessive bleeding in the fourth stage of labor. Include signs and symptoms, treatment, and nursing care.
10. Describe common nursing care provided during labor and birth.

ADMISSION PROCEDURES

Although admission procedures vary from hospital to hospital or birth center, the laboring woman experiences common examinations and she and her family receive the basic care discussed in this chapter.

Admission Consent

All facilities have permission or consent forms for the woman to sign upon admission. These forms authorize the procedures that may be necessary during labor and birth. Whether these consent forms are signed in a centrally located admissions office or in the labor area, the woman and her family need a thorough explanation of what they are signing. (See Pregnant Patient's Bill of Rights in Chapter 1).

Prenatal Records

Ideally a copy of the woman's prenatal records, containing a health history, pregnancy profile, prenatal flow record, and record of what has been taught about birth and parenting, will be sent to the birth site several weeks before the woman's due date. These prenatal records should be reviewed upon admission.

Preadmission Records

It is advisable for people to preregister with the hospital or birth center of their choice before the due date to ensure completion of all necessary forms for identification and financial matters when not under the stress of labor. An additional preadmission form that is very helpful is a *preference profile,* or written birth plan, in which the woman and her family designate what they expect from their childbirth experience. For example, they may request the overhead room light be dimmed at birth, no episiotomy be done, or no student nurses be present in the delivery area. Preference profiles can also give some indication of the type and amount of nurse involvement that the woman wants. Whenever these predesignated preferences do not interfere with the safety of the birth experience, they *must* be respected by nurses and physicians. By having these preferences spelled out clearly in advance of labor, the staff can communicate with the family about any preference listed that might compromise the safety of either mother or baby. In this way problems in matching the desires of the woman and family with the goals and expectations of the nursing and medical staffs can be averted. (See Appendix C for a preference profile.)

If notified in advance of the woman's arrival, the nurse can thoroughly review the prenatal and preadmission records before greeting the woman, thus personalizing and individualizing the greeting and welcome. The nurse should greet the woman, her partner, and family (if present) in a warm and friendly manner, remembering that labor is a crisis time for them. A warm, relaxed, welcoming introduction will do much to reduce anxiety for both the nurse and the laboring woman and family.

Nursing History

While assisting the woman to undress and either put on her own gown or a hospital gown, some basic information can be obtained. If not known by prenatal record, it is important to determine first how many babies she has had and the duration of previous labors. Time may be important in working with a multipara who has a history of rapid labors. Next, the following information is determined:

1. Mother's general condition (frightened? fatigued? relaxed?)
2. When contractions began; their frequency, intensity, and duration
3. Presence of blood-tinged mucus from the vagina (show) or vaginal bleeding
4. Whether membranes have ruptured; time of rupture and color of fluid
5. Due date (EDD); last menstrual period (LMP)
6. Time of last meal; food eaten, including fluids
7. Mother's age and nutritional status
8. Knowledge base; prenatal classes, birth plan
9. Any complications during the pregnancy; any allergies
10. Support system, cultural influences, coping skills

After making these first pertinent observations, the nurse would report any significant deviations from normal immediately.

If the woman is using any preparation for birth techniques to cope with labor, she needs her partner or other family member or friend to remain with her at all times. It can be extremely stressful for her to be without her support person for even a brief examination. In some situations the woman will seek the services of a doula or a professional support person known as a *monitrice.* The doula or monitrice provides emotional support, information and instruction, and physical comfort measures while serving as an advocate for the laboring woman.

Even if the woman has not prepared herself for birth, it may be very important that she not be separated from her family or friend. The nurse can determine this from the preadmission preference profile or simply by asking the woman. When policies, procedures, rules, and regulations seem to get in the way of meeting needs expressed by the laboring woman, it is often helpful to think, "Whose baby is this?"

After making the initial observation the nurse can complete a maternity nursing care history, determining information not previously gathered about the woman and her family. This information will be helpful in deciding on a plan of care during the entire hospital stay. (See Appendix I for an example of a nursing history documentation form.)

At some time during the admission procedures, it is necessary to care for the woman's personal items by labeling all her clothing carefully and listing all her valuables. Many hospitals have a special envelope for valuables, which can be locked in a safe place. If such a service is not available, it is advisable to have a family member take the valuables home.

FIRST STAGE OF LABOR: NURSING CARE

An evaluation of general physical status includes checking the mother's weight, general physical condition, vital signs, and taking blood and urine specimens for laboratory examination.

Physical Examination

The nurse should weigh the mother on admission to determine if there has been a sudden weight gain or loss. A gross examination and systems review will be necessary to rule out any deviations from normal.

Vital Signs

Vital signs are taken and recorded every 4 hours during routine labor or more frequently during abnormal labor. An elevated temperature may mean infection. An elevated pulse rate may mean infection or dehydration. Blood pressure is usually checked and recorded on admission and every 2 hours during labor unless otherwise indicated. If the blood pressure is elevated abnormally (over 140/90), it may be checked and recorded as often as every 15 minutes. An elevated blood pressure may indicate preeclampsia. The nurse should report any abnormalities immediately.

Urine Specimen

A clean voided urine specimen is checked on admission for the presence of blood, sugar, and albumin. If the woman's membranes are ruptured, it may be impossible to obtain a urine specimen free of amniotic fluid. Albumin, blood, or sugar in the urine should be reported immediately. Albumin in the urine specimen may be a sign of preeclampsia.

Timing Uterine Contractions

The nurse records and reports the frequency, duration, and intensity of uterine contractions on admission and throughout labor. As explained in Chapter 7, a uterine contraction has three phases: (1) a period of increasing intrauterine pressure, known as *increment;* (2) a period of peak intensity, called *acme;* and (3) a period of decreasing pressure, known as *decrement.* (See Fig. 7-8, p. 186.) The length of contraction *(duration)* is measured from the increment through the acme and to the end of the decrement. The *frequency* is measured from the beginning of one contraction to the beginning of the next.

The nurse can actually feel the muscular contractions of the uterus by gently touching the fundus. Because the contractions begin at the fundus, there will be a tightening in this area first, which will gradually move down the uterus from top to bottom. At the time of the acme the uterus will be firm all over but tightest at the fundus. Also, the abdominal wall will rise with a contraction and relax again between contractions. Between contractions the uterus will feel soft. With strong uterine contractions the uterine wall cannot be indented by the examiner's fingers. With moderate contractions, the uterus will feel moderately firm. When the uterine contractions are mild, practically no difference in uterine tone can be detected by gentle palpation.

During the first stage of labor the average contraction lasts 40 to 60 seconds. It would be abnormal for a contraction to last longer than 80 seconds or for the uterus not to relax between contractions. Any deviations from normal contractions should be reported immediately.

Abdominal Palpation (Leopold's Maneuvers)

By first determining the position of the fetus, the nurse can locate the fetal heart tones quickly, since they are best heard through the baby's back. Palpating the woman's abdomen to check the baby's position and presentation is called *Leopold's maneuvers* (Fig. 8-1).

Before palpating the abdomen the nurse first inspects it without touching. In most pregnancies the uterus at term is egg shaped with lengthwise enlargement, and the bulk or mass of the fetus is obvious on either the mother's right or left side. The nurse looks for fetal movement, particularly feet and hand movement. The obvious mass is probably the fetal back and the gentle movements are probably the extremities.

With the mother lying on her back with her knees slightly bent and a pillow or a lift to raise her trunk to a 35- to 45-degree angle, the nurse stands at the mother's side facing her and with warm hands palpates the uterine fundus *(first maneuver, A)* to determine what part of the fetus lies in the upper part of the uterus. The fetal head is hard, smooth, and round and can be moved from side to side on the neck. The buttocks (breech) are larger, softer, more irregular, and cannot be moved like the head. The fetal head in the fundus indicates a breech presentation. The fetal buttocks in the fundus indicate a cephalic or vertex (head first) presentation.

To determine on which side of the uterus the long axis (back) of the fetus is located, the nurse's hands move down each side of the uterus at the same time *(second maneuver, B)*. A long, smooth, firm, curved surface is the fetal back. Small irregular bumps and lumps, which often move and kick, are the legs and arms.

Still facing the woman the nurse presses with one hand over the symphysis pubis *(third maneuver, C)*, feeling for the presenting part. The fetal head feels globu-lar and firm. The breech feels soft and irregular. If the fetal head is not engaged, it can be felt like a small, hard, round object above the symphysis pubis. Also, gentle pressure can move it.

For the last maneuver the nurse turns and faces the woman's feet. To confirm that the fetal head is presenting, the nurse presses downward on both sides of the woman's uterus, approximately 2 inches above the symphysis pubis *(fourth maneuver, D)*. In this maneuver the nurse is feeling for the brow of the baby, which should be on the side opposite from where the back was located.

If the fetus is in the left occiput anterior position (LOA), the fetal heart should be heard best in the left lower quadrant. (The head is presenting with the occiput at the left front and the brow facing the right back. The fetal back is on the left.) However, if the fetus is in

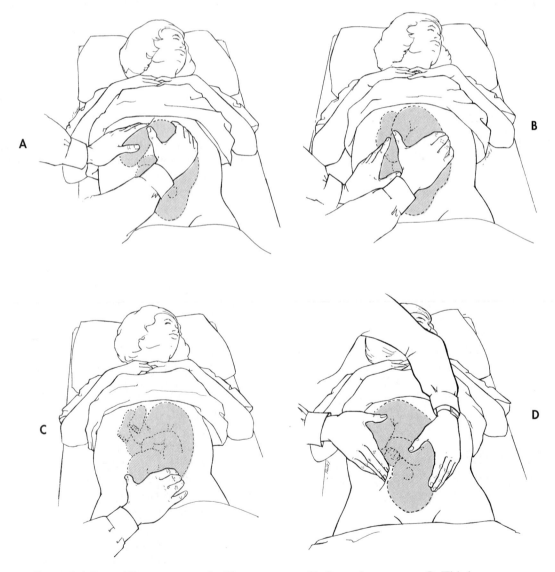

Figure 8-1 Leopold's maneuvers. **A,** First maneuver. **B,** Second maneuver. **C,** Third maneuver. **D,** Fourth maneuver. *(From Bobak IM and others:* Maternity nursing, *ed 4, St. Louis, 1995, Mosby.)*

the left occiput posterior position (LOP), the fetal heart is heard best slightly below the upper outer border of the left hip bone. (The head is presenting with the occiput at the left back and the brow facing the right front. The fetal back is on the right.)

With breech presentations, the fetal heart will be heard at or above the level of the mother's umbilicus: left sacrum anterior (LSA) or right sacrum anterior (RSA) (Fig. 8-2).

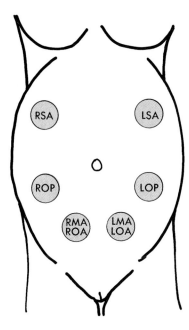

Figure 8-2 Location of fetal heart. Heart tones are best heard through the fetus's back.

Fetal Heart Tones

Auscultation of the fetal heart rate (FHR) has always been important to evaluate fetal well-being during labor and birth. Two techniques of fetal heart rate assessment are auscultation and electronic fetal heart monitoring.

Fetal heart tones are heard with the use of special stethoscopes: a DeLee-Hillis fetoscope (Fig. 8-3) worn on the examiner's head or a Leff stethoscope (Fig. 8-4). An ultrasound fetoscope, or Doppler instrument (Fig. 8-5), is a special electronic device for amplifying the sounds of the fetal heart beat. The normal FHR is from 120 to 160 beats per minute. The FHR is checked and recorded on admission, every 30 minutes during early labor (latent phase), every 15 minutes during active labor, and at least every 5 minutes during the second stage of labor. In addition to this regular checking, the FHR is checked and recorded after any examination or treatment, immediately following rupture of the membranes, and immediately after administration of analgesia or anesthesia.

When listening to the fetal heart with a stethoscope, the nurse should listen for at least a full minute from the acme of the contraction, through the decrement, and into the interval between contractions. Because of the tightened uterine muscle, it is often uncomfortable for the mother when the nurse listens to the fetal heart during the most intense part (acme) of the contraction. Normally the FHR either slows down or speeds up by about 10 beats at the height of the contraction but returns to normal within 10 seconds of the end of a contraction. To be sure that the mother's pulse is not being heard through the stethoscope, the mother's radial

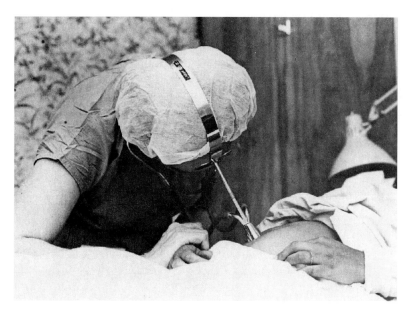

Figure 8-3 DeLee-Hillis fetoscope worn on examiner's head uses bone conduction to amplify the fetal ventricular sounds for counting.

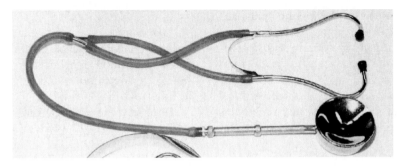

Figure 8-4 Leff stethoscope for auscultation of fetal heart rate. *(From Novak JC, Broom BL:* Ingalls and Salerno's Maternal and child health nursing, *ed 8, St. Louis, 1995, Mosby.)*

pulse can be palpated at the same time the FHR is checked. A comparison of what is being felt at the mother's wrist to what is being heard with the stethoscope will indicate whose heart is being monitored with the stethoscope (Fig. 8-3).

Any abnormalities in FHR (irregular rhythm, rate above 160 or below 120) should be reported immediately.

Continuous Electronic Fetal Heart Monitoring

Electronic fetal monitoring (EFM) uses electronic techniques to continuously monitor FHR and uterine contractions (UCs). The electronic fetal monitor records uterine contractions and fetal heart activity simultaneously, either intermittently or continuously throughout labor (Fig. 8-6). The purpose of electronic fetal monitoring is to pick up early warning signs of fetal distress so that appropriate measures can be taken if necessary.

Baseline Variations

The terminology commonly used when interpreting fetal heart rate patterns is briefly outlined here. *Baseline* is defined as the average FHR in a 10-minute period, noted between contractions, or in the noncontracting uterus. The *normal range* of FHR baseline is between 120 to 160 beats per minute (bpm) in the full-term fetus.

The time line between each beat of the heart varies. The calculated fetal heart rate will therefore change over time. *Baseline variability* is the normally occurring irregularity of FHR, which is due to the interplay of the parasympathetic (cardiodeceleration) and sympathetic (cardioacceleration) divisions of the fetal nervous system as it responds to stress. The fetal heart speeds up under sympathetic stimulation and slows down under parasympathetic stimulation. A sign of a healthy, adapt-

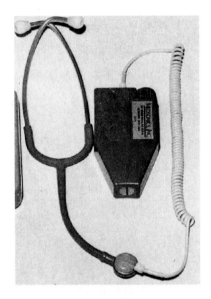

Figure 8-5 Ultrasonic fetoscope operates on Doppler effect, reflecting echoes or sounds from moving interfaces. *(From Novak JC, Broom BL:* Ingalls and Salerno's Maternal and child health nursing, *ed 8, St. Louis, 1995, Mosby.)*

able fetal nervous system is measured by good FHR variability in two aspects: cyclic variations of 2 to 3 beats from one beat to the next, known as *short-term variability* (Stv), which give the fetal heart rate tracing a rough, jagged appearance; and larger fluctuations of 5 to 25 bpm every 2 to 5 minutes, termed *long-term variability* (Ltv) (Table 8-1), which give the baseline a wavy appearance (Fig. 8-7).

Internal fetal monitoring is necessary to assess FHR variability accurately. External electronic fetal monitoring can determine only an average FHR and does not provide information about the subtle changes in true variability. Decreased short-term variability may be due to fetal hypoxia, CNS depressant drugs, parasympathetic drugs, a premature fetus, sleeping fetus, or cardiac and CNS congenital anomalies. A decrease in long-term variability may be due to fetal sleep or certain drugs administered in labor. Marked increase or de-

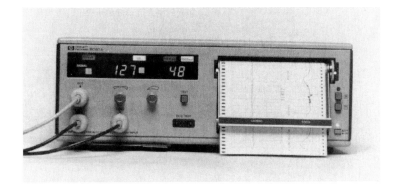

Figure 8-6 Electronic fetal monitor. The monitor tracing illustrates the FHR pattern *(top line)* and uterine contraction pattern *(bottom line)*. *(Courtesy Hewlett Packard, Andover, Mass.)*

TABLE 8-1 Degrees of Variability	
Degree	**Beats per minute**
Absent	0-2
Minimal	3-5
Average	6-10
Moderate	11-25
Marked	>26

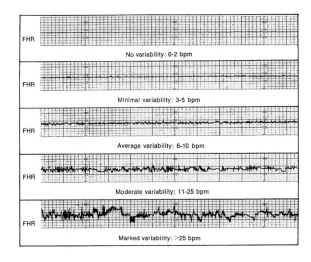

Figure 8-7 Types of fetal heart rate variability. *(From Tucker SM: Pocket guide to fetal monitoring, ed 2, St. Louis, 1992, Mosby.)*

crease in variability as labor progresses, following a previously average reading, could indicate impending fetal distress.

Occasionally *sinusoidal FHR patterns* will be seen. These present as rhythmic, wavelike, long-term variability of 5 to 15 beats per minute every 3 to 5 minutes, with absence of short-term variability. Sinusoidal patterns are seen in severe fetal distress, in the Rh-sensitized fetus, when there is hypoxia of the cardiac center or severe fetal anemia, and as the result of some maternal medications administered during labor. The clinical significance of this pattern is controversial.

Periodic Changes

Because contractions represent sources of repetitive stress to the fetus, signs of fetal response to this stress may first appear as changes in the FHR in relation to the pressure of uterine contractions.

Accelerations are transitory increases in FHR of usually 15 or more beats per minute above baseline that usually last less than 10 minutes. They are associated with fetal movement or contractions and are a sign of fetal well-being. Accelerations occur in response to sympathetic stimulation due to spontaneous fetal movement, uterine stimulation, vaginal examination, or breech or posterior presentation.

Decelerations are decreases in the fetal heart rate from the normal baseline that usually last less than 10 minutes. There are three basic decelerations in FHR in relationship to uterine contractions: early decelerations, late decelerations, and variable decelerations. (See Fig. 8-8 for descriptive illustrations, causes, and nursing actions for each periodic change in rate.) When late or variable decelerations are detected, the following actions should be taken to treat the cause of the distress: (1) The woman's position should be changed to relieve pressure on the umbilical cord and rule out a positional response. If the FHR returns to normal, further interventions may not be necessary. (2) If oxytocin is being administered, it should be discontinued if decelerations are present after positional changes. The oxytocin may be causing the uterus to contract too strongly or not to relax enough between contractions, thus interfering with placental circulation. (3) Oxygen should be administered to the mother by mask. (4) The woman's blood pressure should be taken to rule out hypotension and, if present, maternal hypotension should be corrected.

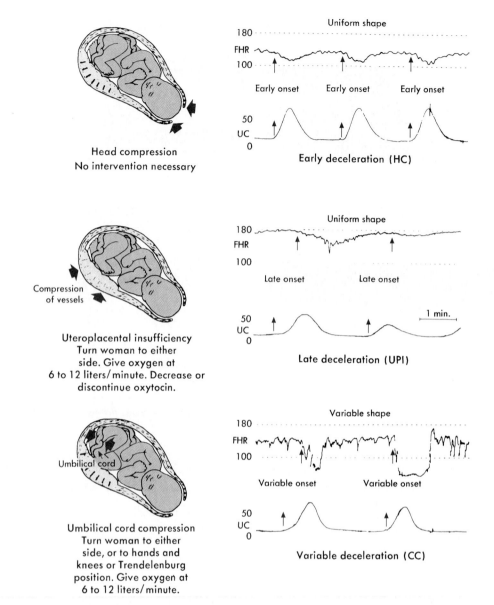

Figure 8-8 Periodic changes in fetal heart rate. *(From Hon EH:* An introduction to fetal heart rate monitoring, *Wallingford, Conn. Corometrics Medical Systems.)*

(5) The umbilical cord should be checked for prolapse, and (6) the fetal scalp should be stimulated.

Tachycardia and Bradycardia

In addition to detecting periodic changes in FHR in relationship to uterine contractions, the fetal monitor can provide other data that could indicate fetal well-being. The monitor will also detect fetal *tachycardia* (baseline fetal heart rate more than 160 beats per minute lasting longer than a 10-minute period) or fetal *bradycardia* (baseline FHR less than 120 beats per minute lasting longer than a 10-minute period) very early in its onset. Both fetal tachycardia and fetal bradycardia may be indicative of fetal distress. (See box on p. 213 for possible causes.)

Interventions for fetal tachycardia include enhancement of uterine blood flood by reducing uterine activity and/or cord compression and providing additional oxygen. Interventions for fetal bradycardia include repositioning the mother, correcting maternal hypotension, discontinuing Pitocin if running, and providing additional oxygen. Always confirm fetal tachycardia or bradycardia by auscultation and comparing the FHR with the maternal heart rate to be sure it is actually fetal and not maternal heart rate being detected.

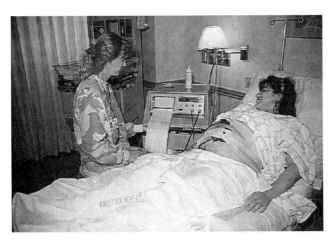

Figure 8-9 External monitoring. Belts allow for attachment of transducers. *(Courtesy Marjorie Pyle, RNC, Lifecircle, Costa Mesa, Calif.)*

Possible Causes of Fetal Tachycardia (>160 bpm for >10 minutes)
Maternal fever
Fetal infection, anemia, arrhythmias
Prematurity
Maternal anxiety
Tocolytic agents given to mother
Maternal hyperthyroidism
Fetal activity
Certain drugs that interrupt vagal response in fetus

Possible Causes of Fetal Bradycardia (<120 bpm for >10 minutes)
Late or profound hypoxia
Maternal hypotension
Prolonged umbilical cord compression
Congenital fetal heart block
Maternal drugs (local anesthetics, beta blockers)

FHR patterns

Assessment of FHR patterns is based on trends, not single occurrences. *Reassuring patterns* include absence of deceleration, accelerations with fetal movement or contractions, and baseline rate and variability within stable normal range. *Suspicious patterns* include progressive increase or decrease in baseline tachycardia of 30 beats per minute over baseline and decreasing baseline variability. *Ominous FHR patterns* include persistent, uncorrectable, late decelerations with loss of FHR variability, variable decelerations accompanied by loss of FHR variability and fetal tachycardia, and sinusoidal FHR patterns.

External EFM

Fetal monitoring can be done by internal or external methods or a combination of both. *External* monitoring consists of two parts: (1) an ultrasound system or microphone amplification technique to pick up the fetal heart and record it on graph paper and (2) a pressure-sensitive transducer that measures the tension on the abdominal wall when the uterus contracts (Fig. 8-9). The advantages of external monitoring are that it does not require rupture of the membranes and that it can be used in early labor or for tests of fetal status such as the oxytocin challenge test (OCT), nipple stimulation test, and the nonstress test discussed earlier. However, external monitoring is much less accurate than internal monitoring and is more difficult to keep in adjustment. The mother's movement is often restricted when adjustment is a problem. (See box p. 214.)

Internal EFM

Internal monitors also consist of two parts: (1) the fetal scalp electrode (FSE), which is attached to the scalp of the fetus to record fetal heart beat; and (2) the intrauterine pressure catheter (IUPC), which is placed inside the uterus to record intensity, duration, and frequency of uterine contractions and resting tone of the uterus (intrauterine pressure between contractions) (Fig. 8-10). Internal monitoring has the advantage of being accurate and easy to adjust. The major disadvantage is that the cervix must be dilated 3 to 4 centimeters and that the membranes must be ruptured, thus making it an invasive technique. Invasive techniques increase the risk of maternal and fetal infections. (See box p. 214.) Also, another disadvantage of internal monitoring is that it restricts the woman's mobility.

Resting tone

The tonus or resting tone of the uterus between contractions can only be measured accurately with internal monitoring using the IUPC. The resting tone of the uterus between contractions is approximately 10-12 mm Hg, during which the fetus is receiving most of its oxygen and nutrients and eliminating waste. Causes for elevation in the resting tone include uterine overdistention (twins); medications (Pitocin); or the mother's pushing, creating expulsion forces.

Telemetry

Wireless fetal monitoring is available that can be used with complete ambulatory freedom for laboring women

Internal Fetal Monitoring (Direct Monitoring)

Advantages

Provides accurate, continuous information

Not subject to artifact

Allows mother to move about in bed

Assesses frequency of contractions and baseline uterine tonus

Assesses FHR variability and periodic changes

Disadvantages

Invasive and thus increases risk of maternal and/or fetal infection

 External Fetal Monitoring (Indirect Monitoring)

Advantages

Noninvasive

Can assess frequency and duration of contractions

Provides continuous information and a permanent record

Disadvantages

Does not assess intensity of contractions

Cannot assess FHR variability

Belts uncomfortable

Subject to artifact

Discourages women from seeking positions of comfort

Cannot assess intensity of contractions or uterine tonus

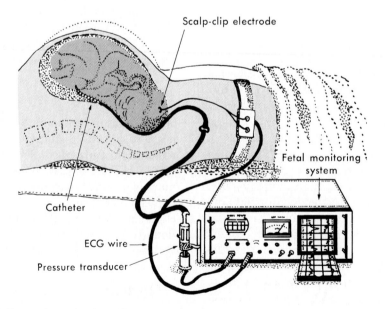

Figure 8-10 Internal monitoring. After the electrode has been attached the lead is secured to a leg plate on the mother's thigh and connected by a cord to the monitor. *(From Novak JC, Broom BL: Ingalls and Salerno's Maternal and child health nursing, ed 8, St. Louis, 1995, Mosby.)*

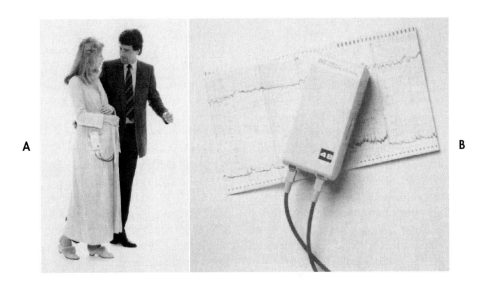

Figure 8-11 A, Mother ambulating with telemetry. A small telemetry transmitter fits in a pocket. **B,** Fetal ultrasound telemetry based on noninvasive, or external, methods of measurement. (*Courtesy Hewlett Packard, Andover, Mass.)*

(Fig. 8-11, *A*). The system is noninvasive and allows accurate fetal monitoring even before the woman's membranes are ruptured. The mother is connected to a lightweight, telemetry transmitter (Fig. 8-11, *B*). Fetal and maternal data are then transmitted to a remote telemetry receiver and processed by a standard fetal monitor. Although not used a great deal in U.S. hospitals, telemetry has the capability of promoting maternal mobility while continuously monitoring the fetus and labor.

It is important for the nurse to recognize that the fetal monitor is only a tool and not a replacement for the nurse. The uses and operation of the monitor should always be explained to the laboring woman and her family.

The American College of Obstetricians and Gynecologists (ACOG) has issued a statement on FHR monitoring in which it was noted that results of research indicate no clear benefit of external fetal monitoring over properly performed auscultation. Thus the method of FHR monitoring selected should be based on consideration of maternal-fetal risk factors and availability of nurses skilled in monitoring techniques.

Because it is beyond the scope of this book to discuss fetal monitoring in detail, the bibliographic sources that are at the end of this chapter are recommended for further study.

Fetal Blood Sampling

If the signs of fetal distress do not respond to treatment as outlined, fetal status can be assessed by obtaining a sample of capillary blood from the presenting part, either the scalp or buttocks. The presenting part of the fetus must be at least to the −2 station and dilation of

the cervix at least 2 centimeters. When membranes rupture, an endoscope is inserted into the vagina. A knife blade with a long handle is used to puncture the fetal scalp or buttocks. Capillary blood is collected in long heparinized glass capillary tubes. A fetal scalp sample with a pH greater than 7.15 to 7.20 is nonacidotic and reassuring of the fetal status. Two successive fetal scalp pH levels of less than 7.15 to 7.20 indicate acidosis and the need for immediate delivery. Some high-risk maternity centers are using sensors that can be attached to the fetal scalp for continuous pH monitoring.

Vaginal Examination

Upon admission and when necessary during labor, a vaginal examination is done to determine the state and progress of labor. Using a sterile glove, antiseptic solution or lubricant, and aseptic techniques, the examiner gently inserts one or two fingers into the woman's vagina to ascertain the cervical dilation and effacement, station, presenting part, position of the presenting part, presence of molding or caput, and status of fetal membranes. In some hospitals vaginal examinations are the responsibility of the physician only, whereas in others vaginal examinations are nursing responsibilities.

Vaginal examinations should not be done if there is excessive vaginal bleeding because if there is a placenta previa or abruptio, a fatal hemorrhage may result.

Rupture of Membranes

Sometimes during a vaginal examination the bag of waters may be found bulging down into the cervix with great pressure. The physician or midwife may decide to rupture the membranes with an Allis's clamp or membrane hook, thus performing an *amniotomy*. There is disagreement over the necessity of this procedure, however, because it is believed that the bulging bag of waters fits into the cervical opening and serves as a hydrostatic wedge to dilate the cervix. Also, with the bag of waters gone the cushioning effect of the waters for the head of the fetus is lost. Those who favor amniotomy believe that labor is accelerated by this procedure, thus reducing the length of time the fetus is stressed. The woman and her family should be told the pros and cons of artificial rupture of membranes (AROM) in birth preparation classes so that they can give informed consent for the procedure.

Whether the membranes are ruptured artificially or spontaneously in labor, the fluid should be clear and colorless. If it is not clear and colorless, the physician should be notified immediately. A yellowish, foul-smelling fluid may be indicative of infection of the amniotic sac *(amnionitis)*. If the presentation is vertex, thick greenish or brownish fluid may mean that the fetus has passed meconium (fetal stool) into the fluid and may be in distress. If the fetus suffers from a lack of oxygen in utero, the anal sphincters may relax and dilate, releasing meconium into the amniotic fluid. With a breech presentation, meconium-stained fluid may be normal.

If a woman suspects possible ruptured membranes, fluid from her vagina can be tested for pH with Nitrazine Paper. A positive result for amniotic fluid turns the paper dark blue because amniotic fluid has a pH of 7.0 to 7.5. With a negative result the Nitrazine Paper would be yellow or brown since vaginal secretions have a pH of 3.8 to 5.5. Blood and some antimicrobial solutions and lubricants could yield false-positive results. Another test for ruptured membranes is the ferning (or arborization) test. In this test a few drops of fluid dry on a clean glass slide, and then the slide is examined microscopically. A positive result would occur when the sodium chloride in amniotic fluid crystallizes on the slide into a fern-like pattern.

The risk of amnionitis may increase as the time the membranes have been ruptured increases. Sometimes if the membranes have been ruptured for 24 hours and good labor has not begun, an induction is started.

Nursing care

The fetal heart must always be checked before amniotomy and immediately after the rupture of membranes. The sheet under the woman's buttocks should be kept clean and dry. Other nursing responsibilities include observing and charting the color, amount, and odor of the amniotic fluid.

Perineal Preparation

Perineal preparation was done in the past because of the belief that it provided a clean field for delivery. An examination of the origin and procedure of perineal shaving has provided evidence that shaving pubic hair to prevent infection is not necessary. In fact shaving compromises the integrity of the skin by inflicting multiple small abrasions. The procedure of perineal shaving is also humiliating and frightening for many women. In addition, shaving irritates the perineum and can increase postpartum discomfort.

Most physicians no longer believe that shaving the perineum is necessary; some scissor-clip the hairs or order a half, or "mini," preparation (perineal area only) if episiotomy repair is necessary and perineal hair is troublesome.

Enema

Either a rectal suppository or a small disposable enema may be given in early labor for women with constipation. An enema is not given if the woman has an unusual amount of vaginal bleeding or is rapidly approaching the second stage of labor. As with perineal preparation, little evidence justifies the routine use of enemas for women in labor. Each case should be evaluated on an individual basis.

Bladder

It is important to keep the laboring woman's bladder as empty as possible because a full bladder mechanically impedes the descent of the fetal head. If the woman is up and about she should be helped to the toilet often. If she is on bed rest she should be offered the bedpan at frequent intervals. A full bladder can be observed and palpated as a soft balloon full of water above the symphysis pubis (Fig. 8-12). If all attempts at voiding fail and the bladder is definitely distended, catheterization is necessary.

Activity

If the woman's membranes have ruptured early in labor and the presenting part is not yet engaged, she should remain in bed because of the possibility of an umbilical cord prolapse. However, if the membranes are intact or if the presenting part is tight against the cervix after membranes have ruptured, she may be more comfortable walking around, taking a warm shower, sitting, or rocking. She should be able to assume a position of comfort even if that means getting on all fours and rocking her pelvis up and down. Never should the woman labor flat on her back because the pressure of the full uterus on the vena cava and other

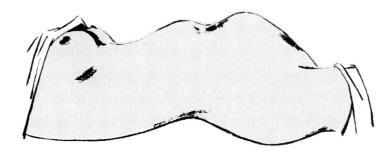

Figure 8-12 Full bladder can be observed and palpated above the symphasis pubis. *(From Lerch C, Bliss VJ:* Maternity nursing, *ed 3, St. Louis, 1978, Mosby.)*

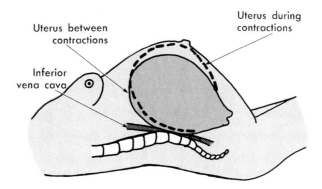

Figure 8-13 Supine hypotensive syndrome.

major vessels can slow down the venous return blood flow to her brain, causing *supine hypotensive syndrome* (Fig. 8-13).

Upright maternal posture and ambulation during labor are not only more comfortable for the woman but also can facilitate labor. When the woman assumes the upright position during labor, gravity enhances fetal descent and rotation. Walking, rather than lying in bed, results in contractions that are less frequent and less painful, but more intense. Thus vertical postures (sitting, standing, and ambulation) can shorten the duration of labor. Greater maternal comfort can be gained as well when women are free to change their own positions to relieve pain. Women in labor are often intuitively aware of what position feels best and if encouraged will find a position of comfort. Also, assisting the woman to assume a comfortable position can help reduce her anxiety about being helpless. It is important to evaluate each woman's labor individually to determine the most comfortable, safe, and efficient positions for her. Labor is not a static process, and neither should the woman's position be static (Fig. 8-14).

Food

The policy of nothing by mouth (NPO) in labor has become standard in many U.S. hospitals. The original reason for the policy was to prevent aspiration of gastric contents should general anesthesia be needed. Recent studies have critically examined this policy and concluded that the routine withholding of food and oral liquids and the consequent use of intravenous fluids lack supporting evidence and pose potential risks to both mother and infant. The undesirable side effects of withholding food and liquids during labor include dehydration, ketosis, hunger, and thirst. Utilization of intravenous fluids to replace oral fluids restricts a woman's movement and adds the potential for fluid overload, both maternal and fetal hyperglycemia with consequent neonatal hypoglycemia.

Many clinical practices are instituting policies to allow and encourage eating and drinking in normal labor. There have been no reported rises in maternal mortality with this policy change; neither have there been any reports of detrimental outcomes for mother or infant. (For further study, see Smith and others, 1993, and Ludka and Roberts, 1993, in bibliography.)

As for the type of food or drink to be taken in labor, the woman herself will usually self regulate what she should consume. Most women eat or drink more in early labor and then taper off once active labor begins. If a woman is in a situation where a cesarean is antici-

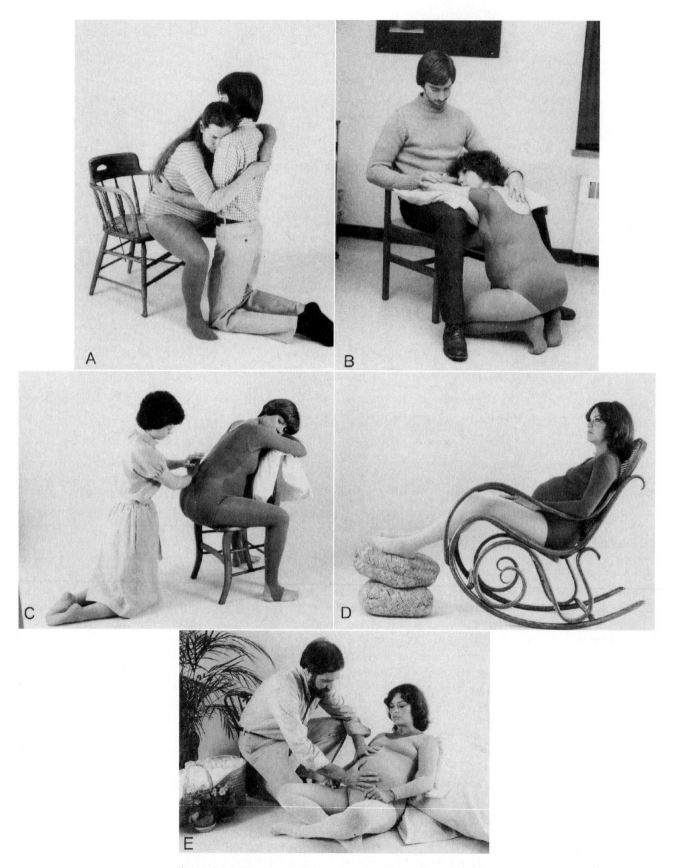

Figure 8-14 Positions for labor. *Copyright 1985 Childbirth Graphics.*

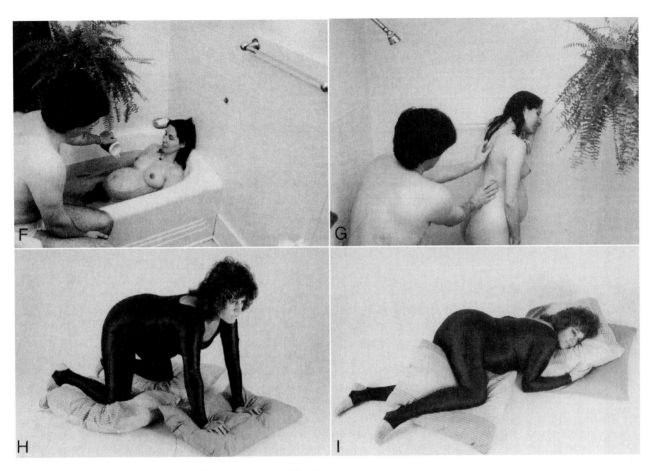

Figure 8-14, cont'd. For legend see opposite page.

pated, she should insist on regional anesthesia if possible.

Comfort Measures

General comfort measures as simple as replacing soiled bed linen are very important. Many of these measures were discussed in Chapter 6. This would be a good time to review that chapter.

Whenever any procedures or examinations are performed, the privacy and comfort of the woman should always be considered. Keeping her covered or draped, explaining all procedures to her, and obtaining her permission to perform them are essential nursing responsibilities. Table 8-2 summarizes nursing care during labor.

SECOND STAGE OF LABOR: NURSING CARE

The second stage of labor begins with complete effacement (100%) and dilation of the cervix (10 cm) and ends with the birth of the baby. Signs and symptoms indicating the approach of the second stage include: (1) an increase in bloody show, (2) nausea and vomiting, (3) diaphoresis, (4) a feeling of needing to defecate, (5) short grunting respirations with bearing down reflex efforts by the mother, and (6) a bulging perineum.

Delivery Room Preparation

More and more women and their families are requesting to deliver in their labor beds or in "birthing beds" (Fig. 8-15); in labor, delivery, recovery rooms (LDRs); or in labor, delivery, recovery, postpartum rooms (LDRPs) to avoid having to move at a very uncomfortable moment in the birth process. If these options are not available, the delivery room can be set up within 2 hours ahead of actual expected delivery time with the delivery table, sterile instrument table, sterile basins, an incubator or an infant warmer unit of some kind, and resuscitation equipment for the baby (Fig. 8-16). All of the sterile linen and equipment can be covered with sterile drapes, which are removed at the time of delivery. Adequate preliminary preparation eliminates last-minute hustle and bustle and subsequent anxieties. The actual moment when a woman is moved from the labor room to the delivery room varies, but generally primigravidas are moved to the

TABLE 8-2
Nursing Care During Labor

Nursing care	Stage 1 of labor — Latent phase	Stage 1 of labor — Active phase	Stage 2	Stage 3	Stage 4
Emotional support	Continuous support, encouragement, reassurance, and information				
Fleets or disposable enema	May be given in early labor if no unusual vaginal bleeding				
Bladder	Encourage woman to void frequently	Void frequently	May have to catherize		Keep bladder empty
Intake	Encourage food and fluids unless contraindicated		Same as stage 1	Same as stage 1	Fluids high in CHO
Activity	Walk, sit, assume position of comfort		Squat or sit up to push		Probably bed rest
Comfort	Wash face and hands with cool water; apply cream, lotion or Chapstick to lips; apply back pressure to a spot on the low back (designated by the woman), encourage relaxation	Cool cloth to face and hands; instruct and assist with bearing down for expulsion; explain what is happening; relieve leg cramps if necessary by forcing the foot upward with pressure on the knee			Check uterus
Temperature, pulse, respiration	Check every 4 hours unless abnormal (temperature >100° F; pulse >100 or <60; respirations >30 or <12)				Check pulse and respirations every 15 minutes (first hour), then every 30 minutes (second hour); check temperature once
Blood pressure	Check every 2 hours unless abnormal: blood pressure over 140/90 is abnormal	If abnormal, recheck frequently		Check before giving oxytocic drugs or any other medication	Check every 15 minutes (first hour) then every 30 minutes (second hour)
Fetal heart tones	Check every 30 minutes (normal, 120-160 bpm)	Check every 15 minutes	Check after every contraction or every 5 minutes		Check every 15 minutes
Measure contractions	Time uterine contractions every 30 minutes; check for intensity, frequency, and duration	Check contractions every 15 minutes	Time each contraction		Check uterus frequently for excessive bleeding; make sure uterus remains firm
Record data		Continuous recording of data; maintain accurate records			

delivery room when the fetal head is visible. Multiparas are moved to the delivery room when fully dilated or, if labor is rapid, when about 7 to 8 centimeters dilated.

LDR/LDRP Preparation

Because the LDR and LDRP rooms serve as labor and delivery rooms, the mother does not have to be transferred for birth. She may remain on the birth bed

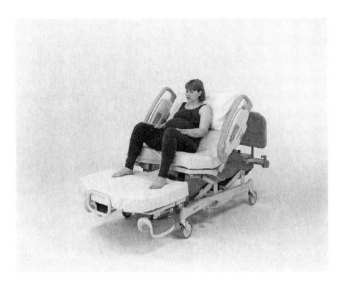

Figure 8-15 Woman in upright position for birth on a birthing bed. *(Courtesy Hill-Rom, Batesville, Ind.)*

on which she labored. These beds offer a range of positions for labor and birth and thus facilitate the process for both mothers and health care professionals.

Delivery Position

Unfortunately, many women and health care providers have been socialized to birth lying down. Also, many health care providers promote the lithotomy position for birth because of its convenience for monitoring FHR, doing and repairing episiotomies, and administering anesthetics and because of its utility for obstetric intervention. Reeducation is necessary for all involved because the disadvantages of the lithotomy position far outweigh the advantages. Disadvantages may include aortocaval compression; risk of venous thrombosis in the legs from the pressure of the stirrups; back pain; decreased pushing ability; rigidity and tightening of the perineum; and fetal distress secondary to maternal hemodynamic changes. In addition, it is difficult for the mother to see and hold her baby, and she has less control of the birth itself.

Numerous studies have been conducted on maternal positions and pushing techniques for second-stage labor, and recently many practitioners are encouraging women to labor and give birth in the positions that they find most comfortable. Squatting is one of several upright positions that may prove to be safer and more comfortable for giving birth than the recumbent posi-

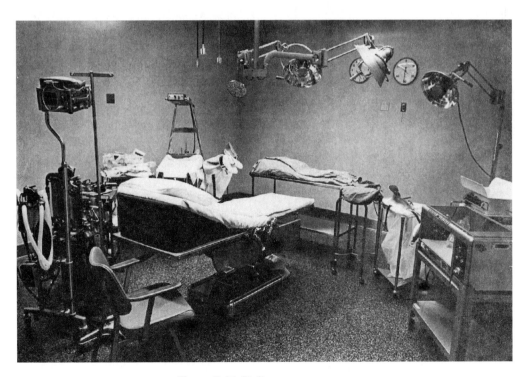

Figure 8-16 Delivery room set-up.

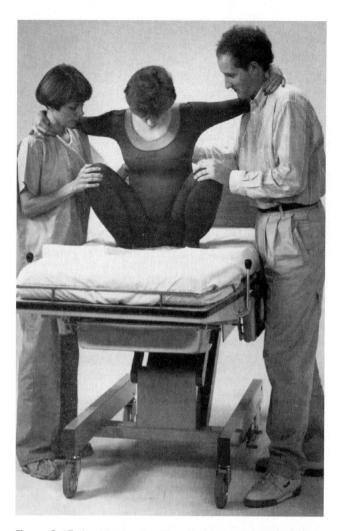

Figure 8-17 A squatting position for birth. *(Courtesy Hill-Rom, Batesville, Ind.)*

tion (Fig. 8-17). A woman giving birth in either the sitting or the squatting position is totally involved in the birth process and can see and touch her baby as the birth occurs.

When women are encouraged to respond to their birthing impulses, not only will they change positions frequently, but they will also push when they feel like it instead of when the nurse instructs them to bear down. Unforced pushing efforts may lengthen the second stage but have not been demonstrated to result in adverse fetal outcome. Although there is no "right way" to ensure the best results in childbirth, evidence suggests encouraging and suggesting positions of comfort and breathing for expulsion as the urge dictates.

Perineal Preparation

Washing the woman's perineum with bactericidal solution is usually done before the actual birth. For this perineal cleansing, the nurse wears a sterile glove.

Birth

As the baby's head crowns the woman should be encouraged to "pant" so that the expulsion of the baby can be controlled. At this point the doctor or midwife may perform an episiotomy if deemed necessary. The nurse notes and records the exact time of the birth of the baby.

The woman's partner, support person, or other family members can be very helpful at this time (Fig. 8-18). However, these persons also need positive reinforcement, recognition, and support from the staff. It is their experience also and can have profound meaning for them. If the family has decided to include young siblings at the birth, a support person should be present for each sibling.

Immediately after birth the baby is dried, and a clear airway is assured using a bulb suction or mechanical suction if necessary. Then the baby is placed on the mother's abdomen. Some mothers want to reach down and help their baby out into the world. The mother can do this "gentle assist" even in a sterile delivery room with the nurse's careful assistance. The cord is usually tied or clamped in two places and cut in between when it stops pulsating. Some physicians give the scissors to the baby's father and encourage him to cut the cord. There is a lot of symbolism in this gesture as he seems to be freeing his child (Fig. 8-19) and thus accepting the responsibilities of parenthood.

Apgar Scoring

The Apgar scoring system is used to evaluate the general condition of the baby at 1 minute of life and again at 5 minutes. Apgar scores are based on five signs: heart rate, respiratory effort, muscle tone, reflex response, and color. Each sign is given the score of 0, 1, or 2 points. A maximum Apgar is 10 at 1 minute and again at 5 minutes (Fig. 8-20). The 1 minute score, if low, indicates the need for active resuscitation. Although the Apgar score is a useful tool to assess the need for resuscitation and treatment in the immediate newborn period, it is not predictive of later performance.

Immediate Care of the Newborn

If the infant is dried, covered with a warm blanket, and placed in skin-to-skin contact with the warm mother or father and is apparently responding and breathing normally, the first 15 or 30 minutes of life can be a family time without interruption by the staff. If there are any deviations from normal, the baby will have to be placed in an incubator or infant warmer for close observation and proper treatment. Fortunately, most infants are well and normal and have Apgar scores of 8 or better and thus can remain with the mother or father. Some mothers like to breast-feed

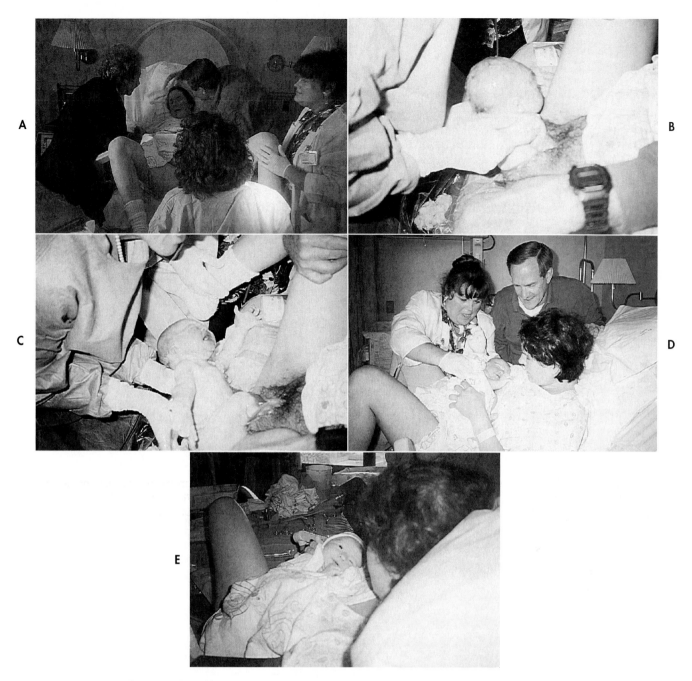

Figure 8-18 A-E, Birth. *(Courtesy Lawrence, Catherine, and Caroline Way, San Francisco, Calif.)*

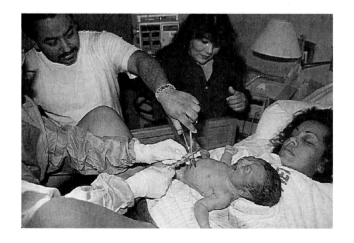

Figure 8-19 Cord cutting is complete. *(Courtesy Marjorie Pyle, RNC, Lifecircle, Costa Mesa, Calif.)*

APGAR SCORING CHART

Sign	0	1	2
HEART RATE	Absent	Slow (below 100)	Over 100
RESPIRATORY EFFORT	Absent	Weak cry, hypoventilation	Good strong cry
MUSCLE TONE	Limp	Some flexion of extremities	Well flexed
REFLEX RESPONSE 1. Response to catheter in nostril (tested after oro-pharynx is clear)	No response	Grimace	Cough or sneeze
2. Tangential foot slap	No response	Grimace	Cry and withdrawal of foot
COLOR	Blue, pale	Body pink, extremities blue	Completely pink

Figure 8-20 Apgar scoring chart. Category condition: 0-3, poor, critical, severely depressed; 4-6, moderately depressed; 7-10, good.

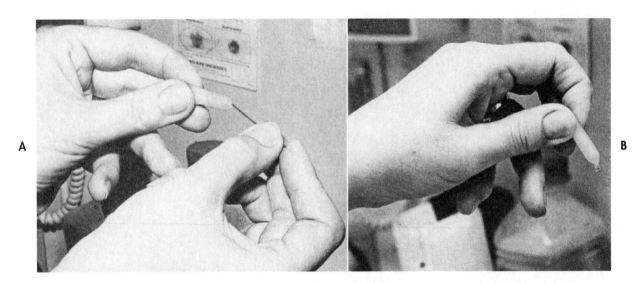

Figure 8-21 Silver nitrate for prophylactic eye treatment for Neisseria gonorrhoeae. **A,** Puncturing wax ampule containing 1% silver nitrate ophthalmine solution with pin. **B,** Squeezing out a drop in each conjunctival sac of newborn.

their babies immediately after birth. If the baby is alert, well, sucking, and wanting to feed, this is an excellent time to begin.

After this initial bonding period, the nurse can weigh and measure the baby, take his or her temperature, remove superficial blood and mucus, and instill two drops of 1% silver nitrate in each conjunctival sac using two ampules, one for each eye. This treatment is still required by law in most states in the United States to prevent blindness (ophthalmia neonatorum) caused by gonococcal organisms that may be present in the vagina.

It is recommended not to irrigate the baby's eyes after the instillation of silver nitrate (Fig. 8-21).

Other acceptable prophylactic agents that prevent ophthalmia neonatorum include the following:

1. Erythromycin (0.5%) ophthalmic ointment or drops in single-dose tubes or ampules.
2. Tetracycline (1%) ophthalmic ointment or drops in single-dose tubes or ampules.

Erythromycin and tetracycline ointment and drops have also been found to prevent chlamydial ophthalmia neonatorum. The American Academy of Pediatrics rec-

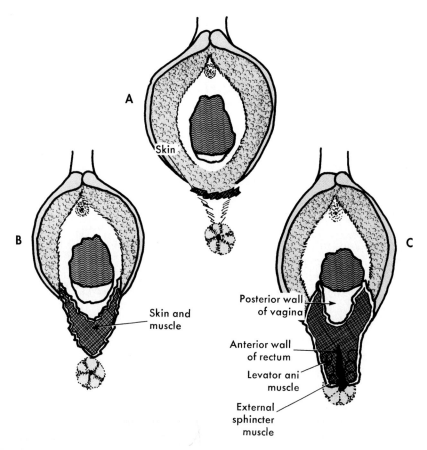

Figure 8-22 Perineal lacerations. **A,** First degree. **B,** Second degree. **C,** Third degree.

ommends instillation of erythromycin or tetracycline ointment into the newborn's eyes shortly after birth in areas of the United States where chlamydial infections are more common than gonococcal infections.

Identification

The mother and baby must be identified quickly after birth. Plastic bands having the same number on them are attached to the mother's wrist and to the baby's wrist and ankle. All three bands contain the baby's sex, date and time of birth, mother's name, and physician's name. Some hospitals footprint the baby and also take the mother's fingerprints; however, these are not legally identifying data.

THIRD STAGE OF LABOR: NURSING CARE

The third stage of labor begins after the delivery of the baby and ends with the discharge of the placenta. The nurse is responsible for recording the time the placenta is delivered. After the placenta is expelled, the physician or midwife inspects it to be sure that it is intact. The physician may order an oxytocic drug after the

placenta is expelled to aid in stimulating contractions of the uterine muscles.

The average blood loss in the third stage of labor is 300 milliliters. The nurse must observe the mother for hemorrhage and shock and massage the uterus if it relaxes. If blood loss reaches 500 milliliters, it is considered a hemorrhage. If this occurs grasp the uterus and massage it gently but firmly until it becomes hard again.

Lacerations

Even in the most carefully controlled delivery, lacerations or extensions of the episiotomy may occur. Usually the same anesthetic used for the episiotomy can be used to repair lacerations. Sometimes a local anesthetic is administered.

Lacerations are classified according to the extent of the tear as first, second, third, or fourth degree. First-degree lacerations are fairly common and involve tearing of the perineal skin and vaginal mucous membrane only. Lacerations involving skin and mucous membrane plus fascia of perineal body are called second degree. Third-degree lacerations involve skin, mucous membrane, muscles, and extend into the rectal sphincter (Fig. 8-22). Fourth-degree lacerations involve all of these structures and the anal wall.

Other lacerations that may occur during vaginal delivery include periurethral tears, occurring near the urethral meatus, and periclitoral tears, occurring near the clitoris. Lacerations can bleed profusely and are usually repaired as an episiotomy is repaired.

Immediate Postdelivery Care

Cleansing the perineal area after the delivery, applying clean perineal pads, covering the mother with warm dry blankets, and, if she is in leg supports, bringing both legs down at the same time are nursing responsibilities.

The woman's blood pressure and pulse, firmness of the uterus, and amount of vaginal bleeding are checked and recorded before she is transferred to the recovery area. It is at this time that the baby may be taken to the nursery in traditional hospital procedures.

If the mother has labored and given birth in an LDR or LDRP, she will not have to be transferred to a recovery room. She will be able to recover from the birth in the same LDR or LDRP. Also, in many maternity programs where the nursing staff is multiskilled, the same nurse will care for the mother and baby together. In these situations the infant may remain with the mother and will not have to be transferred to a nursery.

FOURTH STAGE OF LABOR: NURSING CARE

The first few hours after delivery until the mother's vital signs are stable is called the fourth stage of labor. During this time the nurse checks the woman's blood pressure and pulse every 15 minutes for the first hour and every 30 minutes for the second hour after delivery. The firmness and location of the uterus and amount of vaginal bleeding are also checked frequently. The fundus immediately after delivery should be firm and slightly above the level of the umbilicus.

If the uterus relaxes and bleeds excessively the nurse should massage the uterus until it becomes firm. If the uterus does not contract there may be clots forming at the site of placental separation or there may be retained placental pieces. These clots can be expressed by gentle, firm, downward pressure on the uterus fundus. Overstimulation of the uterus by vigorous massage is not recommended because it may cause uterine relaxation instead of contraction. If massage does not cause the uterus to contract, it may be necessary to "hold" the fundus. This is accomplished by placing one hand over the woman's symphysis pubis, pressing inward and then upward toward her head. The other hand grasps and

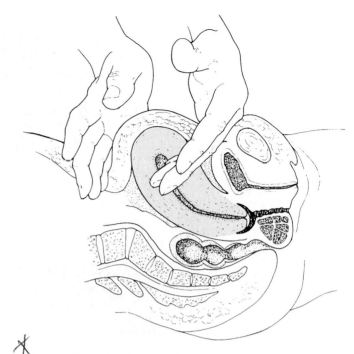

Figure 8-23 Holding the fundus. *(From Bobak IM and others: Maternity nursing ed 4, St. Louis, 1995, Mosby.)*

Pitocin, Syntocin

Available in ampules containing 10 IU per milliliter; 10 to 30 IU added to 500 to 1000 milliliters of intravenous solution and using a controlled infusion device, infused over a period of hours or given intramuscularly

Ergot Derivatives

Ergonovine maleate (Ergotrate): 0.2 mg intramuscularly or orally; Methylergonovine maleate (Methergine): 0.2 mg intramuscularly or orally

---

holds the fundus (Fig. 8-23). Oxytocic drugs may be needed to stimulate the uterus to contract. (See box above.)

Methergine (methylergonovine) and Ergotrate (ergonovine) are not given intravenously because they are powerful vasoconstrictors. If administered intravenously, Methergine and Ergotrate can cause acute hypertensive and cardiac crises, nausea and vomiting, dizziness, headache, tinnitus, dyspnea, diaphoresis, and palpitations.

Because ergonovine has a vasoconstricting effect, it can cause elevated blood pressure. Always take the woman's blood pressure before giving ergonovine. It is never given to women with hypertension or preeclampsia, nor is it ever given before the placenta is expelled

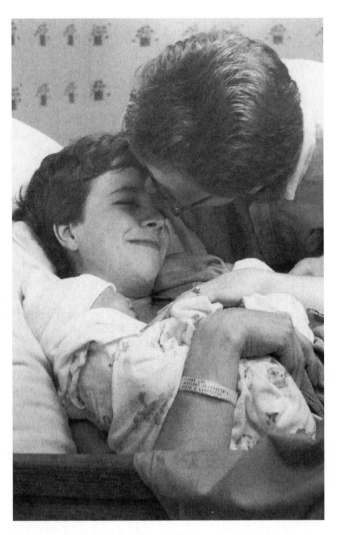

Figure 8-24 Warm support. *(Courtesy The Birthplace at Riverside Medical Center, Minneapolis, Minn.)*

because it can cause the uterus to contract forcibly and thus trap the placenta inside.

Methylergonovine can also raise blood pressure and consequently is never given to a woman with hypertension. Injectable Ergotrate and Methergine must be refrigerated because they deteriorate when exposed to heat and light.

Oxytocic agents, such as Pitocin, are potent drugs and can cause uterine contractions lasting more than 90 seconds *(tetanic contractions.)* The most common method of administering Pitocin is in an intravenous infusion with an infusion pump. Close supervision is necessary.

When the nurse checks the perineal area for vaginal bleeding, any suture line should be checked for possible formation of a *hematoma* (a collection of blood in tissue). Each time the perineal pads are changed, the amount of bleeding and appearance of suture lines should be recorded. Ice compresses applied to sutured areas help to reduce swelling and pain.

Since diaphoresis occurs after birth, the woman may appreciate a sponge bath. Also, after birth the bladder fills up quickly with urine and must be checked for distention frequently. A distended bladder can interfere with uterine contraction and thus cause bleeding.

During the fourth stage of labor the woman's partner and family can offer her warm support and assist with comfort measures (Fig. 8-24). Often this is the time that the new father chooses to telephone anxious family and friends and share the news of the new family member.

SUMMARY

In this chapter common nursing care and procedures for use during the stages of labor and birth were discussed. Step-by-step procedures were not presented since they differ from hospital to hospital. This chapter is a general overview of how the nurse interacts with the intrapartum family when providing basic nursing care. The importance of individualizing care for each family was emphasized.

BIBLIOGRAPHY

American Academy of Pediatrics and American College of Obstetricians and Gynecologists: *Guidelines for perinatal care,* ed 2, Washington, DC, 1988.

Anderson BG, Shapiro PJ: *Obstetrics for the nurse,* ed 6, Albany, NY, 1994, Delmar.

Andrews CM, Chrzanowski M: Maternal position, labor, and comfort, *Appl Nurs Res* 3(1):7-13, 1990.

Bell TA and others: Randomized trial of silver nitrate, erythromycin, and no eye prophylaxis for the prevention of conjunctivitis among newborns not at risk for gonoccal ophthalmitis, *Pediatrics* 92(6):755-759, 1993.

Biancuzzo M: Six myths of maternal posture during labor, *MCN* 18(5):264-269, 1993.

Biancuzzo, M: The patient observer: does the hands-and-knees posture during labor help to rotate the occiput posterior fetus? *Birth* 18(1):40-47, 1991.

Golay J and others: The squatting position for the second-stage of labor: effects on labor and on maternal and fetal well-being, *Birth* 20(2):73-78, 1993.

Guild SD: A comprehensive fetal monitoring program for nursing practice and education, *J Obstet Gynecol Neonatal Nurs* 23(1):34-41, 1993.

Hodnett ED, Osborn RW: A randomized trial of the effects of monitrice support during labor: mothers' views two to four weeks postpartum, *Birth* 16(4):177-183, 1989.

Klaus MH and others: Effects of social support during parturition on maternal and infant morbidity, *Br Med J* 193:585-587, 1986.

Kurokawa J, Zilkoski MW: Adapting hospital obstetrics to birth in the squatting position, *Birth* 12(2):87-90, 1985.

Ladewig PW and others: *Essentials of maternal-newborn nursing,* ed 2, Redwood City, 1990, Addison-Wesley Nursing.

Liu YC: The effects of the upright position during childbirth, *Image* 21(1):14-18, 1989.

Ludke LM and Roberts CC: Eating and drinking in labor: a literature review, *J Nurse Midwifery* 38(4):199-207, 1993.

Lupe PJ and Gross TL: Maternal upright posture and mobility in labor—a review, *Obstet Gynecol* 67(5):727-734, 1986.

Mackey MC, Lock SE: Women's expectations of the labor and delivery nurse, *J Obstet Gynecol Neonatal Nurs* 18(6):505-511, 1989.

Mattson S, Smith JE, editors: Core curriculum for maternal-newborn nursing, Philadelphia, 1993, WB Saunders.

Mayj KA, Mahlmeister LR: *Comprehensive maternity nursing: nursing process and the childbearing family,* ed 2, Philadelphia, 1990, JB Lippincott.

McKay S, Roberts J: Second stage labor: what is normal? *J Obstet Gynecol Neonatal Nurs* 14(2):101-106, 1985.

NAACOG: *Standards for the nursing care of women and newborns,* ed 4, Washington, DC, 1991, The Association.

NAACOG: *Nursing responsibilities in implementing intrapartum fetal heart rate monitoring,* Position Statement, Washington, DC, 1992, The Association.

Seidman D and others: Apgar scores and cognitive performance at 17 years of age, *Obstet and Gynecol* 77(6):875-878, 1991.

Smith MA and others: The rational management of labor, *Am Fam Physician* 47(6):1471-1481, 1993.

Tucker S: *Pocket guide to fetal monitoring,* ed 2, St. Louis, 1992, Mosby.

DEFINITIONS

Define the following terms:

accelerations	diaphoresis
amnionitis	early deceleration
amniotomy	EFM
Apgar score	ergot derivatives
AROM	ferning
artifact	fetal heart rate
aspiration pneumonitis	fetoscope
baseline fetal heart rate	FSE
bradycardia (fetal)	hematoma
decelerations	incubator

IUPC	periodic fetal heart rate
laceration	changes
late deceleration	resting tone
LDR	stethoscope
LDRP	supine hypotensive syn-
Leff stethoscope	drome
Leopold's maneuvers	tachycardia (fetal)
meconium	telemetry
nursing care history	umbilicus
ophthalmia neonatorum	uteroplacental insufficiency
oxytocin	variability
	variable deceleration

LEARNING ACTIVITIES

1. Group discussions.
2. Guests: admissions office personnel or hospital volunteer who helps with maternity admissions to explain procedures.
3. Visit hospital admissions office and observe hospital preadmissions procedures for maternity patients.
4. View audiovisual aids and discuss.
5. Review basic nursing procedure for: enema, catheterization, medical and surgical asepsis.
6. Practice sterile gowning and gloving techniques.

ENRICHMENT/IN-DEPTH STUDY

1. Visit facilities that offer labor, delivery, recovery rooms (LDRs), or labor, delivery, recovery, postpartum rooms (LDRPs). How are these programs staffed; i.e., are nurses multiskilled functioning in labor, birth, and postpartum and newborn care?
2. Review prenatal records of women who will be admitted to your clinical facility for labor and birth within the next month. What deviations from a normal pregnancy course were identified and how were they resolved? What is the probability that these problems will affect the woman's labor and birth experience?
3. Compare external and internal electronic fetal heart rate tracings. How can you tell the difference without reading the woman's chart?

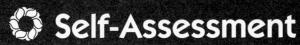

Self-Assessment

1. If the woman preregisters for labor and delivery, what preadmission forms can she complete before hospitalization?

   _____

   _____

   _____

2. When admitting a woman in labor, what information should the nurse gather first?

   a. _____

   b. _____

   c. _____

   d. _____

   e. _____

   f. _____

3. During routine labor, temperature, pulse, and respiration (TPR) are taken and recorded every ____ hours. Blood pressure is taken and ____ every ____ hours.

4. _____ in the urine specimen may be a sign of

   _____.

5. In the first stage of labor it would be abnormal for a uterine contraction to last longer than _____ seconds.

6. Because uterine contractions begin at the fundus, the nurse can monitor the contraction by gently touching the fundus. Describe how to estimate whether the contraction is strong, moderate, or mild: _____

   _____ _____.

7. When performing Leopold's first three maneuvers on a woman in labor, the nurse would stand at the woman's side facing her _____. The first maneuver consists of palpating her _____. The second maneuver determines on which side of the uterus the _____ of the fetus is located. In the third maneuver one hand is pressed over the _____. Before beginning the fourth maneuver the nurse must turn around to face the woman's _____.

8. The normal fetal heart rate is ____ beats per minute.

9. In addition to the regular checking of the fetal heart rate, name three other instances when the heartbeat should be checked:

   a. _____

   b. _____

   c. _____

10. How would you explain the purpose of continuous fetal monitoring to an expectant couple?_____

_____

_____

11. Match Column A with Column B:

Column A

_____ _____ **1** early deceleration

_____ _____ **2** variable deceleration

_____ _____ **3** late deceleration.

Column B

a. late onset

b. carly onsct

c. uteroplacental insufficiency

d. head compression

e. cord compression

f. variable onset

12. The fetal heart rate (FHR) present between uterine contractions is identified as the _____ FHR.

13. Match Column A with Column B

Column A

_____ _____ **1** short-term variability

_____ _____ **2** long-term variability.

Column B

a. fluctuations occurring every 2 to 5 minutes

b. fluctuations of 5 to 25 bpm

c. Stv

d. cyclic variations of 2 to 3 beats from one beat to the next

Circle the correct answers for questions 14 through 20.

14. To accurately evaluate the resting tone of the uterus between contractions, the contractions must be monitored by:

a. external methods

b. internal methods

15. The major disadvantage of internal monitoring is:

a. membranes must be ruptured

b. it is difficult to keep in adjustment

16. Loss of variability or decrease in variability as labor progresses in a previously average reading could be:

a. a good sign

b. an ominous sign

17. Vaginal examinations are done in labor to:

a. determine the state and progress of labor

b. speed cervical dilation

18. Following artificial rupture of membranes (AROM) or amniotomy, the nurse should immediately:

a. listen to and record fetal heart rate

b. perform Leopold's maneuvers

19. The normal appearance of amniotic fluid is:

a. clear and colorless

b. thick and greenish

20. A pregnant woman is being admitted to the hospital in early labor. When preparing to give an enema as ordered, the nurse notices bright-red vaginal bleeding. The nurse would:

    a. cleanse the vaginal area and give the enema as ordered

    b. not give the enema and notify the physician

Fill in the blanks for questions 21 through 32.

21. Describe the significance of the following findings in relation to a woman in labor:

    a. a full bladder _____

    b. the woman lying flat on her back _____

    c. meconium-stained amniotic fluid _____

    d. a woman's complaint of rectal pressure _____

22. What are the signs of the beginning of the second stage of labor?

_____

_____

_____

23. Eye prophylaxsis involves the instillation of _____ into the newborn's eyes.

24. How would you tell expectant parents about the need for newborn eye prophylaxsis? _____

_____

_____

_____

25. Perineal lacerations are sometimes unavoidable. What areas are involved in the following:

    a. First degree: _____

    b. Second degree: _____

    c. Third degree: _____

    d. Fourth degree: _____

26. Complete the following chart for oxytocic drugs used to cause uterine contractions in the third stage of labor:

Drug used	Common dosage	Method of administration
a.		
b.		
c.		

27. The Apgar score assesses the following five signs:

    a. _____

    b. _____

    c. _____

    d. _____

    e. _____

28. Describe the care given to the baby as soon as it is born (immediate needs):

_____

_____

_____

29. In the fourth stage of labor the mother's pulse, respiration, and blood pressure are checked every _____ until stabilized.

30. If the mother begins to bleed excessively in the fourth stage of labor, the first thing to do is _____.

31. When bleeding in the third stage of labor reaches _____ milliliters, it is considered a hemorrhage.

32. Two techniques of fetal heart rate assessment are _____ and _____.

Circle the correct answers for questions 33 through 37.

33. External electronic fetal monitoring produces an average FHR. Therefore external monitoring *cannot* accurately reflect:
    a. fetal hypoxia
    b. FHR variability
    c. a sinusoidal pattern
    d. decelerations in FHR

34. Which one of the following statements about variable decelerations in FHR is true?
    a. Variable decelerations are caused by umbilical cord compression.
    b. Variable decelerations are caused by uteroplacental insufficiency.
    c. Variable decelerations require no intervention.

35. Which one of the following statements about late decelerations in FHR is true?
    a. Late decelerations are caused by uteroplacental insufficiency.
    b. Late decelerations require no intervention.
    c. Late decelerations are reassuring periodic changes in FHR.

36. You note persistent early decelerations on a fetal monitoring strip. Based on your understanding of this pattern, you would:
    a. do nothing; the pattern is normal with fetal head compression
    b. perform a vaginal examination to assess dilation and to determine whether the mother is ready to push
    c. turn the woman to her left side and start to administer oxygen by mask

37. Which one of the following is an advantage of external monitoring?
    a. noninvasive
    b. can assess variability accurately
    c. can measure intensity of contractions
    d. subject to artifacts

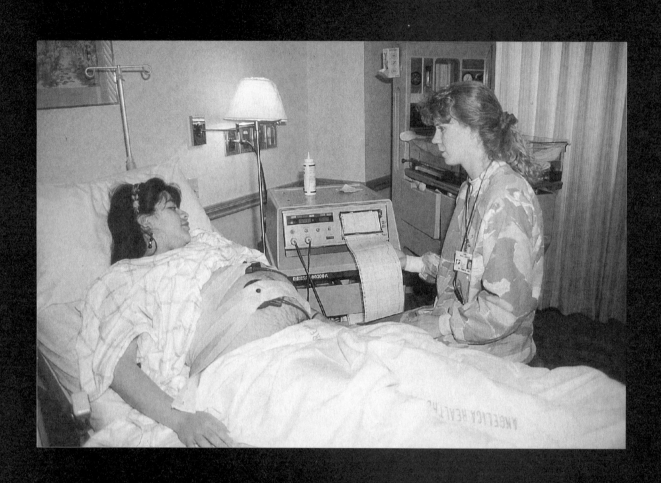

9

THE INTRAPARTUM FAMILY WITH COMPLICATIONS

GOALS

This chapter is designed to provide the reader with information that will:
- develop an awareness of deviations from normal in the intrapartum period.

- explore the nursing role in common complications in the intrapartum period.

STUDENT OBJECTIVES

After studying this chapter, you should be able to:

1. Differentiate between hypotonic and hypertonic labor patterns and discuss the treatment and nursing care for each.
2. Recognize several causes of uterine dysfunction in the latent phase of labor and identify the main cause.
3. Distinguish between the kinds of breech presentations possible, and identify the most common.
4. Identify signs of emergencies during labor and appropriate emergency nursing measures (prolapsed cord, abruptio placentae, placenta previa).
5. Discuss the causes, prevention, treatment, and nursing care for preterm labor.
6. Define postterm pregnancy.
7. Describe postmaturity syndrome and identify the risk to neonates.
8. Describe the three basic types of cesarean

birth, and identify the incision most likely to rupture with a subsequent labor.
9. Discuss nursing care for cesarean birth mothers.
10. Differentiate between forceps delivery and vacuum extraction delivery.
11. Identify women at risk for uterine rupture.
12. Explain the causes of amniotic fluid embolism.
13. Discuss the usual dose, effects, possible side effects for both mother and baby, and nursing care when giving the following analgesics, sedatives, and tranquilizers during labor:
    a. meperidine (Demerol)
    b. sodium pentobarbital (Nembutal)
    c. promethazine (Phenergan)
14. Discuss the mode of administration, the area anesthetized, possible side effects for both mother and baby, and nursing care for the following regional anesthetics:
    a. paracervical block
    b. caudal and lumbar epidural
    c. saddle block (low spinal)

Although labor is a normal and natural process, there are predisposing factors and existing conditions that can complicate the intrapartum experience. In Chapter 5 we discussed the complications apparent in the antepartum period. Those complications that could be predicted would be best cared for in the high-risk perinatal centers described earlier. Statistics have shown that a fetus transported to such a center in utero has a better chance for survival than one transported by ambulance or helicopter following delivery. However, most of the complications explored here do not occur until labor is beginning or has begun.

COMPLICATIONS OF LABOR

✓ Dystocia

Labor begins by the onset of regular, increasingly frequent and increasingly intense, coordinated uterine contractions leading to progressive cervical dilation and descent of the presenting part. The normal labor curve as depicted on a time plot was described in Chapter 7.

According to Emanuel Friedman a *prolonged latent phase* of labor is defined as greater than 20 hours in nulliparas and 14 hours in multiparas. A *protracted active phase* of labor is defined as a dilation rate less than 1.2 centimeters per hour in nulliparas and 1.5 centimeters per hour in multiparas. *Secondary arrest of the active phase* of labor is defined as failure of cervical dilation

for over 2 hours and failure of descent of the presenting part for over 1 hour. These time criteria are useful in identifying the need for further diagnostic effort to determine the cause of abnormal labor but are not necessarily indications for treatment (Fig. 9-1). The term given to difficult, abnormal labor progress is *dystocia.*

It is very sobering to note that dystocia is the largest single cause of the increased cesarean birth rate in the United States. Incorrect utilization of standard labor progression curves can contribute to this increased relationship of cesarean birth and dystocia. The management of abnormal labor depends on the problem and when in the labor the dysfunction occurs. It is important to give significant attention to the management of abnormal labor and not simply cite "failure to progress" as the reason for cesarean delivery when a labor is prolonged.

If the labor pattern does not follow the normal time frame for latent or active phases, it is probably the result of abnormalities in the *powers* of uterine and abdominal muscles, the *passages* (bony pelvis or maternal soft tissue), the *passenger* (fetal malpresentation), or the *psyche* (maternal stress and anxiety).

Dysfunctional Labor Patterns

Normal labor is a dynamic process. Uterine dystocia may be characterized by a hypotonic labor pattern, a hypertonic labor pattern, precipitous labor, or prolonged labor patterns.

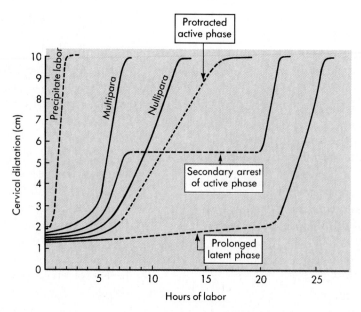

Figure 9-1 Deviations in rate of cervical dilation (as described by Friedman). The prolonged deceleration phase is not pictured. *(From Novak JC, Broom BL: Ingalls and Salerno's Maternal and Child Health Nursing, ed 8, St. Louis, 1995, Mosby.)*

Hypertonic Labor Patterns

Hypertonic labor is manifested by increased frequency and decreased intensity of contractions. Myometrial resting tone is above 15 mm Hg as registered on the electronic fetal monitor. Because the uterine muscle is not relaxing well between contractions, muscle cell anoxia leads to abnormally painful contractions. Fundal dominance is lacking so the contractions, although painful, are not effective in dilating the cervix. Hypertonic labor usually occurs in the latent phase of labor and, if uncorrected, may develop into prolonged labor with fetal distress.

Causes of the hypertonic pattern include maternal stress and anxiety and a disruption in dominance of the contraction pattern, causing colicky, uncoordinated uterine contractions.

Treatment requires a relaxed environment, hydration, reassurance, relaxation, and sleep. Sedation will facilitate sleep. Often after the woman is rested, contractions may begin spontaneously and a normal labor pattern will follow. Another treatment for hypertonic labor is regional anesthesia.

Hypotonic Labor Patterns

Hypotonic labor contractions are weak, irregular, and uncoordinated. The early labor pattern may be within normal limits. However, a pattern of infrequent contractions develops, with mild to moderate intensity, and then slowing or arrest of cervical dilation occurs during the active phase. Myometrial resting tone is less than 8 mm Hg as registered on the electronic fetal monitor.

Causes of a hypotonic labor pattern include oversedation in early labor, an unfavorable cervix, overstretching of the uterus, maternal stress and anxiety, maternal fatigue, or various degrees of cephalopelvic disproportion (CPD). When there is disproportion between the size of the fetus and the birth canal, *fetopelvic disproportion* (often called CPD for cephalopelvic disproportion) exists.

Treatment requires that CPD, abnormal presentations, contracted pelvis, and obstructions be ruled out. It is also important to evaluate the mother's stress and anxiety levels because stress produces neural and endocrine responses that can result in decreased myometrial activity. Dehydration and fatigue may also play a part in hypotonic labor. Assisting the mother with relaxation techniques, massaging her, encouraging ambulation or positions of comfort, ensuring hydration, and promoting rest may facilitate more effective uterine contractions. If these efforts do not improve the labor pattern, intervention is oxytocin augmentation.

Nursing care

The woman and her family may become very worried when their expectations of labor are not met. Consequently, they need a thorough explanation of what is happening. Early recognition of uterine dysfunction is essential so that treatment can begin before the fetus is in distress or the mother is exhausted. Graphing the progression of labor on a labor curve can be helpful in determining labor progress. Because abnormal labor may cause the fetus to be distressed, the nurse must monitor the fetal heart tones often whenever labor deviates from the normal pattern. A woman who is experiencing prolonged labor is at risk for infection; thus the nurse should minimize vaginal examinations and evaluate for signs of infection.

The nurse must be aware that too much medication too soon in labor is the major cause of a prolonged latent phase. Under ordinary circumstances it is wise for the woman to wait until her cervix is dilated at least 3 centimeters before receiving medication for pain.

Providing human companionship and touch and assisting the woman and her partner with relaxation techniques cannot be overemphasized.

Abnormal Fetal Positions

As discussed, the most favorable position for the fetus is either right occiput anterior (ROA) or left occiput anterior (LOA). However, when the fetus is a breech, brow, face, or shoulder presentation, or when the position is right or left occiput posterior (ROP or LOP) (Fig. 9-2), labor can be long and difficult. Face and brow presentations occur less than 0.5% of the time and usually cause prolonged labors. The shoulder presentation (transverse lie) occurs about once in every 500 births. Virtually all shoulder or persistent brow presentations require cesarean delivery because of the high rate of perinatal morbidity with vaginal delivery. For a face presentation a vaginal delivery may occur if labor

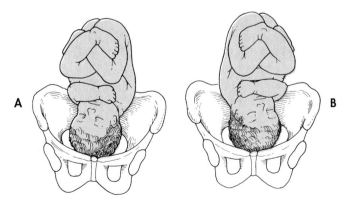

Figure 9-2 Occipitoposterior positions. **A**, Left occipitoposterior. **B**, Right occipitoposterior.

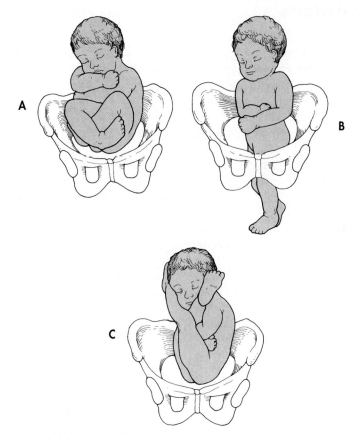

Figure 9-3 Three variations of breech presentation. **A,** Complete breech. The buttocks and feet present and the knees are drawn up. **B,** Footling breech. One or both feet present. **C,** Frank breech. The buttocks present, the legs are extended up and are pressed against the abdomen and chest. This is the most common breech presentation.

happens normally and the pelvis is adequate. A baby born with a face presentation will usually have a swollen and bruised face. The parents need reassurance that this is only a temporary condition. A posterior position causes more contractions because the fetus must rotate through a larger arc (two times the rotation needed for an occiput anterior). A posterior labor is termed *back labor* because the woman experiences severe backache as this long arc rotation occurs.

Approximately 25% of the time the fetal head enters the pelvis with the occiput directed posteriorly. However, during labor anterior rotation occurs spontaneously in 70% of the instances. This rotation can be encouraged by having the mother change position often (every 20 to 30 minutes). Have the mother lie on the side opposite that to which the fetal occiput is directed, or place her in the knee-chest position for three to four contractions at a time. The weight of the baby plus gravity will encourage anterior rotation of the occiput posterior baby. Also, because squatting causes maximal enlargement of the pelvic outlet, this position may provide enough room for an occiput posterior baby to rotate. If rotation does not occur spontaneously, the physician

may rotate the fetal head at the time of delivery, either manually or with forceps.

Nursing Care

Counterpressure on the painful area of the laboring woman will help relieve her back pain. Back massage, cold or hot packs on the low back, and hot showers are helpful. The woman experiencing an occiput posterior labor needs support and encouragement because she and her family will be fatigued and feel frustrated because the labor is longer and more painful.

Breech

About 3% to 4% of all births are breech presentations. There are three varieties: frank (the most common), complete, and footling (Fig. 9-3). Fetal mortality and morbidity rates remain higher among breech compared with nonbreech deliveries. With a breech birth there is a higher fetal risk because the cord can easily prolapse and be compressed. Also, because the head is larger than the buttocks, the buttocks can pass

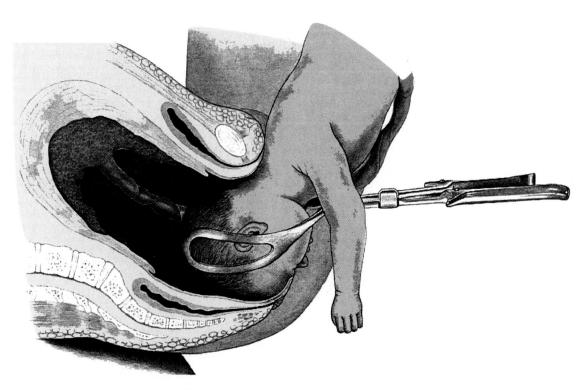

Figure 9-4 Forceps are applied to the aftercoming head. *(From Al-Azzawi F:* Color atlas of childbirth and obstetric techniques, *St. Louis, 1990, Wolfe.)*

through a cervix that is not dilated enough for the head to pass; thus the head can actually become trapped. In recent times a cesarean birth has frequently been the method of choice to deliver a breech baby—particularly if the woman is a primigravida with a large baby. However, there is a growing controversy over whether all breech presentations are best managed by cesarean delivery. Individualization and sound clinical judgment are indispensable in making decisions about the method of delivery for breech presentations. If vaginal birth of a breech is chosen, Piper forceps are commonly used for the controlled delivery of the aftercoming head (Fig. 9-4).

Turning the fetus externally by *external cephalic version* (ECV) is sometimes done in the third trimester. External cephalic version is safe and cost effective. It substantially reduces the cesarean birth rate among breech presentations. Ultrasonography is used to locate the placenta and fetus and to look for abnormalities. Intravenous tocolytic drugs are given to the mother to relax the uterus before the external version. While still floating in the amniotic fluid, the fetus can be manipulated manually and sometimes turned from a breech to a cephalic presentation. Most physicians who have reported recent trials of ECV agree that the procedure is best performed at 36 weeks of gestation. By this time the incidence of spontaneous return to vertex presentation

has declined to a minimum, and the fetus can be delivered if complications occur during the procedure.

Having the woman lie on her back with her buttocks elevated on two or three pillows for 20 to 30 minutes several times a day while the fetus is still floating has been reported to assist the fetus in turning itself from breech to cephalic presentation. Also, the knee-chest position has been used to facilitate fetal turning.

Labor Accidents

Although complications such as placenta previa can be detected before labor begins, some conditions occur during labor without warning.

Prolapsed cord

An obstetric emergency that occurs about once in every 500 births is *prolapse of the umbilical cord*. Prolapse can result in fetal morbidity or mortality and increase maternal risk. Factors that increase the risk of cord prolapse include grand multiparity, hydramnios, abnormally long cord, low implantation of the placenta, breech presentation, transverse lie, unengaged fetal presenting part, multiple gestation, and prematurity. Rupture of the membranes (especially if the presenting part is not engaged) can cause the umbilical cord to lie

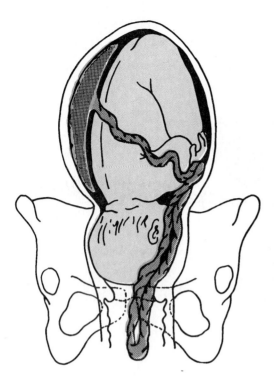

Figure 9-5 Prolapsed cord. *(From Hamilton PM: Basic maternity nursing, ed 6, St. Louis, 1989, Mosby.)*

alongside or below the presenting part after the membranes have ruptured. As a result the oxygen supply to the fetus can be impaired or totally cut off (Fig. 9-5). This is a serious emergency, and the pressure must be relieved from the cord quickly. The main concern in cases of umbilical cord prolapse is to deliver the fetus as fast as possible, vaginally if there is full dilation, but in most cases a cesarean will be required.

Nursing care. Nursing actions include changing the woman's position to take the pressure off the cord by placing her in a knee-chest position or in the Sims' position with her hips elevated on pillows so that they are higher than her chest. She may also be placed in deep Trendelenburg's position. Upward pressure on the presenting part by sterile, gloved fingers in the vagina may keep the cord pulsating until delivery is possible. The woman may become frightened because of the danger to her baby and thus needs constant attendance and reassurance. Oxygen by mask to the mother will probably increase the amount of O$_2$ the fetus receives.

When it is not possible to deliver the fetus quickly, a method using bladder filling and a tocolytic agent has been found useful until an operating room is available. In this procedure the woman's bladder is filled by catheter with 500 to 700 milliliters of saline solution. At the same time a tocolytic agent is administered intravenously by a constant infusion system to prevent pressure on the cord by a strong uterine contraction.

Abruptio placentae

Abruptio placentae and placenta previa were discussed in Chapter 5. (See Figs. 5-4 and 5-5.) These conditions may occur in the antepartum period or may not be apparent until the intrapartum period.

When abruptio placentae occurs in labor, the uterus may feel firm all the time instead of relaxing between contractions. There may also be frequent uterine contractions with elevated uterine resting tone between them. The woman complains of a great deal of abdominal pain and may experience continuous dull back pain also. If the hemorrhage is concealed there may be no vaginal bleeding but the uterus will increase in size. If the hemorrhage is apparent there will be a lot of dark blood from the vagina. The woman may go into shock. The prognosis for major abruption is grave. Fetal mortality averages 30% to 60%. A complication of abruptio placentae is disseminated intravascular coagulation (DIC).

Nursing care. Intravenous fluids and blood replacement must be started quickly, and vital signs, fetal heart tones, urinary output (via Foley catheter), and amount of vaginal bleeding must be monitored closely. Oxygen is administered to the mother by face mask at 8 to 10 L/min. Laboratory studies are performed and vaginal examinations are avoided. Labor is often very rapid when the placenta abrupts; however, if the woman does not deliver quickly, a cesarean birth is in order.

The woman and her family need to know what to expect, and they also need emotional support. They will experience anxiety, confusion, and fear for potential loss of the fetus and even possibly the mother. Reassure them with information about events and efforts of the health care team.

Placenta previa

When a woman with a placenta previa (see Chapter 5) is in labor, the nurse must be alert for any increased bright red vaginal bleeding, a drop in blood pressure, and change in fetal heart tones. It is a good idea to save all perineal and under buttocks pads if the woman bleeds heavily. With the evidence blood loss can be estimated accurately. When blood loss is estimated by weighing pads, 1 gram equals 1 milliliter or on a nonmetric scale 1 ounce equals 29 milliliters. Vaginal examinations are avoided to eliminate the risk of putting an examining finger through the low-lying placenta.

Precipitate labor

A very rapid labor (less than 3 hours) is a *precipitate labor.* These labors usually occur in multiparous women who have very strong contractions. Precipitate labor may also occur in women with large, bony pelves, or soft, pliable genital tissue. Other factors that predispose a woman to precipitate labor may include small fetus in a normal vertex position, previous precipitate labor, and cocaine abuse. The danger in these labors is to the fetus because of the extreme force with which it is propelled through the birth canal. These babies may have bruises on their faces and may have cerebral injuries. There is also a risk of tearing the mother's perineum because of the force with which the baby's head is born. Women who have precipitate labors are at risk for postpartum hemorrhage as a result of a hypotonic uterus.

Preterm Labor

Preterm labor is the onset of rhythmical uterine contractions that produce cervical change, effacement, and/or dilation after fetal viability is established but before fetal maturity is achieved. Subtle symptoms that may herald preterm labor may include menstrual-like cramps, rhythmical low back pain, rhythmical pelvic pressure, change in vaginal discharge, or diarrhea.

Preterm labor usually occurs between the twenty-sixth and thirty-seventh weeks of gestation. A *preterm birth* is any birth that occurs before 37 full weeks of gestation. Preterm labor and delivery continue to be the major causes of perinatal morbidity and mortality in the United States.

The incidence of preterm births is a reflection of the general socioeconomic status of the population, the education level of the parents, the proportion of non-white populations, and whether the mother received prenatal care. Among indigent minority women the incidence of preterm births is more than double the national average. Although the preterm delivery rate varies from institution to institution, it probably falls between 5% and 10% of all births. Health care professionals cannot predict with certainty which women are likely to begin labor prematurely; however, the following factors are known to increase the risk:

1. Socioeconomic factors: lack of prenatal care
2. A previous preterm birth (most important historical risk factor)
3. Multiple gestation (up to 50% preterm labor)
4. Repeated miscarriages or abortions (particularly in the second trimester)
5. Age under 16 or over 40 years
6. Obesity or very low weight (poor nutrition)
7. Cigarette smoking
8. Alcohol or drug abuse
9. Prenatal exposure to diethylstilbestrol (DES)
10. Premature thinning or dilation of the cervix or excessive contractions
11. Maternal medical illness such as kidney infection, liver disease, or heart ailments
12. High blood pressure
13. Strenuous physical work, a long commute, fatiguing child care responsibilities
14. Unusual emotional stress and anxiety
15. Uterine anomalies
16. Polyhydramnios
17. Abdominal surgery and/or cervical cerclage this pregnancy

Identifying women at risk for preterm labor and teaching them life-style modifications and self-examination procedures helps them recognize early danger signals of preterm labor and promotes prompt treatment to stop labor or delay it. The most important components of preterm birth prevention are improving access to care, screening, early diagnosis, and effective therapy. Education about preterm labor should be standard for women at risk for preterm labor, as well as for those with few or no known risk factors.

Management and treatment of preterm labor

Drugs that inhibit uterine contractions are called *tocolytic agents*. Medications, such as ethyl alcohol, prostaglandin synthesis inhibitors, magnesium sulfate ($MgSO_4$), and beta-adrenergic receptor stimulants, have been used to inhibit premature labor, with varying degrees of success. The beta-adrenergic receptor stimulants in use in the United States are isoxsuprine (Vasodilan), terbutaline sulfate (Brethine), and ritodrine hydrochloride (Yutopar). However, the only one of these drugs approved as a tocolytic agent by the U.S. Food and Drug Administration (FDA) is ritodrine hydrochloride (Yutopar). Basically these drugs are smooth muscle relaxants that relax the contracting uterine muscles.

However, ritodrine and terbutaline also stimulate the sympathetic nervous system and can cause the woman to experience side effects of tachycardia, restlessness, anxiety, and nausea and vomiting. Other maternal side effects are cardiac arrhythmias and pulmonary edema. Fetal effects are tachycardia, increased glucose levels, and hypoxia. To reduce the number and severity of side effects, the dose must be low. In the traditional method of administration, terbutaline is given intravenously or subcutaneously, requiring hospitalization. Preinfusion lab work should include ECG, blood glucose, and serum electrolyte determinations. After initial intravenous therapy is successful, oral maintenance or a subcutaneous terbutaline pump may be used.

Magnesium sulfate ($MgSO_4$) also decreases uterine activity by acting directly on the myometrium. $MgSO_4$ is not a hypotensive agent; it *mainly decreases CNS activity* and depresses action of motor nerve impulses. Because it results in some vasodilation, it also decreases blood pressure. Toxic effects are CNS depression, absence of deep tendon reflexes (DTRs), respiratory depression, and respiratory arrest. Adverse reactions generally develop at $MgSO_4$ plasma levels >10-12 mg%; the first sign of toxicity is loss of the patellar reflex.

Contraindications to pharmacological tocolysis include cervical dilation over 4 centimeters, fetal compromise, intrauterine infection, abruptio placentae, fetal death, lethal fetal anomalies, or gestational age over 37 weeks.

Corticosteroids are frequently given at the same time as tocolytic therapy to hasten fetal lung maturity.

Home care treatment of preterm labor is gaining popularity. This may involve hydration, bed rest, oral tocolytics, or use of a subcutaneous terbutaline pump. A variety of home health care agencies provide preterm labor care at home. Women on home therapy perform self-monitoring with a portable tocodynamometer. A home care perinatal nurse visits at least weekly to check blood pressure, pulse, fundal height, and fetal heart rate; do a urinalysis; and perform cervical examinations as indicated. In many cases the home care nurse communicates with the woman daily by phone and interprets daily fetal monitor strips that have been electronically sent to her.

Bed rest with the mother in lateral positions has been shown to be an effective tocolytic. Uterine contractions or irritability may result from dehydration. When women are well hydrated and placed on bed rest with supportive care, preterm labor often ceases.

Nursing care. The family experiencing preterm labor may be under exceptional stress, unprepared for early labor, and grieving for a possible loss of their expected full-term baby. In addition to suffering emotional stress, the woman receiving terbutaline or ritodrine may experience hypotension, tachycardia, nausea, nervousness, sweating, restlessness, and tremors, and should be informed of these expected side effects. Close observation and recording of vital signs, fetal heart tones, intake and output of fluids, and emotional status, in addition to constant and consistent emotional support, are vital nursing actions. Encourage verbalization of the family's feelings and always be realistic with information given. High levels of emotional distress may result in family disruption. Providing anticipatory guidance and offering assistance with problem solving are essential nursing actions.

Postterm Pregnancy

A postterm pregnancy is one that persists for 42 weeks (294 days) or more from last menstrual period (LMP), assuming a 28-day cycle. Currently management of postterm pregnancy falls into three major categories: (1) routine induction, (2) fetal assessment with intervention if there is evidence of fetal compromise,

and (3) no intervention or assessment of the postterm pregnancy.

Although postterm pregnancies represent 7% to 11% of all pregnancies, they account for over 15% of all perinatal mortality.

Postmaturity syndrome is the abnormal condition of a fetus or newborn resulting from declining placental function that occurs in postterm pregnancy. Approximately 20% of postterm babies have this syndrome, which includes dry, wrinkled, peeling skin; staring eyes; creases over the entire surface of the sole of the foot; absence of vernix or lanugo; long fingernails; and meconium staining. The literature is clear regarding the compromised status of most postmature infants. They are at risk for developing serious problems resulting from chronic or acute placental insufficiency and asphyxia at birth, and/or oligohydramnios and umbilical cord compression. The main cause of death in prolonged pregnancy is reported to be cord compression from oligohydramnios (less than 300 ml of amniotic fluid).

Management of the postterm pregnancy requires accurate dating of the pregnancy. (Often postterm pregnancies have been found to be misdated and not truly prolonged pregnancies.) Second, fetal evaluation using fetal movement counting (FMC), nonstress tests (NSTs), contraction stress tests (CSTs), ultrasound to identify pregnancies with reduced amniotic fluid, placental grading, and a fetal biophysical profile will help to determine if the fetus is at risk for the problems associated with postmaturity.

Despite the few documented medical benefits of a policy of routine induction of labor at 42 weeks of gestation, many health care providers believe it is beneficial. Many women also want to end a long, uncomfortable, and frustrating time of waiting. If induction is done, prostaglandin gel may be used for cervical ripening followed by intravenous oxytocin infusion.

Nursing care

Labor should be conducted with the woman in the left lateral position to maximize placental blood flow and with continuous external fetal monitoring. Oxygen should be available, and personnel skilled in handling and intubating newborns should also be available. Passage of fluid stained with meconium during labor is cause for concern, especially if the fetal monitor tracing is not reassuring. If the baby is born through meconium, steps must be taken to prevent meconium aspiration syndrome. (See Chapter 13.) The baby's mouth, nose, and pharynx should be aspirated with a suction device as soon as the head has been delivered. Further examination of the airway by means of laryngoscope, intubation, and suctioning should occur until no more meconium can be removed.

Postterm pregnancy is accompanied by feelings of fatigue, frustration, anger, and disappointment. Many women experience guilt and loss of control. There is fear concerning the baby's well-being and future development. The fetal evaluation itself can become anxiety provoking because it emphasizes concern over fetal well-being. Family relationships can be severely strained. It is important not to ignore, minimize, or treat casually any feelings expressed by the pregnant woman and her family. They need an opportunity to express all feelings in an environment of acceptance and support.

Stimulation of Labor

Induction of labor is causing labor to begin artificially. Prostaglandins (PGE_2; PGF_2) have been used intrave-

nously, orally, sublingually, extraamniotically, intravaginally, intracervically, and by pessary to stimulate labor. However, the best results with the least side effects are obtained by local administration of prostaglandin as close to the cervix as possible.

Oxytocin is a synthetic hormone used to stimulate rhythmic contractions of the uterus and is approved for induction of labor in women for a medical indication only. When a medical indication exists, labor may be induced to protect both mother and/or fetus from serious illness or even death. The most common medical and obstetric indications are listed in the box at left. Authorities disagree on absolute and relative contraindications to induction. Contraindications to uterine stimulation are listed in the box at left, below. However, the risk-benefit ratio for both mother and infant must be considered individually for each case. Oxytocin (Pitocin) is administered by the intravenous route in a diluted solution for inductions.

Cervical ripeness, or maturation, is a very important variable in contemplating induction of labor. The probability for a successful induction is reduced when the cervix is unripe. The Bishop score is utilized to measure the physiological readiness of the cervix. An assessment and measurement of cervical dilatation, effacement, station, consistency, and position is done. In general a Bishop score greater than 8 is indicative of a probable successful induction. (See box below.)

Total possible score is 13. High score indicates a greater chance for successful outcome. Lower scores indicate the cervix is less favorable for induction.

Studies have shown that prostaglandin placed close to the cervix in a suppository or gel can ripen the cervix and induce labor. Often the gel is inserted in the afternoon or evening before a scheduled induction. Prostaglandins biochemically affect cervical ripening and thus act to decrease cervical resistance to dilation. Side effects may include nausea and vomiting, diarrhea, and fever.

Oxytocin causes rhythmic uterine contractions by stimulating uterine muscle. The cervix should be soft (ripe) and Bishop score favorable before an induction

Induction of Labor: Common Indications

Maternal indications
Pregnancy-induced hypertension (PIH)
Premature rupture of membranes after the thirty-sixth week
Intrauterine fetal death
Deteriorating maternal illness
Hydramnios, fetal anomaly incompatible with life
Chorioamnionitis

Fetal indications
Diabetes mellitus
Rh sensitization
Intrauterine growth retardation (IUGR)
Prolonged pregnancy (beyond 42 weeks of gestation)
Anomalies

Contraindications to Induction of Labor

Absolute
Fetal distress
Central placenta previa
Unfavorable fetal position
Proven cephalopelvic disproportion
Active genital herpes infection
Fundal uterine scar

Relative
Overdistended uterus
Grand multiparity (more than five pregnancies)
Breech presentation
Prematurity
Maternal cardiac disease

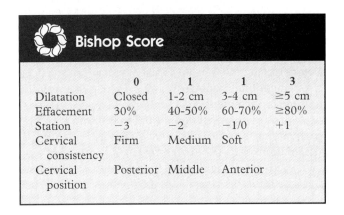

Bishop Score

	0	1	1	3
Dilatation	Closed	1-2 cm	3-4 cm	≥5 cm
Effacement	30%	40-50%	60-70%	≥80%
Station	−3	−2	−1/0	+1
Cervical consistency	Firm	Medium	Soft	
Cervical position	Posterior	Middle	Anterior	

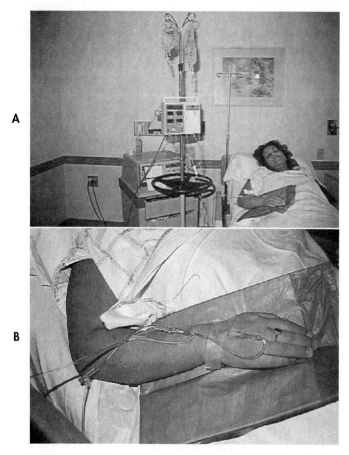

Figure 9-6 Double-bottle set-up. **A,** Secondary line on left contains intravenous solution with oxytocin added. Primary line (closest to mother) contains a plain intravenous solution. **B,** The secondary line is connected as close as possible to the primary intravenous site. *(Courtesy Marjorie Pyle, RNC, Lifecircle, Costa Mesa, Calif.)*

is begun. A double-bottle set-up (the primary line for infusion of a nonoxytocin containing intravenous solution and the secondary line containing intravenous solution with oxytocin added) and an infusion pump are mandatory when induction is via intravenous administration of Pitocin (Fig. 9-6, *A*). The secondary line should be connected as close as possible to the primary intravenous site (Fig. 9-6, *B*).

For stimulation/induction of labor 1 ml (10 U) of oxytocin is diluted in 1000 ml of Ringer's lactate or normal saline. Currently, the ACOG's Technical Bulletin 157: *Induction and Augmentation of Labor*, describes two protocols. One involves an initial oxytocin dose of 1 or 2 mU/min. The oxytocin may be increased every 15 minutes in increments of 1 mU/min. The second protocol involves an initial dose of 0.5 to 1.0 mU/min. The oxytocin may be gradually increased in increments of 1 to 2 mU/min every 30 to 60 minutes. Regardless of protocol used, when the desired frequency of contractions is reached, the rate may be maintained.

If intense, sustained contractions occur (tetanic contractions lasting longer than 90 seconds), the resting period between contractions decreases or disappears, or fetal distress occurs, the intravenous drip containing the oxytocin should be stopped immediately and the plain bottle infused. Oxytocin is broken down in the kidney and liver and has a circulatory half-life of 3 to 4 minutes, whereas the uterine effects last 20 to 30 minutes. For most women the duration of action of the oxytocin is related to its half-life, and thus the stimulus is gone quickly. However, for those few women who are maximally sensitive, the effects of the oxytocin can last longer.

Other ways to start or stimulate labor include nipple or breast stimulation, as discussed in Chapter 5.

Nursing care

Because the woman may experience anxiety related to induction, it is essential that the nurse offer clear explanations for the procedure and maintain a frequent presence. The woman should be continually reassured of fetal status and progress of labor.

Although in utilizing oxytocin for induction the goal is to mimic natural labor, the laboring woman will feel the pain from induced contractions sooner than with naturally occurring labor. Women using prepared childbirth techniques often report experiencing difficulty "staying on top of" oxytocin induced contractions. Thus it is very important for the nurse and support persons to actively support the woman undergoing induction/augmentation of labor.

Because of the antidiuretic effect of oxytocin, the nurse must be alert to signs of fluid overload when high doses of oxytocin are used. It is essential to observe the woman for arrhythmias, oliguria, nausea, vomiting, headache, and hypotension.

During induction continuous electronic fetal monitoring is recommended. Fetal heart tones, blood pressure, pulse, resting uterine tone, and the frequency, duration, and strength of contractions should be checked and recorded at intervals comparable to the dosage regimen; that is, at 15- or 30- to 60-minute intervals when the dosage is evaluated for maintenance increase or decrease. Careful intake and output (I&O) must be followed and documented.

In the event of uterine hyperstimulation (i.e., contractions less than 2 minutes in frequency and greater than 90 seconds in duration) or an elevated resting tone of the uterus, oxytocin should be discontinued immediately. In addition, mainline fluids should be increased, oxygen given by mask, and the physician or midwife notified of your nursing actions and the woman's response.

Augmentation of labor is using amniotomy or intravenous administration of oxytocin to stimulate or regulate ineffective uterine contractions as in a hypotonic labor pattern. Amniotomy for the purpose of augmenting labor is controversial. If amniotomy is not followed by cervical dilatation, oxytocin augmentation may be used. The nursing care for labor augmentation using oxytocin is the same as the nursing care for induction. However, augmentation usually requires lower dose of oxytocin.

Active management of labor

The active management of labor (AML) is a protocol for management of spontaneous labor in the nulliparous woman. AML was first developed in Ireland by O'Driscoll and Meagher to prevent prolonged labor and its complications. Key components of the approach include accurate diagnosis of labor, personal attention throughout the labor (1:1 care by a nurse-midwife), amniotomy when presenting part is engaged, and selective use of oxytocin. The AML is confined to nulliparous women with cephalic presentation of a single fetus in no fetal distress.

The key to the whole program is the diagnosis of labor. Spontaneous labor is defined as regular uterine contractions in association with either cervical effacement or dilation (1-2 cm) and ruptured membranes or bloody show.

Once the diagnosis of labor is made the woman must progress at the rate of at least 1 cm of cervical dilation per hour. The aim of AML is efficient labor and birth without damage to mother or child within 12 hours of admission.

Two important elements of the AML are artificial rupture of membranes (AROM) within 2 hours of admission and the use of oxytocin augmentation if the cervix is not dilating at the rate of 1 cm/hr in the presence of ruptured membranes. The dosage protocol for the oxytocin infusion usually involves beginning oxytocin at 6 mU/min and increasing every 15 minutes until an infusion rate of 36 to 40 mU/min is reached or more than 7 contractions occur in 15 minutes.

The active management of labor as described by O'Driscoll and Meagher is more than an augmentation protocol. It is a comprehensive way of thinking about and facilitating the entire labor experience.

Cesarean Birth

A cesarean birth is the delivery of a baby through an incision made in the abdominal and uterine walls. Cesarean birth rates increased dramatically in the United States from 4.5 per 100 births in 1965 to 22.7 in 1985. In 1987 the cesarean rate was 24.4%; in 1991 the rate was 23.5 per 100 deliveries. Although the frequency of cesarean birth has leveled off in the past 5 years, it re-

mains higher than in most other countries. This high incidence of cesareans is contributing to increased health care costs.

A few factors leading to an increased cesarean rate include (1) reluctance to deliver breech presentation vaginally; (2) better antenatal screening techniques to assess the fetus in utero; (3) an increase in continuous FHR monitoring of low-risk women; (4) a change in attitude of obstetricians concerning treatment of nonprogressive labor (dystocia) so that it is not prolonged unnecessarily; (5) practice of defensive medicine due to rising malpractice claims; (6) increased use of epidural anesthesia; (7) nursing influence; and (8) routine repeat cesareans. The indications for a cesarean birth are cephalopelvic disproportion, malpresentation or malposition, fetal distress, uterine dysfunction, prolapsed cord, abruptio placentae, and placenta previa. Maternal disease such as active herpes genitalis and identified medical need for a repeat cesarean are other indications.

Types

There are three basic types of cesarean birth. (1) The *classic* cesarean is quick and easy to perform. The incision is made in the midline of the abdomen and in the midline of the thick fundus (Fig. 9-7, *A*). However, a normal labor is contraindicated with any subsequent pregnancy because this incision can rupture easily. (2) A *low cervical* cesarean is preferred because the incision is made transversely in the lower uterine segment (Fig. 9-7, *B*). This uterine scar is less apt to rupture with the next pregnancy. (3) In an *extraperitoneal* cesarean the bladder is dissected downward and the peritoneal cavity is not entered. A transverse incision is then made into the lower uterine segment (Fig. 9-7, *C*). Maternal morbidity with cesarean deliveries is two to four times that of vaginal birth. This increased maternal morbidity is largely due to infectious complications.

Nursing care. The woman must be prepared for major surgery and given emotional support. Cesarean birth imposes the physiological stresses of anesthesia, major surgery, physical recovery, and postoperative complications, including infections. Today many families are sharing the cesarean birth experience, with the father present at the cesarean birth. After all, a cesarean is a birth and the beginning of a new family unit just as a vaginal delivery is the beginning of a family. To enhance parent-child attachment after the birth, the parents and infant should spend time together if the infant is not compromised.

Although the family that prepared for a vaginal delivery may be happy and excited about the birth of a healthy baby, the unexpected cesarean may provoke

SKIN INCISION   UTERINE INCISION

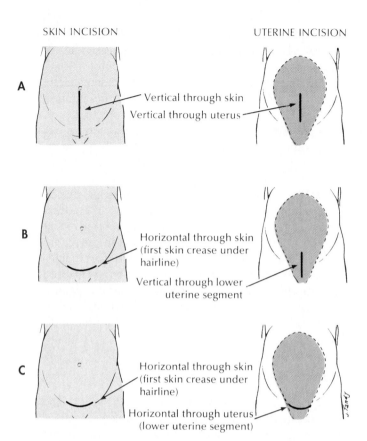

A, Vertical through skin
Vertical through uterus

B, Horizontal through skin (first skin crease under hairline)
Vertical through lower uterine segment

C, Horizontal through skin (first skin crease under hairline)
Horizontal through uterus (lower uterine segment)

Figure 9-7 Cesarean birth: skin and uterine incisions. **A,** Classic: vertical incisions of skin and uterus. **B,** Low cervical: horizontal incision of skin; vertical incision of uterus. **C,** Low cervical: horizontal incisions of skin and uterus. *(From Bobak IM and others:* Maternity nursing, *ed 4, St. Louis, 1995, Mosby.)*

feelings of anger, disappointment, and guilt in the family members. These feelings should not be ignored or minimized. By listening empathetically a nurse can allow the parents to verbalize their feelings and then work through them. The box on p. 247 is a listing of options to facilitate family-centered cesarean births. In many communities there are cesarean birth support groups and preparation classes for couples scheduled for cesarean birth. Cesarean births should also be discussed in prenatal classes for women preparing for vaginal births. Specific information about the incision, pain and discomfort, body image changes, and changes in family interactions should be included in prenatal classes.

Vaginal Birth After Cesarean (VBAC)

It has been shown that careful selection of expectant women and use of proper protocols can make vaginal birth after cesarean safer than repeat elective cesarean delivery. Vaginal delivery offers less maternal and infant morbidity, better opportunities for bonding, and more

successful breast-feeding. According to guidelines published by the American College of Obstetricians and Gynecologists (ACOG), cesarean delivery remains the proper course of action when there is cephalopelvic disproportion, a classic uterine incision, multiple pregnancy, or fetal weight of 4000 grams or more. In the majority of cases, however, a vaginal trial of labor following cesarean birth is now encouraged.

Nursing care

Women planning to undergo a trial of labor have special needs. They must understand the risks and possible complications involved and realize that a trial of labor could result in a cesarean. Preparation for labor with knowledge, relaxation, and breathing techniques is important. Many women who had previous cesareans for nonrecurring problems can experience normal births. Explaining the risks while providing encouragement and support can help to make the difference.

Forceps Delivery

Forceps, skillfully applied, can aid in the safe delivery of a baby. When forceps are applied after the fetal head is crowning, the delivery is termed a *low forceps* or *outlet delivery*. This is the most common forceps application and is chosen by the physician to better control the delivery. When forceps are applied after the head is engaged but has not yet reached the perineal floor, the delivery is termed a *midforceps delivery*. Forceps may be applied in this case because of the mother's inability to push effectively, resulting from exhaustion or regional or general anesthesia. Fetal distress requiring prompt delivery, abnormal presentations, failure to rotate, and arrested fetal descent are other reasons for a midforceps delivery. Application of forceps *(high forceps)* at any time before full engagement of the fetal head is not justified in modern obstetrical practice. To ensure relaxation and prevent pain during midforceps delivery, anesthesia is given to the mother.

Nursing care

The nurse monitors the fetal heart tones before and after the physician applies the forceps. If the FHR decreases after application, the physician must remove the forceps and reapply.

Vacuum Extraction Delivery

Although in the United States forceps delivery is used most of the time when assistance is needed, vacuum extraction has been popular in much of the world for

Options to Facilitate Family-Centered Cesarean Births*

1. Admission to the hospital on the morning of the birth for elective cesareans so that parents can spend the previous night together (provided they have had previous orientation).
2. Father to remain with the mother during the physical preparation, for example, shave, catheterization.
3. The choice of regional anesthesia where possible, and explanation of the differences between regional and general anesthesia.
4. Father in the delivery room when either regional or general anesthesia is the choice (including when anesthesia is started).
5. Mirror and/or ongoing commentary from a staff member for mother and/or father.
6. Photographs or video taken in the delivery room—if even one parent is unable to witness the birth.
7. Mother's hand freed from restraint for contact with husband and baby.
8. Opportunity for both parents to interact with the baby in the delivery room and/or postanesthetic recovery room.
9. Opportunity for breast-feeding in the delivery room or postanesthetic recovery room.
10. Modified Leboyer practices, for example, father to submerge baby in warm water until relaxed and alert in the delivery room or in the nursery, if available for vaginal delivery.
11. Delayed antimicrobials in baby's eyes.
12. If father chooses not to be in the delivery room:
    a. a support person should replace him at the mother's side
    b. father to be given baby to hold en route to nursery
    c. father to have the birth experience relayed to him by a staff member
13. Father to accompany baby to the nursery and remain with infant until both are reunited with the mother.
14. Family reunited in postanesthetic recovery room if possible.
15. Father to be in postanesthetic recovery room to tell his wife about the birth if she has had a general anesthetic.
16. If it is difficult to reunite the family in postanesthetic delivery room, the mother's condition should be judged individually to allow the family to be reunited as soon as possible.
17. Baby's condition to be judged individually so that time alone in an incubator in the nursery can be avoided if possible.
18. Provision of time alone for the family in those first critical hours.
19. Mother-baby nursing as soon as possible, that is, if mother feels well enough she may be able to have mother-baby nursing on the first day.
20. Father to be included in the teaching of caretaking skills.
21. Siblings to be included where possible.

*In an effort to make the cesarean delivery more family centered, the following options should be available where safety permits.
Modified from: Leach L, Sproule V: Meeting the challenge of cesarean births. *J Obstet Gynecol Neonatal Nurs* 13(3):193, 1984.

years. Vacuum extraction involves a disk-shaped cup being applied to the fetal head. A vacuum is then created by a pump that withdraws air between the fetal head and the cup. Traction is applied synchronized with uterine contractions (Fig. 9-8) when the mother needs assistance in the second stage.

There are no known risks to the mother associated with vacuum extraction. In fact advantages may include reduction in injuries to the mother's vaginal walls, bladder, uterus, and bowel. Also, the mother is able to push with her contractions because little or no anesthesia is needed for vacuum extraction.

A disadvantage of vacuum extraction is the swelling of the fetal head tissue, known as a *chignon*, that develops underneath the suction cup. This chignon will generally diminish in size within a few hours after birth and is not known to cause long-term problems. However, other possible risks to the fetus may include cephalhe-

matomas and scalp lacerations. Vacuum extraction is contraindicated with preterm deliveries because of the increased possibility of bleeding in the immature fetal head.

Because practitioners in the United States have been showing an increased interest in vacuum extraction, nurses must be prepared to discuss the advantages, disadvantages, and contraindications with families.

Uterine Rupture

Rupture of the uterus is a rare occurrence. Uterine rupture may occur if a woman has had previous uterine surgery, such as classic cesarean section, myomectomy, salpingectomy, curettage, or manual removal of the placenta; if labor is long and difficult; if a woman has had more than six deliveries; or if oxytocin or prostaglandin is given injudiciously. Rupture of the uterus

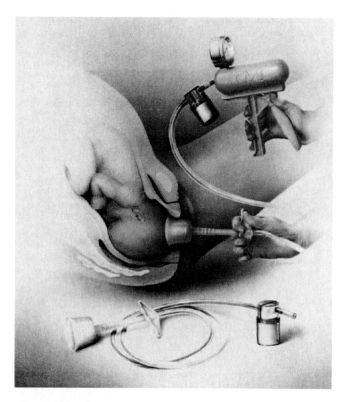

Figure 9-8 Vacuum delivery system. *(Courtesy Columbia Medical and Surgical, Inc, Bend, Oregon.)*

can be incomplete or complete. Incomplete rupture (dehiscence) may go undetected since the uterine wall ruptures but the peritoneum surrounding the uterus remains intact. Complete rupture extends through the uterine wall and the uterine contents are spilled into the abdominal cavity. The thinned-out, lower uterine segment is a common site of uterine rupture. Tears along previous uterine scars can also occur. The risk of rupture of a previous classic cesarean scar is high, but low transverse uterine incisions from previous cesareans are not as likely to rupture. (See Fig. 9-7 for illustrations of uterine incisions.)

The signs of complete uterine rupture are sudden, sharp, abdominal pain; cessation of uterine contractions and fetal heart tones; and signs and symptoms of shock. The mother may complain of feeling a tearing sensation in her abdomen. This is a serious emergency and requires immediate surgical intervention. Often the hemorrhage is into the peritoneal cavity rather than out through the vagina. The maternal mortality rate can be as high as 10%, and the fetal mortality rate can be as high as 50%.

Treatment consists of oxygen therapy, fluid and blood replacement, and the intravenous administration of substances to restore the normal clotting mechanism. The baby may be saved if delivered immediately, but, as indicated, the mother may die. Although this complica-

tion is rare it is important to be aware of it and alert to its signs and symptoms.

Premature Rupture of Membranes

Premature rupture of membranes (PROM) is defined as spontaneous rupture 1 hour or more before onset of labor. The risks are maternal infection (chorioamnionitis), preterm birth, and infection for the baby. Management depends on the gestational age of the fetus and presence or absence of maternal infection. If PROM occurs between 26 and 32 weeks, the woman is treated with prophylactic antibiotics and maintained on bed rest. If PROM occurs between 32 and 35 weeks, the woman is tocolyzed until fetal lungs are mature; bed rest and hydration are maintained; and prophylactic antibiotics are given.

Amniotic Fluid Embolism

The accidental infusion of amniotic fluid into the mother's endocervical veins or into the venous sinuses of the placental site causes a maternal mortality rate as high as 80%. This complication, *amniotic fluid embolism*, is very rare, occurring only once in approximately 65,000 labors. The pathogenesis may include entry of amniotic fluid through lacerations or ruptures of the uterus or cervix; through endocervical veins; and through abnormal uteroplacental sites, such as with placental abruption, placenta previa, or placenta accreta. Although it may occur at any time after the membranes have ruptured, it is most often reported near the end of the first stage of a rapid, vigorous labor. Because the amniotic fluid contains small particles of matter, such as vernix, lanugo, and meconium, multiple tiny emboli may be drawn into the general circulation and in this way reach the pulmonary capillaries, causing obstruction.

Signs and symptoms appear suddenly. The woman experiences sudden dyspnea, cyanosis, chest pain, pulmonary edema, and may cough up blood-tinged mucus before losing consciousness. Uterine relaxation with hemorrhage and profound shock occur. An important complication of amniotic fluid embolism is reduced fibrinogen blood levels and subsequent disseminated intravascular coagulation (DIC). If the woman does not die from the initial respiratory insult, she will have to overcome the severe hemorrhage from the DIC that follows. (See Chapter 11.)

ANALGESIA AND ANESTHESIA

In Chapter 5 we discussed methods of preventing or relieving pain in childbirth without medication. Discomfort in labor can also be relieved by analgesics and anesthesia. *Analgesia* is absence of a normal sense of pain. *Anesthesia* is partial or complete loss of sensation with or without loss of consciousness resulting from administration of a drug. The nurse's understanding of the actions and effects of medication on both the mother and the fetus is very important. Women's responses to drugs are as variable as their responses to labor. Therefore drug therapy should be flexible and individualized. Although any medication used during labor should not endanger the mother or the fetus, every drug has that potential. There is no drug that stops the discomfort of labor completely and is absolutely safe for both the mother and the baby. However, despite the risks involved drugs can reduce the anxiety and pain of labor and delivery and enhance the birth experience for some women. In considering the possible risks involved in using obstetric drugs, one must also consider the benefits. For some women the stress of doing without medication in labor may do more harm than the drugs used. Therefore the nurse must know how and when each medication should be used, the advantages and disadvantages, and possible complications related to the drugs.

There are six groups of medication given for labor and/or birth:

1. Sedatives and tranquilizers, which relieve anxiety and tension in early labor
2. Amnesics, which erase memories of pain and the labor
3. Regional analgesics, which interrupt pain pathways
4. General analgesics, which increase the tolerance of pain
5. General anesthestics, which prevent central perception of pain
6. Local anesthestics, which block pain sensations to a particular area

Sedatives and Tranquilizers (or Ataractics)

Sedative drugs such as the barbiturates secobarbital (Seconal) and sodium pentobaribital (Nembutal) can be useful in relaxing an anxious woman during the early or beginning latent phase of labor when birth is not anticipated for 12 to 24 hours.

Ataractics or tranquilizers such as promethazine (Phenergan), hydroxyzine (Vistaril), and diazepam (Valium) are used in early labor either alone or with barbiturates or analgesics. When given alone these drugs do not affect the pain threshold; however, they potentiate the action of barbiturates and analgesics so that the doses of the barbiturates and analgesics can be reduced when tranquilizers are given with them. These agents also have antiemetic properties that are occasionally desirable.

Sedatives and tranquilizers are never given close to the time of delivery or when preterm deliveries are probable (Table 9-1). These sedative drugs possess no analgesic properties and in some instances may heighten the woman's reaction to pain. In addition, they cross the placenta rapidly and may depress neonatal respiration for long periods.

Amnesics

Scopolamine used to be given to produce amnesia for laboring women. It was frequently combined with morphine sulfate and called "twilight sleep." The laboring woman still had pain but no memory of it or of the birth. Scopolamine given alone causes restlessness and bizarre behavior. When scopolamine is given with analgesics, the restlessness is less severe, but constant attendance is required so that the woman will not harm herself (Table 9-1).

Narcotic Analgesics

Meperidine (Demerol) is the analgesic used most often during labor to relieve pain. The best time to give Demerol is after the cervix is 3 to 4 centimeters dilated (active phase of labor). It is important to understand that the peak action of this analgesic occurs within 40 to 60 minutes of intramuscular administration and 5 to 10 minutes after intravenous administration, and it is effective for 2 to 4 hours. Since Demerol can cause severe respiratory depression in neonates, it should be given at least 2 hours before birth to minimize CNS depression. Neurobehavioral scores show lower levels of activity in such neonates for up to 3 days, although these are subtle changes.

Other narcotic-like drugs used in labor are nalbuphine (Nubain), and butorphanol (Stadol). Stadol and Nubain are synthetic analgesics that relieve moderate to severe pain. All narcotics cross the placenta and may cause neonatal respiratory depression.

Research indicates that analgesic drugs may be linked with "adverse infant outcome" in behavioral and gross motor development. Although the long-term effect of analgesia and anesthesia used in labor on infant learning responses is not known, drugs for labor and birth should not be used indiscriminately (Table 9-1).

Narcotic Antagonists

Narcotic antagonists counteract the respiratory depressant effects of the narcotic analgesics. Levallorphan tartrate (Lorfan) and Naloxone hydrochloride (Narcan) are the most commonly used narcotic antagonists.

TABLE 9-1
Pain-Relieving Drugs for Labor

Drug	Usual dose	Route	When given in labor	Effects
Sedatives (barbiturates)				
Sodium secobarbital (Seconal)	100-200 mg (1.50-3 grains)	PO, IM, rectally	Very early in labor	Lowers perception of stimuli
Sodium pentobarbital (Nembutal)	30-100 mg (1.5-3 grains)	PO, IM, rectally	Very early in labor	Relieves tension Provides rest Produces sleep
Tranquilizers				
Promethazine (Phenergan)	25-50 mg	IM or IV	With narcotic or barbiturate or alone, in early labor	Sedative Relieves anxiety
Hydroxyzine (Vistaril)	5-15 mg	IV or IM		Tranquilizes Enhances physical
Diazepam (Valium)	2-10 mg	IM or IV		mental relaxation
Amnesic				
Scopolamine (Hyoscine)	0.3-0.4 mg (1/200-1/150 grains)	IM	Early in labor	Amnesia Produces drowsiness and sleep
Narcotic analgesic				
Meperidine (Demerol)	50-100 mg or 25-50 mg	IM, IV	After cervix is 3 to 4 cm dilated	Relieves pain, may aid labor progress as cervical relaxation occurs
Nalbuphine (Nubain)	5-10mg 1 mg at 6 to 10 minute intervals	IM IV	In labor	Decreases pain
Butorphanol (Stadol)	1-2 mg 0.5-1 mg	IM IV		
Narcotic antagonist				
Naloxone hydrochloride (Narcan)	Neonate: 0.01 mg/kg of baby's weight Adult: 0.4 mg	IV or sub Q IM or IV	Immediately before, during, after delivery Same as above	Reverses effect of narcotic
Levallorphan tartrate (Lorfan)	Laboring woman: 1 mg	IV	5 to 10 minutes before delivery	Prevents respiratory depression in newborn

Continued.

TABLE 9-1—cont'd
Pain-relieving Drugs for Labor

Possible side effects		Nursing care after administration
Mother	**Fetus and newborn**	
May slow or prolong labor Can cause restlessness, excitement, disorientation May heighten the woman's reaction to pain	Drowsiness for 24-48 hours after birth Respiratory distress; decreased sucking ability	Inform the woman of what she will experience. Use power of positive thinking. Give reassurance and suggestions that drug will relieve pain and cause relaxation. Woman must remain in bed. Put side rails up on bed, and instruct woman not to get out of bed. Provide quiet environment. Observe progress of labor closely. Watch for signs of restlessness and excitement. Check fetal heart tones, respirations frequently.
Maternal hypotension May slow labor May cause dizziness, blurred vision, confusion	Delayed onset of respirations Altered attention span in first 24-48 hours after birth Slow adaptation to feeding	Inform the woman of what she will experience. Use power of positive thinking. Give reassurance and suggestions that drug will relieve pain and cause relaxation. Woman must remain in bed. Put side rails up on bed, and instruct woman not to get out of bed. Provide quiet environment. Check fetal heart tones, respirations, blood pressure frequently. Observe closely for changes in progress of labor.
Extreme restlessness, excitement, disorientation	Respiratory depression; drowsiness	Give constant attendance to the woman. Watch for signs of extreme restlessness and excitement. Check fetal heart tones, blood pressure, respirations frequently.
Hypotension, facial flushing, oral dryness, nausea and vomiting, restlessness Can slow labor if given too early	Respiratory depression; changes in infant behavior first 24-72 hours of life (most serious Neonatal depressions occur if meperidine is given 2 hours before delivery)	Inform the woman of what she will experience. Woman must remain in bed. Put side rails up. Check fetal heart tones, blood pressure, respirations frequently. Watch progress of labor closely. Administer at least 2 hours before birth to minimize CNS depression in newborn.
Does not interfere with labor	Respiratory depression in neonate	Inform the woman of what she will experience. Woman must remain in bed. Check fetal heart tones frequently.
	Baby can be depressed again after drug is metabolized Same as above	Observe continuously.
Effective only against neonatal respiratory depression caused by narcotic analgesics	Prevents rebound respiratory depression in newborn	Observe continuously.

PO = by mouth; IM = intramuscularly; IV = intravenously.

Regional Anesthesia-Analgesia

Regional anesthesia-analgesia provides complete or near-complete pain relief for the mother, allowing her to be awake during the birth, without significant side effects for the fetus, provided no complications occur. Drugs used for regional anesthesia-analgesia include procaine (Novocain), dibucaine (Nupercaine), lidocaine (Xylocaine), tetracaine (Pontocaine), mepivacaine (Carbocaine), chloroprocaine (Nesacaine), and bupivacaine (Marcaine) (Table 9-2).

Paracervical block

Paracervical block is a type of regional anesthesia. Approximately 10 milliliters of local anesthetic is injected into the nerve plexus on each side of the cervix (corresponding to the 3 and 9 o'clock positions) when the cervix is dilated 4 centimeters or more. This injection interrupts the sensory impulses traveling from the uterus to the spinal cord in the paracervical area. Anesthesia relieving the discomfort of uterine contractions develops in 3 to 5 minutes and may last approximately 1 to 2 hours. However, the procedure does not anesthetize the perineum. Most women report considerable benefit. Injections may be repeated depending on the duration of labor. Temporary slowing of the fetal heart rate has been reported. Fetal heart tones should be checked frequently. Maternal blood pressure should also be taken regularly to detect possible medication reactions.

The risk of fetal bradycardia, hypoxia, and acidosis has caused the paracervical block to nearly vanish in modern obstetric practice (Fig. 9-9).

Local infiltration

Local infiltration of the episiotomy site will provide anesthesia for performing the procedure and the repair but little else. Local infiltration anesthesia is produced by injecting dilute solutions of the drug into the skin and subcutaneously into the region to be anesthetized during minor surgery. Repeated injection will prolong the anesthesia as long as needed. (See box on p. 256 for a list of the most frequently used local anesthetics.)

Pudendal block

Pudendal block is local anesthesia into the pudendal nerve centers on the right and left sides of the perineal area (Fig. 9-10). It is probably the safest anesthesia available today for both mother and baby. The injection is made through the vaginal mucosa directly over the ischial spines. With its use an episiotomy may be performed or outlet forceps applied. Although the perineum is blocked to pain, the woman still feels contractions. Used in an otherwise unmedicated childbirth, the advantage is the relief of perineal pain. The disadvan-

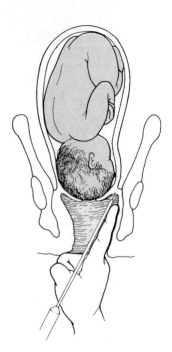

Figure 9-9 Paracervical block.

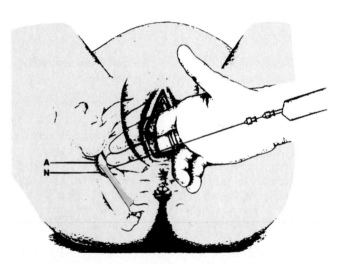

Figure 9-10 Pudendal block. *(From Al-Azzawi F:* Color atlas of childbirth and obstetric techniques, *St. Louis, 1990, Wolfe.)*

tage is the bearing-down reflex is lessened or lost completely. The anesthetic effect is insufficient to permit instrumental vaginal delivery except for low forceps, and it does not allow uterine exploration or manual removal of the placenta.

Caudal and lumbar epidural

Caudal anesthesia is achieved by "blocking" the nerves in the epidural space. It is a type of regional anesthesia achieved by injecting an anesthetic agent into the caudal space of the sacrum. This produces a loss of sensation from the waist down (Fig. 9-11, *B*). When a plastic catheter is inserted above the dural sac, additional anesthetic solution can be added at appropriate intervals. This continuous administration is called a *continuous caudal.*

Lumbar epidural analgesia/anesthesia is another regional block achieved by injecting the anesthetic agent outside of the dura into the extradural space. This epidural space is a potential space outside the spinal dural sac. The space is approached between the third and fourth lumbar vertebrae rather than the caudal area (Fig. 9-11, *A*). As with caudal anesthesia a single injection may be made or a plastic catheter may be threaded into the space to allow continuous epidural administration of medication for labor and delivery.

Epidural analgesia/anesthesia can be administered at any time during labor. However, it is traditionally administered when the primigravida is 5 to 6 cm dilated and the multipara is 3 to 4 cm dilated with regular uterine contractions.

Lumbar epidural is currently the most favored because the catheter is placed very close to the nerve roots conducting the pain of the first stage of labor, thus minimizing the required dosage of drug. Caudal epidural requires a larger volume of local anesthetic during the first stage of labor, although it may provide faster and more intense perineal anesthesia during the second stage of labor.

Today lumbar epidural anesthesia is used more commonly than either spinal or caudal anesthesia because (1) epidural anesthesia provides the greatest degree of flexibility (continuous catheter technique possible; excellent analgesia for all stages of labor and for cesarean sections); (2) caudal anesthesia provides excellent analgesia for the second stage of labor but less so for early labor; and (3) the risk of postdural puncture headache is much higher following spinal anesthesia.

Although epidural anesthesia can be effective for con-

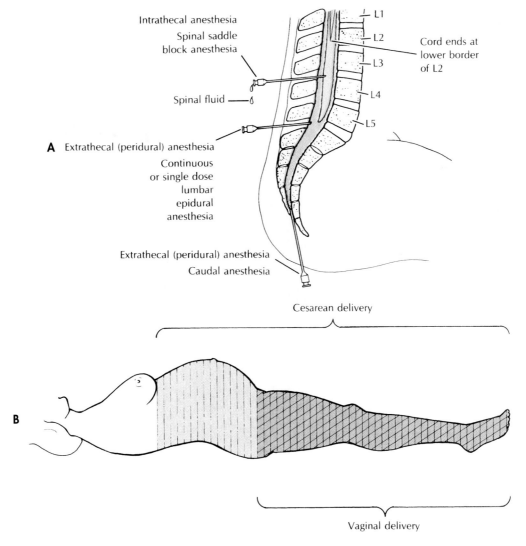

Figure 9-11 A, Regional anesthesia in obstetrics. **B,** Level of anesthesia necessary for cesarean delivery and for vaginal delivery. *(Courtesy Ross Laboratories, Columbus, Ohio.)*

TABLE 9-2
Anesthesia for Labor and Birth

Type of anesthesia	Usual dosage	Administration	Area anesthetized or effects	Possible side effects		Nursing care after administration
				Mother	Baby	
Regional						
Paracervical block	5-10 ml of 1% solution of a "caine" drug	Injection, either side of cervix at 4 cm dilation; may be repeated	Cervix and uterus	Can slow labor	30% incidence of temporary slowing of fetal heart	Close monitoring of fetal heart tones and maternal vital signs and contractions
Pudendal block	5-10 ml of 1% solution of a "caine" drug	Injection into area of pudendal nerves for birth and episiotomy repair	Perineum	None unless allergic to drug	None	Reassurance and explanation; monitor fetal heart tones and maternal vital signs closely
Caudal and lumbar epidural	5-15 ml of 1%, 1.5%, or 2% solution of a local anesthetic agent	Caudal canal Epidural space in active labor	Pelvic region	Hypotension; cannot "push" for delivery May slow labor if started too early	Slowing of fetal heart rate and fetal heart decelerates	Monitor fetal heart tones and maternal vital signs closely; use excellent aseptic techniques

Spinal block	Local anesthetic agent	Injection into spinal fluid in the spinal canal	Abdominal, pelvic, and perineal regions	Maternal hypotension; postspinal headache	None	Close monitoring of maternal vital signs; monitor fetal heart rate; place wedge under right hip to tip uterus off vena cava
Saddle block (low spinal)	1-1.5 ml of solution, concentration depends on "caine" drug used	Injection under dura of spinal cord for birth	Pelvic region	Postspinal headache Hypotension; cannot "push" for delivery	None	Intravenous and O₂ usually used
General Inhalation	Nitrous oxide Halothane Cyclopropane Ethrane, Florane, or other similar agents	Inhaled through mask	Complete body; loss of consciousness	Could aspirate if vomits	Respiratory depression; hypoxia	Be alert and prepared for vomiting (with aspiration of food) and excessive uterine bleeding owing to uterine relaxation
Local infiltration	Mepivacaine (Carbocaine) and lidocaine (Xylocaine) or other local anesthetic	Interstitially; directly into tissue to be repaired	Numbs tissue at site of episiotomy or lacerations	Numbs site	None known	Inform woman of procedure and what she will feel; assess for perineal trauma (swelling, bruising)

Most Frequently Used Local Anesthetics

Anesthetic agent	Characteristics	Individual dose	Cesarean section	Onset of action	Duration of action	Maximum dose	Miscellaneous information
Xylocaine (Lidocaine)	Most versatile local anesthetic, moderate toxicity, intermediate onset and duration, excellent spread.	8-12 ml of a 1% or 1.5% solution	15-20 ml of a 1.5% or 2% solution	5-15 minutes	60-120 minutes	300 mg	Used with increased frequency for epidurals. Essentially devoid of allergic potential.
Nesacaine (Chloroprocaine)	Very low toxicity, most rapidly metabolized with little accumulation, rapid onset but poor spread.	8-12 ml of a 1% or 2% solution	15-25 ml of a 3% solution	5-15 minutes	30-90 minutes	1000 mg	Large inadvertent subarachnoid block associated with neurological residual. May be associated with decreased neonatal tone at birth. May produce allergic reaction in persons sensitive to sulfonamides or thiazide diuretics.
Marcaine (Bupivacaine)	Slow onset, long duration, marked cardiac toxicity, low concentrations give excellent sensory and little motor block.	12 ml of a 0.25% or 0.5% solution 8-15 ml per hour of a 0.125% or 0.25% solution for continuous infusion	20-25 ml of a 0.5% solution	10-20 minutes	120-240 minutes	225 mg	Concentration of .75% not recommended for obstetrics due to cardiac toxicity. Addition of epinephrine does not significantly prolong block. Decreases beat-to-beat variability of fetal heart rate. May be associated with decreased fetal tone at birth. Essentially devoid of allergic potential.

TABLE 9-3
Nonpharmaceutical Pain-relief Methods

	Advantages	Disadvantages	Cost
Biofeedback	Wide applicability outside obstetrics No physician's order needed No devices needed after training	Difficulty in training time is variable Finding a certified biofeedback trainer	Equipment for training costs several thousand dollars. Individual cost is determined by training time.
Transcutaneous electrical nerve stimulation (TENS)	Wide applicability outside obstetrics	Constantly need the device Need physician's order Most effective if introduced before crisis or operation May interfere with continuous electronic fetal monitoring	TENS unit costs approximately $200 to $500.
Acupuncture	Widely used in the Orient for years	Invasive Needles may cause infection Difficulty in finding a qualified professional	Variable, depending on treatments.
Acupressure	Widely used in the Orient for years	Difficulty in finding a qualified professional	Variable, depending on treatments. Could be integrated into nursing treatments.
Therapeutic touch	No devices needed No physician's order needed Noninvasive Nursing background in research and application Self-healing	Not studied well in obstetrics Unknown effect of energy transfer on fetus (two fields involved)	Essentially no cost because it usually is incorporated into nursing care.
Bathing	Low cost High satisfaction No physician's order needed	May cause hyperthermia Continuous electronic fetal monitoring is impossible	Cost of tub and water.

From Brucker MC: Nonpharmaceutical methods for relieving pain and discomfort during pregnancy, *MCN* 2:390-394, 1984.

trol of labor pain, it is not without risks. There is controversy regarding the relationship between epidural anesthesia and cesarean births. Several studies have revealed that almost three times as many first-time mothers with slow labors and epidurals had a cesarean for "failure to progress" than did first-time mothers with slow labors who did not have an epidural. Epidural issues that remain controversial also include increased labor length, increased need for oxytocin augmentation, maternal postpartum urinary retention, and fetal effects such as decreased sucking and responsiveness to surroundings. Other controversies concern epidural contribution to both increasing health care costs and liability of health care providers.

There are studies available today correlating newborn behaviors with the administration of regional anesthesia during delivery. The findings report that as long as 3 days after birth, infants whose mothers received regional anesthesia were more irritable than infants whose mothers were not medicated. Also, the infants of medicated mothers showed decreased motor maturity. Many more studies need to be done on the relationship of anesthesia administration during childbirth to the functioning of the newborn infant.

When all the benefits and risks of epidural anesthesia have been discussed with the woman and her family and she still elects to have an epidural block, the goal of epidural anesthesia should be to provide satisfactory analgesia with minimal motor blockage, which should allow the woman to move her legs and turn in bed. An epidural that results in "heavy legs" and an inability to move causes greater dependence on the staff and results in less control on the part of the woman. This practice should be discouraged.

Spinal anesthesia

Spinal anesthesia is sometimes referred to as a *saddle block* because the anesthetized area is the area that would touch a saddle when riding a horse. This is a regional anesthesia achieved by injecting the anesthetic agent under the dura of the spinal cord (Fig. 9-11, *A*). This provides for a pain-free delivery and does not interfere with uterine contractions. The woman may experience a loss of need to push with contractions so that she will have to be coached to push or delivery will be managed by low forceps. After delivery there is an increased tendency for bladder and uterine atony and spinal headache. When this type of anesthesia is used for cesarean section, it is referred to as a spinal block, and a higher dose of medication is used. The woman must sit for the injection and remain seated for approximately 30 seconds after the injection so that the drug will move downward rather than upward, which could interfere with her ability to breathe.

Nursing Care

Because one of the most common complications of regional analgesia for labor is maternal hypotension, it is important for the nurse to keep constant check on the patient's blood pressure. Before an epidural for labor, an intravenous fluid loading of 500 to 1000 ml of a nonglucose-balanced salt solution (lactated Ringer's or normal saline) is administered. This fluid load compensates for the vascular vasodilation caused by the anesthetic agent. If the mother becomes hypotensive post procedure, immediate action should be taken to restore blood volume to the central circulation. Shifting the woman on her side or elevating and displacing the uterus to the left and administering oxygen at 10 to 12 L/min may restore the blood pressure to normal. Also, the rate of the intravenous infusion should be increased.

Nausea and vomiting are usually the first signs of hypotension and will subside when the woman's blood pressure returns to normal. Administration of oxygen and reassurance of the mother and her family are often very effective in relieving nausea.

The mother may not feel the need to urinate because of the sensory impairment produced by the epidural. A full bladder can slow fetal descent. The nurse must check the mother's bladder every 30 minutes. If she is not able to void, catheterization may be necessary.

Maternal vital signs are monitored every 2 to 3 minutes during the procedure and for the first 20 to 30 minutes post procedure, then every 5 to 15 minutes thereafter. Continuous assessment of fetal heart rate response is necessary. Internal monitoring is preferred.

Complications associated with narcotic agents may include respiratory depression, nausea and vomiting, itching, and urinary retention throughout the labor with regional analgesia-anesthesia. The nurse continuously evaluates for any sign of adverse reaction to the medication utilized. After birth, ambulation is not attempted until full motor and sensory function of the lower extremities is regained.

General anesthesia

General anesthesia is avoided for uncomplicated vaginal birth and used only for specific obstetrical indications, such as breech with entrapped head or shoulder dystocia, with no other anesthesia in place. There is significant risk of regurgitation of gastric contents with pulmonary aspiration and respiratory depression. Light general anesthesia, considered by many to be ideal for cesarean delivery, is achieved with a combination of drugs. Excellent tolerance of the anesthetic is widely reported. Rapid resuscitation of the mother and even small-for-gestational-age and growth-retarded infants can be achieved.

Alternatives to Medication

Nonpharmaceutical approaches to pain relief include biofeedback, transcutaneous electrical nerve stimulation (TENS), acupuncture, acupressure, therapeutic touch, and bathing. (See Table 9-3 for the advantages and disadvantages of these methods.)

With the support of others a prepared woman who has learned to rely on herself can reduce the need for medical intervention with drugs. Prepared childbirth techniques, ambulation, different positions, loving support, and a comfortable environment for birth are low-risk and low-cost alternatives to medication.

SUMMARY

When emergencies occur during the intrapartum period, they are often life threatening; consequently, prompt recognition and response are essential. When the nurse has a firm understanding of the normal labor process, deviations from the process are easy to recognize. Chapter 10 will help you apply your knowledge of the intrapartum period to the actual nursing care of the postpartum family.

BIBLIOGRAPHY

American College of Obstetricians and Gynecologists: Induction and augmentation of labor, *Tech Bull* 157, Washington, DC, 1991.

American College of Obstetricians and Gynecologists: Operative vaginal delivery, *Tech Bull* 196, Washington, DC, 1994.

Anderson BG, Shapiro PJ: *Obstetrics for the nurse,* ed 6, Albany, NY, 1994, Delmar.

Association of Women's Health, Obstetric, and Neonatal Nurses: *AWHONN Practice Resource: cervical ripening and induction and augmentation of labor,* Washington, DC, 1993.

Benedetti TJ, Easterling T: Antepartum testing in postterm pregnancy, *J Reprod Med* 33(3):252-258, 1988.

Brucker MC: Nonpharmaceutical methods for relieving pain and discomfort during pregnancy, *MCN* 2:390-394, 1984.

Clark C: Vaginal birth after cesarean section, *ICEA Rev* 11(3):21-27, 1987.

Confino E and others: The breech dilemma: a review, *Obstet Gynecol Surv* 40(6):330-337, 1985.

Cox JP: Delivery alternatives in the term breech pregnancy, *ICEA Rev* 12(4):21-28, 1988.

Eakes M: Economic considerations for epidural anesthesia in childbirth, *Nurs Econ* 8(5):329-332, 1990.

Galvan BJ, Brockhuizen FF: Obstetric vacuum extraction, *J Obstet Gynecol Neonatal Nurs* 16(4):242-248, 1987.

Gordon SC, Gaines SK, Hauber RP: Self-administered versus nurse-administered epidural analgesia after cesarean section, *J Obstet Gynecol Neonatal Nurs* 23(2):99-103, 1994.

Henrikson ML, Wild LR: A nursing process approach to epidural analgesia, *J Obstet Gynecol Neonatal Nurs* 17(5):316-320, 1988.

Inturhisi M, Camenga CF, Rosen M: Epidural morphine for relief of postpartum, postsurgical pain, *J Obstet Gynecol Neonatal Nurs* 17(4):238-243, 1988.

Isenor L, MacGillivray TP: Intravenous meperidine infusion for obstetric analgesia, *J Obstet Gynecol Neonatal Nurs* 22(4):349-356, 1993.

Mannino F: Neonatal complications of postterm gestation, *J Reprod Med* 33(3):271-276, 1988.

Marshall C: The art of induction/augmentation of labor, *J Obstet Gynecol Neonatal Nurs* 14(1):22-28, 1985.

Mattson S, Smith JE, editors: *Core curriculum for maternal-newborn nursing,* Philadelphia, 1993, WB Saunders.

Miller AM, Lorkovic M: Prostaglandin E$_2$ for cervical ripening, *MCN Suppl* 23-30, Sept/Oct 1993.

Miovech SM and others: Major concerns of women after cesarean delivery, *J Obstet Gynecol Neonatal Nurs* 23(1):53-59, 1994.

Morton SC and others: Effect of epidural analgesia for labor on the cesarean delivery rate, *Obstet Gynecol* 83(6):1045-1052, 1994.

Nichols CW: Postdate pregnancy, part I: a literature review, *J Nurse Midwifery* 30(4):222-239, 1985.

Nichols CW: Postdate pregnancy, part II: clinical implications, *J Nurse Midwifery* 30(5):259-268, 1985.

O'Driscoll K, Meagher D, Boylan P: *Active management of labour,* ed 3, Aylesbury, England, 1993, Mosby Year Book Europe Limited.

O'Neill ML: *Creative childbirth,* Los Angeles, 1993, Papyrus.

Payne P, Nance N: Preterm labor, *ICEA Rev* 12(2):23-26, 1988.

Phelan JP and others: Twice a cesarean, always a cesarean? *Obstet Gynecol* 73(2):161-165, 1989.

Price TM, Baker VV, Cefalo RAD: Amniotic fluid embolism: three case reports with a review of the literature, *Obstet Gynecol Surv* 40(7):462-475, 1985.

Radin TG, Harmon JS, Harmon DA: Nurses' care during labor: its effect on the cesarean birth rate of healthy, nulliparous women, *Birth* 20(1):14-21, 1993.

Reichert JA, Baron M, Fawcett J: Changes in attitudes toward cesarean birth, *J Obstet Gynecol Neonatal Nurs* 22(2):159-167, 1993.

Sala DJ, Moise KJ: The treatment of preterm labor using a portable subcutaneous terbutaline pump, *J Obstet Gynecol Neonatal Nurs* 19(2):108-115, 1990.

Savona-Ventura C: The role of external cephalic version in modern obstetrics, *Obstet Gynecol Surv* 41(7):393-400, 1986.

Scheller JM, Nelson KB: Does cesarean delivery prevent cerebral palsy or other neurologic problems of childhood?, *Obstet Gynecol* 83(4):624-629, 1994.

Shearer MH, Estes M: A critical review of the recent literature of postterm pregnancy and a look at women's experiences, *Birth* 12(2):95-111, 1985.

Taffel SM, Placek PJ, Liss T: Trends in the United States cesarean section rate and reasons for the 1980-85 rise, *Am J Public Health* 77(8):955-959, 1987.

Taylor T: Epidural anesthesia in the maternity patient, *MCN* 18(2):86-93, 1993.

Zhang J, Bowers WA Jr, Fortney JA: Efficacy of external cephalic version: a review, *Obstet Gynecol* 82(2):306-311, 1993.

DEFINITIONS

Define the following terms:

acupuncture	oligohydramnios
AML	oxytocin
analgesia	paracervical block
anesthesia	passage
augmentation	passenger
biofeedback	pessary
Bishop score	Pitocin
breech	posterior
caudal	postmaturity syndrome
cephalopelvic dispropor-tion	powers
cesarean birth	premature rupture of membranes (PROM)
chignon	preterm labor
chorioamnionitis	prolapsed cord
dehiscence	prostaglandins
dystocia	pudendal block
epidural	saddle block
external cephalic version (ECV)	sedatives
fetopelvic disproportion	TENS
hypertonic labor	tetanic contractions
hypotonic labor	therapeutic touch
induction	tocolytic agent
inertia	tranquilizers
labor curve	VBAC
	version

LEARNING ACTIVITIES

1. Group discussions.
2. Guest speakers: a midwife or obstetrician to discuss their

experiences with variations from normal labor; a couple who have experienced a cesarean birth.

3. View audiovisual aids and discuss.
4. Discover what organizations and/or support groups exist in your community for cesarean birth teaching and support.

ENRICHMENT/IN-DEPTH STUDY

1. Draw and label normal labor curves for a primigravida and a multipara.

2. Draw and label the following abnormal labor curves for a primigravida and a multipara: prolonged latent phase and protracted active phase.
3. Working with a fellow student, position that student as you would a woman with a prolapsed cord in the first stage of labor.
4. Discuss the problems of a premature birth for the mother and father and for the baby.

For questions 1 through 3, circle the best answer.

1. Some causes of uterine dysfunction include:

   a. abnormal fetal positions

   b. cephalopelvic disproportion

   c. prolapsed cord

   d. contracted pelvis

   Answer (circle one):

   1. a and b

   2. c

   3. a, b, and c

   4. all of the above

2. Induction of labor is:

   a. causing labor to begin artificially

   b. causing a prolonged second stage

   c. stimulating labor

3. Signs of a complete uterine rupture include:

   a. sudden, sharp abdominal pain

   b. shock

   c. no fetal heart tones

   d. frequent, intense uterine contractions

   Answer (circle one):

   1. a and d

   2. a, b, c

   3. d

   4. all of the above

Supply the correct answer(s) for the following items:

4. Dystocia means _____.

5. The main cause of uterine dysfunction in the latent phase of labor is _____

   _____.

6. When uterine dysfunction occurs, there is a danger of fetal distress; consequently,

   it is very important for the nurse to _____.

7. A fetal indication for cesarean birth would be _____.

8. The cesarean incision most likely to rupture with subsequent labors is _____

   _____.

9. For what reasons may the nurse have to stop intravenous administration of the oxytocin?

_____

_____

_____

10. Five maternal indications for cesarean birth are:

a. _____

b. _____

c. _____

d. _____

e. _____

11. Discuss nursing care of a woman in preterm labor.

_____

_____

_____

12. Below are schematic drawings of the three types of breech presentation. Write the correct name for each one.

A _____ B _____ C _____

13. The majority of breech presentations are of which type?

_____

14. What are the dangers involved in a breech presentation?

a. _____

b. _____

c. _____

15. If the umbilical cord drops down alongside and below the presenting part after the membranes have ruptured, the appropriate emergency nursing measures are:

_____

_____

_____

16. When abruptio placentae occurs in labor, the signs are:

a. _____

b. _____

c. _____

17. When providing nursing care to a laboring woman with placenta previa, the nurse would:

_____

_____

_____

18. There are three basic types of cesarean births. They are:

a. _____

b. _____

c. _____

19. Match Column A with Column B.

Column A

____ ____ **1** hypotonic contractions

____ ____ **2** hypertonic contractions

Column B

a. treatment is usually sedation

b. happens in latent phase

c. happens in active phase

d. treatment is oxytocin

20. Complete the following chart of analgesics, sedatives, and tranquilizers used in labor.

Drugs	Effects	Possible side effects		Nursing care
		Mother	Fetus	
Meperidine (Demerol)				
Sodium pentobarbital (Nembutal)				
Promethazine (Phenergan)				

21. Complete the following chart of regional anesthetics used in labor.

Anesthetics	Areas anesthesized	Possible side effects		Nursing care
		Mother	Fetus	
Paracervical block				
Caudal				
Epidural				
Saddle block				

For questions 22 through 25, circle the best answer.

22. Hypertonic labor patterns are manifested by:

    a. increased frequency and decreased intensity of contractions

    b. fundal dominance

    c. active phase occurrence

    d. infrequent, mild contractions

23. Hypotonic labor patterns can frequently be corrected by:

    a. facilitating relaxation

    b. encouraging ambulation or positions of comfort

    c. oxytocin augmentation

    d. all of the above

24. All except one of the following will relieve the pain of first stage labor. Which is the exception?

    a. intravenous narcotics

    b. paracervical block

    c. epidural anesthesia

25. The process of normal labor is affected by the power, passenger, passage, and psyche. The passenger plays a role in:

    a. frequency of contractions

    b. intensity of contractions

    c. descent and position

    d. pelvic size

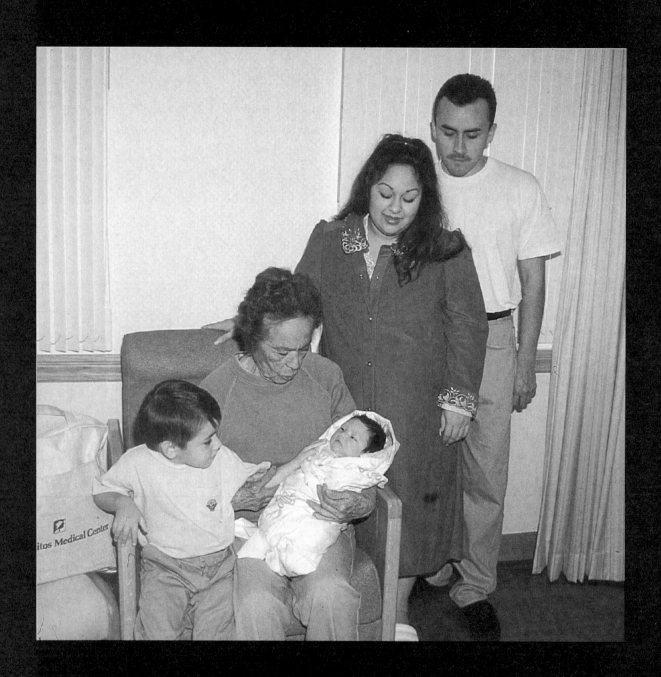

10

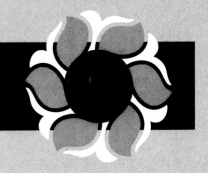

THE POSTPARTUM FAMILY

GOALS

This chapter is designed to provide the reader with information that will:
* promote awareness of the physical and psychological needs of the new mother, her infant, and the family during the postpartum period.

* develop an understanding of the importance of parent/infant interaction during the postpartum period.
* introduce the concept of family planning.

STUDENT OBJECTIVES

After studying this chapter, you should be able to:

1. Define puerperium or postpartum period.
2. Describe taking-in, taking-hold, and letting-go behavior in a new mother.
3. Compare the physiological adaptations that occur in the postpartum mother in each of the following: (a) uterus, (b) lochia, (c) urinary system, and (d) perineum.
4. Compare the time frames when postpartum depression and postpartum psychosis occur.
5. Differentiate between rooming-in and mother-baby nursing.
6. Plan how you would help a new mother cope with the following postpartum discomfort: (a) afterpains, (b) hemorrhoids, (c) episiotomy pain, and (d) constipation.
7. Describe nursing responsibilities in promoting successful infant feeding.
8. List two strategies to correct flat or inverted nipples.

9. Describe correct positioning of the baby at the breast.
10. Differentiate between the time periods when menstruation usually reappears in breast-feeding and nonnursing mothers.
11. Identify the mode of action, effectiveness, contraindications, and side effects of the following temporary methods of birth control: (a) oral contraception, (b) intrauterine contraceptive devices, (c) foam, (d) diaphragm, (e) cervical cap, (f) vaginal suppositories, (g) condoms, (h) implants, (i) injections, and (j) rhythm.
12. Describe the optimal time, procedure, and risks for the following methods of induced abortion: (a) suction curettage, (b) dilation and evacuation using vacuum aspiration, (c) amniocentesis and injection of prostaglandins, and (d) hysterotomy.

DEFINITIONS

The *puerperium* (Latin *puer,* child; *parere,* to bring forth), or postpartum period, begins with the fourth stage of labor and lasts approximately 6 weeks before the reproductive organs return to their approximate prepregnant state by a process known as *involution.* Although healing of the reproductive organs may happen within 6 weeks after delivery, a woman's recovery of full functional ability requires more than 6 weeks (and for cesarean births, considerably longer).

Many texts now identify the first 3 months postpartum as the "fourth trimester," a time of intense learning, need for nurturing, and uniting as a family unit. During this period the woman undergoes significant role changes as she becomes a mother. The man also undergoes role changes in becoming a father, and because of the societal and cultural stereotypes, transition to the fathering role is sometimes the more difficult of the two. Of course other family members, such as siblings and grandparents, also undergo identity changes, which are sometimes complicated by hospital rules and regulations that separate these family members from the mother and baby during the childbearing experience.

The length of the hospital stay postpartum differs greatly from one community to the next—from 6 hours to 2 days for vaginal birth and from 2 to 4 days for cesarean birth. The care this new family receives during the brief postpartum hospitalization is extremely important.

In Chapter 1 we discussed the warm, affectionate tie that can develop between parents and infant during pregnancy and birth. This parent-infant love relationship (attachment) is facilitated by the shared birth experience (see Chapter 7) and when the family is given as much private time as possible during the third and fourth stages of labor. However, as explained earlier, attachment does not occur instantaneously; it is a process occurring over time. Understanding the psychosocial adaptations new parents go through in the postpartum period as they develop their new roles will help you to have a positive influence on the parent-infant relationship (Fig. 10-1).

PSYCHOSOCIAL ADAPTATIONS

The postpartum phases of psychosocial adjustment as described by Reva Rubin, include the "taking-in," the "taking-hold," and the "letting-go" phases.

Rubin found that the *taking-in phase* occurs in the first few days after delivery while physical recovery is also occurring. During this time the mother is passive and dependent, needing to be mothered herself. She is fatigued after the hard work of labor and needs nourishment, rest, and sleep. However, she also needs her new baby so that the acquaintance process can continue. In the first part of this phase women often relive the birth to assimilate it. They want to talk about their experience and resolve any questions or feelings. New fathers and other family members who share the labor and birth need to relive their experiences also. Communication that occurred between the couple during the experience may need discussion, clarification, and resolution. If the new baby is not the sex they wanted, they need to work through disappointment together. It is very seldom that the real baby meets the parents' ex-

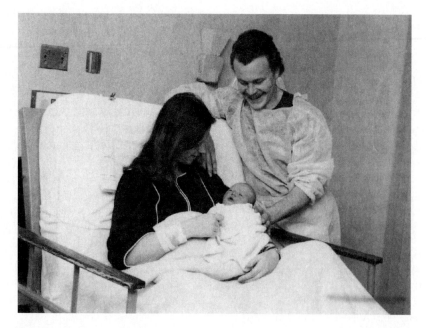

Figure 10-1 Developing new roles. *(Courtesy Valley Hospital and Medical Center, Spokane, Washington.)*

pectations for their perfect fantasized baby. In the taking-in phase the woman is usually passive, doing what she is told, and awaiting invitations from others to begin her own physical care and that of the baby.

During this phase the nurse can be very helpful to the new mother in meeting her needs by offering supportive care, performing mothering tasks, and explaining this phase to her family and friends. "Mothering the mother" is very important in helping her prepare to learn about and nurture her infant. When the mother's needs are met, she will be able to move on to the next phase in her maternal role change. Encouraging the father to talk about the birth experience and including him in infant care instruction will help him to feel comfortable in his new role also. Sex-role stereotyping in our culture has led us to believe that men are not capable of being nurturing and gentle with newborns. Nothing could be further from the truth.

Following the taking-in phase women go through the taking-hold and letting-go phases. It has been generally accepted that these phases last 3 to 7 days each. In the *taking-hold phase* the woman regains control over her body and assumes the mothering role. She has recovered her energy and again asserts her independence and autonomy. Rubin identified the taking-hold phase as "a stage of maximal readiness for new learning."

In the *letting-go phase,* the woman establishes new maternal role patterns, incorporating the necessary changes in personal and family life. While centering on her baby and the baby's needs, she begins to return to her nonpregnant state. The letting-go phase of maternal role attainment begins about 2 weeks into the postpartum period.

Rubin's original research was done in the 1960s when the average length of postpartum hospital stay was double or triple that of today. Subsequent studies support Rubin's classic work in all aspects except the time frames in which the changes are presumed to occur. Taking-in today appears to occur in the first 24 hours after delivery.

Discharge from the hospital setting within 24 hours of birth leaves little time for women to complete Rubin's taking-in phase. Thus in today's hospital environment it is important to stimulate early independent taking-hold behaviors by encouraging women to assume responsibilities of self-care and newborn care shortly after birth. This can be achieved by using the nursing model of mother-baby care described later in this chapter. Also, postpartum follow-up programs are important in facilitating maternal adaptation. Depending on the program of the facility where the birth has occurred, nurses may either telephone or visit the new family 24 to 72 hours after hospital discharge. Programs for continuity of care are discussed in Chapter 14.

In adapting to the fathering role men experience the taking-in phase (passive and dependent) and other phases similar to the woman's taking-hold and letting-go phases. These male phases might be termed the *adjustment* and the *acceptance* phases. In the adjustment phase men resume their day-to-day responsibilities with a new seriousness, aware of the dependency of their new family. This new awareness can be invigorating, causing them to shift career plans or revitalize their current career or job status. However, for some men this new awareness can be very frightening, causing them anxiety and apprehension. Following the adjustment phase is the acceptance phase, in which men accept the intense, intimate relationship between the mother and infant and their new role as fathers.

Couples who have experienced a long and difficult labor, a cesarean birth, or a traumatic birth may have a prolonged taking-in phase. These new parents would profit from group sessions in which they can share their experience and feelings with other couples. In groups there are always one or two others with similar experiences or feelings who can share and offer empathy. All parents who have had a traumatic experience for which they were unprepared need to resolve their feelings about that experience before they can move on to the role changes necessary to parenting.

PARENT-INFANT INTERACTION

How well and rapidly parents go through the postpartum phases is influenced greatly by their interactions with the new baby. The baby's response to the parents' attempts at communication is very important. New parents first touch their babies with fingertips, then palms of the hands, then total hands, and then total body in hand to arm embrace. They frequently hold the infant on the left side close to the chest, near the parents' heart. Eye-to-eye contact is important in this "en face" positioning (Fig. 10-2). Parents talk instinctively to their babies in high-pitched voices, cooing and oohing. Rhythm-reciprocity patterns are often developed: the parent "oohs" and the baby "oohs;" the parent smiles and the baby smiles. When parental-infant bonding is occurring, the behaviors just identified are observable.

The nurse can help the parents in the bonding process by explaining to them that their infant is a unique, distinct individual with a separate personality. Many parents do not understand that their infant can see, hear, and respond to stimuli and is not as fragile as they may believe. The infant's ability to exhibit purposeful movements and to imitate more adult movements never fails to amaze new parents. The nurse can also help parents to understand the phases a newborn goes through and the newborn's states of awareness so that they can

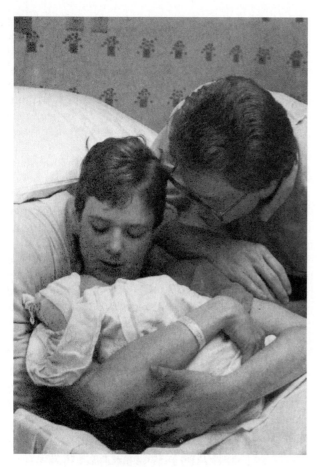

Figure 10-2 Eye-to-eye contact. *(Courtesy The Birthplace, Riverside Medical Center, Minneapolis, Minnesota.)*

truly know their new baby. The normal behavior of the newborn is discussed in Chapter 12.

Assessment of bonding and attachment during all phases of the childbearing experience should be included in the maternity data base. Parents who consistently manifest a lack of these behaviors may require additional care, support, and intervention.

Postpartum Blues

"Baby blues," or maternity blues, are experienced by 50% to 80% of postpartum women. Common symptoms are insomnia, depressed mood or mood ability (rapid changes in mood from depression to elation), headaches, poor concentration, tearfulness, and confusion. These symptoms are usually transient, begin on the third day after childbirth, last 1 day to 2 weeks, and then disappear without treatment.

Women with *postpartum blues* frequently do not know why they feel depressed, will talk of feeling "silly," and will laugh through their tears. This phenomenon may be caused by the extreme drop in hormones that oc-

curs about 72 hours postpartum. Also, many women experience disappointment that they have large, flabby bellies, feel tired, and generally do not look like the gorgeous, well-groomed new mothers on television or in the movies. These women think that they must be failures because they are not perfect. Some women feel extreme disappointment if their labors and births did not go as planned. Others perceive inadequate emotional support from their partners or extreme stress caused by new mothering responsibilities. It is important to let these women talk, cry, and work through their feelings, to explain possible causes for "the blues," and to reassure these new mothers. It is essential that the woman understand that other women experience the blues too—and that perfect mothers exist only in fairy tales.

The family members can be very helpful by giving the mother attention. It is not unusual to find them all admiring the baby, while the mother is left alone. Also, most gifts are for the baby and not for the mother.

Postpartum Depression

Postpartum depression is a mental disorder that has inconsistent acceptance in both the medical and legal communities. Postpartum depression affects about 20% of the women who had the baby blues and begins 2 weeks to 6 months after the birth. This is a form of clinical depression that is not psychotic. These are depressions that last for weeks or months and require medication, psychotherapy, or both. Periods of excessive crying, despondency, feelings of inadequacy, poor self-esteem and inability to cope, insomnia, anorexia, and social withdrawal may signal more than postpartum blues. Many women take great pains to conceal their postpartum depression from families and friends because they feel it is not "womanly," "motherly," or socially acceptable. Treatment of this disorder is especially important because destructive behavior, including suicide, is a possibility. Referral to a mental health professional is important.

Postpartum Psychosis

The last form, which is the most severe form of this illness, is *postpartum psychosis,* or the psychosis that occurs after childbirth. The disorder may become apparent 2 to 3 weeks after the birth to as long as 6 to 12 months. The incidence of postpartum psychosis is estimated to be only 1 or 2 per 1000 birthing women. However, it is a very dangerous psychosis, both to the mother and child, because both suicidal and infanticidal thoughts are present, making the woman dissociated, delusional, and confused. This woman loses her "sense

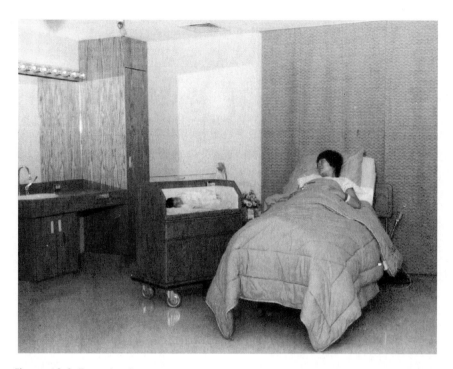

Figure 10-3 Rooming-in. *(Courtesy Valley Hospital and Medical Center, Spokane, Washington.)*

of reality." The distortions of reality involve the pregnancy and birth. Medication and hospitalization may be necessary, and the mother must always be observed in her interactions with the baby when she is symptomatic.

Nursing Care

The single best protective factor is a supportive social network. This usually means a supportive, attentive, and available partner or mate. For single women other family members, friends, or co-workers can offer support. Preparation for the postpartum period with special emphasis on emotional changes should be an important part of prenatal education. Adjustments of parenthood should be discussed and normal feelings of being overwhelmed given credibility. Knowing about the life-style changes to come helps the family to deal with them in the postpartum period.

Nurses can alert women with mild cases of postpartum depression to a counselor familiar with postpartum syndromes or to postpartum depression support groups. It is important that nurses teach families about the symptoms of postpartum depression and reinforce the need for early intervention.

ROOMING-IN

In conventional postpartum care the mother is separated from her baby, who is placed in a separate nurs-

ery and brought to her at designated periods. This practice of separating babies in hospital nurseries began at the turn of the century in this country. Reasons for the introduction of nurseries included a high incidence of maternal sepsis and the frequency of infections in the newborn that could be traced to this source. Also, many mothers received general anesthesia, "twilight sleep," and obstetric intervention during labor and birth and were too incapacitated to care for their babies.

Rooming-in is the term used to designate a hospital arrangement whereby a mother may have her newborn baby in a crib by her bedside whenever she wishes (Fig. 10-3). In the late 1940s some U.S. hospitals started rooming-in units to establish more natural mother-baby relationships. An interesting reason for starting a rooming-in program at Duke University Hospital in Durham, North Carolina was to avoid the possibility of a nursery epidemic of diarrhea. (It is fascinating to note that nurseries that began to prevent infection had become sources of cross-infection themselves). Major advantages cited from these rooming-in programs included reduced hospital costs, improved parenting skills, and reports of parent satisfaction. However, despite these advantages, rooming-in programs have not flourished in the United States.

Although rooming-in was started in an effort to foster development of the parent-child relationship, the actual implementation process often discouraged bonding and attachment. In the institutionalization and development of procedures and routines, the infant was

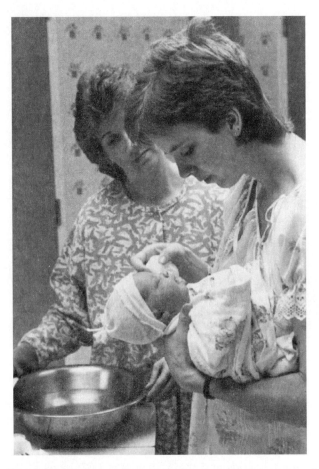

Figure 10-4 Mother-baby nursing is an expanded model of practice. The nurse is role model and educator. *(Courtesy The Birthplace, Riverside Medical Center, Minneapolis, Minnesota.)*

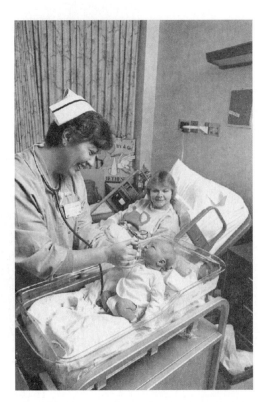

Figure 10-5 For mother-baby nursing to succeed, the major change is attitudinal. *(Courtesy Bethesda Hospital, Zanesville, Ohio.)*

taken to the new mother in her taking-in phase of postpartum adjustment. Often the mother was expected to assume primary responsibility for infant care, with nurses available for assistance or teaching. Because the baby was assigned to the nursery nurse and the mother was assigned to the postpartum nurse, there was confusion in messages and in lines of authority. Some hospital rooming-in protocols would not permit visitors or even allow the baby to be returned to the central nursery at night. Often parents were not prepared for the rooming-in experience and were incapable of basic infant care.

Fatigue in the postpartum period can be extreme. Sleep disruption superimposed on profound fatigue can contribute to feelings of being overburdened. *Real* babies who cry at night and demand feeding every 2 to 3 hours are not like the fantasized babies of the pregnancy. To expect new mothers to assume responsibility for infant care in rooming-in violates everything we know about psychosocial adaptations in the postpartum period, parent-infant interaction, and family beginnings.

MOTHER-BABY NURSING

Mother-baby nursing is not rooming-in. Instead it is provision of both mother and baby care by one nurse providing total care to both the mother and her infant. All policies and procedures are geared toward the new mother as a member of a family unit. This type of nursing care requires combining the roles of nursery and postpartum nurses so that they can give complete care to the mother-baby couplet. It is an expanded role for maternity nurses (Fig. 10-4).

Mother-baby nurses provide infant care at the mother's bedside, guide and teach parenting skills, attend to the mother's physiological and psychological needs, and integrate other family members into this care.

It is sometimes necessary to maintain a newborn nursery staff for transitional observations, special procedures, and care of babies who cannot remain with their mothers. However, these nurses rotate out of the nursery into mother-baby nursing so that mother-baby skills are maintained. Cost savings, parent satisfaction, and improved parent-infant relationships have been reported with mother-baby nursing.

The key words in implementing mother-baby care are *attitude* and *flexibility*. Staff members often fear loss of control and are anxious about the additional learning required. For successful implementation of mother-

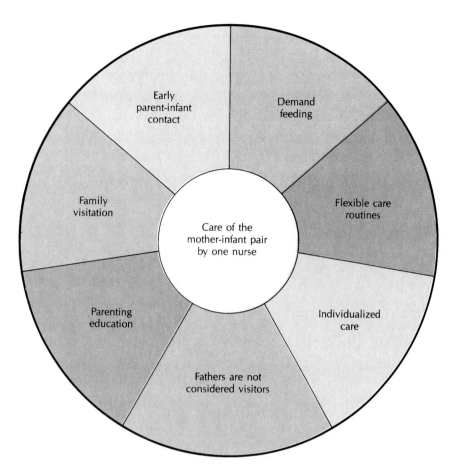

Figure 10-6 The wheel of family-centered postpartum and newborn care. *(Modified from Walters NE: Combined mother-infant nursing care, J Obstet Gynecol Neonatal Nurs 6:480, 1985.)*

baby care, staff members will have to perceive their roles differently. Instead of placing emphasis on tasks, nurses have to value caring for the family as a whole. The major change needed is attitudinal (Fig. 10-5).

In the mother-baby nursing model, pediatricians examine babies at the mothers' bedsides. Mothers are encouraged to ask questions freely and to discuss concerns with the physician, the nurse, or with other mothers. The health care team in mother-baby nursing strives to capitalize on opportunities for the mother to learn how to care for her own baby. The nurse functions as a resource person to the mother, providing guidance and suggestions when appropriate, assistance when needed, and positive reinforcement whenever possible (Fig. 10-6). The box on p. 274 outlines the benefits of mother-baby nursing to families and nurses.

Families need preparation for mother-baby nursing during the prenatal period. It is important to discuss the significance of the postpartum period to parent-infant relationships. Sibling involvement and ways to enhance family adjustment require anticipatory guidance (Fig. 10-7).

FAMILY CARE UNITS

Postpartum programs in self-care, self-administration of medications, early hospital discharge, and home visits by nurses are options that can promote successful adjustment to parenting (Fig. 10-8). In addition, programs that make women responsible for taking their own medications can also free nurses to spend more of their time providing essential instruction and support.

Postpartum care begins prenatally and extends through the labor and birth process, through the postpartum period, and to home follow-up. Maternity nursing is concerned with each family's unique adjustment to the new roles needed in becoming a family.

Further discussion of mother-baby nursing and programs and processes that promote continuity of care can be found in Chapter 14.

PHYSICAL ADJUSTMENTS

Postpartum physical adjustments involve all of the woman's body systems and require a significant expen-

Benefits of Mother-Baby Nursing

Some benefits to the family
1. Families receive consistent information from a single nurse.
2. Continuity and quality of care improves.
3. Mothers can learn by observing the nurse caring for baby.
4. Families have more opportunities to increase their infant caregiving skills.
5. Anxiety about whether the baby is properly cared for is eliminated. The mother *knows* the quality of care because she sees it.
6. Breast-feeding is enhanced because the infant can be truly fed on demand.
7. Baby care is individualized to infant needs.
8. The possibility of infection, especially epidemic infections of the newborn, is reduced.
9. The bonding and attachment process is facilitated.
10. It aids in postpartum involution for the woman.

Results
1. Families become more secure and competent with infant care.
2. Maternal self-esteem is increased.
3. Family satisfaction is increased.
4. There are fewer "panic" calls to the hospital and the pediatrician.
5. There is less infection resulting from nursery epidemics.

Some benefits to the nurse
1. Skills and knowledge base increase, thus making nurses more marketable.
2. Skills become more diversified.
3. Responsibilities for care and teaching are streamlined.
4. Nursing's value to the hospital increases.
5. Nurses are more personally involved and responsible for family care and self-learning.
6. Accountability increases.
7. Communication between the family and the caregiver is improved.

Results
1. Job satisfaction increases.
2. More flexible and unique staffing is provided.
3. A cost-effective model of care is provided.

diture of energy. Some women feel excited, uplifted, and energetic immediately after birth. Others feel exhausted and want to sleep. The nurse needs to thoroughly assess the physical status of the mother. (See box on page 276.)

Uterus

Involution is the return of the uterus to its prepregnant state. Immediately after delivery the uterus weighs about 2 pounds and is usually the size and consistency of a small, firm grapefruit. It can be felt through the abdominal wall at or below the level of the umbilicus, in the center of the abdomen. Within 12 hours of delivery, the fundal height rises to one fingerwidth (1 centimeter) above the umbilicus. On each succeeding post-

partum day the uterus gradually becomes smaller and descends downward into the pelvic cavity (Fig. 10-9). By the tenth day it is at or below the level of the symphysis pubis and can no longer be felt through the abdominal wall. As the uterus descends it should remain firm and contracted to prevent hemorrhage. The height of the fundus indicates the rate of involution. The fundus should be about one fingerwidth lower each day and should always be located in the center of the abdomen.

Contractions of the uterus as it descends are often called *afterpains* and are more pronounced in multiparas than in primiparas. Afterpains are more prominent during breast-feeding. In addition, oxytocic drugs are often given to new mothers to contract uterine muscles during the postpartum period.

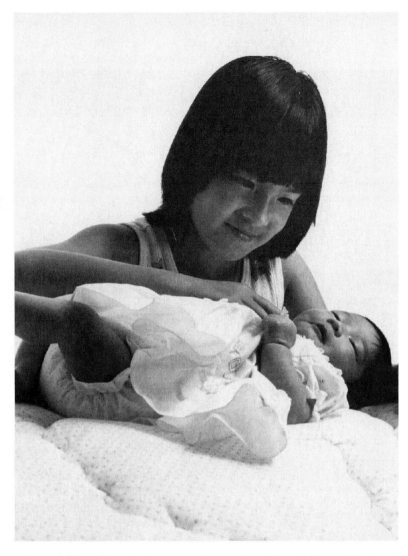

Figure 10-7 Sibling involvement. *(Courtesy Porter Hospital, Denver, Colorado.)*

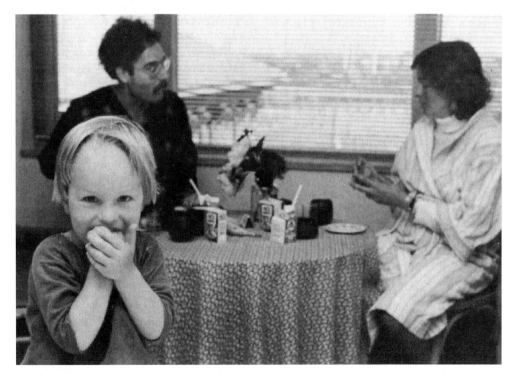

Figure 10-8 Family care unit. *(Courtesy Fairview-Riverside Hospital, Minneapolis, Minnesota.)*

Assessment of the Postpartum Mother

1. Assess vital signs.
2. Palpate breasts for fullness, nodules, and clogged ducts, and inspect nipples for redness and cracks.
3. Assess heart and lung sounds.
4. Palpate uterus for firmness and position.
5. Palpate abdomen for diastasis recti. Inspect incision if cesarean delivery. Question mother about bowel movements, and listen for bowel sounds in all four quadrants.
6. Inspect and palpate bladder for fullness.
7. Assess amount, color, character, and odor of lochia.
8. Observe perineum for bruises or hematoma, intactness and healing of episiotomy repair, and presence of hemorrhoids.
9. Perform Homans' sign.
10. Assess physical comfort level.

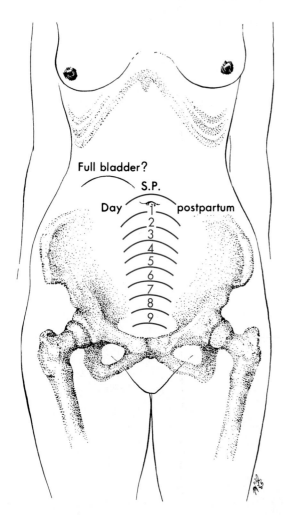

Figure 10-9 Involution of the uterus. *(From Novak JC, Broom BL: Ingalls and Salerno's maternal and child health nursing, ed 8, St. Louis, 1995, Mosby.)*

Medication may be ordered for the discomfort. Analgesics such as ibuprofen may relieve afterpains. Also, warm showers may be helpful in pain relief. The new mother needs to understand the physiological basis of the afterpains. The contractions are useful because they keep the uterus free of clots and promote involution. Lying on the abdomen, relaxation, and slow breathing techniques are helpful in relieving pain. Extreme tenderness of the uterus should be reported immediately because it can indicate intrauterine infection.

Nursing care

The uterus should be palpated for fundal height and firmness and findings should be recorded several times during each postpartum day so that any deviation from normal can be recognized immediately (Fig. 10-10). An elevated or laterally displaced uterus is a common sign of urinary retention after delivery.

So that daily measurements are consistent, the mother should empty her bladder before the uterus is palpated and should lie on her back with her knees bent and her feet flat on the bed. It is important that the new mother understands the process of involution and is taught how to massage her uterus to contract it and also how to recognize when the uterus is not involuting normally.

Lochia

Lochia is the normal uterine and vaginal discharge in the early postpartum period. Lochia consists of blood, shreds of decidual tissue, mucus, bacteria, and epithelial cells from the vagina. Occasionally lochia also contains small clots. Lochia goes through the following three stages as the placental site heals. *Lochia rubra* is the first stage, wherein the lochia is red and bloody for 1 to 3 days. Gradually as the lining of the rest of the uterus sloughs off, the discharge becomes brownish to pinkish in color and is called *lochia serosa*. By the tenth day the lochia turns yellowish-white and is called *lochia alba*. Lochia has a fleshy odor, suggestive of fresh blood. It should not smell foul. Foul-smelling lochia is usually a sign of infection and should be

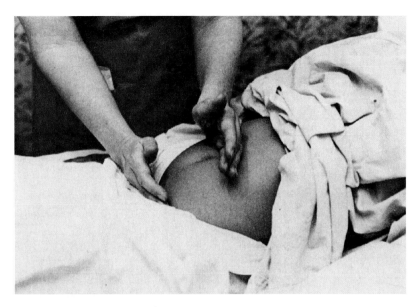

Figure 10-10 Palpating the uterus.

reported immediately. The quantity of lochia is lessened in mothers who are breast-feeding and following a cesarean birth but the stages remain unchanged. A danger sign is the reappearance of bright red blood after lochia rubra has stopped.

Nursing care

The nurse assesses the lochia for color, amount, consistency, and odor and records findings. Teaching the new mother about the normal amount, color, consistency, odor, and progression of lochia is very important. When she is aware of the normal lochia a new mother can report any deviations from normal. Thus an infection could be treated before it becomes serious.

Perineum

If the new mother has had an episiotomy she will experience some discomfort. The tissue around the episiotomy may be edematous, causing pressure on the sutures. Slight separation of the wound edges may occur; however, this is superficial and not serious. The perineum should be kept clean and as dry as possible to prevent infection. Sutures usually dissolve in about 3 weeks. Although procedures for perineal care differ from hospital to hospital, the following basic procedures are common.

1. Remove the perineal pad from front to back to prevent contamination of the vaginal opening from rectal microorganisms. After the perineum is cleansed apply the clean perineal pad tightly from front to back.
2. Cleanse the perineum from front to back by flush-

ing the area with warm water or a mild antiseptic solution after each elimination.
3. Pat the perineum dry with soft tissue or wipes.
4. When bathing use a clean cloth to cleanse the perineal area. Wash the anal area last.

Nursing care

Measures that are very soothing and also facilitate healing of an episiotomy may include cold sitz baths in the first 24 hours, which cause vasoconstriction, reduce edema, and decrease inflammation. After the first 24 hours warm sitz baths, witch hazel compresses, and topical anesthetics are helpful. Emotional support and reassurance that the discomfort will decrease are also necessary. As with any pain, analgesic medication may be helpful.

It is important to inspect the perineum at least once each day to detect any unusual redness, swelling, or discharge around the episiotomy. Any of these signs should be reported. It may be necessary to use a flashlight to visualize the area well, or the woman can turn on her left side and bend her right leg to expose the suture line.

Women who have had an episiotomy find it helpful to contract their buttocks muscles before sitting on a hard surface. This muscular contraction lifts the perineal floor up off the hard surface. Also, the Kegel exercises discussed in Chapter 6 are very helpful in the immediate postpartum period.

Vital Signs

The new mother's pulse may be from 40 to 80 beats per minute on the first and second days postpartum. This slowing of the pulse results from a decrease in cardiac output without a reduction in stroke volume. A rapid pulse may indicate uterine hemorrhage or infection.

The temperature should remain within normal limits. A slight temperature elevation may be caused by dehydration: 36.2° to 38° C (98° to 100.4° F). If this is the case fluid intake should be increased. Any elevation over 100.4° F in any two consecutive 24-hour periods (excluding the first day) is considered significant and potentially serious.

Respiration may be easier and slower because the smaller uterus is no longer pressing on the lungs and diaphragm. Respirations are usually in the range of 16 to 24 per minute. Blood pressure may drop slightly as the amount of circulating blood volume decreases. Of course any abnormal findings in these vital signs should be reported immediately.

Hemorrhoids

Hemorrhoids may appear for the first time as the mother pushes to deliver the baby. These hemorrhoids will usually disappear in several weeks following delivery. Warm sitz baths, cold witch hazel compresses, and elevation of the buttocks on several pillows during rest are helpful remedies. Sometimes topical anesthetics and/or suppositories are ordered. The woman should avoid straining when defecating. Stool softeners, increased fluid intake, and addition of fiber and roughage to the diet are helpful.

Urinary System

After the birth the 50% increase in extracellular fluid that was necessary in the pregnancy is no longer needed. Consequently there is a significant diuresis in the early postpartum period (usually between the second and fifth postpartum days). The urinary output is up to 3000 milliliters per day. Also, the capacity of the bladder increases because of the decreased intraabdominal pressure and the relaxed, stretched abdominal muscles. Overdistention of the bladder can occur along with incomplete emptying. It is important for the new mother to excrete at least 200 milliliters of urine each time she voids. The first voiding should be measured.

The first voiding may be difficult because of trauma on the bladder and urethra during the birth process, causing tenderness, edema, and reflex spasm of the urethra. If the woman has not urinated within 6 hours of birth or the first voids are less than 100 milliliters, catheterization may be necessary. The physician may also order a urine culture and sensitivity test. To encourage voiding the nurse can provide fluids to drink, be sure the woman has privacy, and encourage her to walk to the bathroom if possible. Walking is very helpful, and

the squatting position over a toilet helps to release pressure on the bladder. Sometimes the sound of water running or the actual flow of warm water over the perineum encourages voiding.

Laboratory findings on urinalysis in the first few days and weeks postpartum normally disclose the presence of protein and/or sugar. The proteinuria results from the increased nitrogen content of urine caused by protein destruction in the walls of the uterus as the uterine muscle cells become smaller. The sugar is present in the urine because of lactose absorption from the mammary glands (breasts) into the bloodstream. Normal kidney function returns by 6 to 7 weeks after delivery.

Nursing care

It is important to explain to the mother the possible causes and limited nature of discomfort with voiding. Instruct the mother on the importance of frequent voiding, ambulation, and fluid intake. A full bladder is obvious because it is visible as a soft swelling above the symphysis pubis and feels like a soft balloon full of fluid when palpated. The bladder should be examined for distention at each postpartum check because a full bladder can displace the uterus, thus predisposing to uterine hemorrhage (Fig. 10-11). Pain and frequency of urination are also signs of a urinary tract infection. It is important to differentiate between the normal, frequent urination postpartum that is associated with increased urinary output and urinary tract infection. Symptoms of urinary tract infection include suprapu-

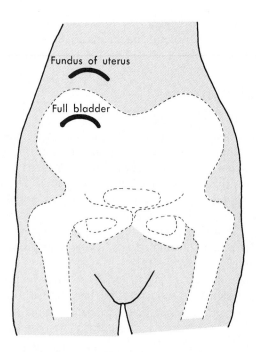

Figure 10-11 Full bladder, uterus displaced.

bic and low back pain, fever, hematuria, and pain on urination.

Bowels

Constipation is a common problem in the postpartum period because of the relaxed abdominal walls and inactivity. Increased levels of progesterone relax smooth muscles and may contribute to bowel hypoactivity. Also, women who have had episiotomies often fear that they may have pain when defecating and consequently hold back their feces. The physician may order stool softeners, laxatives, suppositories, or enemas. However, if the new mother is breast-feeding, laxatives may be excreted in breast milk. Early ambulation, a diet that includes roughage and plenty of fluids, and exercise to tone stretched abdominal muscles are all helpful in reestablishing proper bowel functioning.

Integumentary System

Hormonal changes and the body's attempt to rid itself of extra fluid can cause the woman to perspire profusely (diaphoresis). Often this happens at night, and the woman may wake up drenched in perspiration. It is important that she be told that this is a normal body response. At this time the pigmentation changes that occurred during pregnancy will disappear.

Personal Hygiene

Douching is not necessary in the postpartum period and has been declared medically unsound by the American College of Obstetricians and Gynecologists.

Showers are preferred over tub baths until the lochia stops. The mother may soak in a tub of warm water for suture healing but should not bathe first in the same water.

When bathing the woman should wash her hands first with soap and water and then wash her breasts. The nipples should be washed with plain water, no soap, because soap is drying. She should then wash the rest of her body in the usual manner. After washing her body the woman should use a clean washcloth to cleanse the perineal area, washing the anal area last.

Laboratory Findings

The blood volume and hemoglobin and hematocrit levels usually return to normal within 1 week postpartum. Fibrinogen levels and sedimentation rate remain elevated for approximately 1 week, predisposing the new mother to thrombophlebitis. The white blood cell count is elevated in the first few days postpartum because leukocytosis occurs as the placental site heals.

The white count usually returns to normal within 7 days.

Extremities

Frequently new mothers have varying degrees of varicosities of the lower extremities, thighs, and vulva. It is important to check the extremities for red, hot, painful areas, which could be signs of acute thrombophlebitis and should be reported immediately. When examining the woman's legs, press down gently on her knee (with the legs flat on the bed) and ask her to point her toes toward her face. Pain or tenderness in the calf is a positive *Homans' sign* and an indication of thrombophlebitis. Report this immediately.

Weight

At delivery the woman loses about 12 to 13 pounds (baby, placenta, amniotic fluid, membranes, and blood). Further loss of body weight during the puerperium may be approximately 5 pounds, although this loss does not occur until diuresis begins. Explain to the mother the process of gradual return to prepregnant weight.

Abdomen

The woman's abdominal walls tend to be soft and flabby in the first few weeks after birth because they were stretched during pregnancy. This can be very depressing for the new mother, and she needs reassurance that she will be able to wear her favorite clothing again. She determines to a great deal how soon and how well her muscles will return to their original condition. Exercises to improve the muscle tone of the abdomen may be started as soon as the lochia has stopped. With exercise tone is generally regained in 6 weeks.

Postpartum Exercises

For best results exercises appropriate for the new mother should begin within 24 hours of a vaginal birth and when the physician identifies an appropriate time for the postcesarean mother. The exercise program begins with deep diaphragmatic breathing, diastasis recti (separation of the rectus abdominis muscles) correction, and the Kegel exercise. The woman should begin gradually and be careful not to overexert herself (Fig. 10-12). Vigorous exercise is to be avoided until after lochia has ceased.

HUMAN MILK

The breasts are enlarged and heavy after birth as they change rapidly to prepare for nourishing the baby. The breasts may secrete small amounts of a thin, yellowish

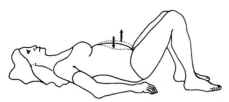

Abdominal Breathing. Lie on back with knees bent. Inhale deeply through the nose. Keep ribs as stationary as possible and allow abdomen to expand upwards. Exhale slowly but forcefully while contracting the abdominal muscles; hold for 3 to 5 seconds while exhaling.

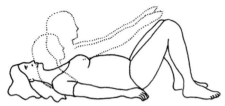

Reach for the Knees. Lie on back with knees bent. While inhaling deeply lower chin onto chest. While exhaling, raise head and shoulders slowly and smoothly and reach for knees with arms outstretched. The body should only rise as far as the back will naturally bend while waist remains on floor or bed (about 6 to 8 inches). Slowly and smoothly lower head and shoulders back to starting position. Relax.

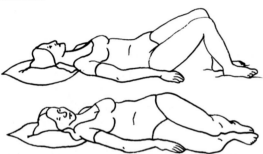

Double Knee Roll. Lie on back with knees bent. Keeping shoulders flat and feet stationary, slowly and smoothly roll knees over to the left to touch floor or bed. Maintaining a smooth motion, roll knees back over to the right until they touch floor or bed. Return to starting position and relax.

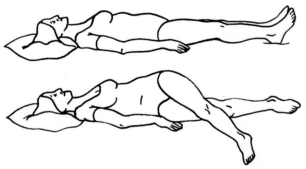

Leg Roll. Lie on back with legs straight. Keeping shoulders flat and legs straight, slowly and smoothly lift left leg and roll it over to touch the right side of floor or bed and return to starting position. Repeat, rolling right leg over to touch left side of floor or bed. Relax.

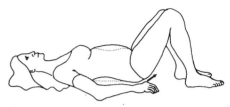

Combined Abdominal Breathing and Supine Pelvic Tilt (Pelvic Rock). Lie on back with knees bent. While inhaling deeply, roll pelvis back by flattening lower back on floor or bed. Exhale slowly but forcefully while contracting abdominal muscles and tightening buttocks. Hold for 3 to 5 seconds while exhaling. Relax.

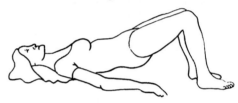

Buttocks Lift. Lie on back with arms at sides, knees bent and feet flat. Slowly raise buttocks and arch back. Return slowly to starting position.

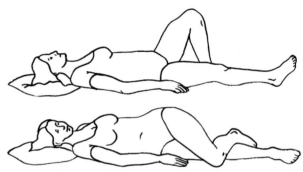

Single Knee Roll. Lie on back with with right leg straight and left leg bent at the knee. Keeping shoulders flat, slowly and smoothly roll left knee over to the right to touch floor or bed and then back to starting position. Reverse position of legs. Roll right knee over to the left to touch floor or bed and return to starting position. Relax.

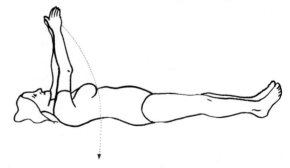

Arm Raises. Lie on back with arms extended at 90° angle from body. Raise arms so they are perpendicular and hands touch. Lower slowly.

Figure 10-12 Postpartum exercises. *(From Bobak IM, Jensen MD: Maternity and gynecologic care: the nurse and the family, ed 5, St. Louis, 1993, Mosby.)*

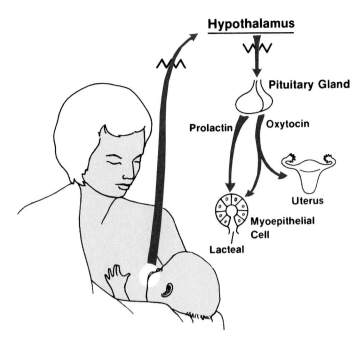

Figure 10-13 Diagram of ejection reflex arc. *(From Lawrence RA:* Breastfeeding: a guide for the medical profession, *ed 4, St. Louis, 1994, Mosby.)*

premilk fluid called *colostrum* during pregnancy, particularly in the last few months. Colostrum is rich in vitamins A and E, protein, and antibodies, and it is thought to have mild laxative properties. Colostrum continues to be secreted for the first 3 to 5 days after delivery, gradually changing to milk. Frequent and early feeding of this colostrum encourages the transitional milk supply by the third to fifth day after birth. By 2 weeks postpartum the milk is mature and the protein content is approximately half that of colostrum.

Lactation Physiology

Lactation is believed to be caused by the pituitary hormone prolactin. During pregnancy the breasts developed to prepare for lactation by the influence of high levels of estrogen and progesterone. It is believed that these high hormone levels inhibited the pituitary gland from producing prolactin during pregnancy. After the placenta is expelled, the woman's blood levels of estrogen and progesterone drop; consequently, the pituitary can produce prolactin to initiate lactation.

Prolactin stimulates the alveolar cells (acini cells) of the breasts and thus promotes milk production. (See Chapter 2, Fig. 2-8). Under the influence of prolactin, milk is secreted continuously into the alveoli of the breasts and remains there until it is ejected or "let down" from the alveoli, through the milk ducts, to the lactiferous sinuses, and then to the baby. This process works on a supply-and-demand basis; the more the mother's breasts are stimulated by the infant suckling

at the nipple, the more prolactin she will have. In the nonnursing mother prolactin drops to prepregnant levels in about 14 days. When the baby sucks at the mother's breasts, sensory impulses are transmitted through the mother's nervous system to her brain, causing the release of oxytocin from her pituitary gland. Within 30 seconds after the baby begins to suck, milk is available. The release of oxytocin from the pituitary causes the myoepithelial cells that surround the outer walls of the alveoli to contract and express the milk. If the breasts are not stimulated regularly, milk production ceases. (See Fig. 10-13 for a diagrammatical outline of the ejection reflex arc.)

Breasts

As the breasts fill up they become larger and firmer to the touch. The veins in the breasts become apparent, and the mother will say that her breasts are heavier, more tender, and warmer to the touch. *Engorgement* is the term given to this swelling of breast tissue and increased blood flow and congestion (Fig. 10-14). At the same time the secretion from the breasts changes from the thin, yellowish colostrum to the thin, bluish consistency of skim milk. Engorgement usually occurs by the third or fourth day postpartum when estrogen levels drop and lasts 24 to 48 hours. Comfort measures for engorgement may include adequate support for the breasts by a supportive brassiere or breast binder. A warm shower (or hot towels placed over the breasts) is often helpful for relaxation and for the promotion of the

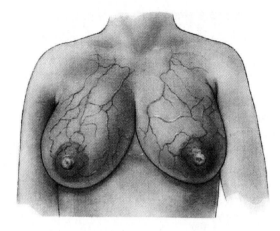

Figure 10-14 Engorgement, predominantly vascular in nature. *(From Lawrence RA:* Breastfeeding: a guide for the medical profession, *ed 4, St. Louis, 1994, Mosby.)*

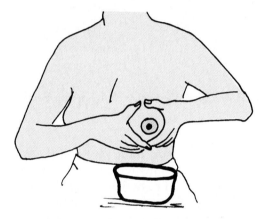 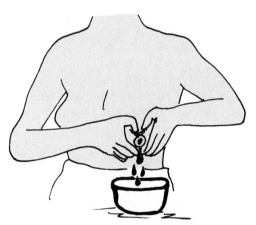

Figure 10-15 Manual expression of milk.

milk ejection reflex, thus softening the breasts. This reflex is involuntary and is stimulated by the anticipation of a feeding, by hearing the baby cry, or by relaxation. The milk ejection reflex causes a tingling sensation accompanied by the leaking of milk from the nipples. Particularly when the breasts are large and hard, bringing the milk from the glands in the breast to the nipple helps the baby drink it more easily. Massaging the breasts between breast-feedings can also help to keep the ducts open. Engorged breasts can cause flattening of the nipple, making it difficult for the baby to grasp. Softening the breast by the let-down reflex or manual expression of milk relieves the hardness around the areola (Fig. 10-15). After feeding, ice packs to the breasts for 5 to 10 minutes can relieve the discomfort of engorgement. However, excessive use of ice packs can contribute to a reduction in milk supply.

Breast Care

To reduce the risk of breast infection it is very important that anyone touching the breasts have clean hands and that the breasts and nipples be kept clean and free of dried secretions. The breasts should be washed with a clean cloth daily during shower or bath. It is not necessary to use soap because it removes the natural oils that protect the skin from drying and cracking, nor is it necessary to wash the nipples before or after breast-feeding. However, it is important to air dry the nipples after feeding and before covering again with the bra. Because damp material against the skin for any time can cause skin breakdown, the mother should not wear bras or pads with plastic liners. If leaking occurs and she wants to protect her clothing from milk stains, the mother may use nonplastic nursing pads, a gauze pad, clean perineal pads cut to fit, clean handkerchiefs, or milk cups. (See Fig. 4-14.) She should also change to a clean bra daily. After feeding, a few drops of breast milk can be applied to the mother's nipples and let dry (breast milk is very healing).

The nurse should inspect the breast-feeding mother's breasts and nipples and teach her how to inspect her own breasts for signs of nipple irritation or skin breakdown. The breasts should also be checked daily for signs

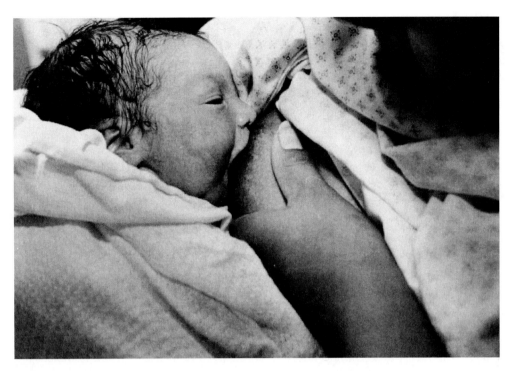

Figure 10-16 Breast-feeding as soon as possible after birth. *(Photo by Jacqueline Capra. From Phillips CR, Anzalone JT: Fathering, ed 2, St. Louis, 1982, Mosby.)*

of *mastitis* (breast infection), such as redness, swelling, tenderness, and fever. All observations should be recorded, and anything unusual should be reported immediately.

Breast-Feeding

Each year scientific evidence provides increasing justification for breast-feeding. Among the key factors influencing the prevalence and duration of breast-feeding are the attitudes and behaviors of health care personnel and the hospital practices. (See Table 10-1 for a listing of hospital practices that influence breast-feeding initiation.) Because most women make decisions regarding infant feeding methods before the third trimester, health care providers are in an ideal situation to influence the choice to breast-feed.

Breast-feeding should be discussed during the prenatal period and dialogue established on the process, advantages, and disadvantages with the expectant mother and family members so that their decision about infant feeding is based on factual information. Mothers should be encouraged to cuddle and put their infants to breast as soon as possible after birth. Thinking of the mother and baby as a unit and caring for the couple in mother-baby nursing encourages the mother to learn about and care for her baby in a supportive environment (Fig. 10-16).

Mother-Infant Nursing

The Baby Friendly Hospital Initiative is a worldwide program developed by UNICEF in 1991 to contribute to the achievement of global breast-feeding for all. This initiative encourages transformation of hospitals into baby-friendly institutions where all of the ten steps to successful breast-feeding are implemented. These ten steps to successful breast-feeding follow.

1. Have a written breast-feeding policy that is routinely communicated to all health care staff.
2. Train all health care staff in skills necessary to implement this policy.
3. Inform all pregnant women about the benefits and management of breast-feeding.
4. Help mothers initiate breast-feeding within a half hour of birth.
5. Show mothers how to breast-feed and how to maintain lactation even if they should be separated from their infants.
6. Give newborn infants no food or drink other than breast milk unless medically indicated.
7. Practice rooming-in—allow mothers and infants to remain together—24 hours a day.
8. Encourage breast-feeding on demand.
9. Give no artificial teats or pacifiers (also called dummies or soothers) to breast-feeding infants.

TABLE 10-1
Hospital Practices That Influence Breast-Feeding Initiation

Strongly encouraging	Encouraging	Discouraging	Strongly discouraging
Physical Contact			
Baby put to breast immediately after birth.			Mother-infant separation at birth.
Baby not taken from mother after delivery.	Staff sensitivity to cultural norms and expectations of woman.	Scheduled feedings regardless of mother's breast-feeding wishes.	Mother-infant housed on separate floors in postpartum period.
Woman helped by staff to suckle baby.			Mother separated from baby because of bilirubin problem.
Mother-baby nursing staff help with baby care *in* room, not only in nursery.			No rooming-in policy.
Verbal Communication			
Staff initiates discussion regarding woman's intention to breast-feed prepartum and intrapartum.	Appropriate language skills of staff, teaching how to handle breast engorgement and nipple problem.	Staff instructs woman to "get good night's rest and miss the feed."	Woman told to "take it easy, get your rest"—impression that breast-feeding is effortful and tiring.
Staff encourages and reinforces breast-feeding immediately after birth.	Staff's own skills and comfort regarding art of breast-feeding and time to teach woman on one-to-one basis.	Strict times allotted for breast-feeding regardless of mother and baby's feeding "cycle."	Woman told she doesn't "do it right," staff interrupts her efforts; corrects her regarding positions and other matters.
Staff discusses use of breast pump and realities of separation from baby regarding breast-feeding.			

10. Foster the establishment of breast-feeding support groups and refer mothers to them on discharge from the hospital or clinic.

When helping a new mother breast-feed, encourage her to hold her baby so that the baby's cheek touches her breast. This stimulates the *rooting reflex* in which the baby's head moves from side to side in an attempt to locate the nipple. The lactiferous sinuses lie underneath the areolar surface, and compression of the milk-filled sinuses extracts milk from the breast. For this reason the entire nipple and some of the surrounding dark tissue (areola) should be inserted into the baby's mouth. If the breast is very full and firm it will have to be compressed slightly beneath the baby's nose. The baby should suck at each breast for each feeding. Stopwatch timing is not necessary. It takes 2 to 3 minutes for the let-down reflex to produce milk in the first days postpartum so the feedings must provide for let-down. Usually infants nurse about 10 to 15 minutes per feeding in the first days of life. Frequent small feedings will provide good stimulation to the breasts without tiring the mother.

To remove the baby from the breast the mother should break the baby's suction by pressing the breast away from the corner of the baby's mouth or by inserting a clean finger into the corner of the baby's mouth. The baby should be burped, or "bubbled," when changing breasts or after the feeding is completed. "Over-the-shoulder," sitting the baby up on the mother's lap and patting the baby's back, or resting the baby on the mother's legs face down and patting the baby's back are all "bubbling" methods. (See Fig. 12-15.) Breast-fed babies may not burp at all because they swallow less air than bottle-fed babies.

Breast-fed babies do not require supplemental formula or glucose water under normal circumstances. If

TABLE 10-1—cont'd
Hospital Practices That Influence Breast-Feeding Initiation

Strongly encouraging	Encouraging	Discouraging	Strongly discouraging
Nonverbal Communication			
Pictures of woman breast-feeding.		Pictures of woman bottle-feeding.	Woman given infant formula kit and infant food literature.
Literature on breast-feeding in understandable terms.			
Staff (doctors as well as nurses) give reinforcement for breast-feeding (respect, smiles, affirmation).		Staff interrupts her breast-feeding session for laboratory tests and other matters.	
Nurse (or any attendant) making mother comfortable and helping to arrange baby at breast for nursing.		Woman does not see others breast-feeding.	Sees official-looking nurses authoritatively caring for babies by bottle-feeding (leads to woman's insecurities regarding own capability of care).
Woman sees others breast-feeding in hospital.	Closed-circuit TV show in hospital on breast-feeding.		
Experimental			
If breast-feeding not *immediately* successful, staff continues to be supportive.			
Previous success with breast-feeding experience in hospital.			Previous failure with breast-feeding experience in hospital.

Modified from Scrimshaw SCM: The cultural context of breast-feeding in the U.S. In report of the Surgeon General's Workshop on Breast-feeding and Human Lactation, U.S. Department of Health and Human Services, June 11, 12, 1984.

the infant is wetting six or eight diapers per day, the skin turgor is good, and the anterior fontanel is not sunken, the infant is receiving adequate nutrition.

The La Leche League International is a national organization dedicated to helping breast-feeding mothers. The address is given in Appendix B. Breast-feeding women should be given the names and phone numbers of community resources before leaving the hospital. Follow-up phone calls and home visits by nurses can continue support and teaching that promote successful breast-feeding.

Working Women

If the breast-feeding mother is returning to work outside the home after the baby's birth, she should be encouraged to hand express her milk or use a breast pump after feedings to increase her milk supply. Flexible ways to combine breast-feeding and bottle-feeding should also be considered.

Returning to work outside the home does not mean that the mother cannot breast-feed (Fig. 10-17). Breast milk can be frozen and the container dated for later feeding.

However, combining breast-feeding and work outside the home will require tremendous support from family, friends, and employer. Changes in the work environment, such as child care services, nursing rooms, and the option of job sharing or part-time employment are needed in the United States. Extended leaves for childbearing or increased flexibility of working hours would also provide encouragement for working women to breast-feed.

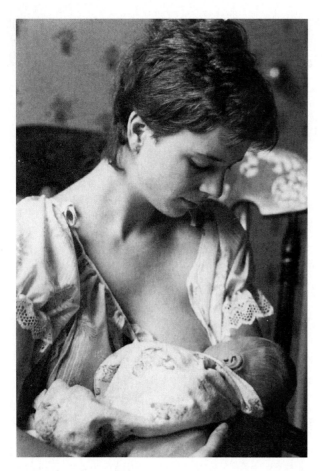

Figure 10-17 Breast-feeding. *(Courtesy The Birthplace, Riverside Medical Center, Minneapolis, Minnesota.)*

Drugs to Avoid While Nursing

Alcohol	Diuretics	Metronidazole
Androgen	Ergotamine	Minor tranquilizers
Antineoplastics	Estrogen	Narcotics
Bromocriptine	Iodine	Radiopharmaceuticals
Chloramphenicol		

Practical Guidelines for Treating the Nursing Mother

Encourage the breast-feeding mother to avoid self-medicating and to take medications only under the supervision of her physician.

Encourage the mother to breast-feed just before taking medication and to delay nursing for at least 4 hours after drug administration.

Alert the mother to possible signs of drug side effects in the infant, and monitor the infant yourself for any possible side effects.

When applicable, use drugs that are minimally absorbed, such as oral inhalation preparations, or choose the drug least likely to be excreted into breast milk.

If possible, select drugs that have been proven safe for infants.

Drugs in Human Milk

Transmission of a drug from the mother to the nursing infant involves blood flow in the mammary gland, the physiological properties of the breast as an organ of transport and metabolism, and the lipid solubility and plasma protein-binding properties of the compound itself. The infant's drug exposure is also dependent on his or her absorption, metabolism, and excretion of the drug. Most drugs ingested by a breast-feeding mother have the potential to enter and be excreted in her milk. Breast-feeding mothers should avoid alcohol, narcotics, and minor tranquilizers, such as barbiturates and benzodiazepines. The box at top right lists other drugs to avoid while nursing. Appendix D has a list of maternal medication usually compatible with breast-feeding and a more complete list of those contraindicated during breast-feeding.

Since a change in the infant is the best sign that a drug taken by a nursing mother is affecting her infant, the nurse should carefully observe the infant for any possible drug effects. If possible confirm the observations of a drug effect by having the mother stop and then restart breast-feeding. Practical guidelines for treating the nursing mother are listed in the box above.

Nonnursing Mother

If the mother is not nursing her baby and her breasts are full, it is important to have the breasts adequately supported with a properly fitted brassiere or a breast binder. Ice packs to each breast for an hour 3 or 4 times a day can reduce discomfort and discourage lactation. Also, analgesics are sometimes prescribed to reduce discomfort. It is important that the woman avoid any breast stimulation or warm water on her breasts, and not remove any breast milk by manual expression or newborn suckling because this encourages further milk production. Occasionally milk may reappear in the breasts in 10 to 12 days, and the same comfort measures are indicated.

If a woman chooses not to breast-feed her baby the physician may prescribe hormones (estrogens) to suppress the milk supply. Because there is much debate over the long-term effects of these hormones, their use

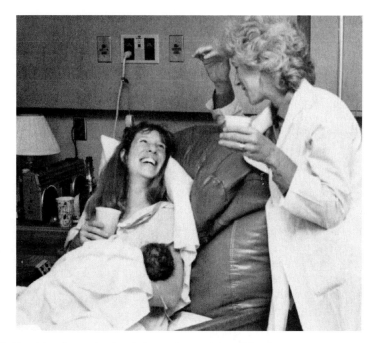

Figure 10-18 Teaching by reviewing information presented in the prenatal period. *(Courtesy Evergreen Hospital Medical Center, Kirkland, Washington.)*

varies greatly. These hormones do not help the rebound engorgement that sometimes occurs 10 to 12 days postpartum. Before these drugs are given the woman should be informed of their potential side effects, and her informed consent should be obtained. After weighing the side effects of estrogens and androgens, many physicians have decided to try nonpharmacological methods first.

MENSTRUATION AND OVULATION

When a woman does not breast-feed any secretion of milk usually stops in 10 to 14 days and menstrual periods usually return in 6 to 8 weeks. Ovulation may occur in this period as well. For breast-feeding mothers menstruation may not return until the third month postpartum or until breast-feeding is stopped. The continued production of prolactin may inhibit the release of the follicle-stimulating hormone (FSH) from the pituitary gland, thus delaying ovulation. However, because the woman may ovulate while she is breast-feeding even though she is not menstruating, breast-feeding cannot be counted on as a contraceptive. If pregnancy is not desired, some form of birth control should be used. Combination birth control pills are not recommended while breast-feeding because they may affect the quality and quantity of the breast milk. The mini-pill (no estrogen) is safe for breast-feeding moth-

ers. However, efficacy is less than with combination pills.

Sexual intercourse can be resumed after the lochia has stopped, the perineum is healed, and the woman and her partner feel ready once again. If the woman is breast-feeding, there can be a milk let-down with sexual activity and particularly with orgasm. This may be perceived as erotic by some couples and as objectionable by others. Because of lowered estrogen levels, the woman may find that her vagina does not lubricate as well as usual, and for comfortable intercourse, some extra lubricant jelly may be helpful. Some women report experiencing feelings of sexual arousal when breast-feeding. The couple needs explanations of these changes and opportunities to discuss their feelings.

TEACHING

With shortened hospital stays for uncomplicated vaginal births, most mothers leave the hospital still in the "taking-in" phase before focusing on the needs of the infant. Also, the stress of labor and birth have been found to affect cognitive function, particularly memory. Therefore new information may be poorly remembered if presented on the first postpartum day. As discussed earlier in this chapter infant care and parenting should be taught prenatally. The postpartum period is a time for *review* of this information and teaching by demonstration and role modeling (Fig. 10-18).

The nurse can teach individually while providing the

mother-baby care discussed in this chapter. In addition, group discussions and classes can be organized in the hospital to review material presented prenatally. All mothers need to be included in teaching even though primiparas usually have the greatest need. It may be several years since a woman had a baby, or she may have a boy this time instead of a girl. When teaching determine what the woman already knows and begin at that point.

Anticipatory Guidance

When reviewing it is important to help the mother understand what she can expect in the 6-week postpartum period and during the fourth trimester. During this "anticipatory guidance" stress the importance of adequate rest to maintain and build up her strength. Morning and afternoon rest periods and 8 hours of sleep at night are very helpful. It may be necessary for her to have help with the work at home or to have help in planning how she will manage so that she will not overwork. Referrals to public health nursing or home care agencies may be necessary, or hospital staff nurses can phone and visit the new family in their home in the first few weeks of the baby's life. This follow-up checks not only on the recovery of the mother but also on the adaptation and development of the baby. Nursing follow-up also provides an opportunity to discuss feelings and any problems. (Discussion of home follow-up programs can be found in Chapter 14.)

An appointment with the physician or midwife is usually recommended for 2 to 6 weeks postpartum. At this time the pelvic organs and breasts are checked for any abnormalities.

Family Planning

An important part of teaching in the postpartum period is reviewing family planning methods with the woman and her partner. (A summary of the various birth control methods is given in Table 10-2.) As the population of the world increases rapidly there has been a deepening concern about the quality of life. In an advanced society such as ours birth control is often seen as enhancing family life. Effectiveness and safety are the major considerations in choosing a method of birth control. For a birth control method to be optimally effective the method should be acceptable to both partners. In the postpartum period the nurse can initiate discussion with both partners concerning all available methods, their action, description, advantages, and disadvantages. Fig. 10-19 illustrates methods of contraception. Fig. 10-20 shows a basal temperature record needed for the rhythm or calendar basal body temperature method. Fig. 10-21 illustrates

A

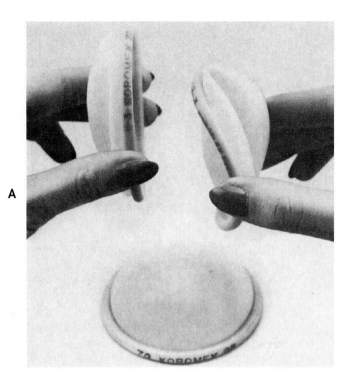

B

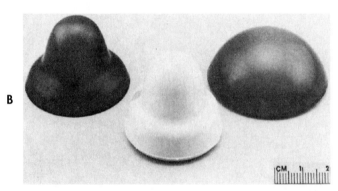

Figure 10-19 Methods of contraception. **A,** Three types of diaphragms: the flat spring, the coil spring, and the arcing diaphragm. **B,** Three types of cervical caps: the Vimule *(left)*, the Prentif cavity-rim *(center)*, and the Dumas, or vault cap *(right)*. *(Courtesy Population Reports, H-7, Population Information Program, Johns Hopkins University).*

the placement of the diaphragm. Fig. 10-22 illustrates the placement of a cervical cap.

Dangers of Birth Control Methods

The intrauterine device (IUD), oral contraceptives, sterilization procedures (tubal ligations), and abortion all carry risks. IUDs have a history of causing increased menstrual bleeding, severe and chronic cramping, and pelvic infections, many of which resulted in permanent sterility. Although most IUDs were withdrawn from sale in the United States in 1986, the copper t380-A (Para-

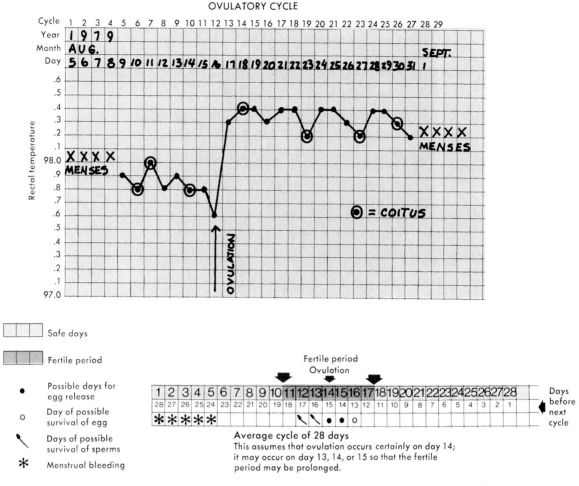

Figure 10-20 Basal temperature method.

Gard) is now available in the United States, as is the IUD Progestasert.

Research has shown that with the current generation of IUDs the risk of infection is mostly in the first few weeks after IUD insertion and to women exposed to sexually transmitted diseases. Most health care providers only recommend IUDs for women who are in stable, mutually monogamous relationships.

Oral contraceptives containing estrogen and progesterone should not ordinarily be prescribed for women with liver disease or diabetes or with a history of thrombophlebitis, hypertension or other cardiovascular diseases, migraine headaches, diabetes, active gallbladder disease or suspected estrogen-dependent malignancies. Pregnancy is also a contraindication, of course. Because the mini-pill contains no estrogen, it may be used by women who are hypertensive or have migraines. Women should be carefully screened to determine their risks for complications before any contraceptive pills are prescribed. Any hormonal method of contraception may be especially risky for smokers over age 35. With oral con-

traceptives periodic follow-up to detect any developing problems is essential.

Most women resume normal ovulatory cycles immediately after contraceptive pills are stopped. Occasionally the first postpill cycle may occur without ovulation. In rare instances—usually in women who had irregular menstrual periods before using the pill—the delay may last several months or more. There is no harm in attempting to conceive immediately after discontinuing the pill.

As with all surgery there is a risk of complications from anesthesia and infection with both sterilization (tubal ligation) and abortion.

THE FUTURE

Biodegradable implants are being developed; they are placed under the skin and eventually dissolve and disappear. These implants are expected to prevent pregnancy for 12 to 18 months.

Injectable microspheres and microcapsules, suspended

TABLE 10-2
Birth Control Methods

Method	Description	How it works	Advantages	Disadvantages
Oral contraceptives	Two categories: Combination contains synthetic hormones, estrogen, and progesterone. Usually taken on 21 consecutive days beginning 5 days after menstruation starts. Mini-pill contains progesterone only. Usually taken every day.	Prevents release of egg from ovary. Progestin-only tablet ("mini-pill") creates unfavorable environment for conception.	Virtually 100% effective when taken according to instructions. Convenient and allows for spontaneity in lovemaking. Reversible; can stop if pregnancy desired. Benefits include decreased risk of endometrial and ovarian cancer.	Not safe for everyone. Possible side effects include nausea, weight gain, headache, depression, blood and circulatory problems (high blood pressure and blood clots). Offers no protection against STDs. Must be prescribed.
Intrauterine device (IUD)	Small plastic device inserted into the uterus by physician or nurse-practitioner. Two types of IUDs available in the U.S.: Copper t380-A (ParaGard) and Progestasert.	ParaGard is a copper-coated device that creates a hostile environment for sperm (effective for 8 yrs). Progestasert releases the hormone progesterone, which thickens cervical mucus (must be replaced every year).	Highly effective (99%). Allows for spontaneity in lovemaking. Can be removed if pregnancy is desired. Usually tolerated well by multiparous women.	Possible side effects: pain, bleeding, vaginal discharge, pelvic inflammatory disease (PID), and subsequent increased chance of infertility. IUD may perforate wall of uterus. Insertion is difficult in nulliparas. IUDs do not protect against STDs.
Diaphragm	Circular rubber device placed over cervix before intercourse; spermicidal jelly or cream placed inside diaphragm to immobilize and kill sperm. Must be fitted by physician or nurse-practitioner.	Acts as a receptacle for spermicidal preparations that immobilize and kill sperm.	Highly effective (81%–95%) if used properly. Very safe; no systemic effects. When no longer used, pregnancy can occur if desired.	Requires highly motivated couple. Some people may find it somewhat "messy" to use. Could be displaced during intercourse. Must be removed, cleaned, and reapplied every 24 hours. Does not protect against STDs.

Method	Description	Advantages	Disadvantages/Risks
Contraceptive foams, creams, suppositories, vaginal contraceptive film (VCF), bioadhesive gel	Chemicals kill or immobilize sperm. Inserted into vagina before intercourse.	Easy to use. No prescription needed. No harmful side effects. No long-term effects on ability to conceive. The efficacy rate is about 82%.	Risks of pregnancy higher than with pill or IUD. Must be used before each act of intercourse. Some couples find this method "messy." Does not protect against STDs.
Cervical cap	A small barrier device that can be filled with spermicidal agent and placed snugly over the cervix. Typically made of soft, pliable rubber or plastic.	Highly effective (82%–94%). Nonhormonal and noninvasive. Does not require daily insertion. Little leakage of spermicide.	Not all women can be safely fitted at present. An extensive learning program is required for the user. May cause an undesirable odor. Does not protect against STDs.
Norplant	Rodlike capsules, 2 inches long, containing progestin. Inserted under skin of upper arm. Contains an ovulation-inhibiting hormone (progestin).	Effective for 5 yrs before must be replaced. Virtually 100% effective. Reversable method.	Initial cost is high ($500-$700) but cost-effective over time (5 yrs). The most common side effect is irregular bleeding. Does not protect against STDs.
Depo-Provera	A contraceptive injection containing a synthetic hormone (a progestin). Prevents pregnancy by inhibiting ovulation.	Highly effective (99%). One injection provides protection for 3 months.	Most common side effect is irregular bleeding and intermittent spotting. Does not protect against STDs.
Male condom	Thin rubber sheath placed over erect penis before intercourse. Acts as mechanical barrier preventing sperm from entering vagina. May be used with vaginal creams or jellies for added protection.	No prescription needed. Easy to use. Inexpensive. Provides some protection against sexually transmitted diseases—including HIV, the virus that causes AIDS—and common vaginal infections. Completely reversible form of contraception. Efficacy 90% when carefully used.	May tear or slip off during intercourse. May diminish pleasurable sensations.

Continued.

TABLE 10-2
Birth Control Methods—cont'd

Method	Description	How it works	Advantages	Disadvantages
Female condom	Polyurethane pouch with two flexible rings at either end.	The condom's inner ring holds it in place inside the vagina; the outer ring covers the outer lips	Reduces risk of STDs.	May slip or tear during intercourse.
Rhythm (calendar-basal body temperature method)	Woman has intercourse only during her "safe" periods, which never include approximately 3 days before and 3 days after ovulation.	By avoiding intercourse during the fertile period. Woman takes her temperature every morning before rising to establish pattern of ovulation. Basal body temperature rises following ovulation and stays up until menstruation.	Accepted by the Catholic church. No physical side effects. Efficacy rate can be as low as 75%.	Not very reliable if menstrual cycles are irregular. Restriction of sexual relations could cause tension in the couple's relationship.
Coitus interruptus (withdrawal)	Man withdraws penis from vagina before ejaculation occurs.	Semen does not enter vagina.	Probably better than nothing.	Requires great self-control. Sperm can be present in lubricating fluid of male before ejaculation. Can limit sexual gratification for both partners.
Ovulation method (cervical mucus method)	Basic changes in cervical mucus occur prior to ovulation.	Slippery mucus usually discharged from vagina 3 days before ovulation; following ovulation mucus becomes sticky.	No mechanical devices needed. Helps woman "tune into" her body.	Requires high level of motivation.
Sterilization tubal ligation (female)	Surgical procedure, cutting and tying off or placing a clip on the fallopian tubes. Outpatient or inpatient procedure with anesthesia.	Ovum cannot get to uterus for fertilization.	Almost 100% effective. No need to use other methods of contraception.	Risk of anesthesia complications and infections (as with all surgery). Permanent in most cases.
Vasectomy (male)	Surgical procedure involving cutting and tying off tubes (vas deferens) that carry sperm to semen. Minor surgical procedure performed in doctor's office under local anesthesia.	Sperm absorbed by body rather than released.	Almost 100% effective. No deaths have been reported following vasectomy. Possible to store sperm in frozen semen banks preserving viable sperm of men who have had vasectomies.	Permanent in most cases.

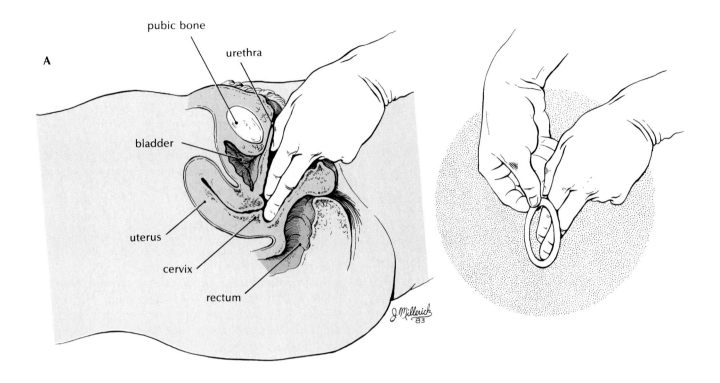

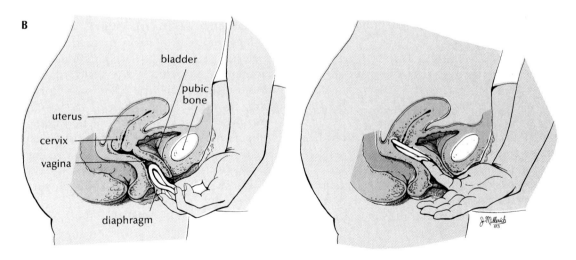

Figure 10-21 **A,** Fitting a diaphragm. **B,** Inserting a diaphragm. *(Courtesy Population Reports, H-7, Population Information Program, Johns Hopkins University.)*

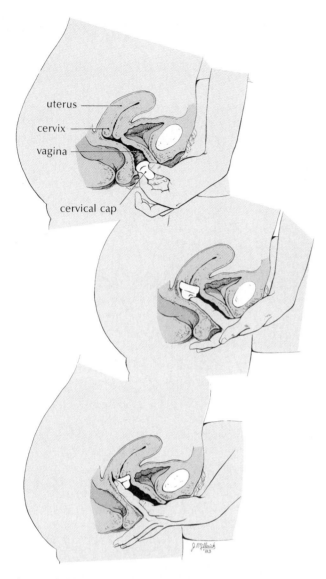

uterus

cervix

vagina

cervical cap

Figure 10-22 Inserting a cervical cap. *(Courtesy Population Reports, H-7, Population Information Program, Johns Hopkins University.)*

in solution and given by hypodermic needle, provide a nearly constant dose of hormones to prevent pregnancy for 1 to 6 months.

Monthly injectables add an estrogen to a progestin to minimize menstrual changes.

A *vaginal ring* is placed by the woman in her vagina, where it gradually releases hormone.

The precursors of these new methods are the long-acting injectable contraceptives: the 3-month Depo-Provera and the 2- to 3-month Noristerat.

Chemical abortion

Mifepristone (RU 486) is a chemically synthesized drug that discourages progesterone from its primary function, which is to prepare the uterus for the reception and development of the fertilized egg.

Roussel-Uclaf, the French pharmaceutical company that makes the drug, says that RU 486 has proved to be 96% effective in inducing abortion in France when followed by a prostaglandin suppository or injection within 48 hours. Medical abortion is as effective as surgical abortion, but it carries fewer risks for the woman. RU 486 can be used to induce early nonsurgical abortions or routinely each month just before menstruation is due. However, the use of RU 486 is controversial in the United States and not readily available for most women.

With further testing and refinement, effective, reversible, long-acting hormonal contraception will one day be available for nearly every couple.

Induced Abortion

Removal, at the choice of the woman, of the products of conception from the uterus before the fetus is able to survive is termed *induced abortion*. Abortion raises the fundamental question about the extent to which the state may interfere with an individual's decision regarding his or her own body. The practice of abortion is probably older than written history.

D&C and D&E

The accepted procedures for performing an abortion are dilatation and curettage (D&C), dilation and evacuation (D&E) using vacuum aspiration, amniocentesis and injection of prostaglandins into the amniotic sac, and hysterotomy. D&E with suction curettage is the preferred technique for early termination of pregnancies up to 12 to 16 weeks of gestation. Under anesthesia (usually paracervical block with intravenous sedation) the cervix is dilated and a vacuum tip is inserted into the uterus. The intense suction at the opening of the cannula separates the products of conception, which are then drawn out through the connecting tubing. The average time for the procedure is 10 minutes. Dilatation of the cervix is the most difficult part of the procedure.

The cervix can be dilated using metal dilators, laminaria (dried sterilized seaweed that expands on contact with moisture) or hygroscopic cervical dilators (Dilapan) inserted into the cervix 10 to 24 hours before the abortion.

Dilatation and curettage (D&C) may be performed toward the end of the first trimester. Under anesthesia (usually paracervical block with intravenous sedation) the uterine contents are removed by scraping with a sharp curette.

Transabdominal Prostaglandin F$_2$ (PGF$_2$)

Starting at the sixteenth week of pregnancy amniocentesis and amnioinfusion procedures are recommended. With prostaglandin injection aspiration of amniotic fluid is not necessary and intravenous administration of oxytocin is usually not necessary. The physician injects prostaglandin into the amniotic sac, and contractions usually begin in 1 to 2 hours. Within 24 hours the abortion is completed by the passage of the products of conception.

Prostaglandin suppositories (PGE$_2$) can be inserted into the posterior vaginal canal to cause abortion after the cervix has been dilated. The use of prostaglandin E$_2$ (PGE$_2$) is the most convenient method with the fewest side effects.

Hysterotomy is performed under spinal or general anesthesia and is comparable to a cesarean delivery. Hysterotomy is rarely performed in the United States.

Nursing Support

Although all patients have a right to care, nurses whose religious, moral, or ethical beliefs do not condone abortion should not be required to care for women undergoing abortion. However, when giving nursing care to these women the primary objective is to give high quality nursing care, and the nurse must take an active role. Remember that the woman is goal oriented—termination of the pregnancy. The nurse will have to take the initiative in making assessments and acting on them. Give the woman a realistic description of the procedure, the surroundings, and the hospital stay. Touching and supportive care are vital.

Before discharge the woman needs to understand signs and symptoms of possible complications and the importance of follow-up care. Also, she may want to discuss contraceptive methods and their use. Often the questions the nurse asks help the woman to face reality. As an example: "Now that your abortion is over, what are you planning to do for contraception?" Remember also that accepting a woman's values and decisions does not mean you must agree with them. Try to understand and be caring. In abortion care nurses can make a unique contribution to the total care of women.

SUMMARY

In this chapter we have discussed the postpartum family and their major physiological and psychosocial adaptations and briefly looked at the subject of family planning. For the first time in this book we have deviated from concern for saving lives to the issue of abor-

tion (terminating life). This is a difficult subject for maternity personnel, whose energies are often concentrated on preserving life at any cost. In the next chapter we will explore complications of the postpartum period.

BIBLIOGRAPHY

Ament LA: Maternal tasks of the puerperium reidentified, *J Obstet Gynecol Neonatal Nurs* 19(4):330-335, 1990.

Anderson GC: Risk in mother-infant separation postbirth, *Image* 21(4):196-199, 1989.

Banton M, Lum B: *Education for the new mother and her family.* In: Littlefield VM, editor: *Health education for women: a guide for nurses and other health professionals,* Connecticut, 1986, Appleton-Century-Crofts.

Beall MH: Breastfeeding: some drug admonitions, *Contemp Obstet Gynecol* 29(1):49-54, 1987.

Blakemore K: Lactation suppression is a matter of choice, *Contemp Obstet Gynecol* 28(5):39-59, 1986.

Conover E: Hazardous exposures during pregnancy, *J Obstet Gynecol Neonatal Nurs* 23(6):524-532, 1994.

Dimino DK: Postpartum depression: a defense for mothers who kill their infants, *Santa Clara Law Review,* 30(1):231-264, 1990.

Donaldson K, Briggs J, McMaster D: RU 486: an alternative to surgical abortion, *J Obstet Gynecol Neonatal Nurs* 23(7):555-559, 1994.

Eidelman AL, Hoffmann NW, Kaitz M: Cognitive deficits in women after childbirth, *Obstet Gynecol* 81(5):764-767, 1993.

Eyer DE: *Mother-infant bonding: a scientific fiction,* New Haven, 1992, Yale University Press.

Hinkle LT: Education and counseling for norplant users, *J Obstet Gynecol Neonatal Nurs* 23(5):387-391, 1994.

Howard FM, Howard CR, Weitzman M: The physician as advertiser: the unintentional discouragement of breastfeeding, *Obstet Gynecol* 81(6):1048-1051, 1993.

Hughes V, Owen J: Is breastfeeding possible after breast surgery? *MCN* 18(4):213-217, 1993.

Jankowski H, Wells SM: Self-administered medications for obstetric patients, *MCN* 12(3):199-203, 1987.

Klaus MH, Kennell JH: *Parent-infant bonding,* ed 2, St. Louis, 1982, Mosby.

LaFay J, Geden EA: Postepisiotomy pain: warm versus cold sitz bath, *J Obstet Gynecol Neonatal Nurs* 18(5):399-403, 1989.

Lawrence RA: *Breastfeeding, a guide for the medical profession,* ed 4, St. Louis, 1994, Mosby.

Martell LK: Teaching about bottlefeeding, *Childbirth Educator,* 34-42, Fall, 1987.

Mattson S, Smith JE, editors: *Care curriculum for maternal-newborn nursing,* Philadelphia, 1993, WB Saunders.

McBryde A: Compulsory rooming-in in the ward and private newborn services at Duke Hospital, *JAMA* 145(9):526-628, 1951.

Monier M, Laird M: Contraceptives: a look at the future, *Am J Nurs* 89(4):496-499, 1989.

Morse JM, Bottorff JL: Intending to breastfeed and work, *J Obstet Gynecol Neonatal Nurs* 18(6):493-500, 1989.

Norr KF, Nacion K: Outcomes of postpartum early discharge, 1960-1986: a comparative review, *Birth* 14(3):135-141, 1987.

OGN Nursing Practice Resource: *Facilitating breastfeeding*, Washington, DC, 1991, NAACOG.

OGN Nursing Practice Resource: *Contraceptive options*, Washington, DC, 1991, NAACOG.

Placksin S: *Mothering the new mother: your postpartum resource companion*, New York, 1994, Newmarket Press.

Ramler D, Roberts J: A comparison of cold and warm sitz baths for relief of postpartum perineal pain, *J Obstet Gynecol Neonatal Nurs* 15(6):471-474, 1986.

Rubin R: Maternal identity and the maternal experience, New York, 1984, Springer.

Tulman L, Fawcett J: Return of functional ability after childbirth, *Nurs Res* 37(2):77-81, 1988.

Ziemer MM, Pigeon JG: Skin changes and pain in the nipple during the first week of lactation, *J Obstet Gynecol Neonatal Nurs* 22(3):247-256, 1993.

DEFINITIONS

Define the following terms:

alveoli	involution
anticipatory guidance	lactation
colostrum	leukocytosis
engorgement	"let-down reflex"
Homans' sign	lochia alba
hypertonic	lochia rubra
induced abortion	lochia serosa

mother-baby nursing	puerperium
PID	rooming-in
postpartum blues	rooting reflex
prolactin	sibling
prostaglandin	

LEARNING ACTIVITIES

1. Group discussions.
2. Visit local agencies concerned with family planning. Report on their facilities, policies, and fees charged.
3. View audiovisual aids and discuss.

ENRICHMENT/IN-DEPTH STUDY

1. If there is a postpartum support group in your community, visit the group. How often do they meet? How long do people usually continue in the group after the baby's birth? Why?
2. Interview new parents. Determine if caring for a new baby is what they thought it would be. What are their main concerns about life-style changes that they have experienced since their baby's birth?
3. You might ask a new mother or new father to cut pictures out of a magazine depicting the baby they thought they would have ("before") and pictures descriptive of their new baby ("after"). Compare the "before" and "after" and discuss.
4. Role play teaching methods of contraception.

Self-Assessment

1. Match Column A with Column B.

   Column A

   _____ 1. "taking-in" phase

   _____ 2. "taking-hold" phase

   _____ 3. "letting-go" phase

   Column B

   a. regains control over body

   b. establishes new maternal role patterns

   c. passive and dependent

For questions 2 through 12, choose the best answers and indicate your choice by circling the answer.

2. What would you suggest for a woman whose episiotomy hurts her?

   a. sitz baths

   b. reassurance

   c. witch hazel compresses

   d. all of above

3. "Afterpains" are caused by:

   a. contractions of the uterus as it gets smaller again

   b. drugs

   c. mental depression

4. Three comfort measures for hemorrhoids are:

   a. warm sitz baths

   b. walking

   c. cold witch hazel compresses

   d. elevating buttocks on several pillows

   Answer (circle one).

   1. a and b

   2. a, b, and d

   3. b

   4. a, c, and d

5. To reestablish proper bowel functioning postpartum, the physician may order:

   a. stool softeners

   b. laxatives

   c. enemas

   d. vitamins

   Answer (circle one).

   1. a and d

   2. all of the above

   3. a, b, and c

6. Immediate weight loss of the mother after delivery is:

   a. 20 pounds

   b. 13 pounds

   c. 7 pounds

7. The milk ejection reflex is involuntary and is stimulated by:

   a. hearing the baby cry

   b. anticipation of a feeding

   c. a and b

8. Breast engorgement usually occurs by:

   a. 1 week

   b. 3 to 4 days

   c. 10 days

9. Menstruation usually reappears in the nonnursing mother:

   a. 2 weeks postpartum

   b. 4 months postpartum

   c. 6 to 8 weeks postpartum

10. Menstruation usually reappears in the breast-feeding mother:

    a. 4 weeks postpartum

    b. 3 to 4 months postpartum or when she stops breast-feeding

    c. 2 weeks postpartum

11. The clean perineal pad is applied from:

    a. back to front

    b. side to side

    c. front to back

12. Douching is contraindicated during postpartum until:

    a. the lochia stops

    b. the 6 week check-up

    c. 6 months postpartum

13. Match Column A with Column B. Each item in Column B may be used once or more than once.

Column A	Column B
____ 1. normal uterine and vaginal discharge postpartum	a. uterus
____ 2. goes through three stages	b. lochia
____ 3. involutes in the puerperium	c. urinary system
____ 4. by tenth postpartum day should be no longer palpable	d. perineum
____ 5. soothing measures include warm sitz baths	e. lochia rubra
____ 6. should be kept clean and dry	f. lochia serosa
____ 7. overdistention of bladder can occur	g. lochia alba
____ 8. significant diuresis early postpartum	
____ 9. brownish in color	
____ 10. red and bloody	
____ 11. yellowish white	

14. The new mother's pulse may be _____ or _____ beats per minute on the first and second days postpartum.

15. A normal postpartum temperature is _____.

16. Blood pressure may _____ slightly in the postpartum period.

17. Respiration may be _____ in the postpartum period.

18. Parent-infant attachment is influenced by the infant's _____.

19. As men adjust to their role as father, they also go through phases. In the adjustment phase men are aware of the _____ of their new family. In the acceptance phase men have to _____ the intense, intimate relationship between the mother and _____.

20. What is the difference between sterilization and contraception?

_____

_____

_____

For questions 21 through 25, select the correct answer.

21. Disadvantages of the IUD include:

    a. depression

    b. pelvic inflammatory disease

    c. swelling of uterus

22. Use of the pill is contraindicated for women who:

    a. have a family history of Parkinson's disease

    b. have never delivered a baby

    c. have a history of blood clotting problems

23. If a new mother complains of tenderness and warmth in her leg and has a fever, you would suspect that she may have:

    a. thrombophlebitis

    b. leg cramps

    c. dehydration and stiffness

24. On palpation of the uterine fundus during the first 24 hours postpartum, if the fundus is boggy you should first:

    a. check the consistency of the fundus again after a 15-minute interval

    b. massage the fundus firmly by cupping your hand around the fundus and rotating gently, placing your other hand just above the symphysis pubis

    c. grasp the fundus between thumb and fingers and hold tight

    d. place the patient in Trendelenberg position

25. The nurse may best aid the new mother in performing a caretaking task by:

    a. interrupting the mother's attempt at diapering and showing her the correct way

    b. initially showing her how to diaper, then allowing her to try

    c. suggesting that the mother watch the nurse diaper the infant several times before she attempts it

Answer questions 26 through 30 true or false.

____ **26.** The fundus is normally found to the right of midline.

____ **27.** Foul-smelling lochia can indicate infection.

____ **28.** Poor "en face" with an infant is a normal, temporary maternal response that does not need further monitoring.

____ **29.** Sitz baths reduce swelling of perineal tissues and can increase the comfort of an episiotomy.

____ **30.** Small infrequent voiding and displaced fundus can indicate an over-distended bladder.

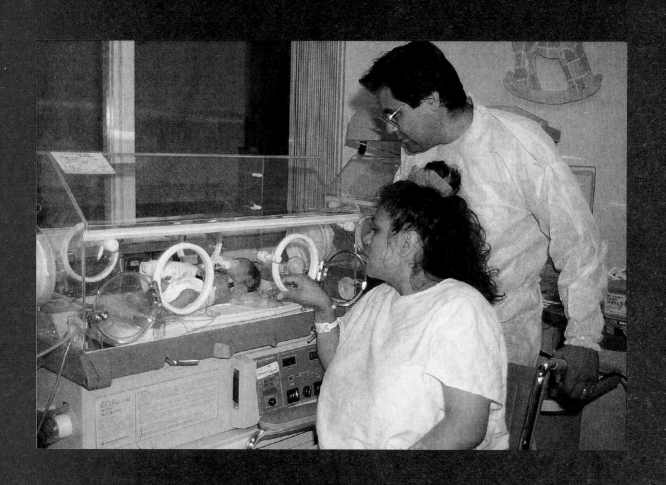

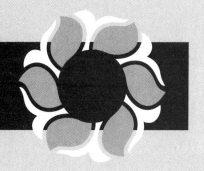

11

THE POSTPARTUM FAMILY WITH COMPLICATIONS

GOALS

This chapter is designed to provide the reader with information that will:
• promote awareness of deviations from normal in the postpartum period.

• explore the role of support persons for grieving families.

STUDENT OBJECTIVES

After studying this chapter, you should be able to:

1. Identify causes, preventive measures, and nursing care for postpartum hemorrhage.
2. Differentiate between early and late postpartum hemorrhage.
3. Identify four obstetric conditions associated with DIC (disseminated intravascular coagulation).
4. Identify the woman at risk for developing a postpartum infection.
5. Explain the treatment for thrombophlebitis.
6. Develop a teaching plan to explain causes and preventive measures for mastitis.
7. Explain how a nurse can detect a uterus that is not involuting properly.

8. List the observations a nurse would make when caring for a woman following a cesarean birth.
9. Design a plan to meet the emotional needs of parents who have been separated from their babies immediately after birth.
10. In lay terms describe how you would counsel the family concerning the expectations for both physical and emotional recovery following a cesarean birth.
11. Formulate a plan of support for a new family whose baby (a) is dead or (b) has a birth defect.

The postpartum period is a time of dynamic changes. During these 6 weeks after birth new mothers may experience complications. Postpartum complications can include hemorrhage, involutional problems, infectious conditions of the genital tract or urinary tract, systemic infection, and emotional disorders.

POSTPARTUM HEMORRHAGE

As emphasized in Chapter 8, after birth the uterus must be kept firm to minimize bleeding. Because of the increased blood supply during pregnancy, a woman can lose from 250 to 350 milliliters of blood at birth without undesirable effects. However, excessive bleeding contributes to postpartum morbidity and can lead to maternal death, the leading cause of which is hemorrhage. Therefore very careful and close evaluation of the uterine fundus height and firmness, vital signs, and amount of vaginal bleeding postpartum is extremely important.

Postpartum hemorrhage is defined as blood loss of 500 milliliters (1 pint) or more following separation and expulsion of the placenta. When the bleeding occurs within the first 24 hours following birth, it is considered *early* postpartum hemorrhage. *Late* postpartum hemorrhage occurs after the first 24 hours post birth, usually at 7 to 14 days of the postpartum period.

Causes of Early Postpartum Hemorrhage

The causes of early postpartum hemorrhage are (1) uterine atony, (2) placental complications (placenta accreta or retained placenta), (3) retention of placental fragments, (4) lacerations and hematomas of the genital tract, (5) ruptured uterus, and (6) inversion of the uterus. Early postpartum hemorrhage occurs in 4% of deliveries.

Uterine atony

In *uterine atony* the uterus does not have good muscle tone and consequently relaxes. Because the large blood vessels are not compressed by tight uterine muscle fibers, the blood vessels bleed freely. Physical findings of uterine atony include a boggy, large uterus, expelled clots, and bright red vaginal bleeding. Common causes of uterine atony include prolonged or extremely rapid labor, an overdistended uterus (multiple pregnancy, a large baby, hydramnios), a uterus displaced by a full bladder, and drugs (general anesthesia, oxytocin, and magnesium sulfate). As discussed in Chapter 8 treatment of uterine atony is vigorous (but not rough) mas-

sage of the relaxed and enlarged fundus, firm expression of accumulated blood clots, fluid/blood replacement, and administration of oxytocics (including Pitocin, Methergine, and/or Prostin) over an extended period.

Placental complications

Retention of placental fragments may be a cause of early postpartum hemorrhage and is also a common cause of delayed or late postpartum hemorrhage. With retained placental fragments the placenta is not delivered intact, the uterus remains large, and vaginal bleeding is bright red. Inspection of the placenta and careful exploration of the uterus are essential to diagnose retention of placental fragments. Dilation and curettage (D&C) may have to be done to remove the placental fragments.

Lacerations and hematoma

These may be the result of difficult or rapid, uncontrolled delivery; breech delivery; large fetal head; use of forceps during delivery or other operative procedures; or vulvar and perineal varices. If the uterus is firm at the umbilicus and in the midline but bright red bleeding persists, a laceration is probably the cause.

When a new mother with a normal temperature complains of severe perineal or pelvic pain that is not relieved by analgesics, suspect a vaginal or retroperitoneal *hematoma*. In this situation blood vessels burst and blood collects in surrounding tissues that remain intact. The hematoma may appear as a bluish, bulging area just under the skin surface. Small hematomas can be watched to be sure they are not enlarging. Large hematomas may be evacuated through an incision in the vaginal wall.

Ruptured uterus

The signs and symptoms of a *ruptured uterus* include localized abdominal pain and tenderness, a tearing feeling, and then hypovolemic shock. The causes of uterine rupture may include a difficult vaginal delivery, a weak uterine operative scar, injudicious use of oxytocin, an obstructed labor, and residual damage from past trauma to the uterus. Emergency surgery to suture the laceration and blood replacement are essential. A hysterectomy may have to be done when a uterus has ruptured.

Inversion

Inversion of the uterus occurs when the uterus is turned inside out. This may be caused by pulling on the umbilical cord before the placenta is separated or by extreme pushing on the uterine fundus in an attempt to assist the delivery. Should this happen the uterus is replaced manually and oxytocic drugs are given to cause it to contract. Antibiotics are also given to prevent infection. If manual replacement of the uterus is inadequate, surgery may be necessary to reposition or remove the uterus.

Causes of Late Postpartum Hemorrhage

Late postpartum hemorrhage is less common than early hemorrhage. It occurs in 0.1% to 1.0% of new mothers. Causes of late postpartum hemorrhage are retained placenta or membranes, subinvolution of the uterus, and *endometritis* (infection of the uterine lining).

SUBINVOLUTION

Subinvolution is a failure of the uterus to return to its normal size following delivery. Two common causes are retention of pieces of placenta and infection of the endometrium *(endometritis)*.

When checking the height of the uterine fundus and the firmness of the uterus daily, it is possible to detect a uterus that is not involuting properly. In addition to finding the uterus too large for the appropriate day postpartum, the lochia will be more profuse and redder than it should be. Once lochia rubra is gone, it should not return. With short hospital stays for birth and inconsistent home follow-up care, the mother must be taught to monitor the height of her uterine fundus postpartum. She must also be taught to recognize abnormal lochia and to report to her care provider if she perceives abnormal uterine involution or lochia.

If late postpartum hemorrhage occurs while the new mother is still hospitalized, treatment may include oxytocics such as Pitocin, Methergine and/or Prostin, intravenous fluids, and surgical intervention. Antibiotics are also prescribed for infection.

If the mother is at home and bleeding is minimal, bed rest and an oral oxytocic such as methylergonovine maleate (Methergine) may resolve the bleeding. Because oxytocics are vasoconstrictive, the mother's blood pressure should be taken before the medication is given. If it is elevated over 140/90, notify the physician before giving the oxytocin. Antibiotics will be prescribed if there is evidence of infection. If the mother is at home and bleeding is heavy, she will be readmitted to the hospital and treated with intravenous fluids, oxytocin, antibiotics, and surgical intervention. Mother-baby care to minimize separation of mother and infant is essential if the mother has to be readmitted to the hospital.

Nursing Care

Blood loss of more than 1000 milliliters can lead to severe postpartum infection, extensive pelvic thrombophlebitis, and hypovolemic shock with its side effects. The signs of shock are a drop in blood pressure; pallor; cold, clammy skin; an increased pulse rate (rapid and weak); anxiety or restlessness; apprehension; and air hunger.

In severe postpartum hemorrhage, transfusions may be given to replace blood lost, and antibiotics are given to prevent infection. In addition to monitoring the administration of blood, the nurse should keep close records of the woman's intake and output and blood loss. Perineal pad counts and weights (1 gram = 1 ml) are helpful in measuring blood loss. If there is an adequate volume of circulating blood, the urinary output should be from 30 to 60 milliliters per hour (monitored with a Foley catheter). Administration of oxygen may also be instituted.

Postpartum hemorrhage is frightening to the woman and her family, and they need constant support. The nurse should explain to the woman the necessity for uterine massage since it can be very painful. It is important that the family be continually informed of what is happening at the same time they are being reassured.

DISSEMINATED INTRAVASCULAR COAGULATION (DIC)

Deficiencies in the blood clotting mechanisms can complicate postpartum hemorrhage. When the elements necessary for homeostasis are depleted, the process is referred to as DIC (disseminated intravascular coagulation). DIC results when some factor (massive tissue injury, cell lysis, bacteremia, etc.) triggers the coagulation cascade. Obstetrical complications that may cause a DIC are abruptio placentae, preeclampsia, eclampsia, incomplete abortion, septic abortion, prolonged retention of a dead fetus, amniotic fluid embolism, sepsis, and tumultuous or hypertonic labor and delivery.

Clinical manifestations of DIC usually begin subtly and become more overt as the disorder progresses. Signs and symptoms range from mild oozing at venipuncture sites to localized bleeding in the form of petechiae. As the condition worsens there will be prolonged bleeding from the gums and possibly bleeding from all orifices.

The nurse must be familiar with various laboratory blood tests that will provide the major basis for diagnosing and managing DIC. The prothrombin time (PT) and partial prothrombin time (PPT) are prolonged in DIC. Platelets are decreased. Clotting time is normal. Fibrinogen levels may be within normal ranges but will be lower than the baseline level.

Treatment for DIC calls for resolution of the underlying condition responsible for the DIC, such as treatment of any existing infection or eclampsia or removal of the fetus and damaged placenta as soon as possible by either vaginal or cesarean delivery. After the source of the DIC condition is removed, the need for further intervention is usually unnecessary. Plasma factors generally return to normal in 24 to 48 hours. Platelet counts return to normal in 5 to 7 days.

In severe DIC blood replacement may be necessary. Also, replacement of blood clotting factors in the form of fresh frozen plasma and replacement of platelets may be indicated.

Nursing Care

Closely monitoring bleeding, measuring and documenting blood loss, and preventing or minimizing blood loss are important facets of nursing care for the woman with DIC. Gentle handling and frequent turning and positioning with pillows will help minimize blood vessel and skin breakdown. Gentle mouth care and medications given intravenously or orally will also decrease unnecessary bruising and hematoma formation. Because these women are at risk of developing shock, they must be monitored closely for the signs of shock.

Overwhelming fear, anxiety, mood swings, depression, and anger may be experienced by the woman with DIC as well as by family members. Understanding and accepting these emotional reactions are essential when providing care. The woman and her family need information about DIC and its treatment, plus information on all tests and procedures performed. Whenever possible, involving the woman and her family in nursing care is helpful because it gives them a measure of control over a very threatening situation.

PUERPERAL INFECTION

A *puerperal infection* is any infection of the genital tract during the puerperium. The identification of the puerperal infection is generally accepted to be a temperature elevation to 100.4° F (38° C) or higher on two or more occasions for more than 24 hours during the first 10 days postpartum (excluding the first 24 hours). However, because antibiotic therapy can mask symptoms, the criterion of an elevated temperature may no longer be valid for all women. Puerperal infection occurs after about 6% of births in the United States.

During labor and delivery the reproductive tract is particularly susceptible to infections. Invasive techniques used in monitoring the progress of labor can introduce new pathogenic organisms into the reproductive tract. Untreated local infections; long, difficult, traumatic labor and delivery; premature rupture of the membranes (PROM); hemorrhage; anemia; and cesarean delivery can also increase the risk of infection. These infections can be caused by bacteria already present in the woman's genital tract or by organisms introduced from other individuals.

Whatever the cause, puerperal infection is a serious postpartum complication. Infections are classified by site. Sites and terms are (1) uterine lining *(endometritis)*, (2) connective tissue around the uterus *(parametritis)*, (3) pelvic cavity *(peritonitis)*, (4) vulva *(vulvitis)*, and (5) vagina *(vaginitis)*. Local infections may invade the lymph channels and the bloodstream, causing *septicemia* (infection of the bloodstream) and *thrombophlebitis* (inflammation of pelvic or femoral veins).

Causes and Symptoms

Common causes are *Streptococcus* organisms, the colon bacillus *Escherichia coli* and other coliform bacteria, *Staphylococcus* and *Bacteroides*.

Symptoms of local infection may include elevated temperature, edema, inflammation, and tenderness of the infected part. Signs and symptoms of a more serious infection may include fever above 100.4° F (38° C), chills, rapid pulse, abdominal tenderness or pain, malaise, foul-smelling lochia, and an abnormally large uterus that is not involuting properly *(subinvolution)*. Any of these signs or symptoms should be recorded and reported immediately so that medical treatment can be started.

Treatment

Treatment includes rest and Fowler's position to promote drainage, a high fluid intake and high protein diet, administration of antibiotics, and administration of oxytocics to keep the uterus contracted to prevent spread of bacteria.

Nursing Care

Comfort measures are taken to relieve the symptoms. Bed rest, increased fluid intake, and elevating the head of the bed to promote uterine drainage are important nursing care measures for the mother with puerperal infection. The nurse should be constantly vigilant for signs of extension of the infection, such as abdominal distention, vomiting, and diarrhea, in addition to the previously listed symptoms.

Because the mother needs rest and sleep to recover from the infection, other caregivers will need to provide most of the care for her baby. Encourage the mother to get well as first priority, but do not separate mother and baby. The bonding needs of mother and baby do not change because of the puerperal infection. Mother-baby nursing is the preferred model of nursing care in this circumstance.

THROMBOPHLEBITIS

Thrombophlebitis is an infection of the lining of a vessel in which a clot attaches to the vessel wall.

Thrombophlebitis in the postpartum period is usually caused by inflammation in the deep pelvic and femoral veins. This condition occurs in less than 1% of all postpartum women. Predisposing factors are increased pressure in the veins of the pelvis and legs that impairs blood return and the possibility of pelvic vein thrombosis from extension of intrauterine infection. The thrombophlebitis may not appear until 10 to 20 days after delivery. The affected leg and thigh may gradually begin to swell, feel tender and warm, and appear discolored. Temperature elevation and chills may be noted. Pain may be experienced behind the knee or in the calf when the woman's leg is extended and pressure is applied to her foot. This physical finding is known as a positive *Homans' sign.*

Treatment consists of bed rest, application of an elastic bandage or support stocking, and elevation of the leg and foot 30 to 45 degrees. Moist or dry heat to the leg may be prescribed. If a portion of a thrombus is dislodged, it is called an *embolus.* An embolus can travel through the bloodstream to the heart and lungs and cause death. Because of the possibility of causing an embolism, the affected leg should never be massaged. Anticoagulants may be prescribed by the physician to lessen the danger of embolism. If an infectious process persists, antibiotics are administered.

✓MASTITIS

Mastitis is an infection of breast tissue. The common organisms involved include *Staphylococcus aureus, Escherichia coli,* and (rarely) *Streptococcus.* Predisposing factors are cracked or fissured nipples, bruising of the breast, and clogged ducts. Thorough cleanliness when handling the breasts has already been emphasized. Dirty hands of hospital personnel or the mother can introduce bacteria through a cracked or fissured nipple. Also, a baby who has acquired the *Staphylococcus* organism in the nursery may carry it to the mother's breasts when nursing. Symptoms of mastitis may include fever; malaise; rapid pulse; and pain, tenderness, and swelling of the affected breast. The affected area of the breast may be red and feel very hard and hot to the touch (Fig. 11-1). The onset is usually sudden and after 10 days postpartum.

Treatment includes rest, fluids, breast support, warm

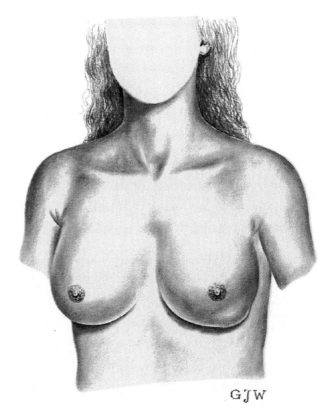

Figure 11-1 Mastitis. *(From Bobak IM, Jensen MD: Maternity and gynecologic care: the nurse and the family, ed 5, St. Louis, 1993, Mosby.)*

wet heat to the affected breast, keeping the breast as empty as possible, analgesics, and antibiotics (usually dicloxacillin or amoxicillin). The mother does not have to discontinue breast-feeding, since the causative organism is possibly already in the baby's nose and mouth. In fact, a breast-feeding mother should nurse her baby frequently to keep the infected breast as empty as possible. It is best to start the infant on the breast on the unaffected side while the breast on the affected side "lets down."

Prevention lies in proper positioning for breast-feeding, frequent feedings, good hygiene, and skin care. Other interventions may include emptying the ducts when feeding, rotating the baby's positions, air drying the nipples, wearing a support bra, and not using soap on the nipples.

CYSTITIS

Cystitis, or inflammation of the bladder, is an occasional postpartum complication. It can be caused by inadequate emptying of the bladder or by trauma from birth or catheterization. The woman should empty her bladder regularly and completely to prevent cystitis. Symptoms of cystitis may include painful, frequent

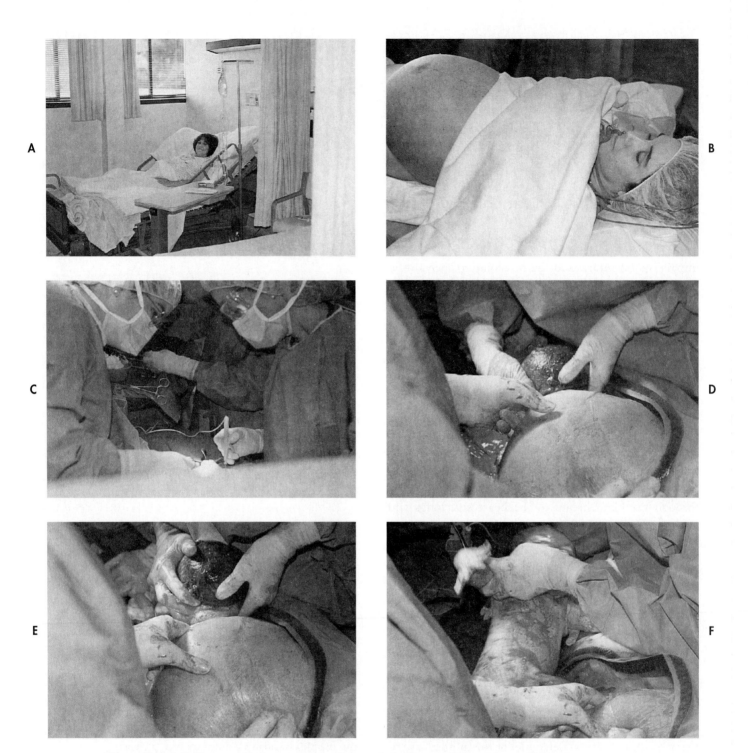

Figure 11-2, A-K Cesarean birth experience. *(Courtesy Curlee, Duncan, Tyler, and Lauren Phillips, Los Angeles.)*

emptying of the bladder, pain over the bladder, and a slight temperature elevation (100° to 101° F) (37.8° to 38.3° C). Upon microscopic examination pus, blood, and bacteria are found in the urine.

Treatment includes an antibiotic drug specific for the causative organisms, increasing fluids, and frequent emptying of the bladder.

CESAREAN BIRTH

Mothers and families who have experienced a cesarean birth as an emergency or after a long and difficult labor have special needs. Women who have experienced cesarean birth have reported feelings of depression, anxiety, guilt, loss of control, less satisfaction with the

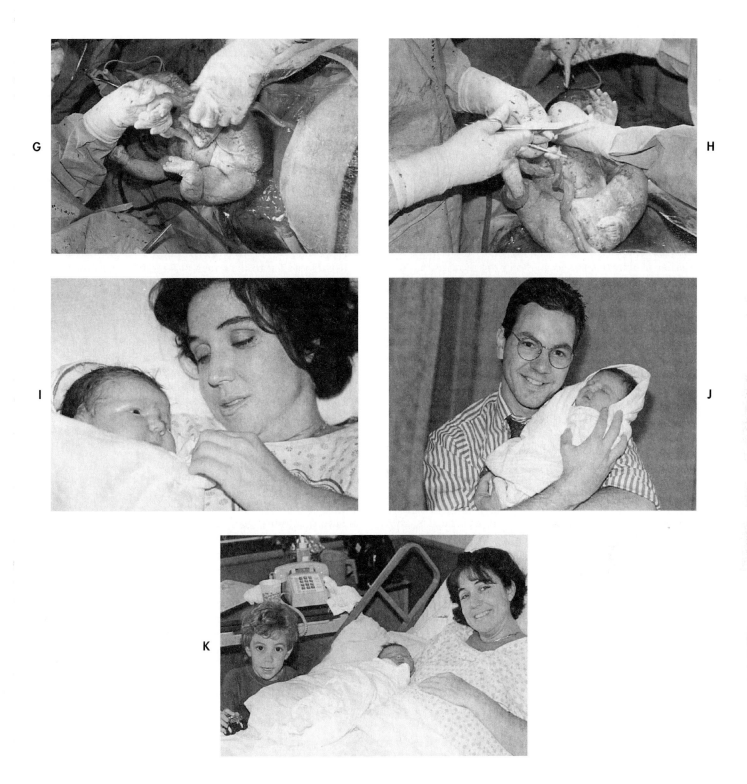

birth experience, and even loss of self-esteem. Mothers and families who undergo planned, scheduled cesareans can sometimes utilize coping mechanisms in preparation for the surgery. Women experiencing an unplanned cesarean do not have this preparation time.

Reasons for a cesarean, the basic types, and emergency preparations were discussed in Chapter 9. In this chapter discussion will focus on the physical and emotional care needed following a cesarean birth. The term *cesarean birth* should be used rather than *cesarean section* (grapefruits are sectioned; women give birth). Whenever possible, therefore, the term *cesarean birth* is used in this text. (See Fig. 11-2 for a birth by cesarean experience.)

Nursing Care

Women who experience an unplanned cesarean birth are at greater risk for infection, including endometritis, bacteremia, and urinary tract and wound infection. An unplanned, emergency cesarean birth can be especially stressful and strain the woman's coping mechanisms. These women need sensitive care that takes into consideration their special needs for information, for the presence of their partners throughout the birth experience, and for contact with their infants.

Following cesarean birth the mother's vital signs should be monitored every 15 minutes for the first 2 hours. Perineal pads and abdominal dressings should be checked frequently for bleeding. The cesarean birth mother usually has less lochia than the mother who experienced a vaginal birth because the placenta and decidua have been manually removed. More than two perineal pads saturated in 1 hour following a cesarean birth indicate excessive bleeding. The uterus must be kept firm; if it should relax, gentle massage and increasing the amount of intravenous oxytocin may correct the problem. Until the woman is able to ambulate, she should turn, cough, and deep breathe every 2 hours to reduce the chance of respiratory compromise. Careful intake and output recording is essential to be sure the urinary system is functioning adequately. A Foley catheter may be used for 24 to 48 hours until the bladder resumes normal function. Because chills are a common postpartum problem, the mother should be covered with a warm blanket.

It is essential to keep the perineum as clean and dry as possible to reduce the risk of pathogenic organisms traveling up the vagina to the uterus. Intravenous fluids must be carefully monitored and regulated; they are usually discontinued when the woman's oral intake is adequate and bowel sounds are present. Medication for pain is prescribed and given judiciously one half-hour before activities that increase discomfort.

Early ambulation is important in preventing thrombophlebitis and in facilitating normal bowel and bladder function. Intestinal gas (flatus) is common after abdominal surgery. Ambulation will help to minimize this gas and the pain that accompanies it. Teaching the woman to splint her abdomen by pressing a pillow against it to cushion the operative area and incision will make moving about and coughing less uncomfortable. Rectal suppositories, a rectal tube, or an enema may be prescribed to alleviate the discomfort. After the initial recovery days, most mothers need only oral analgesics for pain and are able to ambulate well.

For the entire hospital stay, in addition to postsurgical care, a daily postpartum assessment is done, checking breast and nipple condition, amount and character of lochia, height and consistency of the fundus, the abdominal incision, and extremities. Between the second to fourth day post surgery, the mother is discharged from the hospital.

The nurse can help this new mother by pacing care to help her through the "taking in" phase. She will have to work through and resolve her feelings about the unplanned surgery. The woman and her partner and/or family members should be encouraged to share their feelings about the unplanned surgery with each other and with the nurse. Reconstructing the events surrounding the labor and delivery will help to assimilate them. Talking about the surgery and explaining the surgery and healing process will help the mother accept the bodily changes she is experiencing. The new mother must also adjust to the shock of a surgical incision and the pain that accompanies it.

Unplanned separation from siblings remaining at home can be traumatic for both mother and siblings. Siblings should be encouraged to visit mother and new baby in the first hours and days postpartum (Fig. 11-2, *K*). The parents can also send Polaroid pictures of the mother and new baby home to the siblings. Daily phone calls and notes or small gifts from mother can all be used to involve the siblings in the birth event.

Breast-Feeding

In the first few days following a cesarean birth mothers may need extra help with breast-feeding. It is helpful for the woman to lie on her side in a fetal position, splinting her abdomen with a pillow. In this position she can tuck the baby into her body curve and minimize the stretch and any pressure on her incision. When abdominal discomfort is intense, the mother can use the football hold with the infant while breast-feeding in an upright position. Mother-baby nursing is ideal for this mother because it permits her to feed the baby on demand, thus stimulating lactation. During the first few days the mother will need help lifting, positioning, and changing the baby from one breast to another. The father may be the ideal person to help, if his work and home situations permit him to stay in the hospital.

Separation

If the baby born by cesarean is kept in a special care nursery, the mother and father should go to the nursery to interact with their baby whenever possible. If the baby is to be transferred to another facility for special care, the mother should at least touch the baby before transport. Early mother-father-infant contact is very important. Information can be provided about the infant through telephone calls and photos.

Morbidity

Maternal morbidity associated with cesarean birth is higher than that for vaginal delivery, especially for those women who were in labor before the surgery. The main cause of maternal morbidity is postoperative endometritis. Overall, the risk is 5 to 10 times greater after cesarean than after vaginal birth. Serious infections of the uterus are likely to occur following a long labor with ruptured membranes, numerous vaginal examinations during labor, and postoperative anemia.

Common findings include fever (100° to 104° F), uterine tenderness, purulent or foul lochia, peripheral leukocytosis, and absence of another infection site. Nonspecific signs and symptoms, such as malaise, lower abdominal pain, chills, and tachycardia, are also common.

Treatment consists of parenteral antibiotic therapy that provides good coverage of the numerous microorganisms that reside in the genital tract.

Recovery

It is vital that these new mothers and families understand what to expect in the recovery period. Women who have undergone major abdominal surgery instead of vaginal birth may have a need to "prove" they are good mothers by doing all the chores and giving all baby care. They need to understand the importance of rest, fluids, and adequate diet for recovery. The cesarean mother should refrain from driving for several weeks and from lifting and housework for 6 weeks. It will be a minimum of 6 to 8 weeks before physiological recovery. However, it may take 6 months before a woman who has had a cesarean is fully recovered.

Sexual activity can usually be resumed when the vaginal discharge has stopped, the abdominal incision is healed, and the couple is ready. As with vaginal birth, vaginal lubrication may be inadequate and lubricating jellies or creams will be helpful for comfortable intercourse. The woman's sexual partner may be afraid of hurting her or of rupturing the incisions and should be reassured that there is no danger.

Some parents who have experienced cesarean births have organized groups that provide information and help others understand cesarean births. (See Appendix H.) Also, many childbirth education programs include support groups for postcesarean families.

GRIEF AND MOURNING

Although most hospital postpartum units are happy places filled with congratulating families and friends, loss and grief, as well as death and mourning, do invade the happiness of the unit. For a hospital unit and personnel prepared for birth and life, death can be extremely unwelcome. Maternity personnel often feel a sense of failure, helplessness, and even guilt following a stillbirth or the death of a newborn. To be helpful to the parents experiencing the loss of a baby, the nurse must have a basic understanding of grief and mourning.

Bereavement signifies that someone important to a person has died. It is a fact and signifies a loss.

Grief is how the person feels in response to bereavement. Grief is both physical and emotional distress. Grief is an expression of feelings.

Mourning refers to the culturally patterned expressions of a bereaved person's thoughts and feelings. Mourning is a process. Maternal-infant, paternal-infant, and family-infant attachment begin during pregnancy. With perinatal death, a mother and her family lose the "inside baby" of their hopes and dreams. Instead of having someone they remember to mourn, the family has to mourn someone they have not really known.

According to Dr. Elisabeth Kübler-Ross, it is possible to identify five stages of grief and mourning that people experience in coping with death.

1. Shock with denial ("No, not me.")
2. Anger ("Why me?")
3. Bargaining ("If I . . . .")
4. Depression and anticipatory grief ("How can I?")
5. Acceptance ("I can; I must.")

According to Dr. Kübler-Ross the coping mechanisms that people use to deal with death last for different periods, replace each other, or coexist. It is her conclusion that hope persists through all these stages.

Major manifestations of normal acute grief reactions in the working phase include the following:

1. Somatic distress
2. Preoccupation with the image and memories of the dead person
3. Guilt and self-blame while searching for a cause
4. Irritability, impatience, and social withdrawal
5. Inability to maintain normal patterns of conduct and functioning, with insomnia, overactivity, or restlessness

Parents who have grieved have spoken of feeling pain, guilt, anger, and loneliness. Whether parents weep, sob, or scream when grieving depends on their cultural background. Weeping, wailing, and pounding one's chest may be quite natural in some cultures when experiencing grief, whereas in other cultures quiet crying and even silence may be natural. Although the reactions can be extremely different, everyone has some response to grief. Be alert for the parents who appear inappropriately cheerful and seem to focus on external events having nothing to do with the unfortunate events that would normally cause a grief reaction. It is possible that these parents need intervention to help them deal with the reality of the loss.

Remember, nurses often go through the same stages of grief and mourning that the mother and family do. Be aware of what you feel and identify where you are in the grief process. Do not be afraid to cry. Being human is not being "unprofessional." Once you have come to grips with what you feel, you will be ready to be supportive to the mother and the family. (See box at right.)

Death of an Infant

To lose a baby in death is to grieve over someone that parents never had a chance to know, except in fantasy. In the case of stillbirths and neonatal deaths there is often a need for "closure" (to complete the cycle). To accomplish this many parents request to see, touch, and hold their dead infant. If parents do not ask to touch or hold their baby, it could be that they do not know this is possible. Offer this option to them. However, the choice should be theirs. Parents' fantasies about what the baby looks like can be much worse than reality.

Grief needs to be acknowledged and mourning encouraged. If the mother and family wish to see their baby, prepare them first for what the baby looks like. Give them a verbal description of body temperature, color, and any marks or discolorations on the body. Present the mother with her baby, washed and nicely wrapped in a colorful blanket. It is very helpful to point out to the mother the family characteristics and unique characteristics of her baby. Take the time to listen and encourage the mother and her family to verbalize their feelings.

Wanting to have a dead infant baptized, naming the baby (even a stillborn infant), taking photos, and making arrangements for burial are important steps for many parents as they seek closure. It is often very helpful for these parents to talk with others who have lost a baby. Many communities have support groups for parents who experience perinatal loss. (See Appendix G.) Avoid cliches such as "You can always have another baby," "You're still young," or "Everything always works out for the best." The mother and her family need a demonstration of caring about what has happened in the here and now from the nurse, not unrealistic promises.

How the mother and father resolve their feelings in this time of crisis may very well determine the future of their relationship. They also need anticipatory guidance about the extent of grief they will experience for a long time. Many relationships do not weather a crisis such as the death of a baby, particularly when the grief is unresolved.

Fathers can have a particularly difficult time resolving the death of an infant. Many cultures place a heavy burden on men, requiring them to be "manly" and not to cry. They are frequently expected to maintain family stability during the crisis, while they are in great need

 Recommendation for Managing Grief

For obstetric staffs

1. Develop protocols that include the mothers in the decision making.
2. When a stillbirth occurs or an infant dies, ask the mother if she wants to see the baby. Prepare the body as you would a living baby, and wrap it in a blanket.
3. As a precaution against phantom crying, take a picture of the body, and make it a part of the mother's record so that it can be retrieved if needed for therapeutic intervention.
4. Help fathers understand the mourning process, and urge them to join their wives.
5. Avoid cliches. They are disorienting. Nonverbal concern and assurance are reorienting.
6. When the time is appropriate, encourage the mother and father to join a self-help group.

For husbands and relatives

1. Expect the mother to feel the intensity of the mourning for a much longer period than you do.
2. Join the mother in mourning; don't try to do her mourning for her or prevent her from expressing her sorrow.
3. Include the mother in all plans. If she is too tired, postpone the planning.
4. Do not rush home after the death of the child and remove all signs of babyhood from the nursery. The mother will put away the objects when she is ready.

For mourners

1. Let yourself mourn freely and openly.
2. Let yourself be inconsistent.
3. Don't be afraid of bizarre delusions; they are part of the process of being reoriented.
4. Try to involve yourself within 3 months with a group of women who have had a similar experience of losing a baby.
5. Don't try to become pregnant again until you have finished mourning and you have recovered your strength.
6. Help other people, particularly your husband, understand how you feel and how you are processing your disorientation.
7. If you decide to have another pregnancy, plan new names. Each child deserves to be unique and not be a surrogate of a wished-for child.

From Understanding death of the wished-for child, *OGR Service Corporation.*

of compassionate support themselves. Fathers should be able to share the grief experience without limitations on visiting hours. In fact the most difficult time for a grieving father may be the nighttime hours when he is home alone. He should be encouraged to spend the night with his partner should he need her support—and she his.

Siblings and other family members must also be included in the grief process. Siblings sometimes react to the death of a baby brother or sister with nightmares, depression, withdrawal, and guilt feelings. Some siblings feel they have caused the baby to die by feeling jealousy or resentment about the new baby entering the family.

Parents should be encouraged to remain in an area where nurses are skilled in maternity care and able to help parents experiencing perinatal loss. However, for many women who have lost a baby the adjustment is more difficult if they remain on the maternity unit. If possible offer these women a quiet private room away from happy mothers with their babies. This does not mean that the mother wants to be isolated and alone. The opposite is true; she wants and needs human contact. It is simply that the obvious happy interactions of new mothers and babies may be more than she can handle at this time in the grief process.

It is important to mark the mother's chart and room in some distinctive manner to indicate that loss has occurred, thus avoiding uninformed and sometimes hurtful comments from ancillary staff or hospital volunteers.

Infant with a Birth Defect

When faced with the birth of a baby with a defect, the parents are confronted with the loss of their hopes for a perfect baby, the prospect of coping with a lifelong disability, and chronic grief. These parents also go through the stages of grief and mourning. They can exhibit reactions that can range from extreme guilt leading to overprotection and dedication to extreme intolerance leading to denial of the infant. Chronic grief never goes away; each new crisis renews the grief.

As a nurse you must acknowledge what you feel and then you can help the parents. When helping these parents respond to the infant, point out the positive features about the baby, such as pretty eyes, cute nose, and round arms. You can act as a role model, feeding and changing the baby, touching the baby's defect, and cuddling the baby as you would any baby while encouraging the parents to interact with their infant. Often the parents of a baby with a defect express guilt, self-doubt, and feelings of inadequacy and failure and consequently need much support and positive reinforcement. Encourage them to provide the care for their baby and reassure them about how well they are doing.

In making decisions about the long-term care of the infant, the parents need to have all alternatives presented and possible outcomes explored. The final decision must be theirs and not the decision of a physician, midwife, or nurse. Always remember the baby belongs to the parents and not to the hospital or the health care providers. The parents have a right to make their own decision. It is hoped that their decision will be one that will allow them to function and to cope with their situation. Chronic grief does not have to prevent parents from feeling joy, happiness, satisfaction, and accomplishment.

Genetic counseling is very helpful to parents who want to understand the possibility of having another baby with a defect. The nurse can explain genetic counseling and recommend a referral to a counseling center.

Often in their anxiety when first learning of the defect, the parents do not comprehend the explanations given. They may need more thorough explanations later and photographs or descriptive written explanations. If the defect is one that can be corrected surgically, photographs of other babies before and after surgery can be useful. Realistic plans for long-term care plus referral to public health or home nurses and social workers may be needed.

During the hospital stay it is important to provide privacy for the family. There must be a quiet room where they can be comfortable crying or discussing their personal feelings and worries.

Adoption

Mothers who relinquish their babies also experience grief and mourning for they, too, are experiencing a loss. It is hoped that in prenatal care this mother has received help from the physicians, midwives, nurses, social workers, and her family. If she has had this help, by the time of delivery she may have worked through anticipatory grief and be prepared for the loss. However, prepared or not, the actual event of the birth is a crisis for this mother and her family. She will have to decide how much contact, if any, she wishes with her baby. It is thought that interacting with the baby facilitates the grieving process and may be advisable. Just as in coping with the death of a baby, it is difficult to move past the denial phase if the baby is never real. However, the mother needs advance preparation for how she may feel when holding her baby. Feelings of warmth, tenderness, and love for the baby are natural and to be expected. The mother needs to understand that having these feelings does not mean that she has made the wrong decision. If the baby looks like a family member, the mother may be profoundly affected. She needs supportive, nonjudgmental care to help her express her emotions, and she also needs counseling about any guilt feelings.

After the baby's birth some women who are relinquishing their babies prefer not to be with new mothers and babies who are going home together. However, if this mother moves to another unit in the hospital, she still needs follow-up care from the maternity nurses who cared for her during labor and birth. It is important for her to talk about the labor and birth to resolve the experience and facilitate the grieving process. She will also need help in planning her future: going home empty-handed, anniversary depressions, follow-up care, the baby's future, and her own sexuality and birth control.

A woman who relinquishes her baby for adoption can come out of the experience with self-respect and dignity when she is given respect and sympathetic care.

SUMMARY

In this chapter we have discussed complications in the postpartum period. For many women cesarean birth is not a complication but just another way to give birth; it was included here for those times when cesarean birth follows a complication in labor. A brief look at grief and mourning completed this chapter with a discussion of coping with the death of a newborn, a newborn with a birth defect, and relinquishing a baby. In Chapter 12 you will be introduced to the newborn, a truly marvelous being.

BIBLIOGRAPHY

Arms S: *Adoption: a handful of hope,* Berkeley, Calif, 1990, Celestial Arts.

Bastin JP: Action stat! Postpartum hemorrhage, *Nurs 89* 19(2):33, 1989.

Beckey RD and others: Development of a perinatal grief checklist, *J Obstet Gynecol Neonatal Nurs* 14(3):194-199, 1985.

Bobak IM, Jensen MD, Lowdermilk DL: *Maternity and gynecologic care: the nurse and the family,* ed 5, St. Louis, 1993, Mosby.

Carr D, Knupp SF: Grief and perinatal loss: a community hospital approach to support, *J Obstet Gynecol Neonatal Nurs* 14(2):130-139, 1985.

Ferguson H: Planning letter-perfect postpartum care, *Nurs 87* 17(5):50-51, 1987.

Jackson, PL: When the baby isn't perfect, *Am J Nurs* 85(4):396-399, 1985.

Kübler-Ross E: *On death and dying,* London, 1969, Macmillan.

Lake MF, Knuppel RA, Angel JL: The rationale for supportive care after perinatal death, *J Perinatol* 7(2):85-89, 1987.

Lawrence RA: *Breast feeding: a guide for the medical profession,* ed 4, St. Louis, 1994, Mosby.

Mattson S, Smith JE, editors: *Core curriculum for maternal-newborn nursing,* Philadelphia, 1993, WB Saunders.

Mayberry LJ, Forte AB: Pregnancy-related disseminated intravascular coagulation (DIC), *MCN* 10(3):168-173, 1985.

Miovech SM and others: Major concerns of women after cesarean delivery, *J Obstet Gynecol Neonatal Nurs* 23(1):53-59, 1994.

Reichert JA, Baron M, Fawcett J: Changes in attitudes toward cesarean birth, *J Obstet Gynecol Neonatal Nurs* 22(2):159-167, 1993.

Ryan PF, Côté-Arsenault D, Sugarman LL: Facilitating care after perinatal loss: a comprehensive checklist, *J Obstet Gynecol Neonatal Nurs* 20(5):385-389, 1991.

Sullivan PG: Postpartum complications: coping with the unexpected, *The Female Patient* 11:46-53, 1986.

DEFINITIONS

Define the following terms:

anticoagulants	morbidity
atony	mourning
bereavement	parametritis
closure	partial prothrombin time
cystitis	(PPT)
D&C	peritonitis
disseminated intravascular	placenta accreta
coagulation (DIC)	prothrombin time (PT)
embolism	puerperal infection
endometritis	septicemia
fibrinogen	sibling
grief	somatic
hematoma	subinvolution
hemostasis	thrombin
hypovolemic shock	thrombophlebitis
inversion	thrombus
lacerations	vaginitis
mastitis	vulvitis

LEARNING ACTIVITIES

1. Group discussions.
2. Review postcesarean infection control procedures in your hospital.
3. View audiovisual aids and discuss.

ENRICHMENT/IN-DEPTH STUDY

1. Research DIC and write a summary paper for class discussion.
2. Draw a temperature graph representative of a postpartum infection in a woman who has not received antibiotic therapy.
3. Investigate whether a cesarean birth support group exists in your community. If there is such a group, attend a meeting and share your observations with classmates.
4. Interview parents who were separated from their newborns immediately after birth. What were their feelings?
5. Is there a support group for parents experiencing perinatal death in your community? How often does the group meet? Who leads the group?

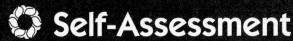
For questions 1 through 6, circle the best answer.

1. If a new mother complains of tenderness and warmth in her leg and has a fever, you would suspect that she may have:
   a. thrombophlebitis
   b. leg cramps
   c. dehydration and stiffness

2. When checking the height of the uterine fundus on the second postpartum day, the fundus should be felt:
   a. at the umbilicus
   b. two fingerwidths below the umbilicus
   c. two fingerwidths above the umbilicus

3. The signs and symptoms of a ruptured uterus include all of the following *except:*
   a. localized abdominal pain and tenderness
   b. a tearing feeling
   c. elevated blood pressure
   d. hypovolemic shock

4. Which of the following are major factors leading to postpartum infection?
   a. prolonged rupture of the membranes
   b. long, difficult labors
   c. hemorrhage
   d. invasive techniques in labor
   e. nothing by mouth during labor
   Answer (circle one):
   1. a and b
   2. a, b, and c
   3. a, b, c, and d
   4. all of above

5. Signs and symptoms of cystitis include:
   a. frequent urination
   b. painful urination
   c. slight temperature elevation
   d. copious amounts of urine
   Answer (circle one):
   1. a and b
   2. all of above
   3. a, b, and c
   4. b

6. If a woman has had an abruptio placentae, the following complication might occur:

   a. DIC

   b. distended bladder

   c. engorged breasts

Supply the correct answer(s) for items 7 through 17.

7. If a breast-feeding mother develops mastitis, will she have to discontinue breast-feeding? Why or why not?

   _____

   _____

   _____

8. Obstetrical complications that may predispose a mother to DIC include the following:

   a. _____

   b. _____

   c. _____

   d. _____

9. If parents must be separated from their infant in the immediate postpartum period because of newborn complications, what can the nurse do to encourage bonding?

   _____

   _____

   _____

10. What kinds of activities are contraindicated for the cesarean mother during her recovery period at home?

   _____

   _____

   _____

11. What are some possible emotional reactions the parents may have following a cesarean birth?

   _____

   _____

   _____

12. According to Dr. Elisabeth Kübler-Ross, it is possible to identify five stages of grief and mourning that people experience when coping with death. These are:

   a. _____

   b. _____

   c. _____

   d. _____

   e. _____

13. Mourning is defined as:

   _____

_____

_____

14. Describe ways in which the nurse can be supportive of a new family whose baby
(1) is dead or (2) has a birth defect.

_____

_____

_____

15. What are the observations you would make when giving nursing care to a new
mother following a cesarean birth?

a. _____

b. _____

c. _____

d. _____

e. _____

f. _____

g. _____

h. _____

i. _____

16. The physician's orders for a new mother with a postpartum infection include bed
rest. How would you position this mother to promote uterine drainage?

_____

_____

_____

Fill in the blanks for questions 17 through 20.

17. The organisms most often responsible for the development of postpartum
infections are _____, _____, and
_____.

18. The cesarean mother usually has _____ lochia than the
woman who experiences a vaginal birth.

19. Early postpartum hemorrhage is defined as blood loss of 500 milliliters or more in
the _____ _____ hours following
delivery.

20. Late postpartum hemorrhage usually occurs _____ to
_____ days following delivery.

For questions 21 through 24, circle the correct answer.

21. What is the _first_ thing to do as a preventative measure if the uterus appears to be
atonic?

a. Have patient put baby on her abdomen.

b. Massage the uterus firmly.

c. Allow baby to nurse.

d. Apply ice to the perineum and abdomen.

22. On the first day after delivery, if the fundus is above the umbilicus and off to one side, the nurse should *first* think of:
    a. a full bladder
    b. poor muscle supports
    c. the presence of clots
    d. retained placental fragments

23. Amy Roberts was home for 8 days after delivery when she began to hemorrhage profusely. The most probable cause of her hemorrhage is:
    a. retained placental parts
    b. subinvolution
    c. uterine atony
    d. excessive activity

24. Which of the following are major factors leading to postpartum infection?
    a. Prolonged rupture of the membranes
    b. Long, difficult labors
    c. Hemorrhage
    d. Nothing by mouth during labor
    Answer (circle one):
    1. a and b
    2. a, b, and c
    3. a, b, c, and d
    4. all of the above

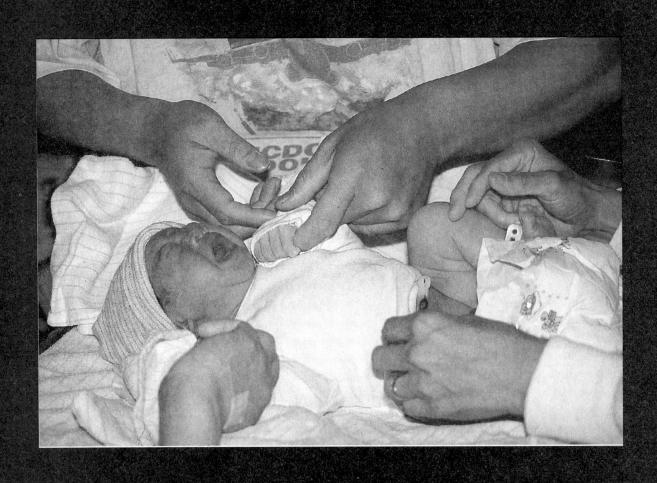

12

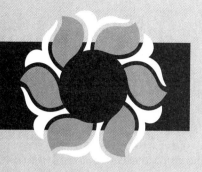

THE NEWBORN

GOALS

This chapter is designed to provide the reader with information that will:
- promote awareness of the newborn's potential for interaction.
- develop a basic understanding of the normal newborn.

STUDENT OBJECTIVES

After studying this chapter, you should be able to:

1. Briefly describe normal behavior of a newborn, emphasizing (a) the four phases of newborn activity in the first 24 hours after birth and (b) the first six "state" cycles.
2. Identify and describe the characteristics of the normal newborn related to the following criteria: average temperature, pulse, and respiration.
3. Define the following terms used when discussing gestational age: (a) AGA, (b) SGA, (c) LGA, (d) preterm, (e) term, and (f) postterm.
4. Describe the physical criteria for determining gestational age (using the clinical form in this book).
5. Demonstrate how to determine gestational age.
6. Identify and describe the characteristics of the normal newborn related to the average measurements for weight, length, chest, and head.

7. Identify and describe the characteristics of the normal newborn related to the following criteria: (a) skin: color, texture; (b) ears: lobe, hearing; (c) face: chin, marks; (d) eyes: color, discharge; (e) nose: smell; (f) mouth: palates; (g) neck: size; (h) breasts: tissue size; (i) chest: breathing; (j) abdomen: shape; (k) cord: condition; (l) genitourinary system (testes or labia); and (m) anus: patency.
8. Describe the following reflexes, their importance, how stimulated, and the approximate time of disappearance: (a) Moro's, (b) rooting, (c) grasp, (d) step, (e) tonic neck, and (f) sucking.
9. Given the following list of common variations in the neonate, (a) define these variations, (b) explain reasons for their occurrence, and (c) state how long they last: caput succedaneum, cephalhematoma, erythema toxicum, "stork bites," milia, subconjunctival hemorrhage, and "epithelial pearls."
10. Discuss the ongoing care of the newborn.

In the United States many normal newborn babies are cared for in a hospital nursery by hospital personnel for the first hours or days of life. Policies concerning length of nursery stay, type of nursery, and infant feeding schedule may differ from hospital to hospital. Some hospitals have a transition or observation nursery where newly born babies are observed closely for the first 6 to 12 hours after birth. When stabilized, and if special care is not required, infants are moved from this transition nursery to traditional nursery care, to rooming-in units, or to mother-baby care. Traditional nursery care may involve a schedule for infant feeding in which the babies are taken to their mothers every 4 hours or "on-demand," in which case the babies are taken to their mothers when hungry. An area of the hospital maternity department may be designated as a rooming-in area where mothers and fathers can keep their babies in their room. Policies for rooming-in can vary from keeping the baby in the mother's room at all times to returning the baby to the nursery whenever the mother wants to sleep.

When a hospital does not have a special nursery set aside for a transition or observation nursery, one particular area of the nursery will usually be designated as the receiving area for newly born babies. This grouping of infants in a nursery according to the type of care they require has been termed *area care*. In area care certain spaces of the nursery are designated for special types of care depending on the needs of the babies. The nursery may be divided into a recovery area, routine observation area, intermediate area, and intensive care area.

In some hospitals there are small, multiple nurseries, housing infants born within a 24 to 48 hour period. In this type of care no new infants are admitted to a nursery until all previous babies are discharged and the nursery has been thoroughly cleaned. This type of care is called a "cohort" system.

In developing family-centered care many hospitals are designing facilities and procedures whereby newborns can be observed closely by nurses without separating the babies from their parents (Fig. 12-1). Close observation and care of the newborn in a room with the parents require nurses skilled in all aspects of maternity care. The nurse who has supported the mother and family through labor and birth may be the same nurse who assesses the newborn and provides necessary care. This is a challenge to nurses who have functioned in only one area (labor and delivery, nursery, or postpartum) for many years. Keeping the baby with the new parents does not negate the fact that the first hours of life are very special transition hours. In fact the parents can be valuable team members contributing to the observation and care of the infant. These parents need to be prepared before the birth for what to expect in the way of normal transition of their newborn.

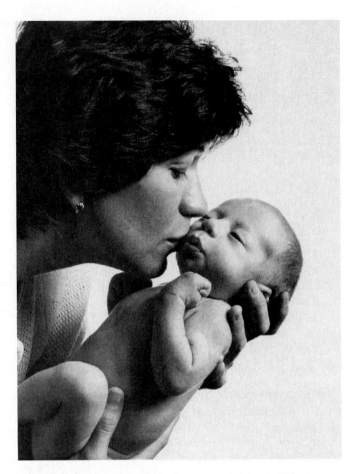

Figure 12-1 Mother and newborn together in the first hours of life. *(Photo courtesy Porter Memorial Hospital, Denver.)*

TRANSITION TO EXTRAUTERINE LIFE

The newborn emerges from a warm, dark, liquid environment to a cool, bright, dry environment filled with noise (Fig. 12-2).

Onset of Breathing

As the fetus passes through the birth canal, its chest is compressed, and approximately one third of the fluid that has filled its lungs in utero is expelled from its mouth. After delivery of the thorax, as the chest cage reexpands air is sucked into the airways. Some childbirth researchers believe that this stimulates the first breath of life. Others believe it is the newborn's reaction to sudden changes in pressure and temperature. Whatever the case may be, the first breath is really a "gasp." The resistant forces of the lung tissue and of the remaining lung fluid are reduced by *surfactant*, a chemical substance within lung air spaces responsible for aiding in lung expansion. Most of the *alveoli* (gas-

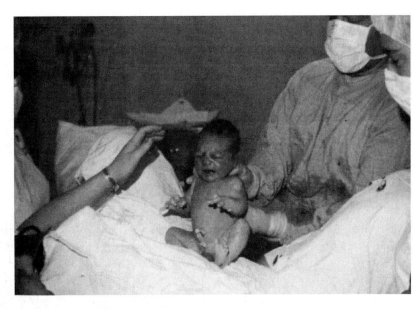

Figure 12-2 Transition to extrauterine life.

	Birth	7 Days of Age	3 Months
Hemoglobin (Hgb) (grams/100 milliliters):			
Average	19.0	17.9	11.3
Range	16.8 to 21.2	53.6 to 68.4	10.4 to 12.2
Hematocrit (Hct)(%):			
Average	61	56	33
Range	53.6 to 68.4	46.6 to 65.4	29.7 to 36.3
Leukocytes:			
Average	18,000	12,000	12,000
Range	9000 to 30,000	5000 to 21,000	6000 to 18,000

exchanging areas of the lung) are expanded within 1 hour after birth. Most lung fluid is removed by absorption and lymphatic drainage within 6 to 12 hours. Thus even with the best delivery the baby will be slightly acidotic immediately after birth but will "blow off" the excess carbon dioxide in 1 to 2 hours.

Closure of Fetal Structures

When the umbilical cord is severed at delivery, closure of the fetal circulatory structures begins. The umbilical arteries and then the umbilical vein contract within a short time after birth. This constriction is initially due to cold temperature and stretching of the umbilical cord but is probably maintained by exposure to rising levels of blood O_2.

The ductus venosus closes within 3 to 7 days after birth, probably passively as a result of reduced blood flow and pressure due to the absence of umbilical vein blood. As the newborn begins to breathe and the blood oxygen levels begin to rise, the lung vessels respond by relaxing their muscular walls and allowing an increase in pulmonary blood flow. More blood flows through the lungs to the pulmonary veins and thus to the left atrium. Left atrial pressure increases as right atrial pressure decreases (because of decreased blood return from the loss of umbilical venous flow), and thus a valvelike fold of tissue snaps shut over the foramen ovale. This tissue fuses with the wall between the atria within 6 to 8 weeks. In many infants the foramen ovale closes incompletely and a small amount of blood is shunted between atria for 1 to 2 months. The ductus arteriosus closes usually within 10 to 15 hours, probably as a reaction to increasing blood oxygen tension and prostaglandin interactions.

Laboratory Values

Normal laboratory values for blood for a term infant are given in the box above. The normal fall in total hemoglobin and hematocrit values, the so-called "physiological anemia of the newborn," is usually fully

Bilirubin (milligrams per 100 milliliters [deciliters])	Age	Normal Range
	Cord	Less than 2 milligrams per deciliter
	0 to 1 day	Less than 6 milligrams per deciliter
	3 to 5 days	Less than 12 milligrams per deciliter
	After 5 days	Less than 1 milligram per deciliter

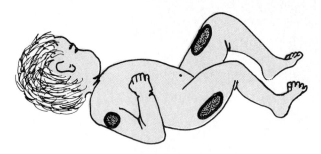

Figure 12-3 Newborn injection sites.

corrected by the age of 6 months, as the infant begins to produce more and more red blood cells.

Gastrointestinal Function

The digestive system and the kidneys begin to function immediately after birth. In the uterus the fetus drank amniotic fluid and urinated normally but did not have a bowel movement.

The newborn's immature liver and gastrointestinal system sometimes cannot provide adequate amounts of vitamin K because their formation is dependent on the presence of bacteria in the intestine. At birth the stomach and bowel contents are sterile and neutral in pH. Vitamin K aids in the formation of prothrombin, which is necessary for blood coagulation. The Committee on Nutrition of the Academy of Pediatrics recommends the administration of 0.5 to 1.0 milligrams of parenteral vitamin K oxide (phytonadione) within 1 hour after birth. In many hospitals vitamin K is given to most newborns intramuscularly in the anterior lateral aspect of the thigh shortly after birth (Fig. 12-3). When the newborn begins to ingest food, normal bacteria will grow in the intestinal tract, and vitamin K will be manufactured by the second week of life.

Jaundice

The number of red blood cells decreases during the first week after birth. Cell breakdown occurs in the spleen and liver; hemoglobin is converted in the liver to bilirubin. Bilirubin is eliminated through the gastrointestinal tract. If the immature liver cannot eliminate all the bilirubin, it will be reabsorbed into the circulation as unmetabolized bilirubin (indirect, unconjugated

bilirubin). This usually happens after the second day of life, and the infant appears jaundiced. This jaundice is known as physiological jaundice *(icterus neonatorum)*. Any jaundice during the first 24 hours of life should be recorded and reported promptly because it is probably not normal physiological jaundice. Normal bilirubin ranges are listed in the box above.

CAPABILITIES OF THE NEWBORN

The newborn has amazing capabilities. The newborn is a socially responsive human being who can probably learn better on the first day of life than ever again. A baby, immediately after birth, will stare intently at the parents' faces and see them. In fact newborns prefer looking at the mother's face, especially the eyes, rather than at other objects. Other capabilities of the newborn include the ability to recognize an approaching object as a threat and to turn away to avoid it and the ability to reach for an object and usually come close to touching it. The newborn also seems to realize that he or she is a human being and will imitate another person's facial expressions such as sticking out the tongue, opening the mouth, and pursing the lips. Newborn babies are active stimulus seekers where repetition and the level of stimulation are important. The baby is actually capable of shutting out stimuli and can even learn to respond by turning its head at the sound of a bell.

Babies are not passive and unresponsive creatures to be hurried off to the hospital nursery after birth. The affectionate bond between mother and child and between father and child begins at the moment of birth (Fig. 12-4). As long as the newborn is responding normally, immediate skin-to-skin contact with the parents is very important in bonding. The newborn will have difficulty opening his or her eyes under bright spotlights but will look around if the lights are dimmed. (It is possible to dim the main lights in the delivery area and still have light focused over the perineum for episiotomy repair or other necessary procedures). Also, shielding the infant's face with one's hands or a blanket will provide enough protection from the light to encourage the baby to open his or her eyes. Objects are in clearest range for the newborn at about 8 to 12 inches. Newborns prefer faces over other patterns. Refraining from using prophylactic eyedrops and weighing and measuring the

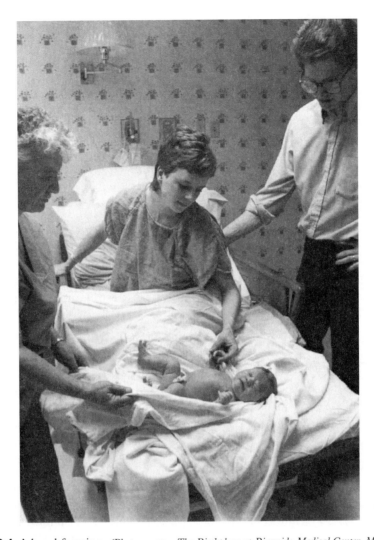

Figure 12-4 A bond forming. *(Photo courtesy The Birthplace at Riverside Medical Center, Minneapolis.)*

baby for 30 minutes to 1 hour after birth will allow the parents time alone with their baby so that the attachment process can proceed without interruption.

The mother may wish to breast-feed in the first hour after birth; the nurse or the father can assist her.

NEWBORN BEHAVIOR

Newborns experience *phases of activity* as they adjust to life outside the uterus. These phases can be measured in time spans as follows:

First reactive phase From birth to 30 minutes of life. In this phase the newborn is alert and responsive to stimuli, searching and inquiring about the new world. Respirations are 60 to 90 per minute; heart rate is 180 beats or more per minute.

Sleep phase From 30 to 60 minutes to 2 hours of life. During this phase the newborn goes into a deep sleep and may secrete large amounts of mucus from the mouth. The infant may also pass a meconium stool. (During this phase it is not unusual for the infant to have periods of apnea.) Heart rate declines to 120 to 140 beats per minute. Respiratory rate declines.

Second reactive phase From 2 to 6 hours of life. During this phase the newborn is again awake and alert. The baby may still be secreting mucus. Body temperature should be normal. Rapid color changes may occur. Heart rate will be labile with wide swings from bradycardia to tachycardia.

Stability phase From 6 to 24 hours of life. During this phase the newborn is successfully making the adjustment to the extrauterine world. The newborn's vital signs should be stable now and color normal. Following this stability phase the newborn sleeps from 18 to 20 hours a day for the first few weeks.

There will be variations in these phases from baby to baby according to the difficulty of the labor and birth and the amount and types of analgesia or anesthesia the mother received.

Crying

The newborn operates with an urgent sense of "now" and is not able to delay physiological needs. Crying is the beginning of vocalization. The most common causes of crying are (1) fatigue, (2) hunger, (3) loneliness, (4) colic pain, and (5) irritability. A normal cry is loud and gusty and neither high pitched nor weak. It is important for a baby to be fed when hungry and not be kept waiting because of an arbitrary feeding schedule. Contrary to the myth that picking up a crying newborn "spoils" the baby, consistent response to the baby's cries for help establishes trust in the caretakers. Research indicates that babies whose mothers responded promptly to their crying cried less when they were a year old. The babies who were allowed to cry for a while (15 to 20 minutes) were likely to be the "crybabies" at 1 year of age. This research would indicate that it is best to respond consistently to a newborn's cry and attempt to meet his or her needs. Responding to the baby's cry helps to establish trust. Most authorities agree that it is impossible to "spoil" a baby by too much rocking or holding during the first few months of life. However, even when responding consistently and meeting the baby's physical and emotional needs, there will still be times when the baby will cry and fret for no apparent reason. When all attempts at comfort no longer work, the baby may just have to cry.

State Cycles

Each baby also has an individual pattern of reactivity in which separate states of awareness can be identified. These are:

Quiet sleep state Respirations are slow and regular, and the infant rarely moves.

REM sleep state Rapid eye movements can be seen through the eyelids. Respirations are irregular and grimaces and other facial expressions are frequent.

Active alert state There is diffuse motor activity involving the whole body. The face may be relaxed or in a cry expression.

Quiet alert state The infant is alert and relaxed, and the eyes are open wide and focusing. It is in this state that the infant is most apt to mimic facial expressions.

Crying state Vigorous diffuse motor activity accompanies crying.

Transitional state In this state the infant may be between any of the preceding states (moving from one to the other).

It is important for the new parents to know about these phases and states of awareness so that they can understand their own babies. Each baby is a separate individual and responds in a unique way. Parents are usually fascinated to learn this because they may have grown up with the myths that babies cannot see or smile

or react to stimuli. Meaningful interaction between infants and parents helps to facilitate bonding.

At the first contact with the newborn after birth, the nurse can reassure the parents that the baby can and wants to see them.

IMMEDIATE NEEDS

Establishing and maintaining an open airway for unobstructed breathing and maintaining a normal body temperature are immediate needs of the newborn. Apgar scoring at 1 and 5 minutes is essential, as is identification of the newborn before leaving the delivery area. (See Chapter 8.) Initial physical and gestational age assessments are vital to recognizing any problems immediately. If the parents are holding the baby, the nurse can make these initial observations without disturbing the parent-infant interaction.

Normal Transition: Respiration

Spontaneous respirations should begin within a few seconds to 1 minute after birth. For most babies gentle aspiration of mucus with a bulb syringe and the help of gravity with the baby in a head-down position are all that is necessary to facilitate respirations.

If the infant does not breathe at birth, the stimulation of a nasal suction catheter or a few breaths of positive pressure by oxygen mask will usually initiate spontaneous respiration. In the severely depressed newborn, resuscitation may be necessary. (See Chapter 13.) For the average baby, holding the baby upside down by the feet and "spanking" on the back are not necessary. Tactile stimuli should be gentle.

Dr. Frederick LeBoyer added an interesting dimension to the childbirth experience with his book, *Birth Without Violence*. In this book he emphasized the "humanness" of the newborn and advocated that this new person be handled with sensitivity and gentleness. The transition from womb to world is indeed harsh, and gentleness is something we can add to that experience.

Heat Production and Heat Loss

A *neutral thermal environment* is one in which an infant's metabolic rate and oxygen consumption are minimal and body temperature remains within normal limits. A newborn of average size maintains a body temperature between 36.5° and 37.0° C (97.7° and 99.0° F) with a minimum use of energy. Neutral thermal range is very narrow for a naked infant.

Adults produce heat by voluntary muscle activity, such as shivering, but newborns do not. Newborns produce heat by chemical or nonshivering thermogenesis. In chemical thermogenesis norepinephrine is released, which initiates a chemical reaction in the brown fat stores of the infant. From 2% to 6% of the body weight of full-term babies consists of brown fat, which is a type of adipose tissue capable of unusual thermogenic activity. This brown fat is found between the scapulas, around muscles and blood vessels in the neck, behind the sternum, and around the kidneys and adrenals. The brown fat contains triglycerides, which break down and oxidize to produce heat. Thermogenesis through this means is limited and requires energy expenditures on the part of the newborn, thus causing an increase in oxygen consumption.

Cold stress

If the baby is unable to meet oxygen needs from room air, it may be necessary to convert to anaerobic metabolism and thus cause an increase in lactic acid production. Metabolic acidosis can then develop. Another consequence of a baby being cold (neonatal cold stress) may be weight loss or failure to gain weight because of increased metabolic consumption of calories. Also, the increased glucose consumption may lead to hypoglycemia.

Whereas *nonshivering thermogenesis* is the principal means of heat production in the newborn, vasoconstriction is the principal means of heat retention. If the mother has been treated with magnesium sulfate for preeclampsia or eclampsia, the baby's vasoconstrictive mechanisms may not be functioning well. Vasoconstriction is not a significant means of heat conservation for the newborn because of the limited supply of subcutaneous fat and large surface area in relation to body mass.

Premature and low-birth-weight babies have less body fat than term infants and consequently are at much greater risk for cold stress. Because of all the problems cold stress may cause, it is important to keep the newborn warm and to provide a neutral thermal environment as quickly as possible after birth.

Prevention of heat loss

To provide this neutral thermal environment, it is important to understand the four major mechanisms by which heat is transferred between the neonate and the environment. Body heat is lost from the skin surface chiefly by (1) radiation, (2) evaporation, (3) convection, and (4) conduction. Loss by *radiation* occurs when heat transfers from the body surface to cooler surfaces or surrounding objects not in contact with infant; that is, incubator wall, room wall, and windows cooled by air conditioners. To minimize heat loss by radiation, bassinets, radiant warmers, and incubators should not be placed near cold outside walls and windows. A plastic

heat shield can be placed in the incubator or Isolette or a double-walled Isolette can be used.

Evaporative heat loss occurs when moisture evaporates from wet skin in a relatively dry atmosphere. A baby wet with amniotic fluid in an air-conditioned room loses body heat rapidly. To minimize heat loss by evaporation, the baby should be dried immediately after delivery with a warm blanket; it is especially important to dry and cover the baby's head. The baby is then wrapped in a second warm, dry blanket before being handed to the parents. If it is necessary to place the baby in an incubator, it should be prewarmed. Any oxygen as well as any solution applied to the infant's skin should be warmed also. The baby should not be bathed until stable and the axillary temperature is 98° F.

Heat loss by *convection* is enhanced by surrounding air currents, cold oxygen, and cold air blown by air conditioners. To prevent convective heat loss, the temperature in rooms where babies are born and in nurseries should be adequate and drafts avoided. Also oxygen should be warmed before administration.

Heat loss by *conduction* occurs by transfer of heat from a warm object to a cooler object by direct contact. To minimize heat loss by conduction, a warm blanket is placed between the infant's body and the cold surface of a scale, x-ray table, or other object. Warming devices (Isolettes, incubators, and open warmers) are warmed before the infant is placed inside.

There is also evidence that babies can be overprotected and kept too warm (hyperthermia) so that they have to increase their metabolic work to cool down. This could also lead to hypoglycemia. Careful regulation of incubator temperatures, not overdressing, and not placing infants too near sunshine or heating ducts will minimize the risk of hyperthermia.

It is possible, simply by minimizing or eliminating heat loss, to keep the average well newborn warm without placing the baby in a heated bed or incubator. Research has shown that term newborns who were thoroughly dried and covered with warm, dry blankets can be held by their mothers after birth without significant temperature loss.

Warming equipment

If for some reason the baby needs resuscitation or other medical attention, it will be necessary to place the baby in a warm servo-control incubator or radiant warmer. Overhead radiant warmers use the principle of radiation. These warmers may have automatic or manual control or both. Infants under manually controlled radiant warmers should be observed continually because it is possible to overheat an infant in a short time if the unit is on full-powered output; however, the low-powered output may be insufficient to warm a cold

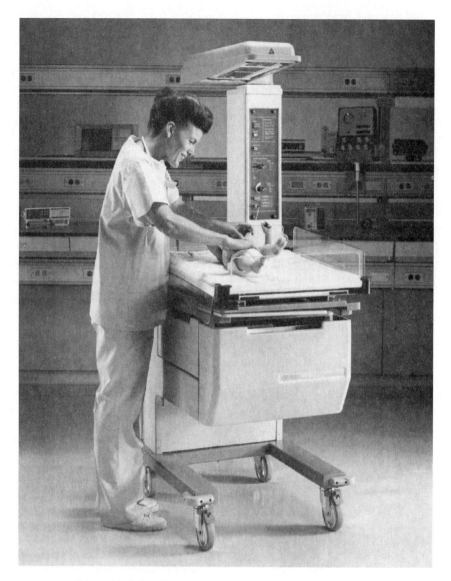

Figure 12-5 Stabilette. *(Photo courtesy Hill-Rom, Batesville, Ind.)*

baby. With an automatic warmer a thermistor (probe) is attached to the infant's abdominal skin to sense the baby's skin temperature (Fig. 12-5). If the baby's skin temperature goes below or above set points, more or less heat will be produced by the warmer and warning systems will be activated. These warning systems may be auditory and/or visual. When using a probe the nurse must be sure that it remains attached to the baby's skin; if it becomes detached, the warmer may continue to heat the baby. Because radiant heat can cause significant water loss, an infant who remains under a radiant warmer more than a few hours will need increased fluid intake. Overhead radiant warmers are valuable because they provide direct and free access to an infant. However, the nurse must remember that a baby under a radiant warmer needs close observation and frequent axillary temperature checks (every 30 minutes) with a thermometer. Because temperature probes can become defective and inaccurate, the nurse should not rely on the skin probe temperature readout alone.

Prewarmed incubators can maintain the baby's temperature very well; however, they do limit access to the baby. Heat is lost whenever the incubator doors or portholes are opened, and radiant heat loss to incubator walls is a potential problem (Fig. 12-6).

NEWBORN INFANT ASSESSMENT

Within a few minutes after birth, careful observation of the infant for obvious anomalies is important. The infant should be observed carefully for general appearance. The infant's *muscle* tone should be firm and strong, *skin* smooth, and *posture* flexed with symmetrical movements of all extremities. The *cry* should be

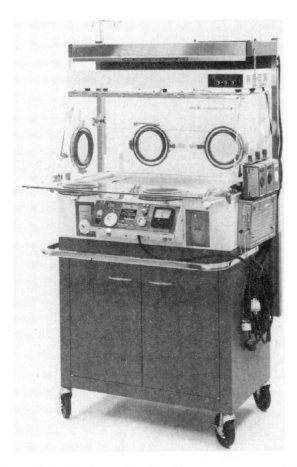

Figure 12-6 Ohio Servo-Care Incubator. *(Courtesy Ohio Medical Products, Madison, Wis.)*

strong and vigorous. The *Moro's reflex* should be elicited easily, and the white newborn's color should be pink or red. Cyanotic hands and feet are common and, in fact, are a healthy response to extrauterine life. The mucosal lining of the mouth of a black baby should be pink or red.

Vital Signs

Vital signs should be checked and recorded. Initial temperature should be taken rectally to check on patency of the anus. After the first temperature, axillary temperature is the most noninvasive way to take a temperature. A temperature range from 97.7° to 99.0° F (36.5° to 37.0° C) (axillary) is within the normal range. The respiratory rate and pattern will often range from 40 to 70 or more in the first hour or so. Most important is noting signs of difficulty: retractions, grunting, flaring of nares, and generalized cyanosis. Any of these signs should be reported to the physician. The preceding vital signs should be checked at least every hour for the first 3 hours or longer if necessary. Initial voiding and meconium should be noted and recorded.

Gestational Age Assessment

Because complications of the neonatal period vary greatly with maturity, an estimate should be made of the infant's maturity. These findings fall into three major categories: (1) *preterm*—before 38 weeks of gestation; (2) *term*—38 to 42 weeks of gestation; and (3) *postterm*—more than 42 weeks of gestation. Within these categories the baby can be classified as AGA (appropriate for gestational age), LGA (large for gestational age), or SGA (small for gestational age). An accurate gestational age assessment helps to differentiate the premature from the small-for-gestational-age baby and the term from the preterm large-for-gestational-age baby. Gestational age can be determined after birth by physical characteristics, neurological examination, and plotting of length, weight, and head circumference on appropriate growth charts.

The physical signs checked are vernix, lanugo, abdominal skin, ear pinna, breast tissue, plantar creases on the feet, and male and female genitalia. The neuromuscular system is checked by estimating the maturity of the following: (1) posture, (2) square window (wrist or ankle), (3) arm recoil, (4) popliteal angle, (5) scarf sign, and (6) heel to ear. Scores are obtained for both physical and neurological examinations conducted within minutes to an hour after birth. A score of 40 indicates a gestational age of 40 weeks. A score of 30 indicates a gestational age of 36 weeks (Fig. 12-7).

The baby's weight, length, and head circumference are measured and charted on the growth charts according to gestational age by examination. The baby's measurements can then be compared with the norms of the chart. Babies whose weight, length, and head circumference fall between the tenth and ninetieth percentiles are classified as appropriate for the gestational age. Those above the ninetieth percentile are classified LGA, and those below the tenth percentile are classified SGA (Fig. 12-7). Babies who are AGA have a better chance for survival than those who are small or large for gestational age. Classification of infants by birth weight and gestational age allows the identification of general risks of a group of infants who would benefit from admission to a special care nursery. The special problems of infants who are large or small for gestational age will be discussed in Chapter 13.

Physical Examination

After the initial observation of the newborn and a quick assessment of gestational age, the parents can safely have their time alone with the newborn. Within the first 2 hours after birth the newborn is either transferred to a nursery or remains in the mother's room (depending on hospital protocols). A physical examination by the nurse at this time is important to detect any ab-

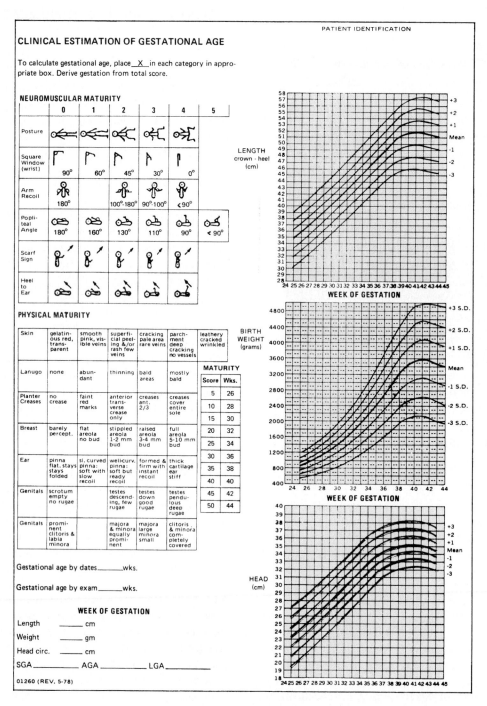

Figure 12-7 Clinical estimation of gestational age. *(Courtesy Ross Laboratories, Columbus, Ohio, Rev May 1978.)*

normalities missed in the initial general observations. This examination does not replace but complements the physician's physical examination. The examination should be done while keeping the infant warm and with adequate lighting. It is preferable to do this initial infant examination at the mother's bedside so that she may learn about her baby's uniqueness. The nurse talks out loud while examining the baby and teaches.

Characteristics of a normal neonate

If the infant is AGA, the nurse should expect to find the following.

Weight. The weight is 2500 to 4000 grams (5 pounds 8 ounces to 8 pounds 13 ounces). Males are slightly heavier than females.

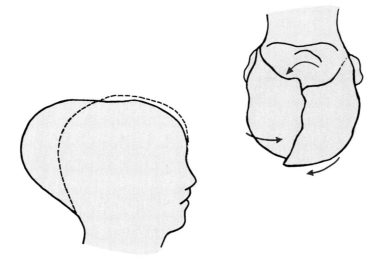

Figure 12-8 Molding. *(From Hamilton MP:* Basic maternity nursing, *ed 6, St. Louis, 1989, Mosby.)*

Length. The average length from head to heel is 20 inches. Eighteen to 21 inches (45.0 to 52.5 centimeters) is a normal range.*

Head circumference. The head circumference is 13 to 14 inches (33.0 to 35.5 centimeters).

Chest circumference. The chest circumference (30.5 to 33.0 centimeters or 12 to 13 inches) is normally about 2 centimeters less than head circumference.

Temperature. The rectal or axillary temperature is 36.5° to 37.0° C (97.7° to 99.0° F).

Respirations. Respirations are regular to irregular, abdominally and synchronously 30 to 60 breaths per minute, with an average of 40. Respirations vary according to the baby's activity. It is normal for newborns to have apneic spells lasting 5 to 10 seconds during sleep.

Pulse. The pulse is 120 to 160 beats per minute, varying according to the baby's activity. For a sleeping baby a heart rate of 80 to 90 beats per minute may be normal. The heart rate is determined using a stethoscope and listening to the apical beat.

Blood pressure. The average blood pressure at birth is 75/42 to 80/46 mm Hg. It should be measured with a one-inch cuff. Although not taken routinely, infant blood pressures are taken on infants in distress and in premature infants.

Head. The head is larger in proportion to the rest of the body and is approximately one third its adult size.

*These measurements are based on white infants in the United States.

In fact the infant's head at birth is one quarter the total length of the body.

The bones of the head are joined together by narrow spaces called *sutures.* Because these bones have not grown together they can overlap, and thus the head can mold to the birth canal. If molding has occurred during labor and birth, the head may be elongated instead of round. This molding will be gone within a few days after birth (Fig. 12-8).

In contrast, the *caput succedaneum* (often called simply the *caput*) is somewhat more firm and ill defined in outline, representing edema of the scalp. This edema, congestion, and petechiae on the scalp (presenting part) crosses the suture lines. It pits on pressure and subsides within 24 to 48 hours after birth (Fig. 12-9, *A*).

A *cephalhematoma* may be present after several hours. This subperiosteal hemorrhage results from trauma during delivery. It will be a localized swelling limited to the boundaries of one cranial bone and may enlarge during the first 2 to 3 days. The cephalhematoma will be absorbed within 6 weeks (Fig. 12-9, *B*) but can cause a rapid increase in the level of bilirubin in the first hours of life as the blood is reabsorbed and excreted.

The *anterior fontanel* is diamond shaped and located between the parietal and frontal bones. Opened 4 to 6 centimeters, it closes by 18 months of age; it feels flat and soft.

The *posterior fontanel* is triangular shaped, located between the parietal and occipital bones, and opened 0.5 to 1.0 centimeter or closed (closes by 3 months of age); it feels flat and soft.

A sunken fontanel may indicate dehydration or decreased intracranial pressure; a bulging fontanel may indicate increased intracranial pressure. A fontanel may bulge slightly while the infant cries or strains. This is

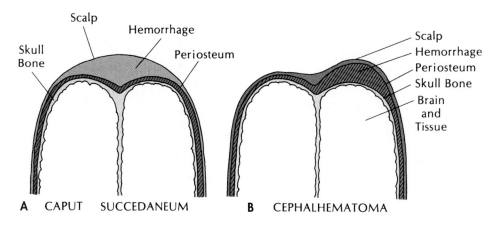

Figure 12-9 A, Caput succedaneum. **B,** A cephalhematoma.

normal. However, if bulging persists when the infant is comforted and stops crying, it should be reported. Washing an infant's head and rubbing the fontanels are not harmful.

Skin. In the full-term baby at birth, *vernix caseosa* (a whitish, cheesy, protective material) may be found in the axilla and groin only. This may be washed off or allowed to remain until it is absorbed or dries and flakes off. The baby's skin is thin, delicate, and velvety smooth and veins may be seen through it. The skin of most babies appears reddish for 6 hours after birth and gradually fades over the next 24 hours. This reddish color is due to the excessive amount of hemoglobin needed to transport oxygen during fetal life. It is normal for a baby's hands and feet to be slightly blue because of poor peripheral perfusion (acrocyanosis). Generalized cyanosis is abnormal.

The infant may have fine downy hair *(lanugo)* on the shoulders, ears, and forehead. Lanugo is more common on preterm infants or dark-haired babies.

A newborn may have a transient, maculopapular rash that appears like wheals surrounded by erythema *(erythema toxicum)*. This is noncontagious and needs no treatment. Small hemangiomas, *"stork bites,"* are common on the eyelids and back of the neck and disappear in 6 to 12 months.

Ears. Earlobes of a full-term baby are stiffened by thick cartilage and tend to stand out slightly from the head. The baby should respond to sounds. Malformation or misplacement of the ears may indicate an abnormality.

Face. The forehead appears to bulge, and the chin appears to recede. There may be tiny white spots called *milia* (which look like "whiteheads") across the baby's nose and forehead. Red marks may appear on the cheeks in front of the ears if forceps were used in deliv-

ery. They will disappear without treatment. Any breaks in the skin should be recorded and reported. The face should be symmetrical (eye creases equal).

Eyes. The structure is normal, although the baby's eyelids may be swollen for 1 to 2 days if silver nitrate has been used for eye care. If pus is present the physician should be notified. The tear ducts may not secrete tears for 2 to 4 weeks. Most newborns have bluish-gray eyes at birth. Permanent eye color is not present until 3 months of age. Subconjunctival hemorrhages may be present. They are caused by pressure during delivery and will disappear within a few weeks. The newborn baby can see, track a moving object, discriminate patterns, and focus on objects at a distance of about 18 inches.

Nose. The newborn breathes through the nose rather than the mouth. There is evidence that the baby can smell breast milk. Drainage from the nose may indicate infection.

Mouth. The mouth should be pink, and the tongue should move freely at the frenulum and should not protrude. The baby should be able to suck strongly. The hard and soft palates should be intact. Large white spots or plaques on the tongue or mucosa of the mouth may indicate *thrush* (a yeastlike fungus infection) and should be reported to the physician. Thrush is not to be confused with the normal "epithelial pearls" (also called Epstein's pearls), which appear in the mouth on the hard palate or gums. These "pearls" are small, white, ricelike epidermal plaques. The newborn's sense of taste is more developed than the sense of sight or hearing. A newborn will react to a sweet taste with a contented sucking.

Neck. The baby's neck is short, weak, and can be flexed. The head seems to settle on the shoulders.

Breasts. In both girls and boys mammary glands may appear swollen because of absorption of hormones from the mother before delivery. This swelling should subside in 2 weeks. The breast tissue should be 1 centimeter or more in diameter.

Chest. The chest is smaller than the head by as much as 2 centimeters and wider than it is long. Movement of the chest and abdomen should be synchronized. Some abnormal respirations and abdominal breathing are normal; however, retractions, grunting, and nasal flaring may indicate respiratory distress. The clavicles should be checked to be sure they are intact and not fractured.

Abdomen. The abdomen appears rounded and large in relation to hips and pelvis. The abdomen should usually move with breathing. Bowel sounds should be present a few hours after delivery.

Umbilicus. There should be two arteries and one vein. The cord is whitish and soft immediately after birth and begins drying until it dries and falls off in 7 to 10 days. Alcohol can be applied three to four times a day to facilitate drying the cord. The diaper should be kept below the umbilicus to expose it to air. Sponge baths should not be given until the cord falls off and the navel has healed. Any drainage or inflammation around the cord may indicate infection and should be noted and reported.

Genitourinary system. Genitals of both sexes will seem large. In the female the labia minora and clitoris are more developed than the labia majora. In the male both testes should be palpable in the scrotum. In the female white caseous discharge, sometimes blood tinged, is normal. This slight, bloody vaginal discharge for 2 to 3 days after birth is the result of hormone action on the lining of the uterus before birth. It will not recur.

Passage of urine may not be noticed for 24 hours because the infant usually urinates at birth. Occasionally the urine appears reddish-tan or "bloody" on the diaper until feeding is well established. This is caused by presence of uric acid crystals and is harmless.

The urethral meatus in the male should be easily visualized at the tip of the penis. The foreskin of the penis may be adherent to the glans.

Anus and bowels. The anus should be open. The infant passes meconium within 24 to 48 hours. The initial meconium stool is dark greenish-black, tarry, and odorless.

The infant may have only one *transitional stool*, beginning with meconium and ending with yellow stool, or

the infant may pass greenish-yellowish material two or three times.

The stools of a breast-fed infant are usually very loose at first, golden yellow, with only a faint sour odor. In 5 to 7 days stools of a breast-fed infant may become pasty and soft but still remain almost odorless. Breast-fed babies may have a stool with every feeding for many weeks. However, breast-fed babies may not have stools for several days.

The stools of formula-fed infants are a paler yellow, are semiformed or contain curds, and have a foul odor. The infant may pass four to six stools a day during the first week or two; following this, the number of stools gradually decreases. Greenish, watery, foamy, mucous, or bloody stools are abnormal and should be reported.

Extremities. The newborn's legs are shorter than the arms at birth. Both arms and legs are flexed when the baby is quiet. Hips are checked by abducting the thighs to the bed and rotating the hips through full range of motion. If a thigh cannot be readily abducted to touch the bed, the hip may be dislocated. When the infant is lying on the abdomen, the buttocks and leg crease should be equal and symmetrical. When the thigh is moved downward and inward with the index finger on the hip, a "click" may also indicate dislocation. In a prone position a preterm infant lies in a "frog" position, whereas a term infant lies with legs flexed (Fig. 12-10).

Mongolian spots (darkened pigmented areas) may be present on the buttocks or lower back. These are most commonly found on dark-complexioned babies and appear like bruises. They will disappear by the time the baby is 3 years old.

Neurological assessment. Numerous reflex reactions can be obtained on examination of the newborn. A crying infant will not provide accurate responses.

The *grasp reflex* is present and strong. The infant will tightly grasp an object placed in its hand. The grasp reflex usually disappears by the age of 3 months.

The *rooting reflex* is present and can be stimulated by gently stroking or touching one of the infant's cheeks. The infant will turn toward the touch with open mouth. This reflex is useful when helping a new mother and infant to breast-feed (Fig. 12-11).

The *sucking reflex* is present, and the infant will suck any object placed in the mouth. The sucking reflex is usually accompanied by the swallowing and gag reflexes, which persist throughout life.

The *step reflex* (Fig. 12-12) is present and can be elicited by holding the infant upright with the feet barely touching a hard surface. The infant will alternate feet as though walking. This step reflex usually disappears by 4 weeks.

The *Moro's reflex* ("startle" reflex) can be elicited by

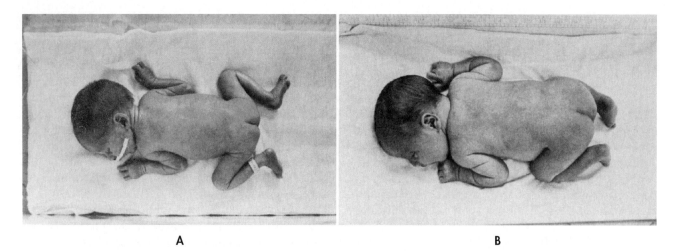

Figure 12-10 Prone position. **A,** Preterm infant lies in a "frog" position. **B,** Term infant lies with legs flexed. *(Courtesy Mead-Johnson Laboratories, Evansville, Ind.)*

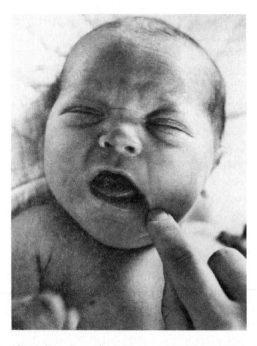

Figure 12-11 Rooting reflex. *(Courtesy Mead-Johnson Laboratories, Evansville, Ind.)*

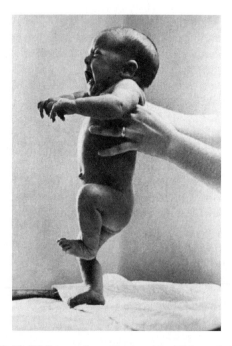

Figure 12-12 Walking reflex. *(Courtesy Mead-Johnson Laboratories, Evansville, Ind.)*

making a sudden, loud noise or a sudden motion. In response the infant throws both arms outward, then brings them together in quivering, embracing movement. The Moro's reflex disappears by the age of 3 to 4 months (Fig. 12-13). The absence of a Moro's reflex usually indicates abnormality.

The *tonic neck reflex* (Fig. 12-14) is a position that most infants usually assume for sleeping. The infant's head turns to one side, and the arm on that side extends while the opposite arm flexes. This resembles a fencing position. The tonic neck reflex disappears at 6 or 7 months of age.

Reflexes vary from baby to baby and also in the same

baby at different times. For instance, immediately after feeding the rooting and sucking reflexes may not be easy to elicit. Absent or poor reflexes should be reported immediately. The persistence of a primitive reflex after the first year or so of life may indicate a neurological problem.

Observation of the infant's behavior is very important in an evaluation of the nervous system. Limpness, poor muscle tone, and decreased activity suggest central nervous system disturbance.

Back. When the infant is turned over on the abdomen and held in the palm of the hand, the back will

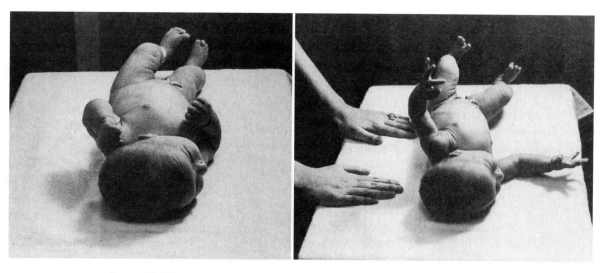

Figure 12-13 Moro's reflex. *(Courtesy Mead-Johnson Laboratories, Evansville, Ind.)*

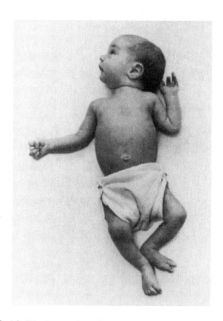

Figure 12-14 Tonic neck reflex. *(Courtesy Mead-Johnson Laboratories, Evansville, Ind.)*

flex slightly. A deep dimple and palpable spinal bone defect should be reported immediately. The spine should be straight and vertebrae symmetrical.

Careful documentation of all the preceding observations is very important to give a baseline for continuing care of the infant. Continued daily observations are also very important. Daily observations should include vital signs, weight (evaluated according to birth weight), color and activity, feeding status, elimination, parent-infant interaction, and health education needs of the parents. If anything abnormal is observed, it should be recorded and reported immediately.

INFANT CARE

Because the baby's temperature-regulating mechanisms will not be functioning for at least a few days after birth, heat conservation is important. The baby's room or nursery temperature should be kept at approximately 75.0° F (24.0° C) with humidity at 50%; the room should be kept free from drafts. Newborns' temperature readings can be taken rectally, axillarily (in the armpit), or tympanically (in the ear). Although the baby's initial temperature is taken rectally to check for a patent anus, subsequent temperatures should be taken in the axilla or the ear to eliminate the danger of irritating or perforating the rectum.

Skin Care

The policies and procedures for bathing a newborn vary greatly. Nursing care of the newborn skin sometimes includes a technique recommended by the American Academy of Pediatrics and referred to as dry skin care. The reasons for this technique may include: (1) the infant is subjected to less heat loss by exposure; (2) skin trauma is diminished; (3) less time is required; and (4) it does not expose the infant to agents with known or unknown side effects. The "dry technique" consists of the following points. (1) Cleansing of the newly born infant should be delayed until the infant's temperature has stabilized after the cold stress of delivery. (2) Only the face, head, and infant's body folds should be cleansed with cotton sponges moistened with sterile water. (3) The remainder of the skin should be untouched unless grossly soiled. There is evidence to indicate that vernix caseosa may serve a protective function, some evidence to indicate it has no effect, and no evidence to indicate it is harmful. (4) For the remainder of the infant's stay in the hospital, the buttocks and peri-anal regions should be cleansed with sterile water and cotton. As an alternative a mild soap with water rinsing may be used as required at diaper changes and more often if indicated. The use of creams, lotions, and emollients should be avoided. There is no single method of cord care that has been proved to limit bacterial colonization and disease. Methods currently in use include local application of alcohol, triple dye, and antimicrobial agents.

If the dry technique is not used and newborns are bathed with soap and water, the initial bath should not be given until the baby's temperature has stabilized. Do not bathe a baby immediately after a feeding because the handling may cause vomiting of the feeding and the possibility of aspiration. When bathing a baby, conserve the baby's heat by uncovering only that part of the body that is being washed. When that body part is washed, promptly cover it again. Wash the cleanest parts first and then proceed to the most soiled areas. Particular care should be given to the cleansing, rinsing, and drying of the scalp, creases of the neck, axillas, hands, under the knees, feet, buttocks, and perineum.

During the bath or during dry skin care, the baby can be observed for any abnormalities. Any deviation from normal should be reported. A tub bath for the baby should be delayed until the cord drops off and the navel has healed (usually 10 days to 2 weeks).

Care of the umbilicus

The umbilicus should be cleaned with rubbing alcohol after each diaper change. Redness or swelling around the umbilicus, a foul odor, or discharge should be reported to the physician.

While caring for the baby at the mother's bedside, the nurse can explain the procedure for a tub bath. Emphasize to the parents the importance of the bath time as a social time. Point out to them the unique characteristics of their infant. Encourage interaction; siblings can help with bath time and enjoy the family togetherness at home. Talk with the parents about ways in which they can include other siblings in infant care.

Tub Bathing

After the cord drops off the skin should be cleansed every other day with a soft, clean washcloth, warm water, and a mild soap. All bathing supplies (see box), equipment, and clothing should be assembled and ready for use in the work area. A large pan or basin can be used for bathing; however, it should be kept *only* for the baby's bath. The bath water should be warm (98° to 100° F). The environment should also be warm (75° to 80° F) and free from drafts.

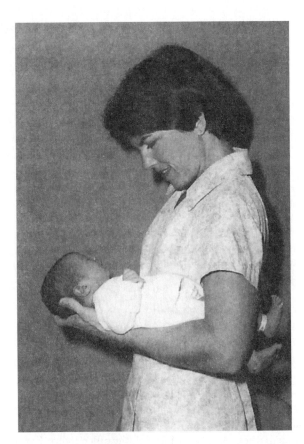

Figure 12-15 Football hold. *(Courtesy Grossmont Hospital, La Mesa, Calif. From Novak JC, Broom BL:* Ingalls and Salerno's maternal and child health nursing, *ed 8, 1995, Mosby.)*

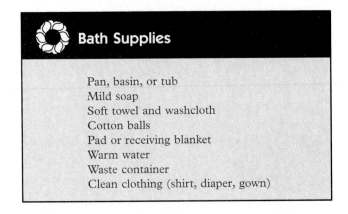

Bath Supplies

Pan, basin, or tub
Mild soap
Soft towel and washcloth
Cotton balls
Pad or receiving blanket
Warm water
Waste container
Clean clothing (shirt, diaper, gown)

Instruct the parents to always wash hands before handling the baby and *never* leave the baby alone when bathing. Other instructions include the following. Wash each eye from the nose outward, using a clean portion of the washcloth for the second eye. Soap the baby's head. Hold the baby securely in a football position (Fig. 12-15), and rinse the head with water. Dry well. Soap the trunk, arms, axillas, and abdomen. Turn the baby over to wash the back. Wash the genitals last. Immerse the baby in the tub to rinse; pat the baby dry. Check all skin creases to be sure they are dry and clean. Dress the baby and brush the baby's hair.

Prevention of Infection

The infant's immature immune system leaves the newborn susceptible to infection, particularly to those organisms with which the newborn has had no previous contact. The most important nursing measure to prevent infection is careful handwashing. When caring for infants at the beginning of the working day and when returning from lunch or dinner, the nurse should scrub hands and arms up to the elbows for 3 minutes with a hexachlorophene or iodophor preparation. After caring for each baby the caregiver's hands should be washed again. Also, nurses should wash their hands after touching any equipment considered "dirty," such as pens, pencils, telephones, charts—anything not specifically used on the baby. The nurse should wear clean scrub clothing or uniform each day. Removing all jewelry from hands and arms and keeping fingernails short and polish-free are also important in preventing infection.

Of course any person (staff or family) with an infectious disease should not handle the baby, and any infant suspected of infection should be isolated from other babies. A space of 2 feet should be kept between infant cribs to separate babies from each other in hospital nurseries. It is advisable to wash the hospital nursery and all nursery equipment with disinfectant each day. All nursery linens are handled separately from the regular hospital linens. Everyone working in a hospital nursery should be familiar with the American Academy of Pediatrics' recommended standards.

Family-centered care practices do not increase newborn infection rates. Well siblings may visit and hold their new baby brother or sister without increasing bacterial colonization in newborns. Family members should be instructed to wash their hands well before handling their baby.

Nutritional Needs

Although some babies do not lose weight, a weight loss of 5% to 10% of the original birth weight can be considered normal for the newborn in the first days of life. The newborn loses this weight because of the meconium, the use of calories to meet metabolic needs, and the loss of more body fluids than taken in. Within 3 to 5 days after birth the baby will begin gaining weight and will reach birth weight by 10 days to 2 weeks of age. By 4 months of life the baby will double the birth weight.

A newborn infant is regulating its internal environment at birth and should be fed within 4 hours of birth to keep blood glucose levels up.

A newborn needs water, calories, protein, carbohydrates, fat, vitamins, and minerals. The amount of fluid a newborn needs is in proportion to body weight; that is, the larger the baby, the greater the fluid need. A newborn cannot conserve water and loses it quickly. Water replacement is particularly important for newborns in hot weather or when they are placed under lights that increase their body temperature. By the third to fourth day of life the term baby needs approximately 140 to 160 milliliters of fluid per kilogram of body weight in 24 hours. (A baby weighing 5 kilograms [10.5 pounds] requires 750 milliliters of fluid intake in 24 hours, providing 150 milliliters per kilogram.) With eight feedings in a 24-hour period, this would translate into 93 milliliters per feeding, or about 3 ounces.

During the first few weeks of life the average baby probably needs about 110 calories per kilogram of body weight. (A 3-kilogram [6.6-pound] baby would require 330 calories per day.) Breast milk and most infant formulas contain 20 calories per ounce. Because of the baby's rapid growth, protein is very important in infant nutrition. Babies need approximately 1 gram of protein per pound of body weight. The newborn needs at least 9 grams of protein per day, although 14 grams per day in the first month is the usual recommendation. This recommendation increases to 15 grams per day in the second month and 16 grams per day from 4 months to 1 year of age. The infant receives its principal protein from lactalbumin in human milk.

Fat is the main source of calories in human milk and is more easily digested than the fat in cow's milk. Thus whole, nonmodified cow's milk should not be given to the infant until after 1 year of age. Because the newborn needs the fat in milk as an important energy source, skim milk is not advised for infants or children under 2 years of age. Skim milk also contains too much salt, ash, potassium, and calcium for infants and young children. From birth to 1 year, breast milk or formula is the food of choice.

Formula-fed infants require vitamin supplementation. Breast milk contains all the vitamins but vitamin D, which must be supplemented. Many formula-fed infants are given formulas fortified with iron; however, iron supplements are given if a nonfortified formula is used. Well babies who are being breast-fed have adequate amounts of iron stores for up to 3 to 4 months past delivery. After that initial 3 to 4 months many physicians recommend adding 1 to 2 milligrams of iron per kilogram of the baby's body weight per day to the breast-fed baby's intake, or iron supplements may be prescribed for the mother's diet. Some physicians prescribe a fluoride supplement for newborns to aid in prevention of dental caries.

Breast-feeding and the pros and cons of both breast- and bottle-feeding were discussed earlier. Helping the

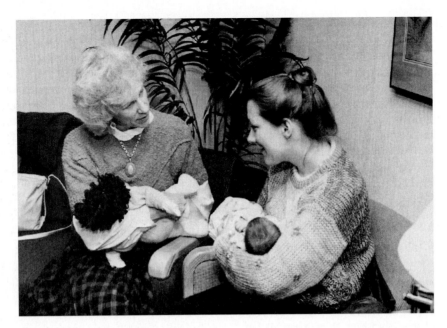

Figure 12-16 Nurse demonstrating holding the baby for feeding. *(Courtesy Evergreen Hospital, Kirkland, Wash.)*

mother who chooses to bottle-feed will be discussed here.

Bottle-Feeding

If a mother chooses bottle-feeding on discharge from the hospital, she is given instructions on the formula to be used for her baby. Often sample formulas and a supply of formula for 2 to 3 days are provided by the company that manufactures the formula. The mother and her family need a thorough understanding of these instructions before going home.

Ready-to-feed formulas and bottles with disposable plastic liners are convenient but often add considerable expense. Commercially prepared formulas are available in liquid or powder form. Nipples and caps need to be carefully washed and rinsed to protect the baby from illness.

Formula preparation

The most common method of formula preparation today is the tap water method. This method uses prepared formula in the form of liquid concentrate or powder. Carefully washed formula bottles and nipples are used and the proper amount of ready-to-use formula liquid or powder is placed in the bottles. Warm water from the tap is added to the bottle according to the directions. The bottle contents can be mixed by shaking. Enough formula for 24 hours can be made in this manner and stored in a refrigerator.

Perhaps the easiest method to prepare formula is the *single-bottle method.* One bottle at a time is thoroughly washed in hot, soapy water, rinsed, and filled with formula. The liquid formula or powder is mixed from fresh tap water. This bottle is given to the baby after preparation, and all unused formula in the bottle is discarded. The nipple is also thoroughly washed in hot soapy water and rinsed both before and after use.

Feeding is done in the semiupright position. Holding the baby is the preferred method of feeding because of the infant's need for emotional warmth during the feeding time (Fig. 12-16). Babies should never be fed lying flat with bottles "propped" because of the danger of aspiration.

Burping, or "bubbling," the infant is done after the first 5 minutes of feeding, in the middle of feeding, and at the end of the feeding to help the baby release the accumulation of air. The infant is held in an upright position and the back is gently patted or stroked.

After feeding, the infant should be placed on the side. In this position, if the baby should spit up, the vomitus will run out of the mouth and lessen the chance of aspiration.

There are various types of nipples used: firm and resistant for babies who suck vigorously and soft, pliable nipples for premature babies who tire easily (Fig. 12-17). The rate of flow through the nipple will vary according to the size and shape of the nipple hole.

Giving water to a baby may be helpful during hot weather or if the baby is constipated. However, never mix honey in the baby's water or formula. Giving either cooked or uncooked honey to a baby under 1 year of age has been associated with infant botulism.

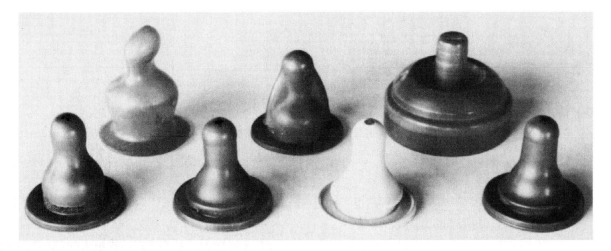

Figure 12-17 Types of nipples. *(From Ingalls AJ, Salerno MC:* Maternal and child health nursing, *ed 7, St. Louis, 1991, Mosby.)*

Diaper Care

Mild laundry soap such as Ivory soap or pure castile soap and moderately warm water should be used to wash the baby's clothing and cloth diapers. Most detergents and clothing softeners should not be used because of the irritating effect on the baby's skin. It is important to rinse the clothing and diapers thoroughly enough to remove detergent residue.

The controversy over cloth versus disposable diapers needs discussion with parents so that they can make an informed decision about which to use. Environmental issues are not simple, and there are environmental consequences to both disposable and cloth diaper use. However, environmentalists believe that cloth diapers may be less damaging to the environment overall.

Infant Position

The American Academy of Pediatrics recommends that healthy infants be placed on their sides or backs to sleep. For premature infants with respiratory distress, for infants with symptoms of gastroesophageal reflux or upper airway anomalies, prone may be the position of choice. This recommendation is based on studies linking the prone position with sudden infant death syndrome (SIDS).

Circumcision

Circumcision is the surgical removal of the foreskin on the penis. The operation is usually performed on the second or third day of life. Circumcision is a ritual in the Jewish religion and is performed on the eighth day of life. At that time the baby is officially named.

The American Academy of Pediatrics reports that newborn circumcision has potential medical benefits

and advantages, as well as disadvantages and risks. Whether the infant is circumcised should be decided by the parents after a thorough explanation of the procedure and discussion of the pros and cons.

There is controversy in terms of whether circumcision is medically necessary. Studies have demonstrated that infants who are not circumcised develop urinary tract infections more frequently than babies who are circumcised. The circumcised penis is easier to clean. Advantages of circumcision include prevention of cancer of the penis in adult men, and inhibition of a variety of sexually transmitted diseases. Circumcision may also influence the rate of cervical cancer in women, which was found to be lower in the sexual partners of circumcised men. Other reasons given for circumcision include avoiding the surgical and psychological risks should the operation be necessary at a later age and aesthetic considerations.

Arguments against circumcision include the fact that it carries risks: hemorrhage, infection, and surgical mishaps. These risks can lead to sutures, transfusions, scarring, and deformity. Another argument against circumcision is that it exposes the newborn to unnecessary pain and trauma. For the operation the infant is restrained on a circumcision board, and the penis is cleansed with soap and water and an antiseptic solution. The baby is draped with a sterile drape that also serves to provide warmth. Sterile surgical instruments are used.

Nursing care

Following the circumcision the penis is covered with sterile gauze saturated with petrolatum. The nurse must observe the newly circumcised baby frequently for abnormal bleeding. The parents need to learn how to observe and care for the newly circumcised baby at home. It will be helpful to observe any bleeding if only one layer of diaper fabric covers the penis. Cleansing the penis with cotton balls moistened in warm water must be gentle. A fresh, sterile gauze with petrolatum dressing should be applied after each diaper change. The parents must understand how to apply gentle pressure to the penis to control bleeding and when to bring the baby back to the hospital or office for an examination by the physician.

Care of the Uncircumcised Penis

It is not necessary to retract any part of the infant's foreskin to wash under it. Daily external washing and rinsing are all that is necessary. The foreskin and glans develop as one tissue. Separation will evolve over time. The foreskin of an infant should never be retracted. Forcing the skin back can cause pain, bleeding, and adhesions. By 3 years of age about 90% of boys have retractable foreskins, and by age 17, 99% do. As the male child learns to bathe himself, he will learn how to clean his penis as well.

DISCHARGE TO HOME

Before discharge, phenylketonuria (PKU)/T_4 testing is performed. (See Chapter 13, p. 362, for discussion of phenylketonuria). T_4 testing is done to rule out primary congenital hypothyroidism, a defect in which the thyroid gland does not produce adequate thyroxine (T_4). If untreated, severe brain damage can result. Treatment consists of thyroid hormone replacement therapy.

In addition, hepatitis B (HB) vaccination is recommended for protection against hepatitis B virus (HBV) infection. Parents are given information and a consent form for HB vaccine.

Hepatitis B vaccine is given in a series of three injections. If a mother does not have HBV in her blood, her baby may get the first injection of hepatitis B vaccine before leaving the hospital. Another option is for the baby to get the first injection at the physician's office or clinic. The next two doses will be given with the other baby shots.

If a mother has HBV in her blood when her baby is born, her baby will need the first injection of hepatitis B vaccine within 12 hours after birth. Hepatitis B immune globulin (HBIG) is also given. The baby will get the next two injections of hepatitis B vaccine as recommended by the physician or clinic.

Whether the infant and new family go home in 12 hours after birth or after several days, health education for the new family is extremely important. Special referrals to public health or visiting nurses or other health care workers may be needed. Follow-up appointments with the physician for mother and baby should be made. In many hospitals today follow-up home visits by hospital nurses are also being made. Whatever the hospital policy, the new parents must learn how to care for their infant.

Parents will also need anticipatory guidance on how to handle sibling relationships and how to take advantage of support systems available. It is important to encourage parents to allow the siblings to share in infant care. A healthy relationship can be encouraged by giving the sibling special attention as an individual needing love and reinforcement of that love.

Support systems are vital to serve as an emotional sounding board and to release the parents of some of the responsibilities of the new family life. Responding to a new baby 24 hours a day can be very tiring very quickly. Parents need support too.

SUMMARY

This chapter has offered an introduction to the newborn. Because safe transition from the uterus to the world outside is so important, it is vital for the nurse to have the knowledge and skills needed to understand and care for the normal newborn.

With a basic understanding of the normal newborn, recognition of deviations from normal becomes possible. Such early recognition of complications and prompt interventions can determine whether the infant survives or with what degree of wellness the infant grows and develops. The next chapter will explore complications in the newborn period.

BIBLIOGRAPHY

AAP Task Force on Infant Position and SIDS: Position and SIDS, *Pediatrics* 89(6):1120-1126, 1992.

Barr RG, Elias MR: Nursing interval and maternal responsivity: effect on early infant crying, *Pediatrics* 81(4):529-535, 1988.

Bell TA and others: Randomized trial of silver nitrate, erythromycin, and no eye prophylaxis for the prevention of conjunctivitis among newborns not at risk for gonococcal opthalmitis, *Pediatrics* 92(6):755-759, 1993.

Bobak IM, Jensen MD, Lowdermilk DL: *Maternity and gynecologic care: the nurse and the family,* ed 5, St. Louis, 1993, Mosby.

Brown MS, Brown CA: Circumcision decision: prominence of social concerns, *Pediatrics* 80(2):215-219, 1987.

Caravella SJ, Clark DA, Diveck HS: Health codes for newborn care, *Pediatrics* 80(1):1-4, 1987.

Dickason EJ, Silverman BL, Schult MO: *Maternal-infant nursing care,* ed 2, St. Louis, 1994, Mosby.

Judd JM: Assessing the newborn from head to toe, *Nurs 85* 19(2):34-41, 1985.

LeBoyer F: *Birth without violence*, New York, 1975, Alfred A Knopf.

Lerner H: Sleep positions of infants: applying research to practice, *Am J Nurs* 18(5):275-277, 1993.

Mattson S, Smith JE, editors: *Core curriculum for maternal-newborn nursing*, Philadelphia, 1993, WB Saunders.

Nurses Association of the American College of Obstetricians and Gynecologists: *Physical assessment of the neonate: OGN nursing practice resource*, October 1986, The Association.

Nurses Association of the American College of Obstetricians and Gynecologists: *Nurse's role in neonatal circumcision: OGN nursing practice resource*, August 1985, The Association.

Novak JC, Broom BL: *Ingalls and Salerno's maternal and child health nursing*, ed 8, St. Louis, 1995, Mosby.

Nurses Association of the American College of Obstetricians and Gynecologists: *neonatal skin care: OGN nursing practice resource*, January 1992, The Association.

Sutton MB, Weitzman M, Howland J: Baby bottoms and environmental conundrums: disposable diapers and the pediatrician, *Pediatrics* 88(2):386-389, 1991.

Task Force on Circumcision: Report of the task force on circumcision, *Pediatrics* 84(4):388-390, 1989.

Wong DL: *Whaley and Wong's nursing care of infants and children*, ed 5, St. Louis, 1995, Mosby.

Wong DL and others: Diapering choices: a critical review of the issues, *Pediatr Nurs* 18(1):41-44, 1992.

Wranesh BL: The effect of sibling visitation on bacterial colonization rate in neonates, *J Obstet Gynecol Neonatal Nurs* 11(4):211-213, 1982.

DEFINITIONS

Define the following terms:

Acidotic	Moro's reflex
AGA	neutral thermal environment
area care	
bilirubin	nonshivering thermogenesis
brown fat	physiological jaundice
caput succedaneum	radiant warmer
cephalhematoma	radiation
circumcision	servo-control incubator
cohort system	SGA
conduction	single-bottle method
convection	sudden infant death syndrome (SIDS)
dry skin care	
erythema toxicum	surfactant
hemangioma	synchronous
hyperthermia	T_4
icterus neonatorum	thermogenesis
iodophor preparation	thermogenic activity
lanugo	thrush
LGA	tonic neck reflex
metabolic acidosis	traditional stool
milia	vernix caseosa
molding	vitamin K
mongolian spots	

LEARNING ACTIVITIES

1. Group discussions.
2. Interview a new mother concerning her baby. Ask if the baby can recognize her in a group of strangers. What does she see as unique about her baby?
3. View audiovisual aids and discuss.

ENRICHMENT/IN-DEPTH STUDY

1. Visit a local pharmacy or grocery store and inspect the prepared formulas for sale. (Composition? Cost?) Price bottles and nipples.
2. Visit a local store and price diapers (cloth) and baby clothing. Then price disposable paper diapers and compare costs of cloth and disposable diapers.
3. Is there a diaper service in your community? What is the cost of this service?

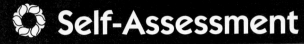

Self-Assessment

1. Circle those laboratory values that suggest anemia on day 1 in the life of a newborn:
   a. Hct 60%
   b. Hct 55%
   c. Hct 40%
   d. Hgb 19.0 grams/100 milliliters
   e. Hgb 16.8 grams/100 milliliters
   f. Hgb 12.5 grams/100 milliliters

2. What is the normal leukocyte count on day 1 of life?
   a. 12,000
   b. 6000
   c. 18,000

3. Normal bilirubin on day 1 of life is under ____ milligrams per deciliter and on day 5 of life is under ____ milligrams per deciliter.

4. When would you expect physiological jaundice to become apparent?

   _____

   _____

   _____

5. Vitamin K aids in the formation of _____, which is necessary for blood _____.

6. What special precautions are necessary when using a manual mode of radiant warmer?

   _____

   _____

   _____

7. A neutral thermal environment is one in which an infant's metabolic rate and oxygen consumption are _____.

For questions 8 through 11, circle the best answer.

8. Average weight loss in the normal newborn in the first days of life is:
   a. 5% to 10% of birth weight
   b. 2% to 4% of birth weight
   c. 12% of birth weight

9. Newborn skin care recommended by the American Academy of Pediatrics is:
   a. hexachlorophene baths
   b. tub baths
   c. dry skin care

10. Newborns cry because they are:

    a. lonely

    b. hungry

    c. in pain

    d. tired

    e. spoiled

       Answer (circle one):

       1. a,b, and c

       2. e

       3. a,b,c, and d

       4. all of the above

11. A newborn's vital signs would be which of the following:

    a. axillary temperature, 99° F; pulse, 110 beats per minute; respirations, 20 per minute

    b. axillary temperature, 98° F; pulse, 120 beats per minute; respirations, 40 per minute

    c. axillary temperature, 100° F; pulse, 200 beats per minute; respirations, 80 per minute

12. Statistics for an average American baby include:

    weight (female) _____ (male) _____

    length _____

    chest circumference _____

    head circumference _____

13. In examination of the normal newborn, briefly note what you would expect to find for each of the following:

    a. skin:_____

    b. ears:_____

    c. face (include nose and mouth):_____

    d. eyes:_____

    e. neck:_____

    f. chest (include breasts):_____

    g. abdomen (include cord):_____

    h. genitals: (male):_____

             (female):_____

14. Match Column A with Column B

Column A	**Column B**
____ 1. meconium	a. pale yellow and semiformed
____ 2. breast-fed stools	b. golden yellow and pasty
____ 3. formula-fed stools	c. black, tarry, and odorless

15. Complete the following chart:

Reflex	Appearance	How stimulated	Time of disappearance
Moro's			
Grasp			
Walking			
Sucking			

16. Match Column A with Column B.

Column A

_____ 1. caput succedaneum

_____ 2. cephalhematoma

_____ 3. erythema toxicum

_____ 4. "stork bites"

_____ 5. milia

_____ 6. subconjunctival hemorrhage

_____ 7. "epithelial pearls"

_____ 8. molding

Column B

a. bleeding into conjunctiva caused by pressure of delivery

b. edema of the scalp

c. tiny white spots on face

d. fine rash of newborn

e. subperiosteal hemorrhage

f. small, white, ricelike epidermal plaques in mouth

g. small hemangiomas

h. uneven and unsymmetrical shape of newborn's head

17. Describe the first reactive phase in the life of a newborn. How long does it last? What are the baby's respirations and heart rate?

_____

_____

_____

18. During what phase of newborn activity does the baby's body temperature return to normal?

_____

_____

_____

19. List the six "state" cycles of the newborn:

a. _____

b. _____

c. _____

d. _____

e. _____

f. _____

20. Match Column A with Column B.

Column A

_____ 1. convection

_____ 2. conduction

_____ 3. evaporation

_____ 4. radiation

_____ 5. nonshivering thermogenesis

_____ 6. vasoconstriction

Column B

a. transfer of heat from a warm object to a cool object

b. newborn's method of producing heat

c. heat loss from wet skin in a dry atmosphere

d. newborn's means of heat retention

e. enhanced by surrounding air currents

f. transfer of heat from body surfaces to cooler surfaces

21. Newborn heat loss by convection can be minimized by _____.

22. Newborn heat loss by evaporation can be prevented by _____.

23. Newborn heat loss by conduction can be minimized by _____.

24. If a newborn baby required extensive life-saving procedures, would you place the baby in a warm incubator or a radiant warmer? Why?

_____

_____

_____

25. Match Column A with Column B.

Column A	Column B
____ 1. SGA	a. before 38 weeks of gestation
____ 2. AGA	b. average for gestational age
____ 3. LGA	c. 38 to 42 weeks of gestation
____ 4. preterm	d. large for gestational age
____ 5. term	e. 42 weeks or more of gestation
____ 6. postterm	f. small for gestational age

26. When determining gestational age (using the clinical form in this book), the nurse checks the following physical characteristics:

a. _____

b. _____

c. _____

d. _____

e. _____

f. _____

g. _____

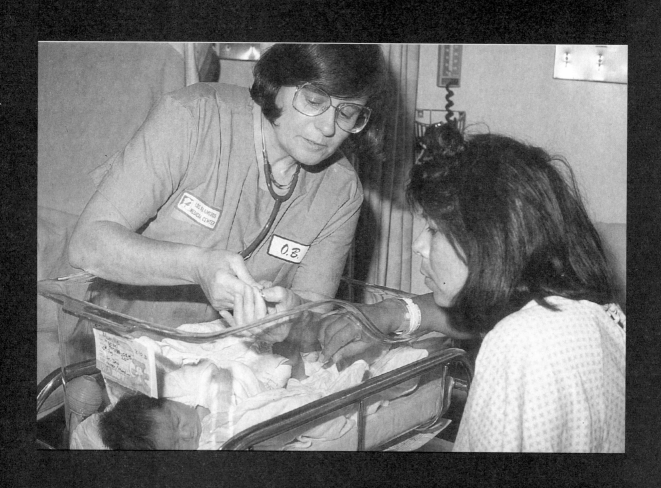

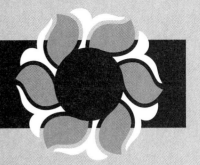

13

THE NEWBORN WITH COMPLICATIONS

GOALS

This chapter is designed to provide the reader with information that will:
- promote awareness of deviations from normal in the newborn period.

- increase awareness of the emotional care of parents, families, and babies requiring neonatal intensive care.

STUDENT OBJECTIVES

After studying this chapter, you should be able to:

1. Distinguish between the resuscitation needs of newborns with Apgar scores of 0 to 3, 4 to 6, and 7 to 10.
2. Describe the special needs for emotional care of the parents of a baby who is in a neonatal intensive care unit (NICU).
3. Discuss the developmental needs of premature and sick babies in a neonatal intensive care unit.
4. Describe the signs of respiratory distress.
5. Compare physiological jaundice and that appearing before the baby is 24 hours old.
6. Name the six major causes of hyperbilirubinemia in the newborn.

7. Design a plan of care for the newborn receiving phototherapy for hyperbilirubinemia.
8. Identify blood sugar (glucose) levels indicating low blood sugar (hypoglycemia) in full-term infants (both before and after 72 hours of age).
9. When given a description of the following conditions, be able to associate the description with the condition: cleft lip and/or palate, hydrocephalus, spina bifida, encephalocele, meningocele, meningomyelocele, anencephaly, Down syndrome, and phenylketonuria (PKU).
10. List five clinical signs of tracheoesophageal fistula with esophageal atresia.

RESUSCITATION OF THE NEWBORN

The average newborn is mildly hypoxic and acidotic at birth. Normal values at birth are as follows: P_{O_2}, 20 to 30 mm Hg; pH, 7.25; and P_{CO_2}, 45 to 50 mm Hg.

For the normal neonate at 24 hours of age, values are as follows: P_{O_2}, 90 to 100 mm Hg; pH, 7.35 to 7.45; P_{CO_2}, 35 to 45 mm Hg.

For most babies breathing begins immediately after birth; for some babies, however, breathing is delayed. These babies require immediate assistance.

Every delivery area should be equipped with newborn resuscitation equipment and staffed with personnel who know how to use it (Fig. 13-1).

Resuscitation equipment

Source of heat for baby (preferably a radiant heater)
Adequate lighting
Infant stethoscope
Bulb syringe for suctioning
Mucus trap with catheter for aspiration of mucus
Suction capabilities
Suction catheters Nos. 5, 6, 8, and 10 FR
Source of 100% oxygen

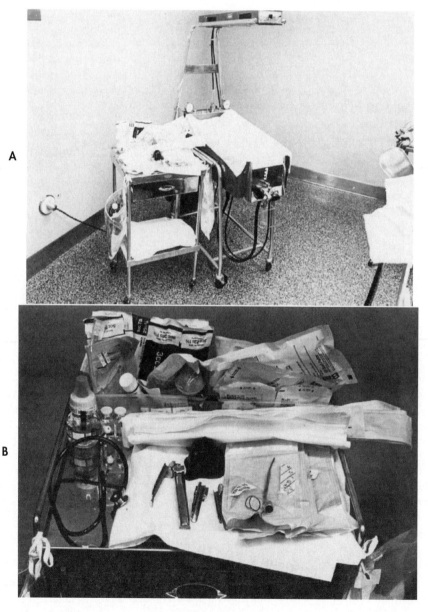

Figure 13-1 A, Resuscitation area. **B,** Resuscitation equipment. *(Courtesy Kaiser Permanente Medical Center, Santa Clara, Calif.)*

Oxygen tubing with and without masks (premature and newborn sizes)

Resuscitation bag that can deliver 100% oxygen and has an adjustable pressure valve

Laryngoscope with spare batteries

Dextrostix (bottle)

Stylet

NS intravenous IV 250 cubic centimeters

D5/w 500 cubic centimeters

D10/w 1000 cubic centimeters

Stopcocks

Laryngoscope blades, size 1 and 0 straight blade, with spare bulbs for laryngoscope

Feeding tubes with syringes

Endotracheal tubes of various sizes (2.5, 3.0, 3.5, and 4.0 millimeters) with adaptors to fit all sizes

Infant airways

Adhesive tape

Warm blankets

Umbilical vein catheters with umbilical catheterization tray

Assorted sizes of syringes and needles

Drugs

Epinephrine 1:10,000

Narcotic antagonist: Naloxone hydrochloride (Narcan)

Sodium bicarbonate ($NaHCO_3$), 0.5 milliequivalents per milliliter

Calcium gluconate, 50 milligrams per milliliter

Heparin sodium 1000 per milliliter

Glucagon 1 unit per milliliter

Isoproterenol (Isuprel) 1:5000

Atropine

Albumin 5%

Before each birth the emergency equipment should be checked to be sure it is all present and in working order.

It is usually possible to identify the fetus that will be in jeopardy before delivery occurs. Intrapartum conditions such as meconium-stained amniotic fluid, maternal hemorrhage and anemia (placental abruption or previa), prolonged rupture of membranes, maternal substance abuse, maternal sedation, prolapse of the cord, and fetal distress without identified cause predispose an infant to require resuscitation. Prematurity and labors associated with medical problems such as diabetes, chronic hypertensive states or pregnancy-induced hypertension (PIH), and postterm gestation can result in both fetal and neonatal asphyxia. Also, cesarean birth for fetal distress frequently results in the need for resuscitation of the newborn.

The Apgar score will give an estimation of a term infant's condition at birth. The infant with an Apgar score of 7 to 10 at 1 minute will not require resuscitation, but an infant scoring 0 to 3 will require resuscitation. The baby scoring 4 to 6 may need only suction, gentle stimulation, and a few whiffs of oxygen. It is important to remember that depressant drugs and anesthesia given to the mother may produce low Apgar scores even though the baby is not asphyxiated. (See Table 13-1 for neonatal resuscitation scores and procedures.)

Although the Apgar score provides guidelines for management of asphyxia, do not wait until the 1-minute assessment time has passed to intervene. When asphyxiated, the infant's oxygen level is low, carbon dioxide level is high, and there is suboptimal ventilation. The infant who is cyanotic and gasping with good muscle tone and heart rate of 100 needs to be kept dry and warm and stimulated and given oxygen. The infant who is born pale, limp, and severely depressed needs immediate resuscitation and intubation. A delay of a minute in starting resuscitation can compromise recovery.

Technique for Resuscitation of Infant

1. Assess infant's status; prevent heat loss. The baby should be placed under a radiant warmer with the head lower than the thorax and should be dried immediately.

2. Establish an airway and stimulate the infant to breathe. The airway must be cleared by gentle suction of the oropharynx to remove meconium secretions. A bulb syringe is usually adequate. Suction mouth, then nose. Too much suctioning with a long catheter in the first few minutes of life can cause laryngospasm. Stimulate the infant by gently rubbing the back or flicking the soles of the feet.

3. Ensure adequate ventilation and oxygenation. Ventilation is assisted by giving oxygen by bag and mask at 20 to 30 breaths per minute (Fig. 13-2).

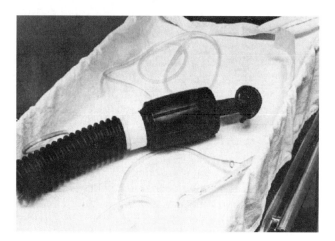

Figure 13-2 Bag and mask.

TABLE 13-1
Neonatal Resuscitation

Apgar score	Baby's condition	Resuscitation procedure
7-10 Normal	Responsive Heart rate normal (>100 per minute) Respirations normal (40 per minute)	1. Clear airway by suctioning mouth and nose with a bulb syringe. Catheter suction may cause bradycardia; if used, do brief, gentle suctioning. 2. Maintain thermal neutrality by drying infant with warm, dry towel and placing infant under a radiant warmer. 3. Routine identification procedures. 4. Neonatal ophthalmic prophylaxis. 5. Brief physical examination.
4-6 Moderately depressed	Poor response Decreased or absent respirations Heart rate less than 100 or normal Decreased muscle tone	1. Routine drying, warming, and suctioning as above. 2. Stimulate to breathe by rubbing up and down spine or slapping soles of feet. 3. Administer warm humid oxygen over the nose and mouth. 4. If infant's condition fails to improve, ventilate with oxygen by bag and mask. 5. If condition improves, continue as for a normal infant. 6. If no response to bag and mask ventilation, proceed to endotracheal intubation as for severely depressed infant below.
0-3 Severely depressed	Unresponsive Depressed or absent respirations Decreased or absent heart rate Pale, flaccid	1. Suction; dry; warm; stimulate. 2. If no response to ventilation with 100% oxygen by bag and mask, intubate with endotracheal tube and ventilate by bag and mask at a rate of 30 to 40 per minute. 3. If heart rate less than 70, administer external cardiac massage. Compress to chest ½ to ¾ of an inch at a rate of 100 to 120 compressions per minute. Maintain a ratio of three compressions per one ventilation. 4. If continued poor response, perform umbilical catheterization and infuse appropriate medication.

To prevent overexpansion of the infant's lungs, the pressure on the bag should be light. If there is a possibility that meconium was aspirated, the baby should be intubated and suctioned before assisted ventilation is begun.

4. A member of the resuscitation team should monitor the infant's heartbeat during this time by tapping a finger in time to the beat. If the heart rate does not increase immediately, intubation will be needed.

5. Intubation should be done by someone experienced in the use of a laryngoscope. Secretions, blood, and meconium are quickly aspirated and an endotracheal tube inserted (Fig. 13-3). Mouth-to-tube or bag-to-tube ventilation is begun at a rate of 30 to 40 per minute. A team member continues to tap out the baby's heartbeat and observe the chest for movement.

6. Ensure adequate cardiac output (circulation). If the baby's heartbeat should fall below 70 beats per minute, cardiac massage is instituted (Fig. 13-4). However, never perform cardiac massage and ventilate at the same time because simultaneous cardiac massage and ventilation can cause pneumothorax. Compress chest ½ to ¾ inch at a rate of 100 to 120 compressions per minute. The ratio of chest wall compression to ventilation is 3:1 (three compressions to one ventilation).

7. Use emergency drugs if necessary. If the baby is still unresponsive at this point, sodium bicarbonate at 0.5 milliequivalents per milliliter concentration, 2 milliequivalents per kilogram, diluted with an equal volume of water, may be given intravenously over a 2- to 5-minute period to combat acidosis.

8. Should the baby continue to be depressed, 0.5 milliliter of 1:10,000 epinephrine can be given by intravenous, intracardiac, or intratracheal methods.

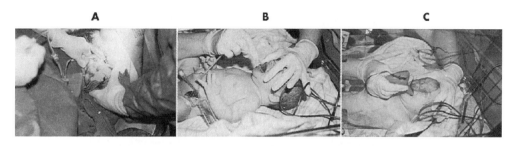

Figure 13-3 Suction equipment. **A,** Suctioning on the perineum with tubing attached to low suction at the wall. **B,** Suction of oropharynx with straight catheter. **C,** Suctioning with bulb syringe. *(Courtesy Marjorie Pyle, RNC, Lifecircle. From Dickason EJ and others:* Maternal-infant nursing care, *ed 2, St. Louis, 1994, Mosby.)*

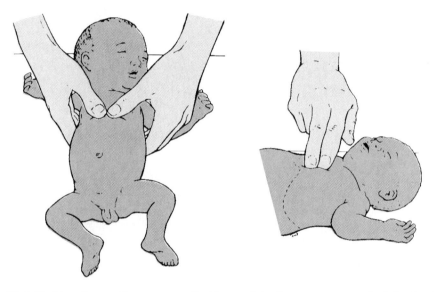

Figure 13-4 Position for cardiac massage. Position at left allows more control of depth of compression. *(From Dickason EJ and others:* Maternal-infant nursing care, *ed 2, St. Louis, 1994, Mosby.)*

Epinephrine is given rapidly and can be diluted 1:1 with normal saline if given intratracheally.

9. Albumin in a 5% concentration may be used to expand blood volume. Dosage is 10 milliliters per kilogram given intravenously, slowly (1 milliliter per minute).

10. Neonatal naloxone hydrochloride (Narcan) may be used as a narcotic antagonist. It is given rapidly intravenously, intramuscularly, subcutaneously, or intratracheally at 0.1 milligram per kilogram for newborns, including premature infants. This dose may be repeated as needed to maintain opiate reversal.

A baby who has been resuscitated will require close management and care and should be transferred to a neonatal intensive care unit. The possibility of brain damage in infants requiring resuscitation at birth is greater than for normal infants.

In Chapter 1 levels of care were discussed (regionalization of perinatal care). Level III (tertiary care) was identified as that level at which neonatal intensive care could be provided. Neonatal intensive care nursing is a fascinating, rapidly changing specialty area of nursing that is beyond the scope of a basic text such as this. In this chapter we will present very basic information on the newborn with complications. Figure 13-5 will give some idea of the equipment in an intensive care unit. One-to-one nursing is usually provided around the clock to the infants in the neonatal intensive care unit (NICU).

CLASSIFICATION OF NEWBORNS

A *preterm* baby is a live infant who is born before the end of 37 weeks of gestation, regardless of the baby's weight. A *low-birth-weight* infant is a baby weighing less than 5.5 pounds (2500 grams) at birth. A low-birth-weight infant may be either preterm or full term but small for gestational age. A *small-for-gestational-age* (SGA) baby is one whose birth weight is below the tenth

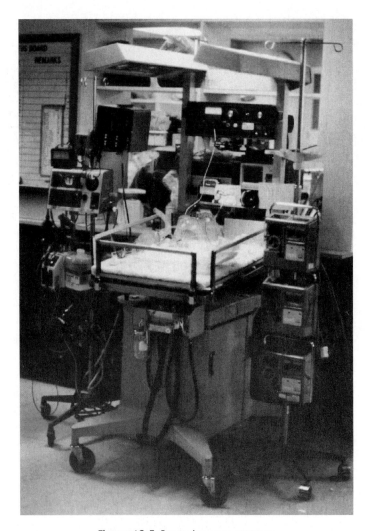

Figure 13-5 Intensive care nursery.

percentile. Some infants are both preterm and growth retarded.

Maternal factors contributing to prematurity may include multiple pregnancy, maternal disease, premature rupture of the membranes, placenta previa, abruptio placentae, incompetent cervix, low socioeconomic status, and maternal age. Maternal characteristics frequently associated with SGA babies include vascular insufficiencies, renal disease, pregnancy-induced hypertension, maternal age under 16 years, nutritional deficiency, cigarette smoking, alcoholism, narcotic addiction, and certain genetic disorders. The majority of infants in the United States who die during the first year of life are either preterm or SGA.

SGA babies are subject to metabolic, nutritional, and neurological disorders. Preterm babies are subject to respiratory, thermal, and neurological problems. (Neonatal risks in preterm and SGA babies can be found in the boxes on p. 355.) The classification of a baby

as either preterm or SGA is based on a number of criteria. (See Chapter 12.)

Preterm Baby

The physical problems of a preterm baby are directly associated with the degree of organ maturity. Prematurity is not a disease but a lack of organ maturity (Fig. 13-6).

The cry of a preterm baby is feeble, and the sucking, gag, and swallowing reflexes are frequently poor or absent, necessitating *gavage feeding.* Tonic neck and Moro's reflexes may be absent or ill defined.

Because of an immature temperature-regulating center and very little subcutaneous fat, the preterm baby has great difficulty maintaining body temperature. A controlled environment (radiant warmer or incubator) that will maintain the baby's optimal body temperature is essential.

Neonatal Risks in Preterm Babies (Regardless of Birth Weight)

Respiratory distress syndrome (RDS)
Recurrent apnea
Hypothermia
Hypoglycemia
Hypocalcemia
Infection
Hyperbilirubinemia and kernicterus
Necrotizing enterocolitis
Intraventricular and pulmonary hemorrhage
Anemia
Patent ductus arteriosus
Feeding difficulties

Neonatal Risks in Small-for-Gestational-Age (SGA) Infants

Hypothermia
Hypoglycemia
Perinatal asphyxia and its sequelae
Polycythemia
Congenital malformations and/or infections

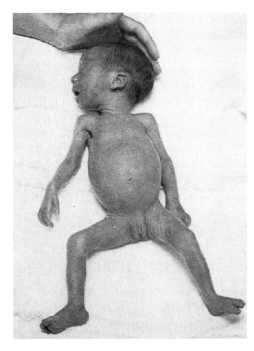

Figure 13-6 Premature infant. *(Courtesy Grossmont Hospital, La Mesa, Calif. From Novak JC, Broom BL:* Ingalls and Salerno's maternal and child health nursing, *ed 8, St. Louis, 1995, Mosby.)*

The preterm baby's skin may be covered by vernix caseosa. The hands and feet may be cyanotic (acrocyanosis). Lanugo (fine hair) is present on the sides of the face, extremities, and back. Generalized edema is present at birth but disappears in a few days, leaving the skin loose and wrinkled with very apparent blood vessels. The ears are soft and small, containing little cartilage. The nipples and areolas are inconspicuous. Heel creases are absent, and the soles of the feet are almost smooth.

Immaturity of the neurological system results in uncoordinated jerky movements. The preterm infant lies in a prone position with the pelvis flat and legs splayed out sideways like a frog. Respirations are shallow and irregular, ranging from 40 to 60 per minute. The infant may experience apnea due to immaturity of the respiratory center. Because the liver is immature and inefficient in conjugating bilirubin, the preterm baby is likely to have hyperbilirubinemia. Because of an immature immunological system, the preterm infant is extremely susceptible to infection, making extreme caution with handwashing and cleanliness vital.

The preterm infant's body systems are too immature to maintain life without a specialized environment and care. An Isolette infant incubator or radiant warmer system with servo-control should always be available to re-

ceive a preterm baby in any hospital where babies are born. In a warming unit the baby wears only a diaper.

Oxygen is not always necessary for preterm babies and will be ordered as needed by the physician in the appropriate concentration. Excessive oxygen may cause retrolental fibroplasia resulting in blindness. If oxygen is required, an oxygen monitor or oxygen analyzer should be used to test the oxygen concentration and thus facilitate keeping it at the desired level. Arterial blood gas measurements accurately record the level of arterial oxygen. If blood gas measurements are not available and an infant has generalized cyanosis, it is usually safe to give just enough oxygen to correct the cyanosis.

Nursing care of the preterm infant includes the following:
1. Conserving the infant's energy
2. Maintaining safety
3. Preventing infections
4. Maintaining body temperature
5. Providing adequate fluid and calorie intake
6. Maintaining airway and adequate oxygen intake

Preterm babies who can suck and swallow are fed with a soft nipple and bottle. The mother can express her breast milk, which can be used to feed the infant. Vitamins and iron supplements are given to preterm babies. Because the baby's growth rate parallels fetal growth rate, the protein and caloric needs are higher than those of the term newborn. However, because the baby's gastric capacity is limited, feedings must be frequent and small.

The infant who has no sucking or swallowing reflexes may be fed by a medicine dropper with a rubber tip or by gavage feeding. The physician prescribes the formula and amount for gavage feeding.

As primary caretakers in the intensive care nursery, nurses are responsible for identifying and reducing stressful stimuli in the newborn's environment. Each infant's unique level of tolerance is assessed, and care is planned to minimize stress without sacrificing the therapeutic value of necessary procedures. Parents are included in planning care and are helped to understand the unique characteristics of their own infant.

Small-for-Gestational-Age Babies

The baby who is small for gestational age frequently requires intensive care during the first 3 to 4 days of life. In contrast to the preterm baby, these babies are alert but give the appearance of being malnourished, with little subcutaneous fat and loose, dry skin (Fig. 13-7). Because the incidence of major congenital anomalies is high in these babies, close inspection and observation are necessary. These small babies are particularly susceptible to hypoglycemia and should not be without food for long periods. These babies are also predisposed to asphyxia and meconium aspiration syndrome resulting from hypoxic episodes in utero. Because of the lack of subcutaneous fat and a disproportionately large surface area, temperature regulation is often difficult in these infants.

The long-term outlook for normal function for premature and SGA babies has improved greatly with the application of intensive care techniques.

Postterm Babies

In most pregnancies there is a progressive increase in placental dysfunction after 42 weeks of gestation. When this happens the infant may appear wasted (Fig. 13-8). The postterm baby's skin becomes dry and cracked after birth and almost has the look of parchment paper. These babies may be stained with the meconium they discharged in utero in response to hypoxic periods. They are also at risk for meconium aspiration syndrome and asphyxia.

Postterm babies do not tolerate the stress of labor very well and are candidates for continuous fetal monitoring.

Neonatal risks in postterm babies may include perinatal asphyxia, meconium aspiration syndrome, pneumothorax, and polycythemia (which causes the hyperviscosity syndrome).

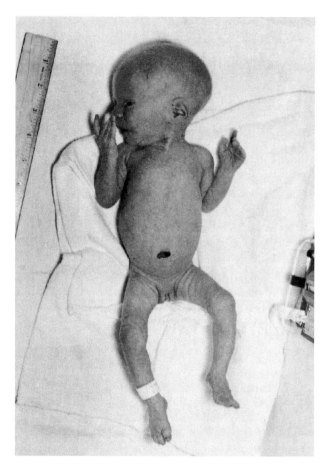

Figure 13-7 Small-for-gestational-age baby. *(From Babson SG, Benson RC:* Management of high-risk pregnancy and intensive care of the neonate, *ed 3, St. Louis, 1975, Mosby.)*

Large-for-Gestational-Age Babies

A large-for-gestational-age baby is one whose birth weight is above the ninetieth percentile. Neonatal risks in LGA infants are listed in the box on p. 357.

EMOTIONAL CARE

Parents/Families

Assuming the role of parent can be very difficult for the parents of a baby in a neonatal intensive care unit (NICU). The holding, touching, and eye-to-eye contact important in establishing a bond between parents and infant often have to be delayed to initiate immediate life-support measures. There is also a period of grieving by the parents for the perfect child they expected but did not have. Preterm labor and delivery happened when the parents were unprepared, and there may be life-threatening consequences for the preterm infant and mother. If the preterm baby has to be transported to an intensive care nursery in another hospital or city,

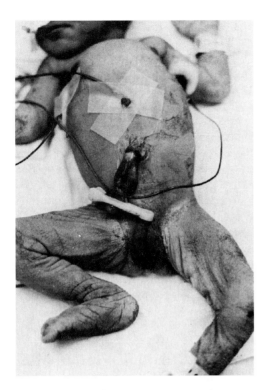

Figure 13-8 Postterm baby. *(From Korones SB:* High-risk newborn infants, *ed 3, St. Louis, 1986, Mosby.)*

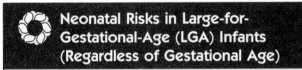

Neonatal Risks in Large-for-Gestational-Age (LGA) Infants (Regardless of Gestational Age)

Birth Injuries
Cervical and brachial plexus palsy
Phrenic nerve palsy
Fractured clavicle or humerus
Cephalhematoma
Subdural hematoma

Infants of Diabetic Mothers (Often LGA)
Respiratory distress syndrome (RDS)
Hypoglycemia, hypocalcemia
Hyperbilirubinemia
Congenital malformations
Renal vein thrombosis
Hyperviscosity syndrome

the separation can be very stressful for the parents. Because the parents may feel that the baby will probably die, they may protect themselves by delaying bonding.

Whenever a baby is in an intensive care unit (whatever the reason), the parents need special nursing care, too. It is very important for the parents to be encouraged to visit their baby in the nursery and to participate in the care. Because the parents will have the re-

sponsibility for providing life-long physical and emotional care, parents and infant must be treated as a unit from the very beginning. Before parents visit the intensive care nursery for the first time, they need to prepare for the unfamiliar environment they are about to enter. The flashing lights and buzzers on the monitors and all of the equipment attached to the baby can be very frightening. Visual aids in the form of photographs of babies in the intensive care nursery plus photographs and descriptions of equipment are very helpful in preparing the parents for what they will see. Sharing information about the infant with the parents is both supportive and critical in their understanding of the situation and may reduce their stress.

Flexible visiting hours in the nursery based on the specific needs of each family are vital. Parents, siblings, and other important family members need encouragement and support to establish a relationship with a baby in the intensive care unit. The parents should scrub their hands and arms with water and an antiseptic soap and cover their street clothes with clean gowns before entering the nursery. The same precautions concerning communicable disease that apply to staff also apply to parents.

Some parents may want to touch or hold the baby on the first visit to the nursery, whereas others may be reluctant. When the outcome for the baby is very uncertain, some parents protect and prepare themselves for the possible death of the baby by withdrawing from contact with the baby. The nurse needs to recognize and accept negative feelings of the family while remaining realistic and not giving false assurances. Encouraging the family to express feelings, concerns, and expectations can be very helpful as they begin to adapt to the new situation. The family can be helped to see their baby as a unique individual. The nurse can point out the baby's specific responses. Bringing baby clothes and toys for their baby and taking photographs to share with siblings are ways to facilitate the attachment process. The baby's first name should be used by all personnel in communicating with the parents. In caring for the family of a preterm or sick baby, the goal should be to send a well baby home as a family member and not as a stranger.

Babies

The developmental needs of premature and sick babies are difficult to meet in an intensive care environment. Loud background noise and intensive light and sleep deprivation associated with NICUs are known to be major stressors for infants. When infants spend up to 3 months or more in these stressful situations, the NICU environment itself may be contributing to delayed cognitive, emotional, physical, neurological, and sensory development.

The nurse's challenge is to minimize the infant's stresses to foster development and optimize outcome. The standard of care in the nursery should include reduction in the intensity of background noise and modification of the intensity of lighting to mimic natural day-night cycles.

An intervention that is developmentally supportive might be to include rocking beds or water beds for an infant younger than 34 weeks of gestation. Another intervention could be skin-to-skin contact between infants and their parents (kangaroo care) for infants who are appropriate candidates.

A developmentally based approach to care in the nursery is a daily challenge for all NICU health care personnel. Nurses must take the lead in achieving the goal of sending home a developmentally supported infant.

COMPLICATIONS

Careful observation of the newborn is a vital nursing responsibility. Such observation coupled with prompt recognition and reporting of variations from normal can assure early initiation of treatment. An introduction to common newborn disorders and complications follows.

Respiratory Distress Problems

During the first hour after birth, tachypnea, retractions, flaring, and grunting may be seen in the normal infant. After the first hour the infant will not exhibit symptoms of respiratory distress because the newborn is absorbing lung fluid and readjusting circulation to the extrauterine environment. Cyanosis, however, is not normal and requires investigation and treatment.

Although there are numerous causes of respiratory distress in the newborn, only the most common problems will be introduced here.

Respiratory distress syndrome

Respiratory distress syndrome (RDS) is also known as idiopathic respiratory distress syndrome, hyaline membrane disease (old nomenclature), surfactant deficiency syndrome, or neonatal atelectasis. RDS primarily involves preterm babies with immature lungs and accounts for about 25% of deaths in the neonatal period and approximately 50% to 70% of all premature deaths.

In these babies there is a relative lack of surfactant in the alveoli in the lungs. This surfactant is a complex of phospholipids in which the phospholipids lecithin, sphingomyelin, and phosphatidylglycerol (PG) can be measured. Without this surfactant, the alveoli collapse and gases cannot be exchanged. It is possible to sample the amniotic fluid by amniocentesis to measure the surfactant levels before birth.

If possible, induction of labor and cesarean birth can be delayed until the ratio of lecithin to sphingomyelin (L/S) is 2 or greater (L/S ratio). An L/S ratio of 2.0 or greater indicates maturity of lung tissue. The presence of phosphatidylgylcerol (PG) confirms maturity and is especially important in the presence of maternal conditions such as diabetes to determine fetal lung maturity.

One of the constant features of respiratory distress syndrome is the early onset of symptoms. Infants who breathe normally in the first 6 to 8 hours of life do not have RDS.

Signs of RDS may include intercostal, subclavicular, and substernal retractions; expiratory grunting; nasal flaring; chest lag on inspiration; decreased or unequal breath sounds; tachypnea; and tachycardia (Fig. 13-9).

Administration of corticosteroids to mothers 24 hours before delivery may reduce the severity and incidence of RDS. Corticosteroids (dexamethasone and betamethasone) accelerate the fetal production of surfactant.

The treatment of RDS includes respiratory support and correction of as many secondary factors as possible. Respirations must be immediately established and adequately maintained. Blood gas sampling is essential for managing a baby with RDS. The course of RDS has been dramatically altered by the use of respirators to prevent alveolar collapse. Continuous positive airway pressure (CPAP) is one of many techniques used in NICUs to treat newborns with RDS. Also, surfactant replacement therapy has shown promising results in the treatment of infants at risk for RDS. The advent of surfactant therapy may significantly reduce the duration of hospitalization of preterm babies.

Transient tachypnea of the newborn (TTNB)

As its name indicates, transient tachypnea of the newborn is a transient condition (affected babies recover). Some babies, particularly those born by cesarean, may have delayed absorption of lung fluid after birth. These babies may have mild to moderate signs of respiratory distress with a respiratory rate of 60 to 140 breaths per minute. There is good air exchange, minimal retractions, and some grunting. Cyanosis is not prominent, but a small percentage of infants may require oxygen to remain pink. This condition is generally not considered pathological and passes within a few days. Nursing care for TTNB is largely supportive.

Meconium aspiration syndrome (MAS)

Meconium is present in the amniotic fluid in 5% to 20% of all births. Some fetuses swallow or aspirate the meconium, which is then inspired more deeply into the

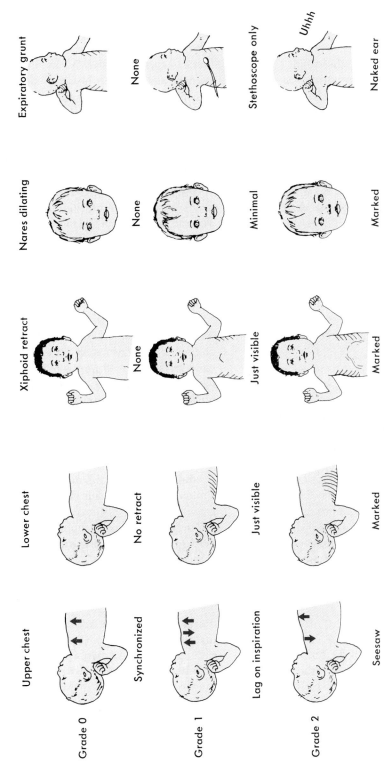

Figure 13-9 Silverman-Anderson index of respiratory distress designed to provide a continuous evaluation of the infant's respiratory status. An index of respiratory distress is determined by values assigned to five criteria: chest lag, intercostal retraction, xiphoid retraction, nares dilation, and expiratory grunt. A score of 0 indicates no respiratory distress; a score of 10 indicates severe respiratory distress. *(From Bobak IM and others: Maternity and gynecologic care: the nurse and the family, ed 5, St. Louis, 1993, Mosby.)*

alveoli with the first breaths. When meconium is present in the amniotic fluid, it is recommended that the baby's airway be cleared by gentle suction as soon as the head is born. This can be accomplished before the chest is delivered to reduce the amount of meconium present in the baby's airway. As mentioned previously, positive pressure breathing should be avoided until most of the meconium has been removed from the infant's lung. Complications of MAS may include pulmonary hemorrhage, pneumonia, severe asphyxia, and infection. A complication of meconium aspiration in 20% to 30% of cases is pneumothorax.

Pneumothorax

Pneumothorax is air outside the lungs and airways, but in the thoracic cavity. A pneumothorax is sometimes referred to as "collapsed lung." It may occur spontaneously, as a result of trauma, or as a result of some other pathological process. Sudden deterioration of the baby's clinical condition follows a pneumothorax. Sudden cyanosis, dyspnea, irritability, and restlessness denoting air hunger are present. The breath sounds over the affected side or lobe diminish, and signs of shock follow. This is an emergency situation requiring immediate medical care.

Apnea

Irregular breathing patterns are common in newborns and particularly in preterm babies. Characteristically these babies will have a cyclical breathing pattern with rapid respirations followed by 5- to 10-second episodes of no breathing (apneic pauses). However, if the periods of apnea are prolonged, they may be the first signs of hypoglycemia, infection, or neurological damage. Close observation and a thorough diagnostic work-up are indicated for infants with apnea.

Gentle physical stimulation of the newborn's extremities can stimulate breathing when apneic pauses occur.

ECMO

Mechanical ventilation and high concentrations of oxygen for neonatal respiratory failure can result in worsening lung disease and barotrauma, which can lead to oxygen toxicity disease or bronchopulmonary dysplasia (BPD) and pulmonary fibrosis. *Extracorporeal membrane oxygenation* (ECMO) is a life-support measure that utilizes a modified heart lung machine to bypass the neonate's blood to an artificial membrane to remove CO_2 and add O_2 to the blood. Thus diseased lungs are allowed a healing period.

In addition to infants with bronchopulmonary dys-

plasia, newborns presenting with meconium aspiration syndrome, congenital diaphragmatic hernia, respiratory distress syndrome, persistent pulmonary hypertension, or sepsis can benefit from the use of ECMO.

Because of the severity of illness before ECMO, neurodevelopmental and medical follow-up are important. Studies to date that have examined the outcomes of infants treated with ECMO have found the majority of ECMO survivors to be developmentally normal. The rate of significant morbidity in infants after receiving ECMO is similar to that of non-ECMO patients with comparably severe illnesses.

CONGENITAL PROBLEMS

Congenital problems are those malformations that occur during intrauterine life. These anomalies are present at and existing from the time of birth.

Cleft Lip and/or Cleft Palate

Cleft lip and *cleft palate* are conditions in which there is failure of growth and union of the bony or soft tissue structures on one (unilateral) or both (bilateral) sides of the midline of the palate and upper jaw. Occurrence of each is approximately 1 in 800 births. It is possible to have a normal lip and defective palate, a defective lip and normal palate, or both defects. These defects are obvious on gross examination and can be corrected by surgical repair. Depending on the severity, the surgerical repair may be immediate or delayed until 2 years of age. Several successive operations may be necessary.

Infants with a cleft lip or palate are difficult to feed. Feeding techniques include use of a palate prosthesis, a rubber-tipped medicine dropper, an Asepto syringe, or a special nipple. Because these babies swallow a lot of air, they need frequent bubbling or burping and should be held in an upright position during feedings to prevent aspiration.

Hydrocephalus

Hydrocephalus is a condition characterized by abnormal accumulation of cerebrospinal fluid within the skull, with enlargement of the head. Hydrocephalus may be caused by an obstruction of the cerebrospinal fluid pathways or by overproduction or defective absorption of the cerebrospinal fluid.

Hydrocephalus may be recognized at birth, or it may not be evident until later. When it is present before birth, the labor can be long and difficult because of cephalopelvic disproportion.

Surgical treatment consists of inserting a shunting device that bypasses the point of obstruction and drains the excess fluid into a body cavity. Many affected infants show brain damage at birth. The shunting procedure often prevents further damage.

Neural Tube Defects

Neural tube defects are common congenital malformations of the central nervous system and include anencephaly, spina bifida, and encephalocele. These defects result from improper development of the embryonic neural tube.

In the United States the frequency of neural tube defects at birth is 1 to 2 per 1000 live births. Elevated alpha-fetoprotein levels in amniotic fluid are associated with the presence of open neural tube defects in the fetus. Thus prenatal detection by amniotic fluid analysis of alpha-fetoprotein is possible for women known to be at high risk for neural tube defects.

In *anencephaly,* the vault of the brain is absent and the brain is rudimentary or amorphous. The appearance of such infants is usually shocking to everyone—parents, nurses, and physicians. Often parents want to see and hold their infants in spite of the appearance. Covering the missing part of the baby's skull with a blanket or cap can make the newborn's appearance less shocking for the parents. Most infants with anencephaly are either stillborn or die within 15 days of birth.

Spina bifida is a spinal malformation in which the bony part of the spinal canal fails to close, presenting an opening through which the spinal meninges and spinal cord may or may not protrude. If the meninges do not protrude and the defect is only of the vertebrae, the spina bifida may present no problems *(spina bifida occulta)*. When the meninges bulge through the opening of the spinal cavity, they form a cystic sac known as *meningocele* (Fig. 13-10). Because no nerve roots are involved, there is no paralysis or lack of sphincter control below the lesion. A meningocele can be corrected by surgical removal of the sac with closure of the skin, and prognosis is excellent.

If nerve fibers as well as the meninges protrude through the defect in bony rings of the spinal canal, the condition is known as *meningomyelocele* (or *myelomeningocele*), in which there may be partial or total paralysis below the lesion. With surgical correction, the neurological deficit can be improved. There is a danger of the sac rupturing and the baby developing meningitis in either of these cases.

Encephalocele is a cranial defect through which meninges and brain tissue protrude. Encephalocele is usually seen in the occipital area, and the affected area is often covered with skin.

Anencephaly and spina bifida account for approximately 95% of neural tube defects, and encephalocele accounts for the remaining 5%.

Nursing care is mainly protective and routine until

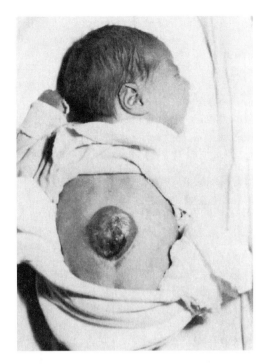

Figure 13-10 Meningocele. *(From Lerch C, Bliss VJ: Maternity nursing, ed 3, St. Louis, 1978, Mosby.)*

surgery can be done. Every effort must be made to protect the sac from pressure and to minimize the danger of infection from urine and feces. Special consideration and support must be given to the parents to help them understand the care and prognosis for their infant's special circumstance.

Imperforate Anus

If a membrane that separates the rectum from the anus is not absorbed in the 8th week of embryonic life, an *imperforate anus* results. The following symptoms are present: no stool is passed, no anal opening is found, and abdominal distention eventually occurs. Surgical correction is needed, and prognosis is good.

Tracheoesophageal Anomalies

Tracheoesophageal fistula with esophageal atresia (TEF/EA) is the most common tracheoesophageal anomaly. An average incidence of 0.15 per 1000 births has been reported in the United States. In this anomaly the esophagus ends in a blind pouch (atresia) with a fistula that connects it to the trachea. Clinical signs of TEF/EA may include excessive drooling, excessive mucus in the upper airway, choking, cyanosis, and regurgitation with feeding. Low birth weight, polyhydramnios, and multiple anomalies are associated with TEF/EA. Although there are reports of familial occurrence, heredity has not been established. Surgical intervention is essential.

Nursing care is directed at preventing aspiration until surgery is performed. Nursing care includes positioning, suctioning, humidification, chest physiotherapy, intravenous fluids, electrolytes, antibiotics, and comforting to keep infant's crying to a minimum. Taking time to communicate with the parents and provide accurate information regarding care is important.

Pyloric Stenosis

The pylorus is the junction of the stomach and small intestine. In *pyloric stenosis*, the musculature of the pylorus increases in size and forms a mass that constricts the opening of the pylorus and impedes emptying of the stomach.

Within 2 to 4 weeks of life the infant begins projectile vomiting, fails to gain weight, becomes dehydrated, and has fewer and fewer bowel movements. Surgical correction is needed, and prognosis is good.

Down Syndrome

Down syndrome results from chromosomal abnormalities. Its most common cause is trisomy of the chromosome 21, making a total of 47 chromosomes instead of the normal 46. This abnormality is most likely to happen when the mother is over the age of 40. The two other types of chromosomal abnormalities that cause Down syndrome are less common. (1) In *translocation* of a chromosome during cell division, the chromosome count is still 46, but 2 chromosomes are misplaced. This can occur in infants born to young women. (2) In *mosaicism*, the least common cause of Down syndrome, the affected infant has a different number of chromosomes in some cells than in others.

The infant with Down syndrome may have physical defects, with deformities most often noticed in the face. The eyes are set close together and slanted, the nose is flat, and the tongue is large and usually protrudes. The level of mental retardation in these babies varies greatly.

Phenylketonuria

Phenylketonuria (PKU) is a congenital inborn error of metabolism that, if not diagnosed and treated within a month or two after birth, will result in permanent mental retardation. In PKU the baby is unable to metabolize the protein phenylalanine, permitting accumulation of phenylalanine and its metabolic products (phenylketones) in body fluids. PKU can be treated by a diet low in phenylalanine.

PKU can be detected within a few days after birth by means of a simple blood test. After 4 to 6 weeks of age, a urine test can be done to detect PKU. Most states

have public health laws requiring that all newborns be tested for PKU by the age of 28 days.

With a simple blood test of the newborn, genetic screening is possible for eight genetic diseases of which PKU is one. The others are galactosemia, maple syrup urine disease (MSUD), homocystinuria (HCU), hypothyroidism, sickle cell anemia, cystic fibrosis (CF), and biotinidase deficiency. (See Table 13-2 for details.)

Umbilical Hernia

An *umbilical hernia* is a protrusion of a portion of the small intestine or omentum through a weak or incompletely closed umbilical ring. Surgical correction is needed.

Disorders of the Blood

Hyperbilirubinemia is an elevated level of bilirubin in the blood; it makes the baby's skin look yellow (jaundice). Bilirubin is expressed in milligrams per 100 milliliters of blood (e.g., 5 milligrams per 100 milliliters; this value would be abbreviated as 5 mg %).

Bilirubin is the end product of hemoglobin breakdown. There are two kinds of bilirubin, indirect and direct. Indirect (unconjugated) bilirubin is the by-product of red blood cell breakdown. Because indirect bilirubin is fat soluble, it cannot be easily excreted in bile or urine. To be excreted indirect bilirubin must be converted (conjugated) to the direct (water-soluble) form of bilirubin by the liver.

Because after birth the infant no longer needs the large amount of hemoglobin needed in utero, the red blood cells begin to break down. Often the infant's immature liver is not able to clear all the bilirubin, and thus the bilirubin is reabsorbed into the infant's circulatory system as unmetabolized bilirubin (indirect or unconjugated). As the circulatory system carries this bilirubin to all body tissues, dilute bilirubin is seen in the skin and sclera as jaundice. Visible jaundice usually occurs when serum bilirubin levels exceed 5 milligrams per 100 milliliters.

Normal physiological jaundice occurs on the second or third day of life in 60% of term babies. Physiological jaundice occurs on the second to ninth day of life in 80% of preterm babies.

Jaundice appearing before the baby is 24 hours old may be *pathological jaundice* usually caused by Rh or ABO incompatibilities. Prematurity, hemorrhage, infection, acidosis, low serum albumin levels, and certain drugs (see Appendices A and D) also predispose an infant to hyperbilirubinemia.

Jaundice associated with breast-feeding can occur as early as the third day after birth. If a breast-fed baby develops jaundice during the first week after birth, the

TABLE 13-2
Eight Genetic Diseases

What diseases can these tests detect?	What causes the disorder?	How often does it occur?	What happens if it is not found and treated?	How is it treated?
Phenylketonuria (PKU) (fee-nil-key'-tone-yer-ee-ah)	The body cannot break down certain parts of proteins (the amino acid phenylalanine).	One in 15,000 newborns	Children become mentally retarded.	A special diet
Galactosemia (gal-ak-toe-see'-me-ah)	The body cannot break down a certain sugar (galactose) found in dairy products.	One in 70,000 newborns	Children become very sick, have liver and eye damage, and become mentally retarded.	A special diet
Maple syrup urine disease (MSUD)	The body cannot break down certain parts of proteins (the amino acids leucine, isoleucine, and valine).	One in 200,000 newborns	Children could become very sick (and may die) or become mentally retarded.	A special diet
Homocystinuria (HCU) (ho-mow-sis'-tin-yer-ee-ah)	The body cannot break down certain parts of proteins (the amino acid methionine).	One in 100,000 newborns	Children may have problems with their eyes, bones, and blood clotting, as well as mental retardation.	A special diet (sometimes a vitamin B_6 supplement)
Hypothyroidism (hi-po-thigh'-roid-ism)	The thyroid gland does not produce enough of a special hormone (chemical) called thyroxine.	One in 4500 newborns	Children do not grow and develop properly, and they become mentally retarded.	Supplement of thyroxine
Sickle cell anemia (sick'-al cell a-knee-me-ah)	The red blood cells have a tendency to change from the normal round shape to an abnormal sickle shape, which may cause a blockage of blood flow to the body's tissues.	One in every 500 black newborns; less common in other ethnic groups	Children have frequent problems with infections, growth, anemia, and recurring episodes of pain.	Treatment can minimize the frequency and severity of problems
Cystic fibrosis (CF) (sis-tick fi-bro'-sis)	Certain glands produce abnormal mucus, and the child has difficulty digesting certain foods.	One in 3000 newborns	Children have problems with growth and lung infections.	Treatment can minimize the frequency and severity of problems
Biotinidase deficiency (bi-o-tin'-e-dase) deficiency	The body cannot properly use a necessary vitamin.	One in 40,000 newborns	Children may have seizures, mental retardation, hair loss, skin rashes, and sudden death.	Supplement of the vitamin biotin

From The Rocky Mountain Regional Newborn Genetic Screening: *Laboratory tests that make sense for your baby.* (Courtesy Colorado Department of Health Laboratory, Denver.)

baby should be evaluated as if not breast-fed. Supplements of formula such as water are not needed unless dehydration can be documented. The mother may continue to breast-feed.

Breast milk jaundice is a separate entity from jaundice associated with breast-feeding. In rare instances (1% to 2% of all breast-fed babies), a substance found in human milk interferes with the metabolism of bilirubin. Such jaundice usually develops during the second or third week after birth. Depending on the level of bilirubin and response of the baby, temporary interruption of breast-feeding is considered. Substituting with formula and using phototherapy for 48 to 72 hours allows the bilirubin to decline, and breast-feeding can be resumed.

Rh incompatibility

Rh incompatibility occurs when an Rh-negative mother gives birth to an Rh-positive baby. If a small amount of the fetal blood has entered the mother's bloodstream during pregnancy, at the time of spontaneous or induced abortion, or at birth, she may have formed Rh antibodies (sensitization). These Rh antibodies may have crossed the placenta, mixed with the blood of her fetus, and begun destroying the fetal red blood cells. Destruction of the red blood cells of the fetus is indicated by increased levels of bilirubin in the blood of the fetus.

When an Rh-negative mother gives birth, a sample of umbilical cord blood is tested to determine (1) blood group, (2) Rh factor, (3) hemoglobin level, (4) results of a Coombs' test, and (5) bilirubin levels. The Coombs' test measures the amount of antibody present in the infant's circulation. A positive Coombs' test indicates that the baby's red blood cells are coated with antibodies. A positive Coombs' test, along with high bilirubin and low hemoglobin levels in the newborn, is an indication of erythroblastosis fetalis, a hemolytic disease of the newborn.

Erythroblastosis fetalis is destruction of the fetal red blood cells by maternal antibodies that cross the placenta and attack fetal red blood cell antigens. Mildly affected infants may have an enlarged liver or spleen at birth, but they look normal. Effects may range from mild hyperbilirubinemia and jaundice to severe anemia, congestive heart failure, and death.

Phototherapy may be used for treatment for mild hemolytic disease. Moreover, because the hemolytic process that began in utero continues after birth, replacing the baby's blood with an exchange transfusion may be necessary. Rh-negative blood is cross matched with the infant's blood, or type O Rh-negative blood is used.

Erythroblastosis is not commonly found in first babies. A specific gamma globulin, RhoGAM, has made erythroblastosis rare. (See Chapter 5.)

ABO incompatibility

When the mother's blood type is O and the baby's blood type is A or B, ABO incompatibility may develop. It is similar to Rh incompatibility but usually not severe because maternal anti-A and anti-B antibodies do not cross the placenta as readily or in as large amounts as the antibodies formed in Rh incompatibility. In ABO incompatibility the first baby may be affected, since previous exposure and sensitization are not required.

Kernicterus

Clinical toxicity of bilirubin in the neonatal period is known as *kernicterus*. This is a syndrome of neurological damage resulting from deposits of bilirubin in brain cells. Kernicterus is a very rare disease, although it does occur in a few preterm babies. Although kernicterus has been associated with unconjugated or indirect serum bilirubin levels over 20 milligrams per 100 milliliters, the "dangerous" level of bilirubin in the infant's blood is dependent on each infant's condition.

Whether and how to treat jaundice in a newborn depend first on the cause of the jaundice. Sepsis (infection) requires prompt identification of the infecting organism and immediate treatment with antibiotics. Most cases of physiological jaundice and of breast milk jaundice require no treatment. However, jaundice in preterm babies or in Rh sensitization may require immediate treatment. The key to treatment is to individualize decision making.

Nursing care. Babies must be observed closely for jaundice in the first days of life. For the most accurate color determination it is best to get the infant into daylight. Blanching the infant's skin by pressing gently on the chest, nose, forehead, or back of the neck and releasing pressure will reveal a yellow color if the baby is jaundiced.

In the screening procedure, called *transcutaneous bilirubinometry,* a hand-held screening device can estimate the amount of bilirubin in the baby's blood. This noninvasive procedure can quickly determine whether the newborn needs further laboratory determination of serum bilirubin levels. In transcutaneous bilirubinometry a spectrophotometric hand-held fiber-optic instrument is held for a few seconds against the baby's forehead. A white light flashes and a meter reads an estimation of the baby's bilirubin level from a window (the size of an adult fingertip). This instrument illuminates the skin and measures the intensity of the yellow color in the skin.

Phototherapy

Although exchange transfusion was formerly the most common treatment, today the most common treatment of hyperbilirubinemia is phototherapy. Exposure to the light's rays causes the unconjugated bilirubin in the infant's circulation to undergo chemical decomposition and to be changed into nontoxic products that are excreted in the urine and feces. The infant is exposed to fluorescent or incandescent lights that emit light at the appropriate wavelength. The effectiveness of phototherapy depends on the amount of radiant energy (not brightness) that strikes the infant's skin. This dose-response theory of phototherapy explains why the radiant flux of phototherapy lights should be measured frequently. Phototherapy lights should be changed when the irradiance falls below the level that is considered therapeutic for that particular light.

The infant's clothing is kept to a minimum, and preferably not even a diaper is worn. The eyes of the infant are shielded with patches during phototherapy. Vital signs must be checked every 2 hours, and the infant must be turned frequently. Temperature control and adequate fluid intake are important because the infant's body temperature can rise in response to the heat of the lights. Complications of phototherapy may include increased insensible water loss and dehydration; skin rash; and loose, green stools. Weight loss, lethargy, and tanning have also been reported. Parents should be informed about these side effects and supported when they occur. The lights should be turned off for eye care and blood samplings. Home phototherapy is an excellent alternative to hospitalization if the baby is well enough to be discharged to home care.

In standard phototherapy parents are not able to hold their babies except to feed them. However, a new method of phototherapy based on fiber-optic technology allows parents to handle their jaundiced newborns normally without concern over interfering with the light therapy. The light blanket or wrap is portable and literally wraps the baby in uniform, high-intensity light. The filtered fiber-optic light source eliminates ultraviolet and infrared radiation, thereby reducing the risk of skin and eye damage as well as the hazards of hyperthermia and dehydration. The blanket phototherapy allows the treated infant to be swaddled, held, and even nursed with continuous phototherapy treatment.

Sepsis Neonatorum

Sepsis neonatorum is a disease of infants less than 1 month of age who are clinically ill and who have positive blood cultures. Generally the incidence is only 1 in 1000 in full-term infants but can be as high as 1 in 250 in preterm infants. The first signs of sepsis may be vomiting, tachypnea, lethargy, failure to feed, inability to maintain body temperature, and gray or mottled skin color. The diagnosis of sepsis neonatorum is made by recovery of the pathogen from blood cultures. The septic baby should be cared for in a high-risk nursery. Antibiotics specific for the cultured organisms are used in treatment.

Hypoglycemia

For a term, normal-weight newborn the lower limit of blood glucose in the first 72 hours of life is 30 milligrams per 100 milliliters. After the first 3 days of life the lower limit is 40 milligrams per 100 milliliters. Low-birth-weight infants are considered to be hypoglycemic if the blood sugar level is less than 20 milligrams per 100 milliliters within the first 72 hours of life and 30 milligrams per 100 milliliters after 72 hours. Infants at risk for developing hypoglycemia are (1) small-for-gestational-age infants, (2) infants of diabetic mothers, and (3) severely stressed infants. A low blood glucose level is reflected by central nervous system dysfunctions, such as tremors, convulsions, apnea, lethargy, limpness, jittery or tremulous movements, and irregular respirations.

Early recognition and treatment of hypoglycemia in the newborn are vital because neurological impairment may occur if the brain is deprived of glucose.

Most hospitals treat low glucose levels by administering glucose. Asymptomatic infants who can be fed should be breast-fed or given glucose or formula as early as it is safely possible. Symptomatic infants and babies too sick or unable to feed may require continuous intravenous infusions of glucose. The rate of intravenous glucose is adjusted and tapered over time until blood glucose levels have been stable at 40 milligrams per 100 milliliters for 18 to 24 hours and the oral intake is sufficient to meet caloric needs.

Screening for hypoglycemia can be done by obtaining a drop of blood from the infant's heel and testing it for glucose level with reagent strips. In some hospitals this screening is a routine nursing procedure for all infants classified at risk for developing hypoglycemia.

SUMMARY

This chapter has presented only a brief introduction to the newborn with complications. If you are interested in the care of the newborn with complications, the sources listed at the end of this chapter will give you a place to begin your study.

BIBLIOGRAPHY

Avery G: *Neonatology: pathophysiology and management of the newborn*, ed 3, Philadelphia, 1987, JB Lippincott.
Blackburn S, Lowen L: Impact of an infant's premature birth

on the grandparents and parents, *J Obstet Gynecol Neonatal Nurs* 15(2):173-178, 1986.

Bobak IM, Jensen MD, Lowdermilk DL: *Maternity and gynecologic care: the nurse and the family,* ed 5, St. Louis, 1993, Mosby.

Cohen FL: Neural tube defects: epidemiology, detection, and prevention, *J Obstet Gynecol Neonatal Nurs* 16(2):105-115, 1986.

Dickason EJ, Schult MO, Silverman BL: *Maternal-infant nursing care,* ed 2, St. Louis, 1994, Mosby.

Drosten-Brooks F: Kangaroo care: skin to skin contact in the NICU, *MCN* 18:250-253, 1993.

Emergency drug doses for infant and children and naloxone use in newborns: clarification, *Pediatrics* 83(5):803, 1989.

Estrada EA: ECMO for neonatal and pediatric patients: state-of-the-art and future trends, *Pediatr Nurs* 18(1)67-73, 1992.

Gennaro S, Brooten D, Bakewell-Sachs S: Postdischarge services for low-birth-weight infants, *J Obstet Gynecol Neonatal Nurs* 20(1):29-36, 1991.

Gerraughty AB: ECMO: the artificial lung for gravely ill newborns, *Am J Nurs* 87:655A-658F, 1987.

Graven SN and others: The high-risk infant environment, Part 1. The role of the neonatal intensive care unit in the outcome of high-risk infants, *J Perinatol* 12(2):164-171, 1992.

Harrison LL, Twardosz S: Teaching mothers about their preterm infants, *J Obstet Gynecol Neonatal Nurs* 15(2):165-172, 1986.

Hughes M-A, McCollum J: Maternal stress and coping in the NICU: an exploratory study, *ACCH Advocate* 1(1):57-61, 1993.

Hughes M-A and others: How parents cope with the experience of neonatal intensive care, *Children's Health Care* 23(1):1-14, 1994.

Jones MB: A physiologic approach to identifying neonates at risk for kernicterus, *J Obstet Gynecol Neonatal Nurs* 19(4):313-318, 1990.

Koller CD: Medicine, machines, and magic tricks: parental perceptions of the benefits of family-centered care, *ACCH Advocate* 1(1):43-47, 1993.

Korones S: *High-risk newborn infants: the basis for intensive nursing care,* ed 4, St. Louis, 1986, Mosby.

Krause KD, Younger VL: Nursing diagnoses as guidelines in the care of the neonatal ECMO patient, *J Obstet Gynecol Neonatal Nurs* 21(3):169-176, 1992.

Langer VS: Minimal handling protocol for the intensive care nursery, *Neonatal Network* 9(3):23-27, 1990.

Lynam LE: Surfactant replacement therapy: a second look, *Neonatal Network* 9(3):79-81, 1990.

Mattson S, Smith JE, editors: *Core curriculum for maternal-newborn nursing,* Philadelphia, 1993, WB Saunders.

Miller EP, Armstrong CL: Surfactant replacement therapy: innovative care for the premature infant, *J Obstet Gynecol Neonatal Nurs* 19(1):14-17, 1990.

Nathan L and others: Meconium: a 1990s perspective on an old obstetric hazard, *Obstet Gynecol* 83(3):329-332, 1994.

Newman CB, McSweeney M: A descriptive study of sibling visitation in the NICU, *Neonatal Network* 9(4):27-31, 1990.

Newman TB, Klebanoff MA: Neonatal hyperbilirubinemia and long-term outcome: another look at the collaborative perinatal project, *Pediatrics* 92(5):651-657, 1993.

Novak JC, Broom BL: *Ingalls and Salerno's maternal and child health nursing,* ed 8, St. Louis, 1995, Mosby.

Parilla BV and others: Iatrogenic respiratory distress syndrome following elective repeat cesarean delivery, *Obstet Gynecol* 81(3):392-395, 1993.

Roberts PM, Jones MB: Extracorporeal membrane oxygenation and indications for cardiopulmonary bypass in the neonate, *J Obstet Gynecol Neonatal Nurs* 19(5):391-400, 1990.

Rose BS: Phototherapy: all wrapped up? *Pediatr Nurs* 16(1):57-58, 1990.

White-Trout RC and others: Environmental influences on the developing premature infant: theoretical issues and applications to practice, *J Obstet Gynecol Neonatal Nurs* 23(5):393-401, 1994.

DEFINITIONS

Define the following terms:

acidosis	lecithin
anencephaly	low-birth-weight baby
apnea	L/S ratio
barotrauma	meconium aspiration syndrome (MAS)
breast milk jaundice	
bronchopulmonary dysplasia	meningocele
	meningomyelocele
cleft lip and palate	phenylketonuria (PKU)
CPAP (continuous positive airway pressure)	phosphatidylglycerol (PG)
	phototherapy
Down syndrome	pneumothorax
ECMO	preterm baby
encephalocele	sphingomyelin
endotracheal tube	spina bifida
erythroblastosis fetalis	surfactant
gavage feeding	tachypnea
hydrocephalus	tracheoesophageal fistula
hyperbilirubinemia	transcutaneous bilirubinometry
hypoglycemia	
intubation	transient tachypnea of the newborn (TTNB)
kangaroo care	
kernicterus	
laryngoscope	

LEARNING ACTIVITIES

1. Group discussions.
2. Visit a neonatal intensive care nursery (NICU) for observation. What equipment is in use?
3. Is there a transport service available for sick newborns in your community? Where is the closest NICU?
4. View audiovisual aids and discuss.

ENRICHMENT/IN-DEPTH STUDY

1. Interview a family whose baby received care in a neonatal intensive care unit. What are their feelings about the experience?
2. Do you know a child born with a congenital defect? Have there been changes in the family's life-style because of this birth?

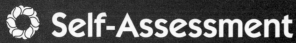
For questions 1 through 10, circle the best answer.

1. The infant with an Apgar score of 4 to 6 at birth will:

    a. probably require resuscitation

    b. not require any assistance

    c. need only gentle stimulation

2. A preterm baby is a live born infant whose:

    a. weight is less than 5 pounds

    b. gestation period is less than 38 weeks

    c. mother is sick

3. A small-for-gestational-age baby is one whose:

    a. birth weight is below the tenth percentile

    b. weight is less than 5 pounds

    c. gestation period is less than 38 weeks

4. A preterm baby is extremely susceptible to infection because of:

    a. an immature liver

    b. immature temperature-regulating mechanisms

    c. an immature immunological system

5. In stabilizing the preterm newborn, nursing care should include specialized care and environment because:

    a. the preterm infant has little chance of survival

    b. the preterm infant needs oxygen

    c. the preterm infant's body systems are immature

6. Signs of respiratory distress in the newborn include all but one of the following. Which of the following is *not* a sign of RDS?

    a. tachypnea

    b. nasal flaring

    c. elevated temperature

    d. expiratory grunt

    e. retractions

    f. cyanosis in room air

7. Babies with respiratory distress lack adequate surfactant in their lungs. Surfactant is needed to:

    a. clean the lungs

    b. produce amniotic fluid

    c. prevent alveolar collapse

8. Infants at risk for developing hypoglycemia are:

    a. full-term normal infants

    b. infants of diabetic mothers

    c. infants with PKU

9. The first evidence of sepsis in the newborn may be:

    a. flushing of the skin

    b. inability to maintain body temperature

    c. respiratory distress

10. Which one of the following breathing patterns in the newborn is pathological:

    a. transient tachypnea

    b. irregular breathing

    c. prolonged apneic spells

Supply the correct answer(s) for items 11 through 21.

11. The Silverman-Anderson index of respiratory distress is determined by values assigned to what five criteria?

    a. _____

    b. _____

    c. _____

    d. _____

    e. _____

12. Physiological jaundice is caused by _____.

13. Jaundice appearing before the baby is 24 hours old may be pathological and is usually caused by _____ and _____ incompatibilities.

14. List six causes of jaundice in the newborn:

    a. _____

    b. _____

    c. _____

    d. _____

    e. _____

    f. _____

15. The treatment of RDS includes _____ support and correction of as many secondary factors as possible.

16. What is a complication of meconium aspiration syndrome?

_____

17. The cry of a full-term baby is lusty and loud, and the cry of the preterm baby is _____ and _____.

18. What does nursing care of the infant receiving phototherapy for hyperbilirubinemia include?

_____

_____

_____

19. Explain what you would do for an infant who has an Apgar score of 3 at 1 minute of life. There was no meconium in the amniotic fluid.

_____

_____

_____

20. A preterm baby has just been transported by ambulance to a high-risk nursery. Explain to the parents what the high-risk nursery looks like and what care their baby will receive there.

_____

_____

_____

21. What could you do to offer support for these parents?

_____

_____

_____

22. Match Column A with Column B.

Column A

_____ 1. cleft lip and/or palate

_____ 2. hydrocephalus

_____ 3. spina bifida

_____ 4. Down syndrome

_____ 5. phenylketonuria

Column B

a. abnormal accumulation of cerebrospinal fluid

b. results from chromosome abnormalities

c. defective growth and union of bony and soft tissue structure

d. spinal malformation

e. inborn error of metabolism

23. Match Column A with Column B.

Column A

_____ 1. postterm baby

_____ 2. SGA baby

Column B

a. hypoglycemia

b. meconium aspiration

24. Match Column A with Column B.

Column A

Lower limits of normal for blood glucose

_____ 1. Term infants: before 72 hours of age

_____ 2. Term infants: after 72 hours of age

Column B

a. 30 milligrams per milliliter

b. 20 milligrams per milliliter

c. 40 milligrams per milliliter

d. 50 milligrams per milliliter

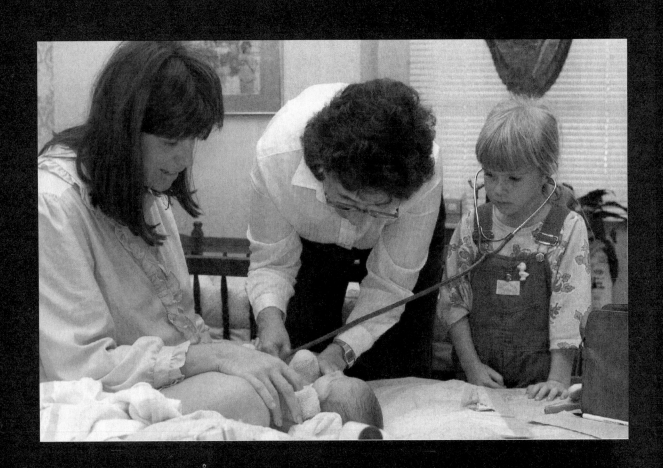

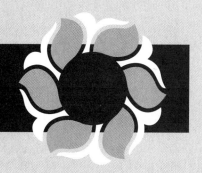

14

CONTINUITY OF CARE

GOALS

This chapter is designed to provide the reader with information that will:
- develop awareness of the need for continuity of care for the childbearing family in an era of short-stay maternity.
- serve as a framework for a continuity of care management model for the childbearing years.

STUDENT OBJECTIVES

After studying this chapter, you should be able to:

1. Discuss the evolution to short-stay maternity care and perinatal home care from a historical perspective.
2. List the pros and cons of short-stay maternity programs.
3. Identify the components of short-stay maternity programs.
4. Identify nursing skills needed for quality postpartum care of mothers and babies in their home.
5. Describe postpartum nursing care for the mother, infant, and family in the home.
6. List common problems found in both mother and baby during postpartum home visits.
7. List five care management tools.
8. Explain how case management can be utilized in the provision of maternity care.

INTRODUCTION

Maternity care, like most of health care, is going through dramatic shifts. Lengths of stay have been shortened, and many services have been moved from inpatient to outpatient care. Today a mother and her newborn may go home in 24 hours or less after a vaginal birth and in 48 hours following a cesarean birth.

In order to provide safe, quality maternity care in a 24-hour or less period of hospitalization, the hospital must extend its walls into the community, focus on prevention and wellness, and view the childbearing event as a continuum. A hospital stay of 24 hours for normal birth is only one small piece of the childbearing year. To move women and their families quickly and safely through the brief hospital experience, it is essential that the childbearing year be managed in a coordinated fashion by multidisciplinary teams (Fig. 14-1).

Short-Stay Maternity

Often what short-stay means to hospital maternity staffs is not enough time. What it really means is greater intensity of the hospital experience that is only one part of a short-stay program beginning in the community and following the family home again. A great deal of the work should be done before the expectant family arrives at the hospital. The hospital stay itself must maximize the short postpartum time with nonseparation of mother and baby through the provision of mother-baby nursing care and then follow-up by telephone or home visits to support the transition to parenting.

Philosophy

The basic philosophy behind short stay is a belief in the normalcy of childbearing and family formation. When health care providers perceive birth as a transition to parenting, they understand that childbirth is more than a physiological event requiring medical and nursing skills. They understand the importance of this event to families having a developmental and situational

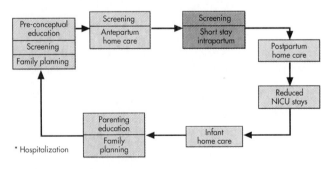

Figure 14-1 Care management for the childbearing year.

crisis and, as a result, develop maternity programs that include services needed throughout the entire childbearing year: prenatal, intrapartum, and postpartum. These programs are designed to promote the integrity of the family.

The normal processes of physiological restoration and psychological adaptation of the mother and physiological adaptation of the baby require assessment, support, nurturing, and teaching. In many instances new mothers are discharged early from hospitals without adequate follow-up.

Evolution to Short Stay

After World War I there was a decrease in the availability of family members or friends who could provide domestic help, so women stayed in the hospital for up to 2 weeks when their babies were born. During World War II the length of stay for childbirth decreased to 10 days. This was not for medical reasons but for social reasons; that is, there was a shortage of nurses was due to increased demand for nursing in military facilities and on the battlefields.

In the 1950s hospital stays for childbirth decreased again—this time to 7 days—because of a shortage of hospital beds and staff. In 1962 the first major study on safety of short stay for maternity was conducted by Hellman. At that time the average length of stay for childbirth was 6 days. Because there were not enough beds in the hospital where he worked, Hellman sent selected babies home in 24 to 48 hours and found the practice to be safe for both the mothers and babies chosen for early discharge.

During the alternative birth era (1970s) the primary reason U.S. hospitals favored early discharge was to offer alternatives to traditional hospital labor and delivery care and to attract parents who might opt for home birth. In the 1980s with the pressure on cost containment, programs of home care were provided for most mothers and babies who were discharged from hospitals early (2 to 3 days). And now in the 1990s the length of stay for well mothers and babies is shortening to 12 to 24 hours postpartum. Once again, the driving force is not medical but social; that is, the need for hospitals to control health care costs in an era of managed care and health care reform.

Literature Review

As data have become available about how new mothers and their babies respond to short-stay maternity programs, it has been demonstrated that most low-risk mother-baby pairs, with adequate follow-up, tend to do just fine. Since 1943 in articles published related to early discharge, the topics of medical safety, consumer satisfaction, and cost savings have been addressed. A brief summary of programs for short stay as reported in the literature follows.

Program development

Multidisciplinary teams, literature reviews, and input from present community practices and from consumers were considered imperative during the planning of short-stay obstetrics (OB) programs.

Criteria for participation

Each program had established criteria for participants, and most programs had an enrollment procedure. Participants were able to enroll anytime during pregnancy. Another important criterion for the programs was that the family planned before delivery for supportive help at home following discharge. This plan was reviewed and discussed by the family and nurse before hospital admission. Finally, most programs had physical criteria established for mother and baby that were followed closely before an early discharge was considered. In all programs final approval for discharge was made by a physician or certified nurse-midwife (CNM).

Program phases

The phases of most short-stay maternity programs discussed in the literature were as follows: antepartum planning and education, in-hospital postpartum assessment, support, education, home visit or telephone follow-up, and program evaluation. One program had a home visit before hospital admission; another had an interview with the consumer to assess the home situation and educational needs before hospitalization. Most of the programs had prenatal classes established for both early discharge program participants and traditional care consumers.

Postpartum care

In-hospital postpartum care ranged from 12 to 48 hours following delivery. Continuous assessment of mother and baby using established physical criteria for discharge was a part of all programs. Several programs had systematic approaches for education of families before discharge from the hospital. In one program worksheets were filled out by the staff as the knowledge level of the family was assessed related to competence in self-care for mother, care of infant, and feeding techniques. This worksheet then followed the family home to be used as a beginning point for in-home education.

Home follow-up

The home follow-up process varied. In some programs visits were made each day through the fourth postpartum day, then a last visit was made 2 weeks later. Another approach consisted of visits made on the second or third postpartum day, with another visit made a week later. In several programs in which the initial visit was not made the day following discharge, a telephone call was made to the home within 24 hours of discharge. The families always went home with telephone numbers to call if help was needed. In most of the programs the home visit staff were "on call" for 24 hours a day, 7 days a week for families in the program.

In all programs medical safety was demonstrated. Readmissions were very limited, with most of the readmissions for babies with hyperbilirubinemia. Complications in the mothers were handled by the home visit staff and were not related to the early discharge.

Evaluation

In the majority of the programs consumer satisfaction was determined by surveys completed by the new mothers following discharge from the program. Most of the time these women reported they would recommend the program to their friends.

Economic feasibility was another form of evaluation. In the programs that addressed economics, a substantial savings over costs for normal length of stay was shown.

Numerous studies have concluded that (1) early discharge of selected mother-baby pairs is safe, (2) consumers are satisfied, and (3) cost savings for hospitals have resulted from short-stay maternity programs.

Pros

In addition to early discharge being safe and satisfying for low-risk mother-baby pairs, it has been recognized that an early return home may help minimize the disruption in family life created by hospitalization for childbirth. Parent-infant interactions can be enhanced in the familiar environment of the family's home. In leaving the hospital environment early both mother and baby have decreased exposure to hospital pathogens, thus reducing the risk of nosocomial and iatrogenic complications.

A benefit to all of short-stay programs for maternity care is that shorter hospital stays reduce health care costs. In journal articles definite savings of 30% to 40% are described. These benefits are significant in a time of dwindling financial resources for health care.

Cons

Many caregivers express ambivalence and frustration about early discharge because they are concerned about the potential for undetected parenting problems: inadequacy, abuse, neglect, etc. There is also a concern about the possibility for under diagnosis or delayed diagnosis of medical conditions in the newborn, and even over diagnosis of medical conditions after the family has returned home, resulting in readmissions of babies for hyperbilirubinemia, weight loss, and to rule out sepsis.

In addition, there is the concern for the psychological safety of the mother who is experiencing maternity blues at home without professional support. Since early discharge has the mother returning home with limited breast-feeding experience, there is also concern about the lack of professional support and education she will receive for lactation.

In a March 1994 position statement, the Association of Women's Health, Obstetric and Neonatal Nurses (AWHONN) cited the following position:

AWHONN believes that mothers, newborns, and families need professional nursing care during the early postpartum period. Therefore, AWHONN supports the development of comprehensive maternity-care programs that include creative methods to deal with the fiscal issues, while addressing the physical, educational, and emotional needs of mothers, newborns, and families. After discharge from the hospital, opportunities for continuing perinatal care should be available through out-patient, ambulatory, and community-based nursing services.

The current information on short-stay maternity indicates that the advantages of early discharge outweigh the disadvantages, provided no compromise is made with mother and infant safety. Family education, preparation for short stay, health surveillance through postpartum phone or home follow-up, and close collaboration among physicians and nurses are all needed for short-stay maternity programs to provide safe, quality care. The focus is on CONTINUITY OF CARE throughout the childbearing year.

Goals

Short-stay maternity programs focus on providing the family with the skills/tools they will need to grow and take responsibility for their own health and that of their children. The goal is to help the childbearing family make the transition to their new roles safely and with

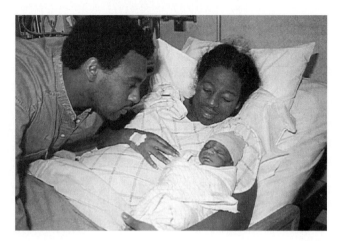

Figure 14-2 Transition to new roles. *(Courtesy Marjorie Pyle, RNC, Lifecircle, Costa Mesa, Calif.)*

optimum outcomes in a cost-effective program (Fig. 14-2). To achieve this goal the nurse functions in an expanded role as educator, facilitator, advocate, and care provider. Care changes from a paternalistic style to one of joint participation.

PROGRAM DEVELOPMENT

The optimum way to assure safety in early hospital discharge following childbirth is through short-stay programs that include sufficient antepartum planning and education, risk screening with appropriate referrals and care, postpartum mother-baby nursing care, and home follow-up.

Antepartum Planning/Prenatal Evaluation

The first component is antepartum planning with prenatal education that emphasizes preparation for short stay. Well defined risk screening criteria for both mother and baby are needed, and the focus is on collaborative care with health professionals and the family as a team.

Prenatal education that enhances family awareness and emphasizes their responsibility for self-care is important. In providing this education the goal is to prepare families for what to expect during pregnancy, childbirth, the postpartum period, and first weeks home. As a result they will be more receptive to early discharge from the hospital.

It is believed that most fathers who participate in the prenatal period are more likely to support the mother throughout the childbearing experience. Thus father's participation is encouraged unless his involvement violates cultural taboos or expectations. When prepared to participate together in the childbearing experience, most families will receive satisfaction from making the birth a shared family experience and will have increased self-confidence in their parenting roles.

Prenatal contact with the hospital staff provides an opportunity for families to develop a trusting relationship with interested staff who will provide care for the family during the birth and postpartum period. In addition to infant care and childbirth/prenatal classes, prenatal preparation can be assisted with pregnancy and parenting newsletters delivered at separate intervals throughout pregnancy, instructional videotapes, support groups, and reading materials.

Prenatal risk screening can identify women at risk for pregnancy complications and begin appropriate prenatal care. When problems are identified early, life-style behaviors that contribute to pregnancy risk can be lowered. If the pregnancy is at risk due to medical problems, corrective treatment can begin early in pregnancy, thus lowering the woman's risk and significantly reducing costs for hospitalization of herself and her baby.

Criteria

In *Guidelines for Perinatal Care,* AAP and ACOG (1988), recognizing that the average length of stay for normal OB has been shortened to 1 or 2 days, special exclusion criteria for early discharge were no longer cited. The emphasis was placed on follow-up assessments instead. Maternal and neonatal follow-up care was described to include the following components:

1. A structured discharge plan
2. An assessment of the physical and psychosocial status of both mother and neonate
3. A discussion between the physician or another health care professional and the mother (and father if possible) about any expected perinatal problems and ways to cope with them
4. A plan for future care, both immediate and long range

Thus in *Guidelines,* plans for continuity of care and adequate follow-up care of both the mother and the baby are the focus, and interdisciplinary efforts are encouraged.

Antepartum home monitoring and nursing home care programs for high-risk pregnant women have demonstrated improved outcomes. Therefore antepartal risk screening and appropriate home care and home monitoring are changing thoughts about excluding even at-risk patients from early discharge. With education, antepartal home care, and preparation for birth and parenting, some women who were previously not considered to be candidates for short stay may now qualify.

In-Hospital Postpartum Care

Postpartum hospitalization is no longer a time for the new mother to simply rest. She will have to do that at home after her brief hospitalization. Instead, during short stay postpartum health care providers observe the mother and baby long enough to identify most maternal and neonatal complications. They also provide professional assistance to the family unit during this time of great adjustment and maternal discomfort. Through role modeling and facilitating care to the mother-baby couplet, they provide adequate teaching so the parents may return home capable of maternal self-care as well as providing basic care to the newborn.

Mother-baby nursing

With length of stay for postpartum women and infants shortened to 12 to 24 hours, nursing care provided to the postpartum mother and newborn needs to be adjusted to the decreased amount of time available. The nursing model that can optimize mother-infant care and teaching is mother-baby nursing.

Mother-baby nursing is not rooming-in. Instead, mother-baby nursing is a form of primary nursing care. Also known as couplet care or dyad care, mother-baby nursing utilizes one nurse to care jointly for both a postpartum mother and her newborn as a single unit. Both physiologically and psychologically the newborn infant and postpartum mother are viewed as an interdependent couplet with mother-baby nursing. Mother-baby nursing can be defined as the delivery of safe, quality health care while recognizing, focusing on, and adapting to both the physical and psycho-social needs of the new mother, the family, and the newborn. The emphasis is on the provision of maternal and newborn care that fosters family unity while maintaining physical safety. Because this type of nursing differs from the conventional model of maternity nursing that utilizes subspecialties, the mother-baby nursing model requires reorganization. (See Chapter 10.)

Cross-training

For the transition from traditional maternity nursing care to mother-baby care to be accomplished, a merger of postpartum and well baby nursery staff must occur. This requires additional educational preparation for each nurse involved. Postpartum nurses must be oriented to the fundamentals of newborn care; nursery nurses must be oriented to the fundamentals of postpartum care. In this process the nursery and postpartum staffs are combined to form one mother-baby unit, and the new mother-baby model of nursing care is implemented.

Care

Care for the mother-baby couplet is individualized by the nurse responsible for care of the couplet (Fig. 14-3). This care includes assessment of both mother and baby; establishment of mother-baby care plans or following an established care path; physical care (e.g., baths, linen changes, I and O, sitz baths, treatments), vital signs, medication, feedings, weights, stools, voidings, Dextrostix, Hct, cord care, etc.; individual and group teaching and discharge planning; referrals to home care as necessary; charting on mother's and baby's charts at the bedside; and mother-baby report to on-coming staff (utilizing care plan and critical path).

While carrying out responsibilities, individual instruction is provided as needed to promote family togetherness. This teaching is streamlined; using a self-assessment tool (see the box below), the mother identifies what she "needs to know." Although this is often not what the nurse would "like her to know," a mother's self-assessment of learning needs allows the nurse to focus on what is most important for each woman in a short period postpartum.

It is important to utilize teaching aids in the form of videos, booklets, and individualized specific written instructions on printed handouts. In mother-baby nursing the nurse teaches through demonstration and role modeling while caring for mother and baby together.

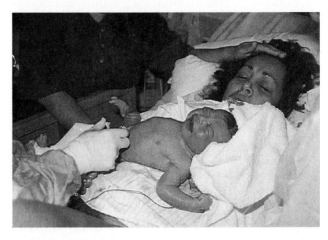

Figure 14-3 The mother-baby couplet. *(Courtesy Marjorie Pyle, RNC, Lifecircle, Costa Mesa, Calif.)*

Self-Assessment

We want to help you to take good care of yourself and your baby, so we have provided a list of topics that are important to new mother and baby care. Please feel free to check the boxes for topics you want to review with your mother-baby nurse, and return this list to your nurse as soon as possible.

Needs: Mother
- ☐ Rest and activity
- ☐ Breast care
  1. Breast-feeding
  2. Bottle-feeding
- ☐ Medications
- ☐ Exercises
- ☐ What foods to eat
- ☐ Birth control

- ☐ Body changes after delivery
- ☐ When to call your physician

- ☐ Dieting
- ☐ Sexual activity
- ☐ Baby blues and fatigue
- ☐ Pain control
- ☐ Adjustment of your other children
- ☐ Other _____

Needs: Baby
- ☐ Breast-feeding
- ☐ Bottle-feeding
- ☐ Bathing
  1. Cord care
  2. Circumcision care
  3. Uncircumcised care
  4. Skin care
- ☐ Calming the fussy baby
- ☐ Normal sleep patterns
- ☐ Using a pacifier
- ☐ Diapering and clothing
- ☐ Urine
- ☐ Diaper rash

- ☐ Safety
- ☐ When to call baby's physician
- ☐ Car seat safety

- ☐ Taking a temperature
- ☐ Protection from accidents
- ☐ Immunizations/baby shots
- ☐ Constipation or diarrhea
- ☐ Baby products
- ☐ Other_____

Discharge instructions

Before discharge the mother is given instruction to notify her physician as soon as possible for any of the following:

- Fever above 100.4° F for several hours
- Frequent or burning urination
- Heavy bleeding—more than a heavy menstrual period and soaking a pad in 2 hours or less
- Fainting
- Pain, tenderness, redness, or swelling of the leg
- Foul smelling discharge from vagina
- Headache or visual disturbance
- Pain in lower abdomen/perineum (stitches)
- Sore, red area on breast that doesn't go away with moist hot packs

She is also instructed to notify the baby's physician of any of the following:

- Refusing food for several feedings in a row
- Baby listless (hard to awaken) or crying continuously
- Loose, watery bowel movements—more than three in a row
- Grunting sounds when breathing or difficulty breathing
- Vomiting—not just spitting up small amounts
- Skin color change—yellow or dusky
- Temperature >99.6° or <96° F
- Not urinating or abnormal color or odor to urine

Discharge criteria

For most short-stay maternity programs, the antepartum, intrapartum, and postpartum course for both mother and infant should be uncomplicated and expected to remain so. Hospitalization is usually a minimum of 6 hours post delivery and an average of 24 hours.

Neonate

Minimum stay is usually 6 hours. The neonate is examined by a physician and assessed to be normal. Thermal homeostasis, stable vital signs, and successful feeding are present before discharge. Needed laboratory data are obtained, and required laboratory testing is arranged. The mother demonstrates ability in basic infant care.

Mother-vaginal birth

Minimum stay is usually 6 hours. The mother is able to walk and care for herself and infant. There are no complications that require further observation as determined by the physician, and the mother's postpartum course is normal.

Mother-cesarean birth

In addition to the above, the cesarean mother has bowel sounds and a plan for suture or clamp removal. Minimum hospitalization is 48 hours post surgery.

HOME CARE

Antepartum Home Care
Goal

The goal of antepartum home care is to enable the woman to maintain a safe pregnancy at home with minimal family disruption and to achieve optimum pregnancy outcome for both mother and baby in an era of cost containment.

Objectives

Objectives of a home visit program are to provide skilled antepartum and postpartum home nursing care and evaluate outcomes, readmission rates, family satisfaction, and cost-effectiveness.

Agencies

Although public health nursing has contributed to improved health for mothers, infants, and children since the early 1900s, in the past decade state and federal cost control measures have reduced the availability of home visit services for childbearing families. The number of hospitals and private agencies providing antepartum home care is increasing. A hospital may provide perinatal home care by maternity unit nurses or its own health care program. Sometimes a hospital contracts with community agencies such as Visiting Nurses Association (VNA) to provide home care. National and community-based companies also provide home care, sometimes with direct contracting with the woman's employer.

When providing antepartum nursing care in the woman's home, it is essential that the home care nurse understands the stressors that an antepartum family may be experiencing due to the pregnancy complications. Role relation disturbances between the woman and her partner and even her children are normal in these situations, but may be perceived by the woman to be very troublesome and even guilt provoking. By acknowledging and discussing these problems while in the home, the nurse can help the family to cope.

Patient education is integrated into each antepartum home care visit. Topics discussed may include nutritional needs of pregnancy; discomforts, especially related to long-term bed rest; preparation for birth; and care of babies with special needs. If preterm birth is a possibility, discussion of neonatal intensive care is important. The focus of antepartum home care is to provide necessary assessments, education, and reassurance, as well as to plan interventions with the woman and her family.

The basic nursing assessment completed on antepartum visits includes evaluation of emotional status and learning needs; vital signs measurement; urine check for ketones, sugar and albumin; maternal heart and lung sounds; measurement of fundal height; monitoring of fetal heart tones and uterine contractions; medications; nutrition; fluid intake; and activity level. The home nurse makes sure that the home environment is safe and that the mother has help with child care and housework if needed. With a physician order the nurse may also do cervical examinations, collect specimens for laboratory testing, and administer medications. Antepartum non-stress tests may also be done at home.

Careful documentation is essential in home care. Consultation with other members of the health care team is very important, with the physician apprised of the woman's status after each home visit. All communications and records are confidential.

Postpartum phone calls

When postpartum follow-up is made via the telephone, these follow-up phone calls are made within 6 to 24 hours after discharge. Phone call evaluation is documented on a hospital postpartum follow-up log with copies sent to care providers for mother and baby. The phone call will assess the mother's physical status; the infant's status regarding feeding, voiding and stooling, jaundice, appearance of cord, umbilicus and circumcision, and general appearance and behavior; and any concerns of the parents.

The new mother and her family are prepared postpartum to take part in their own assessment after discharge by learning how to measure fundal height, describe lochia, and examine breasts. Mothers are also taught to evaluate their babies by taking their temperatures, examining and describing urine and stools, identifying feeding problems, describing skin color, feeling fontanels, and examining and describing the umbilicus and genitals.

Postpartum home care

Postpartum home visits following short stay are usually made during a period of high stress for the family. Mothers are transitioning to new roles; they are also tired from the labor and birth experience, and sleep deprived from night feedings of their newborn. Their hospital stay was so short that there was inadequate time to work through the birth experience by recall and discussion with hospital nurses. Also, the new mother may be experiencing postpartum blues, pain from epi-

Referral Agencies of Assistance to Mother and Infant Appropriate to Each Community

List name of person, agency, phone number, and address of services available and accessible to each home care nurse.

1. City, county, and state public health nursing services
2. Childbirth education and support groups
3. Community agencies
   - Child protective services
   - Drug information
   - Family and children's services
   - Social service agencies (religious denominations; city, county agencies)
   - Family counseling
   - Legal aid
   - Homemakers' services
   - Health centers and services, mothers/infants
   - Neighborhood clinics
4. County welfare
   - Child support
   - Day care
   - Emergency financial aid
   - General assistance
   - Medical assistance
   - AFDC (Aid for dependent children)
   - WIC (Women-infant nutrition)
5. Economic resources—private sector
   - Clothing/household goods
   - Church and community resources
6. Aftercare services
   - Parenting education and support programs
   - Doulas
   - Home care agencies
   - Visiting nurses
7. Breast-feeding counseling service
   - Lactation consultants
   - Electric breast pump rental
   - Support groups

siotomy/laceration, backache, uterine cramping, breast or nipple soreness, and breast engorgement.

Sometimes new mothers may be reluctant to have the home care nurse visit if the household is upset because they are not used to having "guests" in such circumstances. It is also possible that the family may be uncomfortable and concerned about a "stranger" entering their home. Other women may welcome any and all help to clean up the house. Each family is unique, and all home situations and home visits are different.

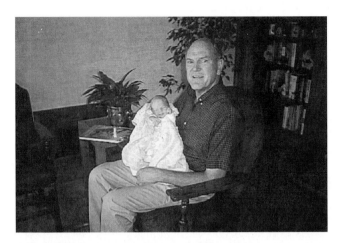

Figure 14-4 Visiting in the home, the nurse can assess the home environment and the support available. *(Courtesy Roger Phillips, Santa Cruz, Calif.)*

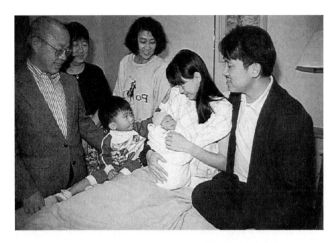

Figure 14-5 Incorporating the whole family into care. *(Courtesy Marjorie Pyle, RNC, Lifecircle, Costa Mesa, Calif.)*

The key components of the postpartum home visit are health assessment of both the mother and newborn and family guidance and teaching. Before leaving the home, the home visit nurse should make appropriate referrals to community resources and write down all instructions. (See the box on p. 378.) The home visit nurse should dress in a professional manner and furnish needed supplies for home care.

Home visits

Home visits by qualified nurses provide individualized teaching with family members present. During a home visit of from 1 to 1½ hours, the nurse can assess the home environment and the support available (Fig. 14-4). Physical examination of the mother includes vital signs, perineum, breasts, lochia, uterine involution, elimination, nutritional status, activity, fatigue, emotional status, and identification of any deviations from normal parameters. Physical examination of the baby includes vital signs, eyes, fontanels, umbilicus, skin color, voiding, stooling pattern, circumcision, feeding, and identification of any deviation from normal.

Assessment of mother-baby interaction, the home environment, and psychological support will help the nurse determine the level of family functioning. Observation of breast- or bottle-feeding is important in helping the mother feed her baby successfully. A review of teaching that occurred in the postpartum hospitalization and new teaching can occur as necessary. Referrals to community agencies/resources can be made as appropriate.

With 24-hour postpartum discharge the best time for home visits is 24 to 72 hours after discharge. Since bilirubin levels peak on the fourth day, collecting specimens for laboratory testing can be done at this time.

Common problems found on postpartum home visits

Mother:
- Pain
   - Episiotomy
   - Cesarean
   - Breast engorgement
   - Back pain
   - Hemorrhoids
- Constipation
- Potential for infection
- Psychological needs
- Fatigue

Baby:
- Feeding problems
   - Breast
   - Bottle
- Hyperbilirubinemia
- Weight gain
- Stool cycles

Home health care responsibilities

The mother who is caring for her baby full time at home is probably more ready to learn than she was in the hospital. The home visit can offer a unique chance to instruct the whole family (Fig. 14-5). The care provider who goes into a family's home is not there to take over and control; instead, the care provider is a guest in the family's home. To gain entrance nurses need to establish trust and rapport quickly. Along with professional responsibilities a special relationship is shared between the care provider and the childbearing family. More than simply providing physical assessment and tasks, the care provider coordinates the care planned with family needs and wants, focusing on family whole-

How Home Care Differs From Care in Formal Hospital Settings

- Nurse is a guest.
  —Setting for care is borrowed.
- Entrance is granted, not assumed.
  —Trust and rapport are needed.
- Control belongs to the family.
  —Power base changes.
- Practice is solitary.
  —Accountability is essential.
- Intimacy is fostered.
  —Socializing is part of visit.
- Family issues become more visible.
  —Behavior is more natural.
- Sending a message of caring is essential.
  —Validate the family's situation.

ness and well-being. This requires the ability to be flexible. Also, as a guest in the family's home, a care provider must be trustworthy, competent in providing care, and dependable.

Home care nursing differs from hospital nursing in its independence. (See the box above.) The home care nurse is alone in the home without access to another nurse for help or consultation, which would be possible in a hospital setting. Thus home care nurses need confidence in their skills and in their critical decision-making abilities. Strong communication skills and the ability to coordinate care with other members of the interdisciplinary health care team are also needed.

Necessary criteria for short-stay maternity to be successful include the following: participation by the expectant parents in prenatal education; collaboration between physicians (obstetricians, pediatricians, and family practice doctors), nurse-midwives, and nurses; a support person at home to provide usual home and family services such as cooking and cleaning for new mother and infant; monitoring criteria for success/failure with specific guidelines for home care and good documentation; guidelines for team relationships between doctors, nurses, and families; and home health supervision by well-prepared nurses.

CARE MANAGEMENT

Care management or case management is the process of organizing, managing, and guiding a patient's care through a hospital stay or through an episode of illness. Throughout this process the emphasis is on physician-nurse-patient/family health care team communication.

Care Management Tools
Case management plan

Case management plans are tools for tracking patient progress in care management.

The case management plan contains patient care standards for specific DRGs or case types, expected patient outcomes, timelines, processes/activities, and cost/utilization of resources. It is multidisciplinary in scope.

Critical paths

A critical path or patient care "road map" could be thought of as a visualization of the patient care process. The critical path is a clinical management tool that outlines in sequence the *key tasks* that must be performed in a predictable and timely fashion by all disciplines involved for a particular case type to achieve an appropriate length of stay. The following eight functional areas are included in the critical path: consultations and assessments, tests, treatments, medications, diet, activity or safety, teaching, and discharge planning.

There is confusion in terms used to describe care management and its tools. Other terms used for care management are case coordination, continuing care coordination, service integration, continuity coordination, and service coordination. In some hospitals critical paths are also known as practice guidelines/parameters, clinical guidelines, clinical protocols/algorithms, patient pathways, key processes, clinical paths, outcomes, quality improvement, etc.

In 1985 Zander described the pioneering nursing case management model developed at the New England Medical Center hospitals in which the model "design" utilized "Case Management Plans and Critical Paths." This design has evolved to the "Care Maps", which is the trademark and concept of the Center for Case Management, South Natick, Massachusetts.

The Care Map

The Care Map is a standardized plan of care for patients that has added quality indicators and patient care standards. The Care Map consists of the critical path and a patient problem list with predictable problems outlined and patient-centered outcomes identified within a time frame achievable at least 75% of the time for a particular DRG. The Care Map is used by the nurse or case manager to explain to the patient what will most likely happen during a hospitalization. It can be translated into lay terms and can be used as a patient guide.

Variance Analysis

Whenever there is a deviation from the care identified by the map or critical path, a variance or "detour," which may be positive or negative, has occurred. Earlier than predicted discharge to home is a positive variance. Delayed discharge due to failure to perform a laboratory test is a negative variance.

Variances are classified into three categories: practitioner, system, and patient. An example of a patient variance is a patient who does not progress through the critical pathway because of physiological complications. Examples of a system variance are delays in scheduling or orders not completed on time. An example of a practitioner variance is delay in writing of physician orders for a treatment the patient needs to advance through the critical path.

Determining Variances

Once each shift, each nurse looks for variances in her patient's progress and identifies the underlying causes—for example, patient noncompliance or staff scheduling problems. The nurse then develops a plan to put the patient back on track.

Clinical pathway

A clinical pathway is a plan for patient care that contains all possible elements of care that may be considered. It can be used to track care for an extended period when care is complex; that is, pre-hospitalization, hospitalization, and home care post hospitalization. A clinical path is a standard, detailed pathway that includes the entire continuum of care.

Practice parameters

In response to concerns about the quality and cost of medical care, the American Medical Association (AMA) and numerous professional organizations (both national and state) are working cooperatively to help in the development and implementation of scientifically sound, clinically relevant practice parameters linked to national and regional norms. Practice parameters are strategies for patient management, developed to assist clinical decision making. Although extremely valuable in enhancing care, practice parameters do not substitute for professional judgment when assessing the health care needs of each person as an individual.

Antepartum Case Management

Case management is ideal for enhancing pregnancy outcomes as insurers, utilization review companies, the U.S. government, and independent health practitioners all focus on minimizing hospital stays. There is no question that women who receive prenatal care during pregnancy have better pregnancy outcomes than women who have little or no prenatal care. When a woman has been identified as having increased risk for poor pregnancy outcomes, a case management approach to her care throughout pregnancy can produce substantial cost savings. Studies provide evidence of the effectiveness of a regular schedule of home nursing visits in achieving the goals of prenatal care among women at increased social or medical risk.

Antepartum team

The antepartum case management team is multidisciplinary and includes perinatal nurses, physicians, CNMs, clinical nurse specialists, parent educators, parent-infant specialists, perinatal social workers, occupational therapists, physical therapists, home health aides, and LVNs/LPNs. Everyone providing the direct care at home requires specialized preparation and supervision by a case manager.

High-risk care

High-risk maternity case management programs include the following:
- Providing expectant mothers with a phone consultation service through which they can receive advice from physicians or registered nurses.
- Referring women to appropriate care providers as risk status changes.
- Providing home uterine monitoring for the preterm labor patient with use of a home monitoring device and daily assessment by nurses.
- Maintaining the preterm labor patient in her home with tocolytic therapy.

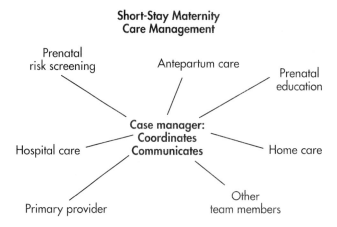

Figure 14-6 Short-stay maternity care management.

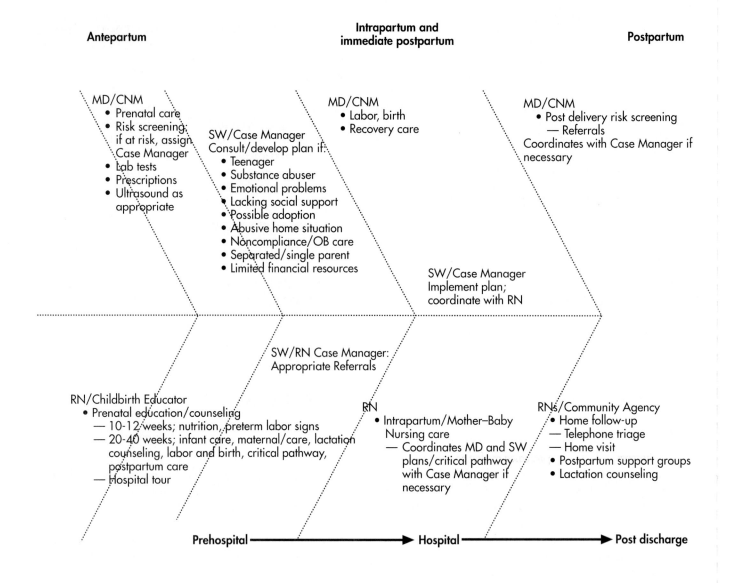

Antepartum

MD/CNM
- Prenatal care
- Risk screening; if at risk, assign Case Manager
- Lab tests
- Prescriptions
- Ultrasound as appropriate

SW/Case Manager
Consult/develop plan if:
- Teenager
- Substance abuser
- Emotional problems
- Lacking social support
- Possible adoption
- Abusive home situation
- Noncompliance/OB care
- Separated/single parent
- Limited financial resources

RN/Childbirth Educator
- Prenatal education/counseling
  — 10-12 weeks; nutrition, preterm labor signs
  — 20-40 weeks; infant care, maternal/care, lactation counseling, labor and birth, critical pathway, postpartum care
  — Hospital tour

Intrapartum and immediate postpartum

MD/CNM
- Labor, birth
- Recovery care

SW/Case Manager
Implement plan; coordinate with RN

SW/RN Case Manager:
Appropriate Referrals

RN
- Intrapartum/Mother–Baby Nursing care
  — Coordinates MD and SW plans/critical pathway with Case Manager if necessary

Postpartum

MD/CNM
- Post delivery risk screening
  — Referrals
Coordinates with Case Manager if necessary

RNs/Community Agency
- Home follow-up
  — Telephone triage
  — Home visit
- Postpartum support groups
- Lactation counseling

Prehospital ⟶ Hospital ⟶ Post discharge

Clinical Pathway
Child Bearing Year

- Assessing fetal well-being with non-stress tests (NSTs) in the comfort of the woman's home.
- Providing home oxygen therapy for the antepartal patient whose diagnosis may require additional oxygen.
- Providing in-home nursing care for conditions such as PIH (pregnancy-induced hypertension), gestational diabetes, preterm labor, and hyperemesis gravidarum.
- Providing nutritional support services.
- Providing homemaker services to new mothers following short-stay hospitalization for birth.
- Caring for postoperative cesarean mothers' special needs following early hospital discharge. These needs may include an array of infusion and/or antibiotic therapies, hydration therapies, and wound care.

- Providing home phototherapy for neonatal hyperbilirubinemia.
- Providing care for growing premature babies at home, including apnea and pH monitoring.

Case Management Program

A case management program for maternity care begins with prenatal risk assessment in the physician's or certified nurse-midwife's (CNM) office or in the clinic setting. Level of risk is quantified as low, at risk, or higher risk. A nurse case manager is assigned for higher-risk women and a clinical pathway is designed. (See Fig. 14-6 for case manager role.)

Text continued on p. 393.

EXAMPLES OF CARE MANAGEMENT TOOLS
LABOR CARE

Patient Name: _____

M.D.: _____

Initiated by: _____

Date and Time Developed: _____

Dx: Vaginal Delivery
Without Complicating Dx

Expected LOS: 8-16 hrs.

Spontaneous Vaginal Delivery Care Plan

NURSING DIAGNOSIS	OUTCOME CRITERIA			
	STAGE I OF LABOR	STAGE II OF LABOR	STAGE III OF LABOR	STAGE IV OF LABOR
Potential for lack of progress in labor	Patient will dialate to 10 cms ❑	Delivery of infant will occur ❑	Delivery of placenta will occur ❑	Will experience no complications in recovery ❑
Potential for maternal/ fetal compromise R/T process of labor	Maternal/fetal well-being will be obvious ❑	⟶ ❑	⟶ ❑	⟶ ❑
Knowledge deficit R/T labor process	Woman and significant other will verbalize process of labor ❑ Woman and significant other will use comfort techniques as desired ❑	⟶ ❑ Will exhibit effective push efforts ❑ ❑	⟶ ❑ ❑ ❑	⟶ ❑ Will demonstrate fundal massage ❑ Demonstrates no signs of discomfort ❑
Pain R/T uterine contractions	Patient will verbalize increased comfort or tolerable pain level ❑	⟶ ❑	⟶ ❑	⟶ ❑
Anxiety R/T childbirth process	Patient will verbalize diminished anxiety ❑	⟶ ❑	⟶ ❑	⟶ ❑
High risk for fluid volume deficit R/T altered intake and physiological process of labor	Intake will balance with output ❑ Will exhibit no signs and symptoms of hemorrhage, dehydration, or fluid overload ❑	⟶ ❑ ⟶ ❑	⟶ ❑ ⟶ ❑	Will maintain adequate circulating fluid volume ⟶ ❑ ⟶ ❑

Spontaneous Vaginal Delivery Critical Path

Consults	Notify attending physician ❑ Notify pediatrician or neonatologist prn ❑ Notify OB anesthesiologist ❑	⟶ ❑ ⟶ ❑ ⟶ ❑	⟶ ❑ ⟶ ❑ ⟶ ❑	⟶ ❑ ⟶ ❑ ⟶ ❑
Tests (as ordered)	Routine lab ❑ H&H ❑ CBC ❑ Urine Dipstick ❑ UA w/micro ❑ UA w/o micro ❑ Drug screen if indicated ❑		Cord blood ❑ Blood gas as ordered ❑	Lab as ordered ❑

Continued.

	STAGE I OF LABOR	STAGE II OF LABOR	STAGE III OF LABOR	STAGE IV OF LABOR
Activity	Physiological positioning ❏ Ambulation ❏	——→ ❏ ——→ ❏	——→ ❏ ——→ ❏	——→ ❏ ——→ ❏
Tx	IV ❏ TW enema, or Fleets prn ❏ Cath prn ❏ Vag exam prn ❏	IV ❏ Catheter prn ❏ Vaginal exam prn ❏	IV ❏ Catheter prn ❏	IV ❏ Catheter prn ❏ Massage fundus prn ❏
Monitoring	Admission Assessment ❏ Nursing care per standards: I&O ❏ VS ❏ Palpate abdomen for ctx ❏ EFM ❏ Ultrasound ❏ Transducer ❏ Electrode ❏ Catheter ❏	—————→ ——→ ❏ ——→ ❏ ——→ ❏ ——→ ❏ ——→ ❏ ——→ ❏ ——→ ❏ ——→ ❏	I&O ❏ VS per standard ❏	I&O ❏ VS per standard ❏ Check of fundal height, lochia, and incisional bleeding ❏ Attachment ❏ Breast-feeding ❏
Meds	Nursing care per standards: O₂ @ 10 L prn for decels ❏ Sedation ❏ Pitocin ❏ MgSO₄ ❏ Other:_____ Epidural, if ordered ❏ Antibiotics ❏ Prostin ❏	——→ ❏ ——→ ❏ ——→ ❏ ——→ ❏ ——→ ❏ ——→ ❏ ——→ ❏ ——→ ❏ ——→ ❏	——→ ❏ ——→ ❏ ——→ ❏ ——→ ❏ ——→ ❏ ——→ ❏ ——→ ❏	——→ ❏ ——→ ❏ ——→ ❏ ——→ ❏ _____ Hepatitis vaccine if necessary ——→ ❏ ——→ ❏
Diet	Ice chips and popsicles ❏ NPO ❏ Clear liquid ❏	——→ ❏ ——→ ❏ ——→ ❏	❏ ❏ ❏	——→ ❏ ——→ ❏ Regular diet ____ ❏
Teaching	Orientation to unit ❏ Labor progress ❏ Breathing and relaxation technique ❏ Reinforce childbirth education ❏ Discuss Care Plan and Critical Path ❏	——→ ❏ ——→ ❏ ——→ ❏ ——→ ❏	——→ ❏ ——→ ❏ ——→ ❏ ——→ ❏	Breast-feeding ____ ❏ Self Fundal Massage ____ ❏ Basic infant care ❏ ——→ ❏

Fill in ❏ with initials if outcomes met. If action/outcome inappropriate for this patient, mark ❏ N/A and initial. Boxes not marked with initials are variances. Explain variances here:

_____

_____

_____

Reviewed with Patient/Family

_____ _____ _____
Date   Time   Initials

EXAMPLES OF CARE MANAGEMENT TOOLS
NORMAL NEWBORN

Patient Name: _____

M.D.: _____

Mother's Name: _____   Dx: Normal Newborn

Initiated by: _____

Date and Time Developed: _____   Expected LOS: 24 hrs. after birth

Normal Newborn Care Plan

NURSING DIAGNOSIS   **OUTCOME CRITERIA**

	1-8 HOURS AFTER BIRTH ___ to ___	9-16 HOURS AFTER BIRTH ___ to ___	17-24 HOURS AFTER BIRTH ___ to ___
Altered health maintenance R/T physical adjustment to extrauterine life	Stable VS ❏	Infant will maintain temp in open crib and have VS WNL Temp 36.5-37.5°C (97.2°-99.9°F) ❏ HR 120-160 ❏ RR 40-60 ❏ BG 40-90% ❏	⟶ ❏
Altered nutrition: Less than body requirements; more than body requirements	Baby able to initiate and sustain suck and swallow coordination with normal color and respiratory effort ❏	⟶ ❏	⟶ ❏
High risk for infection	Newborn is free from signs of infection; no drainage or odor to umbilical cord; no skin lesions ❏	⟶ ❏	⟶ ❏
Potential for altered patterns of urinary and bowel elimination	Meconium is passed within 24 hrs after birth and beginning of a normal stool cycle is evident ❏ Baby voids within first 24 hours ❏	⟶ ❏ ⟶ ❏	⟶ ❏ ⟶ ❏
Alteration in family process R/T newborn care and parenting	Family demonstrates attachment to newborn ❏	⟶ ❏	⟶ ❏
Knowledge deficit R/T newborn care skills, safety/security	Mother verbalizes understanding of newborn care ❏ Identification bands on mother and newborn match, and mother verbalizes visitation and infant safety polices ❏	⟶ ❏ ⟶ ❏	Demonstrates newborn care skills ❏ ⟶ ❏

Normal Newborn Critical Path

| Consults (as needed) | Social Services _____ ❏
Lactation Consultant _ ❏
Public Health _____ ❏
WIC _____ ❏
Home _____ ❏
Other _____ ❏
M.D. notified of birth _ ❏ | ⟶
⟶
⟶
⟶
⟶
⟶
Initial M.D. exam ❏ | ⟶
⟶
⟶
⟶
⟶
⟶
M.D. dismissal exam ❏ |

Continued.

	1-8 HOURS AFTER BIRTH ____ to ____	9-16 HOURS AFTER BIRTH ____ to ____	17-24 HOURS AFTER BIRTH ____ to ____

Tests	Routine lab ❏
	Cord gases ❏
	Cord blood studies
	  Coombs' ❏
	  ABO ❏
	  Rh ❏
	Urine and/or meconium
	for toxicology ❏
		Lab values within normal
		range for age ❏
			⟶ ❏

Activity/Safety	Infant identified with bracelets ❏ Security procedures in place and explained to mother ❏	⟶ ❏ ⟶ ❏	Photo taken before discharge ❏ ID and discharge ❏

Treatments/Monitoring	Admission nursing
	Assessment/document ❏
	Weight ❏
	Measurements ❏
	Muscle tone, reflexes ❏
	Vital signs
	T, HR, R q 1° x 2 until sta-
	ble, then
	q 4° for 8° ❏
	Eye care prn ❏
	Cord care after initial bath
	and then every diaper
	change ❏
	Chemstick protocol for
	blood glucose screening on
	admission, <5 lb. or
	>9 lb. ❏
	
	Observe infants for signs of
	distress (cyanosis, temp. >97°
	and <99° jitteriness, poor
	feeding, or respiratory ❏
	distress)
	— On admission and at any
	  time infant exhibits signs
	  of distress: obtain Dex-
	  trostix, if <45 mg %, send
	  for serum glucose ❏
	— If Dextrostix 45 mg %,
	  continue observation
	  and feedings ❏
	— Notify M.D. if serum
	  glucose is less than 40
	  mg % or if the baby is
	  symptomatic at any time ❏
	Trim fingernails prn ❏
	Circumcision ❏
		
		Vital signs per nursing
		standards ❏
		Eyes clear, no discharge ❏
		Cord dry and healing, no
		odor ❏
		
		⟶
		Blood glucose stable, infant
		feeding ❏
		
		Hyperbilirubinemia
		assessment ⟶ ❏
		
		No bleeding/hematoma ❏
			
			⟶ ❏
			⟶ ❏
			Remove clamp when dry
			(approx. 24 hrs.) ❏
			
			⟶ ❏
			
			⟶ ❏
			
			PKU and T4 prior to DC ❏
			No excessive swelling ❏

Medications	Aquamephyton (IM) ❏ Erythromycin Ophthalmic Ointment (OU) ❏ Triple Dye or Alcohol to cord ❏ Bacitracin with diaper change (with circumcision) ❏ Other _____ ❏	Hepatitis B vaccine ❏ HBIG ❏ ⟶ ❏ ⟶ ❏ _____ ❏	 ⟶ ❏ ⟶ ❏ _____ ❏

	1-8 HOURS AFTER BIRTH ___ to ___	9-16 HOURS AFTER BIRTH ___ to ___	17-24 HOURS AFTER BIRTH ___ to ___
Nutrition/Breast-feeding	To breast within first hour ❑	Breast on demand ❑	No difficulty feeding or excessive fussiness ❑
Formula/Type	Feeds as soon as awake and stable ❑	Feed every 2-4 hrs., $^1/_2$-1 oz. ❑	❑
Teaching/Discharge Planning (All teaching includes mothers and significant others)	Discuss care plan and critical path ❑ Orientation to infant care/treatments/and safety standards ❑ Use of bulb syringe for suction of orophayrnx and nasopharynx ❑ Verbalizes under-standing of metabolic screen/abnormal hemoglobin screen ❑ Successful infant feeding ❑ Maintains infant positioning for feeding and sleeping ❑ Takes axillary temp. and verbalizes understanding of normal interventions ❑	❑ ❑ ❑ Coordinated suck and swal-low, rooting, latch-on, removal ❑ Discuss: Jaundice ❑ Bonding/Attachment ❑ Normal newborn characteristics ❑ Hydration ❑	❑ ❑ Weigh <10% of birth weight ___ lb. ___ oz. ❑ ❑ Performs routine care: Eye care ❑ Cord care ❑ Bath ❑ Circumcision/care ❑ Growth and develop-ment, sibling issues ❑ Home safety ❑ Car seat/safety ❑ Acknowledges need to learn CPR ❑ Give written d/c instructions. Verbalizes and demonstrates understanding of newborn care and d/c instructions. ❑ Review of signs of illness, first office visit, appropriate person to call for problems/questions. ❑
Elimination		Voiding 4-6 times/day ❑ No abdominal distention ❑	❑ Meconium stool before discharge ❑

Please fill in ❑ with initials if outcomes met. If action/outcome inappropriate for this patient, mark ❑ N/A and initial. Boxes not marked with initials are variances. Explain variances here:

_____

_____

_____

Reviewed with Patient/ Family

_____	_____	_____
Date	Time	Initials

EXAMPLES OF CARE MANAGEMENT TOOLS
MOTHER (AFTER VAGINAL BIRTH)

Patient Name:_____   Dx: Vaginal Delivery
Without Complicating Dx

M.D.:_____

Initiated by:_____

Date and Time Developed:_____   Expected LOS: 24 hrs. after birth

Mother Postpartum Care Plan

NURSING DIAGNOSIS	OUTCOME CRITERIA		
	1-8 HOURS AFTER BIRTH ___ to ___	**9-16 HOURS AFTER BIRTH ___ to ___**	**17-24 HOURS AFTER BIRTH ___ to ___**
Family coping: potential for growth, related to the perceived need to learn infant care	Patient/family will demonstrate appropriate coping mechanisms ❏ Patient/family will demonstrate bonding and attachment behaviors ❏ Patient/family will discuss issues relative to birth, role change, and siblings ❏	❏ ❏ ❏	Patient/family can identify appropriate resources and support system and interact with infant ❏ Patient/family will learn to successfully care for the infant ❏
Knowledge deficit R/T self-care after delivery	Mother/family verbalizes postpartum care plan and critical path ❏	❏	Mother can demonstrate self-care ❏
Altered physiological status R/T vaginal delivery	Mother will achieve a stable postpartum state: BP-below 140/90 ❏ (systolic rise less than 30mm; diastolic rise less than 15 mm) P-60-90/min ❏ R-15-30/min ❏ +97°F - 100°F po ❏ Fundus firm at midline ❏	❏ ❏ ❏ ❏ Progressive uterine involution ❏ Lochia appropriate and no foul odor ❏	❏ ❏ ❏ ❏ Patient/family can verbalize process of involution and lochia changes ❏
Potential for altered patterns of urinary/bowel elimination	Patient will void q 4° or more	❏ Patient will diuress ❏	Patient can empty bladder ❏ Bowel sounds are present ❏
Pain R/T vaginal birth, episiotomy, hemorrhoids, uterine cramping, breast engorgement, nipple soreness	Patient will verbalize pain or discomfort to nurse ❏ No hematoma ❏	Patient will experience relief from pain ❏	Patient will experience minimal pain at d/c ❏
High risk for infection R/T birth process	Mother is free of infection and has stable vital signs.	❏	❏

Mother Postpartum Critical Path

	1-8 HOURS AFTER BIRTH ___ to ___	9-16 HOURS AFTER BIRTH ___ to ___	17-24 HOURS AFTER BIRTH ___ to ___
Consults (if indicated)	Social Services_____ ❑ Lactation Consultant____ ❑ Health Dept._____ ❑ WIC_____ ❑ Home Care_____ ❑ Other_____ ❑	→ → → → → → →	→ ❑ → ❑ → ❑ → ❑ → ❑ → ❑
Test	Rubella and Hepatitis prep. status ❑ Hct ❑ CBC ❑ Hgb ❑		H&H done ❑
Activity	Ambulate with assistance ❑ ADL with assistance ❑	Ambulate without assistance ❑ ADL without assistance ❑	→ ❑ → ❑

Treatments/Monitoring	Nursing assessment
	• Observe bonding process ❑
	• Output ❑
	• Ice packs to perineum ❑
	• Pericare ❑
	• OB check: ❑
	   lochia ❑
	   fundus ❑
	   perineal area
	   P, R, BP q15 min x1°, then q 30" x2, then q 4°
	• Temp q 4° ❑
	• Phlebitis check ❑
	• Breast care ❑
	• Catheter, if fundus displaced or increased bleeding ❑
	• Empty bladder at least q 4° (criteria=normal fundal check) ❑
		Shift assessment ❑
		
		→ ❑
		
		Sitz bath prn ❑
		→ ❑
		Fundus firm and involuting ❑
		
		Vital signs per nursing standard ❑
		
		Bra worn → ❑
		
		→ ❑
		
		No bladder distention ❑
			→ ❑
			
			→ ❑
			
			→ ❑
			→ ❑
			→ ❑
			Episiotomy incision clean and dry → ❑
			Vital signs normal → ❑
			No signs/symptoms of phlebitis
			→ ❑
			
			→ ❑
			
			Emptying bladder with each void ❑

Medications	IV with Pitocin ❑ Demerol ❑ Tylenol ❑ Other_____ ❑ Anusol HC/_____ ❑ Witch Hazel/_____ ❑ Phenergan_____ ❑ Other_____ ❑ ❑	Discontinue IV when stable ❑ → ❑ → ❑ → ❑ → ❑ → ❑ → ❑	RhoGAM, if indicated ❑ → ❑ → ❑ → ❑ → ❑ → ❑ Rubella, if non-immune ❑ Rx filled or given to take home ❑
Nutrition	Regular diet ❑ Encourage po fluids ❑	→ ❑ → ❑	→ ❑ → ❑

Continued.

EXAMPLES OF CARE MANAGEMENT TOOLS—*cont'd*
MOTHER POSTPARTUM CRITICAL PATH

	1-8 HOURS AFTER BIRTH ___ to ___	9-16 HOURS AFTER BIRTH ___ to ___	17-24 HOURS AFTER BIRTH ___ to ___
Teaching/Discharge/Planning (all teaching includes patient and significant others)	Verbalizes understanding of unit/safety standards for infant and self-care Discuss care plan and critical path • Pericare, sitz baths, perineal meds ❑ • Involution, bleeding fundus ❑ • Breast care ❑ • Handwashing ❑ Provide mother with "self-assessment of learning needs" • Instruct to review and select items she wants discussed ❑	Teach breast pump and manual expression ❑ Give written discharge instructions, introduce videos (as appropriate) per "self-assessment" ❑ Verbalizes understanding of: Diet ❑ Activity/rest, ❑ elimination ❑ Birth control ❑ Hormonal changes ❑ Role changes ❑	Verbalizes/demonstrates understanding of discharge instructions: danger signals, of maternal complication, first office visit, appropriate, person to call for problems and questions. ❑

Please fill in ❑ with initials if outcomes met. If action/outcome inappropriate for this patient, mark ❑ N/A and initial. Boxes not marked with initials are variances. Explain variances here:

_____

_____

_____

Reviewed with Patient/Family

_____   _____   _____

Date   Time   Intitials

EXAMPLES OF CARE MANAGEMENT TOOLS
CESAREAN BIRTH

Patient Name: _____

M.D.: _____

Initiated by: _____

Date and Time Developed: _____

Dx: Cesarean Section Without
    Complicating Dx

Expected LOS: 3 days after cesarean

Cesarean Birth Care Plan

NURSING DIAGNOSIS　　　　　　　　　　　　　**OUTCOME CRITERIA**

NURSING DIAGNOSIS	PREPARATION PHASE PRE-OP PHASE	POST-OP PHASE 1-4 HOURS ___ to ___	4-24 HOURS ___ to ___	DAY 1 ___	DAY 2 ___	DISCHARGE DAY
Coping, ineffective, R/T surgical intervention, perceived loss of birthing experience and fatigue	Understands and verbalizes present fears/ concerns; surgery			Verbalizes feelings R/T childbirth ❏ No signs of inability to cope ❏ Increases the amount of interaction and ❏ care of newborn daily	→❏ →❏ →❏	→❏ →❏ →❏

Infection, potential for, R/T delivery and secondary surgical incision		VS stable ❏
		No signs of infection ❏
		  Abdominal incision ❏
		  Uterus ❏
		  Bladder ❏
		  Breasts ❏
		  Perineum ❏
			→❏
			→❏
			→❏
			→❏
			→❏
			→❏
			→❏
				❏
				❏
				❏
				❏
				❏
				❏
				❏
					❏
					❏
					❏
					❏
					❏
					❏
					❏
						→❏
						→❏
						→❏
						→❏
						→❏
						→❏
						→❏

Alteration in comfort: pain R/T incision or uterine cramping		Pain relieved with meds and comfort measures ❏	→❏	Ambulates, experiencing minimal pain ❏ Handles baby safely and with ease ❏	→❏ →❏	→❏ →❏
Potential alteration in parenting R/T difficulty in bonding with neonate		Able to feed infant ❏	States positive feelings towards baby ❏ Bonding with infant ❏	Spontaneously touches, holds, and makes eye contact with baby ❏	Mother/family members demonstrate attachment behaviors ❏	Realistically discuss parenting role ❏
Knowledge deficit R/T postpartum course, care of newborn, and implications for subsequent pregnancies				Verbalizes understanding of emotional changes after birth ❏	Verbalizes understanding of guidelines for repeat cesareans and for VBACs ❏	Verbalizes/demonstrates knowledge of care for self and baby • Breast care ❏ • Activity/exercise ❏ • Elimination ❏ • Diet/vitamins ❏ • S/S of complications ❏ • Post c-section care ❏

Continued.

EXAMPLES OF CARE MANAGEMENT TOOLS—*cont'd*

Cesarean Birth Critical Path

	PREPARATION PHASE / PRE-OP PHASE	POST-OP PHASE 1-4 HOURS___to___	4-24 HOURS___to___	DAY 1___	DAY 2___	DISCHARGE DAY
Tests/Treatments	CBC ❑ UA ❑ VDRL ❑ Rubella ❑ HBSAG ❑ T&S ❑ Foley catheter inserted ❑	Hemovac, measure and record ❑ Catheter draining clear urine, 30-60 cc/hr ❑ EKG strip WNL ❑ Pulse Oximeter: O_2 sat WNL ❑	Check RhoGAM/Rubella status ❑ DC catheter as ordered ❑	H&H WNL ❑ Emptying bladder each void ❑	⟶ ❑	⟶ ❑
Medications	Antacids (Na carry citrate, etc.) ❑ IV started ❑	Pain/nausea meds as ordered ❑ PCA pump ❑ Epidural meds @ ___ ❑ IV with Pitocin ❑	Pain controlled by meds as ordered ❑ PCA pump ❑ RhoGAM ❑ ⟶ ❑	HS med _____ ❑ Stool softener _____ ❑ PO analgesic for pain ❑ Pitocin IV may be stopped ❑	Rubella ❑ Stool softener ❑ PO analgesic for pain ❑	⟶ ❑ ⟶ ❑
Activity/Safety		Bedrest in R or L lateral position ❑	Dangle within 12 hrs ❑ Ambulate with assistance in room and to chair ❑	Ambulate without assist ❑ Shower ❑	⟶ ❑ ⟶ ❑	⟶ ❑ ⟶ ❑
Assessment/Monitoring/Interventions	Prepared for surgery per policy/procedure ❑ EFM for baseline monitor strip ❑	Assess bowel sounds—none to hypoactive ❑ Abdominal dressing dry and intact ❑ VS every 15 min for 1 hr, then every 30 min for 1hr., then every 4 hrs. (WNL) ❑ Fundus firm ❑ TEDs if ordered ❑	⟶ ❑ Remove abdominal dressing as ordered ❑ VS every 4 hrs. (WNL) ❑ ⟶ ❑ Negative Homans' ❑ ⟶ ❑ Bonding with baby ❑	Hypoactive to active bowel sounds ❑ ⟶ VS every 8 hrs. (WNL) ❑ ⟶ ❑ ⟶ ❑ Remove and reapply TEDs ❑ Bonding progressing ❑	Flatus/bowel movement ❑ Incision clean and dry ❑ ❑ ⟶ ❑ ⟶ ❑ ⟶ ❑	⟶ Staples removed, Steri Strip per order ❑ ❑ ⟶ ❑ ⟶ ❑ ⟶ ❑
Teaching/Consults/Discharge Plan	Preop teaching ❑ Cesarean/anesthesia care path for postpartum ❑	Lungs clear ❑ Turn, cough, and deep breathe, incisional splinting every hour while awake ❑ Breast-feeding with assistance ❑	⟶ ❑ Tri-flow breather as ordered ❑ If appropriate: Bottle-feeding ❑ Lactation suppression ❑ Social services consult if indicated ❑	⟶ ❑ ⟶ ❑ Pericare ❑ Breast-feeding, positioning of baby ❑ Newborn care ❑ Lactation consultant ❑ ⟶ ❑	⟶ ❑ ⟶ ❑ Diet, rest, activity ❑ Psychological issues related to cesarean birth ❑ Infant safety, care seat, etc. Home visit referral if needed ❑ ⟶ ❑	⟶ ❑ When to call M.D. for self and/or baby ❑ Teaching booklet ❑ Contraception ❑ Medications/Rx to take home ❑ ⟶ ❑
Diet	NPO ❑	Sips of H_2O/Ice chips with no nausea or vomiting ❑	Clear liquids; advance as tolerated ❑	⟶ ❑	Regular diet ❑	⟶ ❑

EXAMPLES OF CARE MANAGEMENT TOOLS—*cont'd*
Cesarean Birth Critical Path

Please fill in ❏ with initials if outcomes met. If action/outcomes inappropriate for this patient, mark ❏ N/A and initial. Boxes not marked with initials are variances. Explain variances here.

_____

_____

_____

Reviewed with Patient/Family

_____	_____	_____
Date	Time	Initials

Recognizing that risk status can change at any time during pregnancy, a nurse consultant can be assigned to women classified as low or at risk. This consultant is available by phone to answer the woman's questions and be involved in teaching prenatal classes.

A clinical pathway is utilized to provide the care of low- or at-risk women as well as high-risk women. This clinical pathway follows the patient through the child-bearing year—from antepartal care through the intrapartum stay and home follow-up by telephone or home visit. An example of a clinical pathway for an uncomplicated vaginal birth is on p. 382.

Case Management/Hospital

In an OB case management model the clinical pathway developed antepartally follows the patient into the hospital setting. The clinical pathways for hospitalization become the "road maps" for care. However, all care that preceded hospitalization is reviewed for its impact on the hospital care. Development of clinical pathways, critical paths, and nursing care plans requires organizing the clinical detail that will make outcome measurement possible.

Examples of critical paths and nursing care plans begin on p. 383. These are provided as examples only. Each multidisciplinary team of care providers must develop the care management tool that is appropriate in their own practice setting.

SUMMARY

In the delivery of care to new mothers and babies, nurses and physicians have always worked interdependently but in parallel structures rather than in formal collaborative practice with shared protocols. There have been nursing care plans and medical care plans with little or no cross-over. Care management provides the opportunity to develop collaborative, cost-effective practices in maternity care. As physicians and nurses work together in this collaborative practice, nurses are empowered.

The examples of care management tools presented here for normal labor and vaginal birth, cesarean birth without complications, and normal newborns are not all inclusive. They are simply presented to offer a framework for understanding care management of the most common needs for normal, healthy mothers and babies.

BIBLIOGRAPHY

American Academy of Pediatrics, American College of Obstetricians and Gynecologists: *Perinatal care services: guidelines for perinatal care,* Evanston, Ill, 1983, AAP.

American College of Obstetricians and Gynecologists: *Standards for obstetric-gynecologic services,* ed 6, Washington, DC, 1985, The College.

American Medical Association, Office of Quality Assurance and Medical Review: *Directory of practice parameters, titles, sources, and updates,* 1994, The Association.

American Medical Association, Office of Quality Assurance and Medical Review: *Practice parameter updates,* May 1994, The Association.

American Nurses' Association: *Nursing case management,* ANA Pub No N5-32, Kansas City, Mo, 1988, The Association.

Arnold LS, Bakewell-Sachs S: Models of perinatal home follow-up, *J Perinat Neonatal Nurs* 5(1):18-26, 1991.

Avery D and others: An early postpartum hospital program: implementation and evaluation, *J Obstet Gynecol Nurs* 11:233, 1982.

Avery M, Fournier L, Jones P and others: An early postpartum hospital discharge program: implementation and evaluation, *J Obstet Gynecol Nurs* 12(4):233-235, 1982.

AWHONN, Position Statement: *Shortened maternity and newborn hospital stays,* March 1994, The Association.

Barkauskas VH: Effectiveness of public health nurse home visits to primarous mothers and their infants, *Am J Public Health* 73(5):573-580, 1983.

Beck CT: Early postpartum discharge programs in the United States, *Women Health* (17):125-138, 1991.

Brider P: Who killed the nursing care plan? *Amer J Nurs,* 91(5):35-39, 1991.

Britton HL, Britton JR: Efficacy of early newborn discharge in a middle-class population, *AJDC* 138:1041-1046, 1984.

Brooten D, Brown LP, Munro BH, and others: Early discharge and specialist transitional care, *Image* 20(2):64-68, 1988.

Bull M, Lawrence D: Mothers' use of knowledge during the first postpartum weeks, *J Obstet Gynecol Neonatal Nurs* 315-320, 1985.

Carty EM, Bradley CF: A randomized, controlled evaluation of early postpartum hospital discharge, *Birth* 17:4, Dec 1990.

Coffey RJ and others: An introduction to critical paths, *Qual Manag Health Care* 1(1):45-54, 1992.

Cohen EL, Cesta TG: *Nursing case management: from concept to evaluation,* St. Louis, 1993, Mosby.

Cohen EL: Nursing case management: does it pay?, *JONA* 21(4):20-25, 1991.

Dahlberg NL: A perinatal center based antepartum homecare program, *J Obstet Gynecol Neonatal Nurs* 17(2):30-34, 1988.

Declercq ER: Where babies are born and who attends their births: findings from the revised 1989 United States standard certificate of live birth, *Obstet Gynecol* 81(6):997-1004, 1993.

DeZell AV, Comeau E, Zander K: *Nursing care management: managed care via the nursing case management model:* Patients and Purse Strings II: Schreubel JC, editor: National League for Nurses Pub No 20-2191:253-267, 1988.

DiFlorio I: Mothers' comprehension of terminology associated with the care of a newborn baby, *J Pediatr Nurs* 17(2):193-196, 1991.

Dineen K and others: Antepartum home-care services for high-risk women, *J Obstet Gynecol Neonatal Nurs* 21(2):121-124, 1991.

Droste S, Keil K: Expectant management of placenta previa: cost-benefit analysis of outpatient treatment, *Amer J Obstet Gynecol* p 1254-1257, 1994.

Eidelman AI, Hoffmann NW, Kaitz M: Cognitive deficits in women after childbirth, *Obstet Gynecol* 81(5):764-767, 1993.

Erkel EA: The impact of case management in preventive services, *JONA* 23(1):27-32, 1993.

Etheredge MLS, editor: *Collaborative care nursing case management,* The Center for Nursing Case Management, New England Medical Center Hospital, 1989, American Hospital Association.

Evans CJ: Description of a home follow-up program for childbearing families, *J Obstet Gynecol Neonatal Nurs* March/April, 113-117, 1991.

Gage M: The patient-driven interdisciplinary care plan, *JONA* 24(4):26-35, 1994.

Ghilarducci E, McCool W: The influence of postpartum home visits on clinic attendance, *J Nurse Midwifery* 38(3):152-158, 1993.

Gillerman H, Beckham MH: The postpartum early discharge dilemma: an innovative solution, *J Perinat Neonatal Nurs,* 5(11):9-17, 1991.

Gjerdingen DK, Chaloner KM: The relationship of women's postpartum mental health to employment, childbirth, and social support, *J Fam Pract* 38(5):465-472, 1994.

Goldenberg RL, Cliver SP, Bronstein J, and others: Bed rest in pregnancy, *Obstet Gynecol* 84(1):131-135, 1994.

Goodwin DR: Critical pathways in home healthcare, *Nurs Adm* 22(2):35-40, 1992.

Hampson SJ: Nursing interventions for the first three postpartum months, *J Obstet Gynecol Neonatal Nurs* March/April, 116-122, 1989.

Hellman LM, Kohn SG: Early hospital discharge in obstetrics, *Lancet* 1:227-232, 1962.

Jansson P: Early postpartum discharge, *Am J Nurs* p 547-550, 1985.

Larson C: Efficacy of prenatal and postpartum home visits on child health and development, *Pediatrics* 66(2):191-197, 1980.

Lemmer CM: Early discharge: outcomes of primiparas and their infants, *J Obstet Gynecol Neonatal Nurs* p 230-236, 1987.

Lukaco A: Issues surrounding early postpartum discharge: effects on the caregiver, *J Perinat Neonatal Nurs* 5(1):33-42, 1991.

Lyon JC: Models of nursing care delivery and case management: clarification of terms, *Nurs Econ* 11(3):163-169, 1993.

McGregor LA: Short, shorter, shortest: improving the hospital stay for mothers and newborns, *MCN* 19:91-96, 1994.

McIntosh ID: Hospital effects of maternity early discharge, *Med Care* 22(7):611-619, 1984.

Mehl L and others: Outcomes of early discharge after normal birth, *Birth Fam J* 3:101-106.

Moore ER, Bianchi-Gray M, Stephens L: A community hospital-based breast-feeding counseling service, *J Pediatr Nurs* 17(4):383-389, 1991.

Nagey DA, Bailey-Jones C, Herman AA: Randomized comparison of home uterine activity monitoring and routine care in patients discharged after treatment for preterm labor, *Obstet Gynecol* 82(3):319-323, 1993.

Norr KF, Nacion KW: Outcomes of postpartum early discharge, 1960-1986: a comparative review, *Birth* 14:3, Sept 1987.

Norr KF, Nacion KW, Abramson R: Early discharge with home impacts on low-income mothers and infants, *J Obstet Gynecol Neonatal Nurs* 133-141, March/April 1989.

Olds DL, Kitzman H: Can home visitation improve the health of women and children at environmental risk? *Pediatrics* 86(1), 1990.

Power DJ, Wolf E, Van Coenerden De Groot HA: Early discharge from maternity units in Cape Town, *S Afr Med J* p 896-895, 1980.

Powers KA, McCloskey CR: The childbearing experience: a

prototype for the study of continuity of care, *Issues Compr Pediatr Nurs* 5:53-66, 1981.

Rohrer KS, Poppe M, Noel L: On the scene: managed care at the Johns Hopkins Hospital, *Nurs Adm Q* 17(3):54-79, 1993.

Rubin R: Maternity nursing stops too soon, *Amer J Nurs* 75(10):1680-84, 1975.

Scupholme A: Post-partum early discharge: an inner city experience, *J Nurs Midwifery* 26(6):19-22, 1981.

Sheehan F: Assessing postpartum adjustment: a pilot study, *J Obstet Gynecol Neonatal Nurs* 11(1):19-23, 1981.

Siegel SB: Telephone follow-up programs as creative nursing interventions, *J Pediatr Nurs* 18:86-89, 1992.

Sterling YM, Noto EC, Bowen MR: Case management roles of clinicians: a research case study, *Clin Nurs Spec* 8(4):196-201, 1994.

Sterns TE: An early discharge program: an entrepreneurial nursing practice becomes a hospital-affiliated agency, *J Perinat Neonatal Nurs* 5(1):1-8, 1991.

Stulginsky MM: Nurses' home health experience, part I: the practice setting, *Nurs Health Care* 14(8):402-407, 1993.

Stulginsky MM: Nurses' home health experience, part II: the unique demands of home visits, *Nurs Health Care* 4(9):476-485, 1993.

The American College of Obstetricians and Gynecologists: *Quality assessment and improvement in obstetrics and gynecology*, Washington, DC, 1994, The College.

Thompson DG: Critical pathways in the intensive care & intermediate care nurseries, *MCN* 19:29-32, 1994.

U.S. Department of Health and Human Services, Public Health Services—Health Resources and Service Administration, Maternal and Child Health Bureau: *Healthy children 2000*, 1992, Jones and Bartlett.

Williams LR, Cooper MK: Nurse-managed postpartum home care, *J Obstet Gynecol Neonatal Nurs* January/February 1993.

Yanover NJ and others: Perinatal care of low risk mothers and infants: early discharge with home care, *N Engl J Med* 294(13):702-705, 1976.

Zander K, McGill R: Critical and anticipated recovery paths: only the beginning, *Nurs Manag* 25(8):34-40, 1994.

Zander K, McGill R: Nursing case management: resolving the DRG Paradox, *Nurs Clin North Am*, 23(3):503-520, 1988.

Zander K: Focusing on patient outcome: case management in the 90s, *Dimension Crit Care Nurs*, 11(3):127-129, 1992.

DEFINITIONS

Define the following terms:
care management
Care Map
case management
case manager
case type
clinical pathway
critical path
cross training
practice parameters
variance analysis

LEARNING ACTIVITIES

1. Group discussions.
2. Guest speakers: a nurse case manager employed by a home health agency.
3. View audiovisual aids and discuss.

ENRICHMENT/IN-DEPTH STUDY

1. Research what resources are available for home postpartum care services in your community. How does a family acquire these services? What is the cost?
2. Research what peer support groups are available for women seeking breast-feeding help in your community. How does a woman find out about these groups?

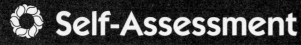
Supply the correct answers for questions 1 through 6.

1. The phases of most short-stay maternity programs discussed in the literature were: antepartum planning and _____; in-hospital postpartum assessment, support, and _____ home visit; _____ follow-up; and program evaluation.

2. The current information on short-stay maternity indicates that the advantages of early discharge outweigh the disadvantages, provided no compromise is made with _____ and _____ safety.

3. The nursing model that can optimize mother-infant care and teaching is _____ _____ nursing.

4. Case _____ is essential in home care.

5. The key components of the postpartum home visit are health assessment of both the mother and newborn as well as family guidance and _____.

6. Home care nursing differs from hospital nursing in its _____.

For questions 7 through 10, determine if each statement is true or false. Fill in the space to the left of the statement with T for true and F for false.

____ 7. The following eight functional areas are included in a critical path: consultations and assessments, tests, treatments, medications, diet, activity or safety, teaching, and discharge planning.

____ 8. Care management tools include case management plans, critical paths, care plans, clinical pathways, and practice parameters.

____ 9. A clinical pathway is a plan for patient care that contains only critical elements of care that may be considered.

____ 10. Practice parameters are strategies for nursing care developed to assist nurses in planning care.

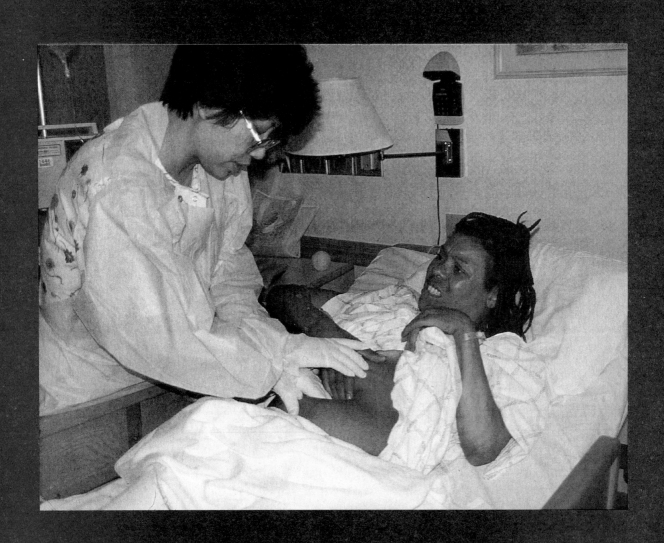

15

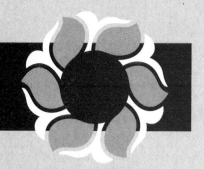

CLINICAL APPLICATION

The objectives that follow have been designed to help you use your clinical time effectively. Although the opportunity to complete these objectives will depend on the clinical experiences available, utilize all available resources to prepare yourself to meet these objectives whenever possible.

ANTEPARTUM CLINICAL OBJECTIVES

Clinical objective	Discussed and/or demonstrated	Learning activities and comments
1. Demonstrate a broad and basic understanding of the female bony pelvis and external and internal genitalia.		Review Chapter 2. Diagram the female external and internal genitalia, identifying the basic structures. Inspect a female bony pelvis in an anatomy laboratory or locate a drawing of a female bony pelvis in a text. Compare the female and male bony pelvis.
2. In antepartum clinic or office, when examining an expectant mother, demonstrate the following skills: a. Calculation of estimated date of delivery (EDD) b. Evaluation of fetal heart tone c. Abdominal palpation and inspection using Leopold's maneuvers		Review Chapters 4 and 8.
3. Interview an expectant mother and assess her need for instruction in the antepartum period in regard to: a. Diet b. Rest c. Elimination d. Exercise e. Hygiene f. Clothing g. Smoking h. Ingesting medications or alcohol i. Sexuality in pregnancy		Review Chapter 4. What instruction booklets are available in the antepartum clinic or office for use by childbearing families? What audiovisual aids are available? What classes are available?

Continued.

ANTEPARTUM CLINICAL OBJECTIVES—cont'd

Clinical objective	Discussed and/or demonstrated	Learning activities and comments
4. Distinguish between the psychological and physiological changes in pregnancy.		Review Chapter 4. Interview a pregnant woman during the third trimester of pregnancy and have her describe changes that occurred during the pregnancy. How did she know she was pregnant? How did she feel in each trimester: Physically? Emotionally?
5. Analyze a family's instructional needs for the following: 　a. Preparation for baby 　b. Sibling rivalry		Interview an expectant family. What are their plans for incorporating the new baby into their family?
6. Examine the adjustments involved in making the decision whether to bottle-feed or breast-feed.		Review Chapters 2 and 4. Describe the advice you would give to an expectant mother who is debating between breast- and bottle-feeding her infant. Evaluate a LaLeche League meeting in your community (group support, group strengths, and group weaknesses).
7. Evaluate a prenatal class relative to: 　a. Physical environment 　b. Emotional environment 　　(1) Support 　　(2) Discussion 　c. Use of audiovisual aids 　d. Demonstrations 　e. Group participation		Review Chapter 6. What group strengths were observed? What group weaknesses were observed? How were anxieties manifested?
8. Facilitate decision making for expectant parents who announce they plan to deliver at home.		Review Chapter 14. Ask them why; ask yourself why. Do not impose your value system. What are the pros and cons?
9. Discuss measures appropriate for the various minor discomforts of pregnancy.		Review Chapter 4.
10. Plan a basis for nursing action in the following deviations from normal in the antepartum period: 　a. Rh incompatibility 　b. Abortion 　c. Ectopic pregnancy 　d. Bleeding problems 　e. Hyperemesis gravidarum 　f. Diabetes 　g. Heart disease 　h. Pregnancy-induced hypertension (PIH)		Review Chapter 5.
11. Design an information booklet for expectant parents, identifying the danger signs that could indicate complications of pregnancy.		Review Chapter 4.
12. Explain the rationale for and demonstrate the ability to perform: 　a. Nonstress test (NST) 　b. Contraction stress test (CST) 　c. Assist with oxytocin challenge test (OCT)		

INTRAPARTUM CLINICAL OBJECTIVES

Clinical objective	Discussed and/or demonstrated	Learning activities and comments
1. Demonstrate basic understanding of psychological, emotional, sexual, and sociocultural factors in labor.		Review Chapter 7. Talk with families in early labor. Did they take any prenatal classes? What are their expectations? What are their past experiences?
2. Demonstrate basic understanding of fetopelvic relationships.		Review Chapter 7. When admitting a woman in labor, try to palpate the baby's back and small parts.

3. Demonstrate ability to admit a laboring woman and determine status of labor:
  a. Review history and all prenatal records
  b. Perform admission assessment
    (1) Vital signs: blood pressure, temperature, pulse, respiration, height, and weight
    (2) Urine specimen: sugar and albumin
    (3) Assess frequency, length, and quality of uterine contractions
    (4) Accurately auscultate FHTs with both the doppler and the fetoscope (during and between contractions)
    (5) Check deep tendon reflexes (DTRs)
		Review Chapters 7 and 8.
		In addition to the information on the woman's history records, what other information do you need to proceed with care?

4. Demonstrate providing nursing care to laboring women and their families:
  a. Verification of suspected rupture of membranes by use of Nitrazine test
  b. Assistance with artificial rupture of membranes (AROM)
  c. Evaluation of contractions
  d. Administration of medication
  e. Maintenance of an empty urinary bladder
  f. Maintenance of hydration
  g. Position changes and comfort measures
		Review Chapter 8.
		
		Review Chapter 7.
		
		Review Chapters 7 and 9.
		
		Review Chapter 9.
		
		Review Chapter 8.

5. Demonstrate an understanding of and an ability to give supportive nursing care for a woman and her family who are using prepared childbirth techniques.		Review Chapter 6. What type of prenatal class did this family attend (Lamaze, Bradley, Yoga, or other)? Did they read any books on birth?

6. On printouts of electronic fetal monitoring, evaluate:
  a. Baseline fetal heart rate
  b. Early decelerations
  c. Late decelerations
  d. Flattening of baseline (fetal heart tone)
  e. Variable decelerations
  f. Tachycardia
  g. Bradycardia
		Review Chapter 8.
		Examine fetal monitoring records of patients who have been discharged. Compare and contrast the "strips" from three or four such records.

7. Demonstrate assisting with application of internal fetal monitor.		Observe a nurse assisting the physician first. Role play procedure with help of fellow student.
8. Demonstrate an understanding of medical and surgical asepsis.		Observe a nurse or an instructor prepare delivery equipment.

Continued.

INTRAPARTUM CLINICAL OBJECTIVES—cont'd

Clinical objective	Discussed and/or demonstrated	Learning activities and comments
9. Design a plan for nursing action in each of the following at-risk and high-risk conditions:		Review Chapter 9.
a. Preterm labor		Review Chapter 9.
b. Prolapsed cord		
c. Placenta previa		Review Chapter 8.
d. Abruptio placentae		Review Chapter 5.
e. Irregular fetal heart tone or fetal distress		Review Chapter 9.
f. Convulsions or eclampsia		
g. Oxytocin induction or augmentation of labor		
h. Meconium-stained amniotic fluid		
10. Prepare a woman for cesarean birth:		Review Chapter 9.
a. Abdominal preparation		
b. Foley catheter		
c. Presurgical paper work		
d. Necessary equipment for baby		
e. Emotional support (mother, father, and family)		
f. Pre-op medication		
g. Pre-op lab work		
11. In preparation for delivery examine all equipment in the delivery area.		How does the delivery table or birthing bed operate?
		Can you use the resuscitator? Suction? Oxygen?
		Where is the infant resuscitation tray?
		What are the emergency codes?
		Review Chapter 8.
12. Demonstrate giving appropriate nursing care during delivery:		
a. Support mother		Review Chapter 7.
b. Support father		Review Chapter 8.
c. Administer medications		Review Chapter 8.
13. Demonstrate general care of newborn following delivery:		Watch a nurse assign an Apgar score to a newborn at birth and 5 minutes after birth. Do you agree with the score?
a. Bulb, DeLee-Hillis, or electric suction		
b. Warmth, drying, and cap		
c. Apgar scoring		
d. Identification		
14. Provide for interaction that will facilitate bonding in immediate postdelivery period.		Review Chapters 1 and 8.
15. Provide recovery care for the new mother and family in the immediate postpartum period.		Review Chapter 8.
a. Vital signs		
b. Bladder care		
c. Fundus check		
d. Perineum/episiotomy check		
e. Vaginal bleeding monitoring		
16. Plan a basis for nursing action in the following deviations from normal:		Review Chapter 8.
a. Perineal lacerations		
b. Postpartum hemorrhage		Review Chapter 8.
c. Resuscitation of a neonate with a low Apgar score		Review Chapter 13.

NEWBORN CLINICAL OBJECTIVES

Clinical objective	Discussed and/or demonstrated	Learning activities and comments

1. Demonstrate to your instructor the different nursing actions necessary in caring for the following infants:
  a. Apgar score 7 to 10
  b. Apgar score 4 to 6
  c. Apgar score 0 to 3
		Review Chapter 13.
		Turn on and operate infant stabilization crib. At what pressure would you operate the suction? How would you suction a newborn?
		How does the laryngoscope work?
		With a fellow student to assist you, role play resuscitation of a newborn.
		Do you know how to give cardiac massage to a newborn?
		Do you know how to use bulb suction? When do you compress the rubber suction bulb?

2. Receive a newborn after birth and make appropriate nursing observations and interventions.		Review Chapter 12. Observe a nurse receiving a newborn after birth. What does the nurse do? What can you do to conserve the newborn's body heat? When should the eye prophylaxis be administered?

3. Demonstrate caring for a newborn:
  a. Vital signs (temperature, pulse, and respiration)
  b. Weighing
  c. Identification
  d. Observe for anomalies
  e. Measurements (length, head, and chest)
  f. Gestational age assessment
  g. Observations (color, cry, and activity)
  h. Charting
		Review Chapter 12.
		Observe a nurse admitting a newborn.
		Complete *Observation of a Newborn* form.

4. Identify the three stages of activity immediately following birth (term infant):
  a. Alert/active phase (Stage I)
  b. Quiet phase (Stage II)
  c. Alert/active phase (Stage III)		

5. Identify sleeping and waking states:
  a. Sleep states
    (1) Regular
    (2) Irregular
  b. Wake states
    (1) Drowsiness
    (2) Alert inactivity
    (3) Waking activity
    (4) Crying		

6. Demonstrate nursing actions in regard to safety and important care techniques while bathing a newborn:
  a. Eye care
  b. Cord care
  c. Skin care
  d. Circumcision care
  e. Elimination
		Observe a nurse giving care to a newborn.
		
		Review Chapter 12.
		
		Review Chapter 12.
		Review Chapter 12.

7. Administer medications to newborns as ordered.		Review Chapter 12.

Continued.

NEWBORN CLINICAL OBJECTIVES—cont'd

Clinical objective	Discussed and/or demonstrated	Learning activities and comments
8. Explain to your instructor how you can differentiate among newborns when describing normal observations.		Review Chapter 12. Always wash your hands before touching any baby. Look at three different babies. What is their color when crying? Not crying? What are their respirations like? How are their heads shaped? What is the relationship of the head to body size? What is the average weight and length? How does the cry sound? How have you seen newborns express their individuality?

9. Demonstrate teaching and assisting a new mother to breast-feed.
  a. Breast engorgement
  b. Breast care
    (1) Lactating mother
      (a) Presence or absence of milk
      (b) Positioning of infant
      (c) Length and frequency of nursing and burping
      (d) Nipple care
      (e) Use of Lanolin or vitamin E
      (f) Breaking suction
      (g) Colostrum/milk
      (h) Engorgement prevention/care
      (i) Supportive bra
      (j) Breast pads
      (k) Supply and demand: use of manual/electric breast pump/collection and storage of milk
      (l) Hand expression
		Review Chapters 10 and 12.
		Check the charts of breast-feeding mothers. How do you expect the medication given in labor and delivery to affect the babies?
		Notice the attitude of the mother; how she handles her infant and positions herself; and the baby's alertness, sucking ability, and interest.

10. Demonstrate teaching and assisting
  a. A new mother to bottle-feed
  b. Lactation suppression
		Review Chapter 12.
		Does the mother understand formula preparation?
		What are the types of formula available commercially? Where? How much do they cost?

11. Demonstrate the ability to effectively communicate with families regarding their infant's health maintenance and well-being. Complete a demonstration baby bath.		Review Chapter 12. Select a family that is in need of teaching.

12. Compare the preterm infant with the normal newborn in relation to:
  a. Cry
  b. Size
  c. Weight
  d. Skin
  e. Activity
		Review Chapter 13.
		Visit the neonatal intensive care unit to observe preterm babies.
		Read charts of preterm infants. Note how their Apgar scores may vary. Note their progress.

13. Design a plan to assist the parents in coping with the death of a newborn.		Review Chapter 11.
14. Design a plan to assist the parents in coping with a sick neonate.		Review Chapter 11.

NEWBORN CLINICAL OBJECTIVES—cont'd

Clinical objective	Discussed and/or demonstrated	Learning activities and comments
15. Design a plan for nursing action in each of the following deviations from normal: a. Hyperbilirubinemia b. Sepsis c. Respiratory distress syndrome d. Hypoglycemia 16. Assess educational needs of mother/infant/partner: a. Infant care b. Infant nutrition: breast-feeding/formula-feeding c. Infant states, state-related behaviors, and individual differences d. Infant stimulation e. Infant growth and development f. Parenting g. Birth control/family planning h. Infant safety needs i. State-required lab tests 17. Discuss newborn care with family: a. Nutritional needs b. Growth and development c. Cord care d. Circumcision care, if indicated e. Bathing f. Diapering g. Taking a temperature h. Signs and symptoms to report to health care provider i. Environmental safety		Review Chapter 13.

POSTPARTUM CLINICAL OBJECTIVES

Clinical objective	Discussed and/or demonstrated	Learning activities and comments

1. Evaluate the condition of the fundus, lochia, breasts, extremities, episiotomy, voiding, and vital signs of a woman on the first postpartum day; report and record findings.
  a. Uterine involution
    (1) Fundus height/position
    (2) Firmness
    (3) Lochia
      (a) Type
      (b) Amount
      (c) Color
      (d) Clots
  b. Bladder function
  c. Hematoma development and treatment
  d. Symptoms of infection and hemorrhage
  e. Hemorrhoid care
  f. Neurological assessment (DTRs, clonus)
  g. Homans' sign
		Review Chapter 10.
		Check postpartum charts. How are these findings recorded?

2. Perform and instruct the new mother concerning perineal care.
  a. Perineal hygiene
    (1) Wash and wipe front to back
    (2) Sprays and ointments
		Review Chapter 10.

3. Examine the attitude of a new mother toward her baby.		Review Chapter 10. Ask for permission to stay with a mother and her baby during a feeding. Look for maternal attitudes and interactions. Complete one *Mother-Infant Observation* form.
4. Examine the attitude of a new father toward his baby.		Review Chapters 1 and 10. Observe a father interacting with his baby. Complete one *Father-Infant Observation* form.

5. Demonstrate making three observations during your first visit to a postpartum mother following a cesarean birth that would be different from observations you would make for a mother following a vaginal delivery.
  a. Breasts
  b. Fundus
  c. Incision
  d. Lochia
  e. Extremities
  f. Abdomen
  g. Pain
  h. Vital signs
  i. Voiding
  j. Bowel sounds/abdominal distention
		Review Chapter 11.
		A cesarean birth is major abdominal surgery. What observations would you make in the first hours after surgery? Remember that this cesarean patient is also a new mother.

6. Demonstrate helpful postpartum exercises.		Visit hospital physiotherapists. What exercises do they recommend? Review handout on postpartum exercises given in the hospital unit and those given by physicians.

POSTPARTUM CLINICAL OBJECTIVES—cont'd

Clinical objective	Discussed and/or demonstrated	Learning activities and comments
7. Describe the purpose of the postpartum checkup by the physician or midwife.		Ask physician what happens at postpartum checkup. Visit clinic; ask nurses what happens at postpartum checkup. Arrange a visit to a postpartum clinic and assist with postpartum checks.
8. Demonstrate helping a new mother recognize her change in emotionals.		Ask multiparous mothers to identify what worried them after they went home. Meet the newborn's father and/or woman's family. Note the relationships. What is said and how is it said? Complete the *Postpartum Family Assessment Guide.*
9. Compare attitudes of mothers who have had vaginal deliveries with those of mothers who have had cesareans.		Visit mothers who have had both vaginal and cesarean births. Talk with the fathers. Were they present at the cesarean? Would they like to have been? Why? When did they hold their baby for the first time?
10. Design a plan for therapeutic nursing care for the mother of a preterm infant.		Review Chapter 11. Visit the mother of a preterm infant. What are her special worries? Note the Apgar score of the baby.
11. Design a plan for nursing action in each of the following deviations from normal in the postpartum period: a. Puerperal infection b. Thrombophlebitis c. Mastitis (How can you help this mother and family?) d. Postpartum hemorrhage		Review Chapter 10. Review Chapter 11.
12. Administer medications as ordered: a. RhoGAM b. Rubella vaccine c. Postpartum medicines		Review Chapter 10.
13. Demonstrate knowledge of grieving process of families with neonatal loss and provide appropriate intervention.		Review Chapter 11.
14. Assess psychosocial needs of new mother and family: a. Taking-in/taking-hold stages b. Mother-infant acquaintance process c. Parent-infant attachment d. Family integration/social situation e. Knowledge of grieving process of families with fetal loss f. Coping skills		
15. Identify criteria and demonstrate referral to: a. Social worker b. Home health		

Continued.

POSTPARTUM CLINICAL OBJECTIVES—cont'd

Clinical objective	Discussed and/or demonstrated	Learning activities and comments

16. Discuss maternal self-care with new mother:
  a. Perineal care
  b. Hemorrhoids
  c. Breasts and nipples
  d. Activity limitations
  e. Nutrition
  f. Need for balance of exercise and rest
  g. Sexuality and contraception
  h. Psychosocial aspects of postpartum period
  i. Signs and symptoms of complications to report to health care provider
17. Discuss support person(s) and extended family adaptation:
  a. Transition to new roles
  b. Communication among mother, support person(s), and family—expectations vs. reality
  c. Siblings
    (1) Possible age-appropriate regression
    (2) Strategies for meeting sibling needs
18. Provide community resource information for short- and long-term maternal and newborn follow-up.		

MOTHER-INFANT OBSERVATION
Directions

1. Obtain the following information from the chart before meeting the mother:

Age _____ Para _____

Gravida _____ Abortions _____

Ages of other children _____

Postpartum day _____

Bottle-feeding _____

Date and time last analgesic drug given _____

2. Ask the mother if you may observe her and her baby together. Be sure the mother understands that you are interested in their normal interactions and not in a "good show." Determine if the mother has any physical discomfort. How is she feeling emotionally (happy, tense, worried, relaxed)?

_____

_____

_____

3. Observe verbal and nonverbal actions and interactions of the mother and her baby. Also observe any other interaction that takes place in the room (for example, staff, other family members, roommate). Focus on these interactions, keeping in mind the process of bonding and the postpartum phases: taking-in, taking-hold, and letting-go.

4. After 20 minutes report to the conference area. Record your observations.

   a. What were the mother's nonverbal actions? How did she hold the baby?

   _____

   _____

   _____

   b. What did the mother say to the baby? What was her tone of voice?

   _____

   _____

   _____

   c. What were the baby's actions and responses?

   _____

   _____

   _____

   d. What were the mother's interactions with you or others in the room?

   _____

   _____

   _____

The conference will be designed to promote an understanding of the mother-infant interaction you have observed.

FATHER-INFANT OBSERVATION

This is a tool to help you assess fathering capabilities. Select a father to interview. First study the mother's chart. Review prenatal care, labor, and delivery.

1. Is this her first child with this man?
2. How long have they been together?
3. Is he a father for the first time? If not, what was his previous childbirth experience?
4. How old is he?
5. What is his educational background?
6. What is his ethnic background?

Next, interview the father.

Data Gathering:

1. During pregnancy, did the father experience any physiological or psychological reactions or concerns similar to those the mother experienced?

_____

_____

_____

2. What were the high points of the pregnancy for him?

_____

_____

_____

3. Did the father attend prenatal classes? What did he learn there? Why did he attend?

_____

_____

_____

4. Was the father present during labor? What was his role during labor (that is, passive observer or active participant)? Did he think the staff was helpful to *him* during labor?

_____

_____

_____

5. Was the father present during birth? What does he remember of the actual delivery (for example, responses, feelings, touching, holding)? If answer to No. 5 is no, when did he first see and/or hold his infant?

_____

_____

_____

6. Did he have a preference for a boy or girl?

_____

_____

_____

7. What does he see as his role or responsibility in infant and child care?

_____

_____

_____

Observe the Baby and Father Together. Observe the Father for the Following.

1. Visual awareness of the newborn and father's verbal response:

    a. Does he enjoy looking at his baby?

_____

_____

_____

    b. Does he see his baby as pretty, beautiful, or ugly?

_____

_____

_____

    c. What does he say?

_____

_____

_____

    d. Does he call the baby by name?

_____

_____

_____

2. Tactile awareness of the newborn:

    a. Does he want to pick up his baby?

_____

_____

_____

    b. How does the baby's skin feel to him?

_____

_____

_____

    c. Describe how he touches and holds his baby (for example, close to him, stiff, rough, gentle, hesitant, assured).

_____

_____

_____

3. Awareness of distinct characteristics of newborn:

    a. Can he distinguish his own baby from others?

_____

_____

_____

b. Does he feel that his baby looks like him or the mother?

_____

_____

_____

c. Does he perceive his infant as "perfect"?

_____

_____

_____

d. What aspects of the infant's behavior have impact on the father (for example, baby opening eyes, grimacing, grasp reflex)? Write down his answers.

_____

_____

_____

e. Do you feel that this father is forming a bond with his newborn? What leads you to feel this?

_____

_____

_____

POSTPARTUM FAMILY ASSESSMENT GUIDE

Date _____ Postpartum day _____ Marital status _____

Ethnic group _____ Religion _____ Age _____

Gravida _____ Para _____ Abortions _____

Weeks of gestation _____ Pregnancy planned? Yes _____ No _____

Education/occupation: Mother _____

Father _____

Antepartum

Preparation classes? _____ Did both attend? _____ Reading? _____

Physical preparation (exercises, breasts) _____

Mother's blood type _____ Rh _____

Father's blood type _____ Rh _____

Medications taken during pregnancy:

_____

_____

_____

Significant family, personal, OB history:

_____

_____

_____

Labor

Length of labor: stage one _____ stage two _____ stage three _____ stage four _____

Medications (drug, dose, route, and time) _____

_____

_____

Continuous fetal monitoring _____

Fetal distress _____

Rupture of membranes (artificial or spontaneous) _____

Anesthesia or analgesia _____

Labor complications _____

Delivery

Type of delivery _____

If cesarean, what was indication for surgery? _____

Date and time of delivery _____

Episiotomy or cesarean incision _____

_____

Estimated blood loss _____

Admission hematocrit _____

Postpartum hematocrit _____

Infant

Apgar score (1 minute) _____ (5 minutes) _____

Sex _____ Weight _____ Length _____

Feeding: breast _____ bottle _____

Cry (frequent, strong, weak) _____

Activity level (alert or lethargic) _____

Complications _____

_____

Postpartum

	Maternal physical condition		
	Day 1	Day 2	Day 3
Vital signs			
Bladder			
Fundus			
Breasts and nipples			
Lochia (color, odor, number of pads)			
Episiotomy or cesarean incision			
Hemorrhoids			
Legs			
Elimination: Urinary			
Bowels			

Family-Infant Interaction

Mother

Appearance _____

Feelings about labor and delivery _____

_____

Physical complaints _____

_____

Activity level (passive, initiates activity, nervous, or lethargic). Would you say she is in the taking-in, taking-hold, or letting-go phase? Why? _____

_____

_____

_____

_____

Father

Appearance _____

Feelings about labor and delivery _____

_____

Involvement in infant care (passive or active) _____

_____

Siblings

Appearance _____

Feelings about new baby _____

Interaction with parents _____

_____

Grandparents

Appearance _____

Involvement in infant care _____

_____

Attitudes about birth experience and recovery _____

Interaction with new parents _____

Communication

	Mother:	Father:
Calls baby by name		
Calls baby "it"		
Looks at baby		
Holds baby close to body		
Holds baby stiffly away from body		
Immediately meets baby's needs		
Explores baby		
Makes eye contact with baby		
Is satisfied with sex of baby		
Physically overstimulates baby (slaps, hits, shakes, or pokes)		
Says baby stinks		
Focuses more on own needs		

Infant

Behaviors in response to:

Mother _____

_____

Father _____

_____

Sleep patterns _____

Breast-feeding: Patterns _____

Problems _____

Information Needs:

Knowledge of baby care

	Mother:	Father:
Bath/cord care		
Circumcision care		
Diapering		
Temperature		
Diaper rash		
Pediatric follow-up		
Infant safety		
Infant states, state-related behaviors and individual differences		
Infant stimulation		
Infant growth and development		
Parenting		

Knowledge of infant feeding

	Mother:	Father:
Bottle		
Rooting reflex		
Type of formula		
Amount per feeding		
Preparation		
Burping		
Vitamins and iron		
Introduction of solid foods		
Feeding schedules		
Breast		
Rooting reflex		
Nipple care		
Let-down reflex		
Supportive bra		
Positioning		
Length of feeding		
Techniques for expressing milk		
Medications and breast-feeding		
Diet		
Smoking		

Nutrition

Typical diet at home _____

_____

_____

Approximate caloric intake _____

Fluid intake _____

Birth control

Understands time for resumption of sexual activity _____

Type of contraception _____

Understanding _____

Exercise

Type _____

Understanding _____

Personal hygiene

Bathing _____

Showering _____

Douching _____

Help at home (grandparents, other children)? _____

_____

Layette? _____

_____

What follow-up would you recommend (family resources, community resources)? _____

_____

_____

_____

Has a referral been made for home care and/or telephone calls?

_____

_____

_____

OBSERVATION OF A NEWBORN

Select a newborn infant for observation.

1. Review the mother's chart:

   Gravida _____ Para _____ Expected date

   of delivery _____

   Estimated gestational age _____ Small for gestational age _____

   Average for gestational age _____ Large for gestational age _____

   Rh _____ Length of labor: first stage _____

   second stage _____

   Type of delivery: vaginal _____ cesarean _____

   Analgesia and anesthesia: _____

2. Review the infant's chart:

   Apgar score at 1 minute _____ 5 minutes _____ Birth weight _____

   Loss or gain _____ Type feeding _____

3. Complete Column 1 of the following guide with textbook information from
   Chapter 12 of the norms to be expected.

4. Providing warmth for the infant, observe the infant. Complete Column 2.

5. Date: _____

6. Time of examination: _____

Observations	COLUMN 1 Textbook information from Chapter 12	COLUMN 2 Observation of infant
General Appearance:		
1. Posture, body align- ment, and symmetry		
a. Sleeping		
b. Awake (quiet)		
c. Crying (loud, strong, weak, high- pitched)		
2. Respirations		
3. Apical pulse rate		
4. Length		
5. Weight		
6. Axillary temperature		
Assessment of Head and Neck:		
7. Head		
a. Circumference		
b. Size in relation to rest of body		
c. Size compared with adult		
d. Symmetry		
e. Molding		
f. Cephalhematoma		

Observations	COLUMN 1 Textbook information from Chapter 12	COLUMN 2 Observation of infant
8. Fontanels (size, shape, consistency)		
a. Anterior fontanel		
b. Posterior fontanel		
9. Skin		
a. Color		
b. Rash		
10. Ears		
a. Response to sound		
b. Position and shape		
c. Location of ears		
11. Face		
a. Chin		
b. Milia		
12. Eyes		
a. Color		
b. Condition (clear, discharge, swelling)		
c. Eye movement		
13. Nose		
a. Patent		
b. Blocked		
c. Drainage		
14. Mouth		
a. Palate (intact or abnormal)		
b. Mucosa (pink or white patches or cyanotic)		
15. Neck		
a. Length		
b. Mobility		
c. Presence of webbing and/or fat pad		
16. Breasts		
a. Size of areola		
b. Fullness		
c. Engorgement		
d. Discharge		
17. Chest		
a. Symmetry		
b. Type of respiration (shallow, irregular, grunting)		
18. Abdomen condition (soft, hard, distended)		
19. Umbilicus		
a. Color		
b. Odor		
c. Condition		
20. Genitourinary system		
a. First passage of urine		
b. Female (condition of external genitalia)		
c. Male (testes)		

Observations	COLUMN 1 Textbook information from Chapter 12	COLUMN 2 Observation of infant
21. Anus and bowels		
a. Stool (first)		
b. Daily stools (color, consistency)		
c. Anus, patent		
22. Extremities		
a. Symmetry		
b. Number of fingers and toes		
c. Rotation of hips		
d. Buttocks and leg creases		
23. Nervous system		
a. Grasp reflex		
b. Rooting reflex		
c. Sucking reflex		
d. Walking reflex		
e. Moro's ("startle") reflex		
f. Tonic neck reflex		
24. State of awareness		
a. Deep sleep		
b. Rapid eye movement sleep		
c. Crying		
d. Transitional		
e. Quiet alert		
f. Active awake		

Answers to Self-Assessments

CHAPTER 1

1. True
2. False
3. True
4. True
5. True
6. True
7. True
8. True
9. False
10. True
11. True
12. False
13. 2. a, b, c, and e
14. c. both a and b
15. b. fingertip to palm to increased body contact
16. 1. a and d
17. a. 21st
18. a. 50%
19. a. ACNM
20. b. they are not certified
21. a. disinterest in infant
    b. parents not touching infant
    c. anger and noncommunication between parents
22. a. Reexamine our priorities and change goal to alleviating prematurity and low birth weight.
    b. Encourage consumer input into planning maternity care.
    c. Support regionalization of maternity care.
23. a. respiratory distress syndrome
    b. intraventricular hemorrhage
    c. necrotizing enterocolitis
    d. sepsis
24. a. infant cared for primarily in mother's room
    b. individualized care provided
    c. open visitation for family and friends as the mother wishes
25. attitudinal
26. education
27. dignity
28. responsibilities
29. one third

CHAPTER 2

1. Examine Fig. 2-1.
2. Examine Fig. 2-15.
3. Examine Fig. 2-2.
4. Examine Fig. 2-8.
5. Examine Fig. 2-9.
6. Examine Fig. 2-14.
7. a. It serves as sphincter to close openings.
   b. It serves as a hammock or sling.
8. b, d, and e
9. c
10. d
11. c
12. a
13. a
14. b
15. a
16. middle layer
17. a. to provide sexual gratification
    b. to produce hormones
    c. to reproduce
18. a. coccyx
    b. sacrum
    c. innominiate bone
    d. pubis
19. a. proliferative phase
    b. ovulatory phase
    c. secretory phase
    d. menstrual phase
20. a. follicular phase
    b. luteal phase
21. 1. c
    2. b
    3. a
    4. d
    5. d
22. 1. c
    2. b
    3. d
    4. a
    5. e
    6. f
23. estrogen and progesterone
24. proliferative
25. secretory
26. linea terminalis
27. efferent (motor) and afferent (sensory)
28. Examine Fig. 2-17, *B*.
29. Examine Fig. 2-17, *A*.
30. a. tubules
    b. seminal vesicles
    c. prostate gland

CHAPTER 3

1. True
2. False

3. True
4. False
5. True
6. True
7. True
8. False
9. True
10. False
11. True
12. False
13. False
14. True
15. True
16. d
17. 1
18. a
19. b
20. c
21. c
22. a
23. c
24. d
25. c
26. a
27. a
28. 1. b
    2. c
    3. a
    4. c
    5. a
29. 1. c
    2. a
    3. b
30. Examine Figs. 3-8 and 3-9.
31. age
32. congenital anomalies
33. embryo
34. birth
35. growth and development
36. a. respiratory
    b. metabolic
    c. excretory
37. T for toxoplasmosis
    O for "other" (hepatitis B)
    R for rubella
    C for cytomegalovirus (CMV)
    H for herpes simplex virus (HSV)
38. foramen ovale
39. six
40. a. Wear gloves for all contact with moist body substances, nonintact skin, and mucous membranes.
    b. Wear masks and protective eyewear during procedures where splashes to eyes, nose, or mouth are likely.
    c. Wear gowns or plastic aprons during procedures that are likely to generate splashes of body fluids.
    d. Wash hands if contamination with body fluids occurs and immediately after gloves are removed.
    e. Carefully dispose of needles and sharps. Avoid recapping.
    f. Use ventilation devices to avoid mouth-to-mouth resuscitation.

CHAPTER 4

1. False
2. True
3. False
4. True
5. c
6. c
7. b
8. a
9. c
10. d
11. d
12. d
13. b
14. a
15. b
16. b
17. 4
18. c
19. c
20. b
21. a. Protect and support optimal health of unborn baby.
    b. Protect and promote physical and emotional health and well-being of expectant mother.
    c. Assist expectant father and other family members to adapt to new roles.
22. a. easily digested
    b. offers immunity
    c. creates closeness
23. number of pregnancies
24. number of deliveries of infants a woman has had
25. a. hematocrit >38%, hemoglobin >12 grams
    b. (1) negative; (2) negative
26. a. What the mother sees when she is pregnant influences how the baby will look.
    b. Heartburn means curly hair.
    c. Sex is determined by how mother carries baby.
    d. Activity of fetus in uterus indicates how well the baby will sleep.
27. Assess the family's needs and attempt to meet them.
28. Elevate legs during rest periods.
29. a. 4
    b. 4
    c. 4
    d. individual
    e. 3

30. Increase calcium intake.
31. a. washing nipples daily without using soap
    b. nipple exam to detect flat or inverted nipples
32. a. Mother can take oral contraceptives.
    b. Mother can return to work.
    c. Mother can be nutritionally adequate.
33. a. bleeding from vagina
    b. swelling of face and fingers
    c. severe, continuous headache
    d. blurring of vision
    e. pain in abdomen
    f. persistent vomiting
    g. chills and fever
    h. scant urine
    i. sudden escape of large amount of fluid from vagina
34. 1. h
    2. a
    3. d
    4. e
    5. b
    6. g
    7. i
    8. f
35. 1. d
    2. b
    3. a
    4. c
36. backache
37. dependent edema
38. rule out preeclampsia
39. soap
40. increases, decreases
41. 5, 4, 1
42. 11.0 g/dl

CHAPTER 5

1. a
2. c
3. b
4. a
5. fetal activity
6. full
7. ultrasonography
8. fetal death
9. amniocentesis
10. intrauterine transfusions
11. titer
12. blood transfusion
13. RhoGAM
14. inducing end of pregnancy
15. termination of pregnancy before fetus has become viable
16. rest
17. overdistention of uterus
18. 17, 35, 6
19. a. hemorrhage
    b. hypertension

20. diabetes, heart disease
21. after, before
22. to help the mother and family to work through the grief process of denial, anger, bargaining, depression, and acceptance
23. to carefully regulate insulin dosage and dietary management
24. gestational diabetes
25. a. Recognize fears about uncertain pregnancy outcome.
    b. Make sure each woman who should get RhoGAM is treated.
    c. Explain causes of Rh incompatibilities to families.
26. a. abortion
    b. ectopic pregnancy
    c. GTN
27. a. placenta previa
    b. abruptio placentaelanguage barriers
28. a. inaccessibility
    b. high cost
    c. language barriers
29. a. Encourage her to express her fears.
    b. Encourage her to control her own environment (i.e., plan her daily care).
    c. Offer anticipatory guidance.
30. It is possible.
31. a. edema
    b. proteinuria
    c. elevated blood pressure
32. a. quiet room
    b. weigh daily
    c. intake and output
    d. medication
    e. eclamptic precautions
    f. check for albumin AM and PM
    g. collect laboratory specimens
    h. monitor fetus
    i. check patellar reflexes 4 times a day
33. a. marginal
    b. complete
    c. partial
34. 1. e
    2. a, b
    3. c, d
35. 1. b
    2. d
    3. c
    4. e
    5. a

CHAPTER 6

1. a. relaxation and breathing techniques
   b. physical exercises (squatting, tailor sits, pelvic rock, etc.)
   c. physical happenings and emotional responses of pregnancy
   d. second-stage coping techniques and pushing techniques

e. good posture and body mechanics

f. genital and pelvic floor awareness and exercises

2. b
3. b
4. d
5. c
6. b
7. c
8. c
9. c
10. (demonstration to instructor)

CHAPTER 7

1. c
2. a
3. c
4. complete dilation
5. 8 to 10; 3 to 5
6. birth
7. 30 minutes to 2 hours; 5 to 30 minutes
8. placental
9. 5 to 30 minutes
10. birth, until vital signs are stable
11. 1 to 2 hours
12. station
13. fear, happiness, increased anxiety, seriousness, heavy perspiration, restlessness, and elation
14. True: regular and dilate cervix
    prelabor: irregular and do not dilate cervix
15. A
16. 10 centimeters
17. 1 centimeter
18. 10 centimeters
19. a. perspiration
    b. chills
    c. hiccups
    d. nausea and vomiting
20. This is a normal experience.
21. The pelvic inlet's widest diameter is transverse, and the widest diameter of outlet is anterior-posterior.
22. a. engagement
    b. descent
    c. flexion
    d. internal rotation
    e. extension
    f. restitution
    g. expulsion
23. a. cephalic
    b. breech
    c. shoulder
    d. face
    e. brow
24. 200 to 500 milliliters
25. a. to facilitate delivery when fetal distress occurs

b. to relieve prolonged pressure on fetal head

c. to enlarge vaginal outlet

d. because a clean cut is easier to repair than a laceration

26. second stage
27. firm
28. a
29. longitudinal
30. cephalic presentation
31. a. LOA
    b. LOT
    c. LOP
    d. ROA
    e. ROT
    f. ROP
32. 1. d
    2. b
    3. c

CHAPTER 8

1. preference profile, identification, and financial arrangements
2. a. when contractions began, frequency, and duration
    b. vaginal discharge
    c. membranes
    d. EDD
    e. time of last meal
    f. general condition of mother
3. 4, recorded, 2 hours
4. albumin, preeclampsia
5. 80
6. With strong uterine contractions the uterine wall cannot be indented by the examiner's fingers.
7. head, fundus, back, symphysis pubis, feet
8. 120 to 160
9. a. after any procedure
    b. after membranes rupture
    c. after medicating the mother
10. The purpose is to pick up early warning signs of fetal distress.
11. 1. b, d
    2. e, f
    3. a, c
12. baseline
13. 1. c, d
    2. a, b
14. b
15. a
16. b
17. a
18. a
19. a
20. b
21. 1. can slow down descent of fetus
    2. can cause supine-hypotensive syndrome

3. may mean fetal distress

4. may mean complete dilation

22. increased bloody show, urge to move bowels, vomiting

23. silver nitrate or erythromycin ointment

24. Explain that it is required by law and why.

25. a. skin and mucous membrane
    b. skin and muscles
    c. skin, muscles, and rectal sphincter
    d. skin, mucus, muscles, rectal sphincter, and anal wall

26. a. Ergotrate 0.2 milligrams by mouth or intramuscularly
    b. Methergine 0.2 milligrams by mouth or intramuscularly
    c. Pitocin 10 to 40 units intravenously by infusion in 500 to 1000 ml of intravenous solution

27. a. color
    b. reflex response
    c. heart rate
    d. respiratory effort
    e. muscle tone

28. warmth, open airway, identification

29. 15 minutes

30. massage the uterus

31. 500

32. auscultation and electronic fetal heart monitoring

33. b

34. a

35. a

36. a

37. a

CHAPTER 9

1. 3

2. a

3. 2

4. difficult labor

5. maternal stress and anxiety and disruption in dominance of contraction pattern

6. monitor fetal heart tone closely

7. fetal distress

8. classical

9. hypertonic uterine contractions or fetal distress

10. a. failure to progress in labor
    b. previous cesarean birth
    c. uterine dysfunction
    d. abruptio placentae
    e. placenta previa

11. close observation and recording of vital signs, fetal heart tone, intake and output, and emotional status, plus constant and consistent emotional support

12. a. complete
    b. footling
    c. frank

13. frank

14. a. prolapsed cord
    b. cord compression
    c. head trapped

15. Take the pressure off the cord and keep it pulsating.

16. a. tense uterus
    b. uterus does not relax
    c. pain

17. Be alert for any increase in bright red vaginal bleeding, a drop in blood pressure, and change in fetal heart tones.

18. a. classic
    b. low cervical
    c. extraperitoneal

19. 1. c, d
    2. a, b

20. See Table 9-3.

21. See Table 9-4.

22. a

23. d

24. b

25. c

CHAPTER 10

1. 1. c
   2. a
   3. b

2. d

3. a

4. 4

5. 3

6. b

7. c

8. b

9. c

10. b

11. c

12. a

13. 1. b
    2. b
    3. a
    4. a
    5. d
    6. d
    7. c
    8. c
    9. f
    10. e
    11. g

14. 40, 70

15. 98.6° F

16. drop

17. easier and slower

18. response to the parents

19. dependency
    accept
    baby

20. Sterilization is final; contraception is temporary.

21. b

21. c
22. a
23. b
24. b
25. False
26. True
27. False
28. True
29. True

CHAPTER 11

1. a
2. b
3. c
4. 3
5. 3
6. a
7. No. It is important to drain the ducts.
8. a. abruptio placentae
   b. eclampsia
   c. incomplete abortion
   d. sepsis
9. a. Send photos of infant.
   b. Have parents name infant.
   c. Have parents send clothing for infant.
   d. Speak of infant by name.
10. She should refrain from lifting, housework, and driving for several weeks.
11. disappointment if they expected a vaginal delivery, or relief that baby is all right
12. a. shock and denial
    b. anger
    c. bargaining
    d. depression
    e. acceptance
13. a process that expresses bereaved persons' thoughts and feelings
14. Allow them to grieve; be open and honest.
15. a. Check vaginal flow.
    b. Check fundus.
    c. Check dressings.
    d. Check chest (turn, cough, and deep breathe).
    e. Check intake and output.
    f. Check catheter.

g. Check breasts.
h. Check abdomen for distention.
i. Check extremities.
16. Elevate head of bed.
17. *Streptococcus, Bacteroides,* colon bacillus, *Staphylococcus*
18. less
19. first 24
20. 24 hours; 3
21. b
22. a
23. a
24. 2

CHAPTER 12

1. c and f
2. c
3. 6 milligrams per deciliter, 12 milligrams per deciliter
4. after 24 hours of life
5. prothrombin, coagulation
6. close observation because overheating is possible
7. minimal
8. a
9. c
10. 3
11. b
12. 2500 to 4000 grams (5 lb 8 oz to 8 lb 13 oz); 20 inches; 12 to 13 inches; 13 to 14 inches (33.0 to 35.5 centimeters)
13. a. may have vernix in creases
    b. stand out slightly from head
    c. milia, nose breather, strong suck
    d. baby can see, focuses at 18 inches
    e. short and can be flexed
    f. smaller than head by up to 2 centimeters
    g. appears rounded and large in relation to hips and pelvis
    h. appear large
14. 1. c
    2. b
    3. a
15. See chart below.

Reflex	Appearance	How stimulated	Time of disappearance
Moro's	Present at birth	Sudden noise or motion	3 months
Grasp	Strong at birth	Object to hand	3 months
Step	Present at birth	Feet barely touching surface	4 weeks
Sucking	Strong at birth	Object to mouth	Never

(See pp. 333-334.)

16. 1. b
    2. e
    3. d
    4. g
    5. c
    6. a
    7. f
    8. h
17. lasts from birth to 30 minutes of life; respirations are 60 to 90 per minute, heart rate is 180 or more; baby is alert
18. second reactive phase
19. a. quiet sleep
    b. REM sleep
    c. active alert
    d. quiet alert
    e. crying
    f. transitional
20. 1. e
    2. a
    3. c
    4. f
    5. b
    6. d
21. avoid drafts
22. drying baby
23. a warm blanket between baby and cold surface
24. radiant warmer because there is more room to work
25. 1. f
    2. b
    3. d
    4. a
    5. c
    6. e
26. a. skin
    b. lanugo
    c. plantar creases
    d. breast
    e. ear
    f. genitals (male)
    g. genitals (female)

CHAPTER 13

1. c
2. b
3. a
4. c
5. c

6. c
7. c
8. b
9. b
10. c
11. a. chest lag
    b. intercostal retraction
    c. xiphoid retraction
    d. nares dilation
    e. expiratory grunt
12. hyperbilirubinemia
13. Rh and ABO
14. a. prematurity
    b. hemorrhage
    c. infection
    d. acidosis
    e. certain drugs
    f. low serum albumin levels
15. respiratory
16. pneumonia
17. soft, feeble
18. vital signs every 2 hours, turning infant frequently, adequate fluid intake, temperature control
19. Resuscitate infant.
20. Show photos of a neonatal intensive care nursery; explain equipment and care.
21. Listen; offer anticipatory guidance.
22. 1. c
    2. a
    3. d
    4. b
    5. e
23. 1. b
    2. a
24. 1. a
    2. c

CHAPTER 14

1. education, postpartum, telephone
2. mother, infant
3. mother-baby
4. management
5. teaching
6. autonomy
7. True
8. True
9. False
10. False

APPENDIX A

Joint Position Statement on the Development of Family-Centered Maternity/Newborn Care in Hospitals*

PREAMBLE

The Interprofessional Task Force on Health Care of Women and Children endorses the concept of family-centered maternity care as an acceptable approach to maternal/newborn care. The Task Force believes it would be beneficial to offer further comment and guidance to facilitate the implementation of such care. To this end, the organizations constituting the Task Force have participated in a multidisciplinary effort to develop a joint statement regarding the rationale behind and the practical implementation of family-centered maternity/newborn care. The effort has resulted in the development of this document, which the parent organizations believe can be helpful to those institutions considering or already implementing such programs. A description of potential components of family-centered maternity/newborn care is presented to assist implementation as judged appropriate at the local level.

DEFINITION: FAMILY-CENTERED MATERNITY/NEWBORN CARE

Family-centered maternity/newborn care can be defined as the delivery of safe, quality health care while recognizing, focusing on, and adapting to both the physical and psychosocial needs of the client-patient,

*From Interprofessional Task Force on Health Care of Women and Children, June, 1978.

the family, and the newly born. The emphasis is on the provision of maternity/newborn health care which fosters family unity while maintaining physical safety.

POSITION STATEMENT

The Task Force organizations, The American College of Obstetricians and Gynecologists, the American College of Nurse-Midwives, The Nurses Association of The American College of Obstetricians and Gynecologists, the American Academy of Pediatrics, and the American Nurses' Association, endorse the philosophy of family-centered maternity/newborn care. The development of this conviction is based upon a recognition that health includes not only physical dimensions, but social, economic and psychologic dimensions as well. Therefore, health care delivery, to be effective and satisfying for providers and the community alike, does well to acknowledge all these dimensions by adhering to the following philosophy.

- That the family is the basic unit of society;
- That the family is viewed as a whole unit within which each member is an individual enjoying recognition and entitled to consideration;
- That childbearing and childrearing are unique and important functions of the family;
- That childbearing is an experience that is appropriate and beneficial for the family to share as a unit;

429

- That childbearing is a developmental opportunity and/or a situational crisis, during which the family members benefit from the supporting solidarity of the family unit.

To this end, the family-centered philosophy and delivery of maternal and newborn care is important in assisting families to cope with the childbearing experience and to achieve their own goals within the concept of a high level of wellness, and within the context of the cultural atmosphere of their choosing.

The implementation of family-centered care includes recognition that the provision of maternity/newborn care requires a team effort of the woman and her family, health care providers, and the community. The composition of the team may vary from setting to setting and include obstetricians, pediatricians, family physicians, certified nurse-midwives, nurse practitioners, and other nurses. While physicians are responsible for providing direction for medical management, other team members share appropriately in managing the health care of the family, and each team member must be individually accountable for the performance of his/her facet of care. The team concept includes the cooperative interrelationships of hospitals, health care providers, and the community in an organized system of care so as to provide for the total spectrum of maternity/newborn care within a particular geographic region.[1]

As programs are planned, it is the joint responsibility of all health professionals and their organizations involved with maternity/newborn care, through their assumptions and with input from the community, to establish guidelines for family-centered maternal and newborn care and to assure that such care will be made available to the community regardless of economic status. It is the joint concern and responsibility of the professional organizations to commit themselves to the delivery of maternal and newborn health care in settings where maximum physical safety and psychological well-being for mother and child can be assured. With these requirements met, the hospital setting provides the maximum opportunity for physical safety and for psychological well-being. The development of a family-centered philosophy and implementation of the full range of this family-centered care within innovative and safe hospital settings provides the community/family with the optimum services they desire, request and need.

In view of these insights and convictions, it is recommended that each hospital obstetric, pediatric, and family practice department choosing this approach designate a joint committee on family-centered maternity/newborn care encompassing all recognized and previously stated available team members, including the community. The mission of this committee would be to develop, implement, and regularly evaluate a positive and comprehensive plan for family-centered maternity/newborn care in that hospital.

In addition, it is recommended that all of this be accomplished in the context of joint support for:

- The published standards as presented by The American College of Obstetricians and Gynecologists, The American College of Nurse-Midwives, The Nurses Association of The American College of Obstetricians and Gynecologists, The American Academy of Pediatrics, and the American Nurses' Association.[2-7]
- The implementation of the recommendations for the regional planning of maternal and perinatal health services, as appropriate for each region.
- The availability of a family-centered maternity/newborn service at all levels of maternity care within the regional perinatal network.

POTENTIAL COMPONENTS OF FAMILY-CENTERED MATERNITY/NEWBORN CARE

No specific or detailed plan for implementation of family-centered maternity/newborn care is uniformly applicable, although general guidance as to the potential components of such care is commonly sought. The following description is intended to help those who seek such guidance and is not meant to be uniformly recommended for all maternity/newborn hospital units. The attitudes and needs of the community and the providers vary from geographic area to geographic area, and economic constraints may substantially modify the utilization of each component. The detailed implementation in each hospital unit should be left to that hos-

[1]Committee on Perinatal Health, The National Foundation—March of Dimes. *Toward Improving the Outcome of Pregnancy: Recommendations for the Regional Development of Maternal and Perinatal Health Services,* 1976.

[2]The American College of Obstetricians and Gynecologists. Standards for Obstetric-Gynecologic Services, 1974.

[3]American College of Nurse-Midwives. Functions, Standards, and Qualifications, 1975.

[4]The Nurses Association of The American College of Obstetricians and Gynecologists. Obstetric, Gynecologic and Neonatal Nursing Functions and Standards, 1975.

[5]American Academy of Pediatrics. Standards and Recommendations for Hospital Care of Newborn Infants, 1977.

[6]American Nurses' Association. Standards of Maternal-Child Health Nursing Practice, 1973.

[7](a) The American College of Obstetricians and Gynecologists, the American College of Nurse-Midwives, and The Nurses Association of The American College of Obstetricians and Gynecologists. Joint Statement on Maternity Care, 1971. (b) The American College of Obstetricians and Gynecologists, The American College of Nurse-Midwives, and The Nurses Association of The American College of Obstetricians and Gynecologists. Supplement to Joint Statement on Maternity Care, 1975.

pital's multidisciplinary committee established to deal with such development. In addition to the maternal/newborn health care team, community and hospital administrative input should be assured. In this manner, each hospital unit can best balance community needs within economic reality.

The major change in maternity/newborn units needed in order to make family-centered care work is attitudinal. Nevertheless, a description of the potential physical and functional components of family-centered care is useful. It remains for each hospital unit to implement those components judged feasible for that unit.

I. **Preparation of families:** The unit should provide preparation for childbirth classes taught by appropriately prepared health professionals. Whenever possible, physicians and hospital maternity nurses should participate in such programs so as to maximize cohesion of the team providing education and care. All class approaches should include a bibliography of reading materials. The objectives of these classes are as follows:

   A. To increase the community's awareness of their responsibility toward ensuring a healthy outcome for mother and child.

   B. To serve as opportunities for the community and providers to match expectations and achieve mutual goals from the childbirth experience.

   C. To serve to assist the community to be eligible for participation in the full family-centered program.

   D. To include a tour of the hospital's maternity and newborn units. The tour should be offered as an integral part of the preparation for childbirth programs and be available to the community by appointment. The public should be informed of a mechanism for emergency communication with the maternity/newborn unit.

II. **Preparation of hospital staff:** A continuing education program should be conducted on an ongoing basis to educate *all levels* of hospital personnel who either directly or indirectly come in contact with the family-centered program. This education program may include:

   ▪ Content of local preparation for childbirth classes.

   ▪ Current trends in childbirth practices.

   ▪ Alternative childbirth practices: safe and unsafe, as they are being practiced.

   ▪ Needs of childbearing families to share the total experience.

   ▪ Ways to support those families experiencing less than optimal outcome of pregnancy.

   ▪ Explanation of term "family" so that it includes

any "significant" or "supporting other" individual to the expectant mother.

   ▪ The advantages to families and to the larger society of establishing the parenting bond immediately after birth.

   ▪ The responsibilities of the patients toward ensuring a healthy outcome of the childbirth experience.

   ▪ The potential long-term economic advantage to the hospital for initiating the program and how this could benefit each employee.

   ▪ The satisfaction to be gained by each employee while assisting families to adjust to the new family member.

   ▪ How the family-centered program is to function and the role each employee is to perform to ensure its success.

III. **Family-centered program within the maternity/newborn unit:** The husband or "supporting other" can remain with the patient throughout the childbirth process as much as possible. Family-newborn interaction immediately after birth is encouraged.

   A. *Family Waiting Room* and Early Labor Lounge, attractively painted and furnished, should be available in or near the obstetric suite where:

      1. Patients in early labor could walk and visit with children, husbands, and others.

      2. The husband or "supporting other" person could go for a "rest break" if necessary.

      3. Access to light nourishment should be available for the husband or "supporting other."

      4. Reading materials are available.

      5. Telephone/intercom connections with the labor area are available.

   B. *Diagnostic-Admitting Room* should be adjacent to or near the Family Waiting Room where:

      1. Women could be examined to ascertain their status in labor without being formally admitted if they are in early labor.

      2. Any woman patient past 20 weeks' gestation could be evaluated for emergency health problems during pregnancy.

   C. *"Birthing Room":*

      1. A combination labor and delivery room for patient and the husband or "supporting other" during a normal labor and delivery.

      2. A brightly and attractively decorated and furnished room designed to enhance a home-like atmosphere. A comfortable lounge chair is useful.

3. Stocked for medical emergencies for mother and infant with equipment concealed behind wall cabinets or drapes, but readily available when needed.
4. Wired for music or intercom as desired.
5. Equipped with a modern labor-delivery bed which can be:
   a. raised and lowered.
   b. adjustable to semi-sitting position.
   c. moved to the delivery room if the need arises.
6. Equipped with a cribbette with warmer and have the capacity for infant resuscitation.
7. Appropriately supplied for a normal spontaneous vaginal delivery and the immediate care of a normal newborn.
8. An environment in which breastfeeding and handling of the baby are encouraged immediately after delivery with due consideration given to maintaining the baby's normal temperature.

D. *Labor Rooms:*
   1. The husband or "supporting other" can be with a laboring patient whether progress in labor is normal or abnormal.
   2. Regulation hospital equipment is available.
   3. An emergency delivery can be performed.
   4. Attention is given to the surroundings which are attractively furnished and include a comfortable lounge chair.

E. *Delivery Rooms:* Should be properly equipped with standard items but, in addition, should have delivery tables with adjustable backrests. An overhead mirror should be available. The delivery rooms should accommodate breast-feeding and handling of the baby after delivery with due consideration to maintaining the baby's normal temperature.

F. *Recovery Room:* Patients may be returned from the delivery room to their original labor rooms, depending upon the demand, or to a recovery room. Such a recovery room should have all the standard equipment but also allow for the following options:
   1. The infant to be allowed to be with the mother and father or "supporting other" for a time period after delivery with due consideration given to the infant's physiologic adjustment to extrauterine life. Where feasible, postcaesarean section patients may be allowed the same option.

2. The husband or "supporting other" to be allowed to visit with the new mother and baby with some provision for privacy.
3. A "pass" to be given to the father or "supporting other" of the baby to allow for extended visiting privileges on the "new family unit."

G. The Postpartum *"New Family Unit"* should:
   1. Contain flexible rooming-in with a central nursery to allow:
      a. Optional "rooming-in."
      b. Babies to be returned to the central nursery for professional nursing care when desired by the mother.
      c. Maximum desired maternal/infant contact especially during the first 24 hours.
   2. Have extended visiting hours for the father or "supporting other" to provide the opportunity to assist with the care and feeding of the baby.
   3. Have limited visiting hours for friends since the emphasis of the family-centered approach is on the family.
   4. Contain a family room where:
      a. Children can visit with their mothers and fathers.
      b. Professional staff are available to answer questions about parenting and issues regarding adjustments to the enlarged family.
      c. Cafeteria-like meals can be served and eaten restaurant-style by the mothers.
   5. Have group and individual instruction provided by appropriately prepared personnel on postpartum care, family planning, infant feeding, infant care, and parenting.
   6. Allow visiting and feeding by the mothers in the special nurseries such as:
      a. Newborn, intensive care nursery.
      b. Isolation nursery.
   7. Allow for breastfeeding/bottle feeding on demand with professional personnel available for assistance.

H. Discharge planning should include options for early discharge. If this option is desired, careful attention to continuing medical and/or nursing contact after discharge to ensure maternal and newborn health is important. Potential for utilization of appropriate referral systems should be available.

APPENDIX B

1. *The Pregnant Patient has the right*, prior to the administration of any drug or procedure, to be informed by the health professional caring for her of any potential direct or indirect effects, risks or hazards to herself or her unborn or newborn infant which may result from the use of a drug or procedure prescribed for or administered to her during pregnancy, labor, birth or lactation.

2. *The Pregnant Patient has the right*, prior to the proposed therapy, to be informed, not only of the benefits, risks and hazards of the proposed therapy but also of known alternative therapy, such as available childbirth education classes which could help to prepare the Pregnant Patient physically and mentally to cope with the discomfort or stress of pregnancy and the experience of childbirth, thereby reducing or eliminating her need for drugs and obstetric intervention. She should be offered such information early in her pregnancy in order that she may make a reasoned decision.

3. *The Pregnant Patient has the right*, prior to the administration of any drug, to be informed by the health professional who is prescribing or administering the drug to her that any drug which she receives during pregnancy, labor and birth, no matter how or when the drug is taken or administered, may adversely affect her unborn baby, directly or indirectly, and that there is no drug or chemical which has been proven safe for the unborn child.

4. *The Pregnant Patient has the right*, if Cesarean section is anticipated, to be informed prior to the administration of any drug, and preferably prior to her hospitalization, that minimizing her and, in turn, her baby's intake of nonessential preoperative medicine will benefit her baby.

5. *The Pregnant Patient has the right*, prior to the administration of a drug or procedure, to be informed if there is NO properly controlled follow-up research which has established the safety of the drug or procedure with regard to its direct and/or indirect effects on the physiologic, mental, and neurologic development of the child exposed, via the mother, to the drug or procedure during pregnancy, labor, birth, or lactation— (this would apply to virtually all drugs and the vast majority of obstetric procedures).

6. *The Pregnant Patient has the right*, prior to the administration of any drug, to be informed of the brand name and generic name of the drug in order that she may advise the health professional of any past adverse reaction to the drug.

7. *The Pregnant Patient has the right* to determine for herself, without pressure from her attendant, whether she will accept the risks inherent in the proposed therapy or refuse a drug or procedure.

8. *The Pregnant Patient has the right* to know the name and qualifications of the individual administering a medication or procedure to her during labor or birth.

9. *The Pregnant Patient has the right* to be informed, prior to the administration of any procedure, whether that procedure is being administered to her for her or her baby's benefit (medically indicated) or as an elective procedure (for convenience or teaching purposes).

10. *The Pregnant Patient has the right* to be accompanied during the stress of labor and birth by someone she cares for, and to whom she looks for emotional comfort and encouragement.

11. *The Pregnant Patient has the right* after appropriate medical consultation to choose a position for labor and for birth which is least stressful to her baby and to herself.

12. *The Obstetric Patient has the right* to have her baby cared for at her bedside if her baby is normal, and to feed her baby according to her baby's needs rather than according to the hospital regimen.

13. *The Obstetric Patient has the right* to be informed in writing of the name of the person who actually delivered her baby and the professional qualifications of that person. This information should also be on the birth certificate.

14. *The Obstetric Patient has the right* to be informed if there is any known or indicated aspect of her baby's care or condition which may cause her or her baby later difficulty or problems.

15. *The Obstetric Patient has the right* to have her and her baby's hospital medical records complete, accurate, and legible and to have these records, including Nurses' Notes, retained by the hospital until the child reaches at least the age of majority, or, alternatively, to have the records offered to her before they are destroyed.

*Prepared by Doris Haire, Chair., Committee on Health Law and Regulation, International Childbirth Education Association.

The Pregnant Patient's Bill of Rights*—cont'd

16. *The Obstetric Patient,* both during and after her hospital stay, *has the right* to have access to her complete medical records, including Nurses' Notes, and to receive a copy upon payment of a reasonable fee and without incurring the expense of retaining an attorney. It is the obstetric patient and her baby, not the health professional, who must sustain any trauma or injury resulting from the use of a drug or obstetric procedure. The observation of the rights listed above will not only permit the obstetric patient to participate in the decisions involving her and her baby's health care, but will help to protect the health professional and the hospital against litigation arising from resentment or misunderstanding on the part of the mother.

The Pregnant Patient's Responsibilities*

In addition to understanding her rights the Pregnant Patient should also understand that she too has certain responsibilities. The Pregnant Patient's responsibilities include the following:

1. The Pregnant Patient is responsible for learning about the physical and psychological process of labor, birth and postpartum recovery. The better informed expectant parents are the better they will be able to participate in decisions concerning the planning of their care.
2. The Pregnant Patient is responsible for learning what comprises good prenatal and intranatal care and for making an effort to obtain the best care possible.
3. Expectant parents are responsible for knowing about those hospital policies and regulations which will affect their birth and postpartum experience.
4. The Pregnant Patient is responsible for arranging for a companion or support person (husband, mother, sister, friend, etc.) who will share in her plans for birth and who will accompany her during her labor and birth experience.
5. The Pregnant Patient is responsible for making her preferences known clearly to the health professionals involved in her case in a courteous and cooperative manner and for making mutually agreed-upon arrangements regarding maternity care alternatives with her physician and hospital in advance of labor.
6. Expectant parents are responsible for listening to their chosen physician or midwife with an open mind, just as they expect him or her to listen openly to them.
7. Once they have agreed to a course of health care, expectant parents are responsible, to the best of their ability, for seeing that the program is carried out in consultation with others with whom they have made the agreement.
8. The Pregnant Patient is responsible for obtaining information in advance regarding the approximate cost of her obstetric and hospital care.
9. The Pregnant Patient who intends to change her physician or hospital is responsible for notifying all concerned, well in advance of the birth if possible, and for informing both of her reasons for changing.
10. In all their interactions with medical and nursing personnel, the expectant parents should behave toward those caring for them with the same respect and consideration they themselves would like.
11. During the mother's hospital stay the mother is responsible for learning about her and her baby's continuing care after discharge from the hospital.
12. After birth, the parents should put into writing constructive comments and feelings of satisfaction and/or dissatisfaction with the care (nursing, medical and personal) they received. Good service to families in the future will be facilitated by those parents who take the time and responsibility to write letters expressing their feelings about the maternity care they received.

All the previous statements assume a normal birth and postpartum experience. Expectant parents should realize that, if complications develop in their cases, there will be an increased need to trust the expertise of the physician and hospital staff they have chosen. However, if problems occur, the childbearing woman still retains her responsibility for making informed decisions about her care or treatment and that of her baby. If she is incapable of assuming that responsibility because of her physical condition, her previously authorized companion or support person should assume responsibility for making informed decisions on her behalf.

*By members of the International Childbirth Education Association.

Preference Profile

Preference Profile

Mother's name _____ Age _____

Father/labor partner's name _____ Age _____

Grav _____ Para _____ Age of children _____

Due date _____ Caregiver _____

Other support person? _____

Prenatal classes _____ Yes _____ No _____ What kind? _____ Where? _____

Baby care classes _____ Yes _____ No _____ What kind? _____ Where? _____

Desire to restrict visitors? _____

Whom do you want with you in labor? _____ For birth? _____

Type of childbirth expected: _____

Do you desire anesthesia for birth? _____

Do you have any medical problems or allergies? _____

Do you have any strong feelings about the following?
1. Episiotomy _____
2. Breast-feeding _____
3. Bottle-feeding _____
4. Circumcision _____
5. Cutting of umbilical cord _____
6. Lighting at birth _____
7. Medications for mother or baby _____
8. Fetal monitor—use of or type _____
9. Intravenous fluids _____
10. Partner's presence at cesarean birth _____

Do you want the baby to go to a nursery or stay with you in mother-baby nursing? _____

Is there something special you would like to learn or do while in the hospital? _____

How can the medical and nursing staff help you to achieve your preferences for labor and delivery? _____

Signed _____
      Signatures of mother and labor partner and dates

APPENDIX D

Transfer of Drugs and Other Chemicals into Human Milk

Since the first publication of this statement, much new information has been published concerning the transfer of drugs and chemicals into human milk. This information, in addition to other research published before 1983, makes a revision of the previous statement necessary. In this revision, lists of the pharmacological or chemical agents transferred into human milk and their possible effects on the infant or on lactation, if known, are provided (Tables 1 to 7). The fact that a pharmacological or chemical agent does not appear in the tables is not meant to imply that it is not transferred into human milk or that it does not have an effect on the infant, but indicates that there are no reports in the literature. These tables should assist the physician in counseling a nursing mother regarding breast-feeding when the mother has a condition for which a drug is medically indicated.

The following questions should be considered when prescribing drug therapy to lactating women. (1) Is the drug therapy really necessary? Consultation between the pediatrician and the mother's physician can be most useful. (2) Use the safest drug; for example, acetaminophen rather than aspirin for oral analgesia. (3) If there is a possibility that a drug may present a risk to the infant (e.g., phenytoin, phenobarbital), consideration should be given to measurement of blood concentra-

TABLE 1
Drugs That Are Contraindicated During Breast-Feeding

Drug	Reported sign or symptom in infant or effect on lactation
Bromocriptine	Suppresses lactation
Cocaine	Cocaine intoxication
Cyclophosphamide	Possible immune suppression; unknown effect on growth or association with carcinogenesis; neutropenia
Cyclosporine	Possible immune suppression; unknown effect on growth or association with carcinogenesis
Doxorubicin*	Possible immune suppression; unknown effect on growth or association with carcinogenesis
Ergotamine	Vomiting, diarrhea, convulsions (doses used in migraine medications)
Lithium	$\frac{1}{3}$ to $\frac{1}{2}$ therapeutic blood concentration in infants
Methotrexate	Possible immune suppression; unknown effect on growth or association with carcinogenesis; neutropenia
Phencyclidine (PCP)	Potent hallucinogen
Phenindione	Anticoagulant; increased prothrombin and partial thromboplastin time in 1 infant (not used in USA)

*Drug is concentrated in human milk.

TABLE 2
Drugs of Abuse That Are Contraindicated During Breast-Feeding*

Drug	Effect
Amphetamine	Irritability, poor sleep pattern
Cocaine	Cocaine intoxication
Heroin	
Marijuana	Only one report in literature; no effect mentioned
Nicotine (smoking)	Shock, vomiting, diarrhea, rapid heart rate, restlessness; decreased milk production
Phencyclidine	Potent hallucinogen

*The Committee on Drugs believes strongly that nursing mothers should not ingest any of these compounds. Not only are they hazardous to the nursing infant, but they are detrimental to the physical and emotional health of the mother.

TABLE 3
Radiopharmaceuticals That Require Temporary Cessation of Breast-Feeding*

Drug	Recommended alteration in breast-feeding pattern
Gallium-67 (^{67}Ga)	Radioactivity in milk present for 2 wk
Indium-111 (^{111}In)	Small amount present at 20 hr
Iodine-125 (^{125}I)	Risk of thyroid cancer; radioactivity in milk present for 12 days
Iodine-131 (^{131}I)	Radioactivity in milk present 2 to 14 days depending on study
Radioactive sodium	Radioactivity in milk present 96 hr
Technetium-99m (^{99m}Tc), ^{99m}Tc macroaggregates, ^{99m}TcO$_4$	Radioactivity in milk present 15 hr to 3 days

*Consult nuclear medicine physician before performing diagnostic study so that a radionuclide with the shortest excretion time in breast milk can be used. Before study the mother should pump her breast and store enough milk in freezer for feeding the infant; after study the mother should pump her breast to maintain milk production but discard all milk pumped for the required time that radioactivity is present in milk.

TABLE 4
Drugs Whose Effect on Nursing Infants Is Unknown but May Be of Concern

Drug	Effect
Psychotropic drugs	Special concern when given to nursing mothers for long periods
Antianxiety	
Diazepam	None
Lorazepam	None
Prazepam*	None
Quazepam	None
Antidepressant	
Amitriptyline	None
Amoxapine	None
Desipramine	None
Dothiepin	None
Doxepin	None

*Drug is concentrated in human milk.

TABLE 4
Drugs Whose Effect on Nursing Infants Is Unknown but May Be of Concern—cont'd

Drug	Effect
Imipramine	None
Trazodone	None
Antipsychotic	
Chlorpromazine	Galactorrhea in adult; drowsiness and lethargy in infant
Chlorprothixene	None
Haloperidol	None
Mesoridazine	None
Chloramphenicol	Possible idiosyncratic bone marrow suppression
Metoclopramide* K	None described; potent central nervous system drug
Metronidazole	In vitro mutagen; may discontinue breast-feeding 12 to 24 hr to allow excretion of dose when single-dose therapy is given to mother
Tinidazole	See metronidazole

*Drug is concentrated in human milk.

TABLE 5
Drugs That Have Caused Significant Effects on Some Nursing Infants and Should Be Given to Nursing Mothers with Caution*

Drug	Effect
Aspirin (salicylates)	Metabolic acidosis (dose related); may affect platelet function; rash
Clemastine	Drowsiness, irritability, refusal to feed, high-pitched cry, neck stiffness (one case)
Phenobarbital	Sedation; infantile spasms after weaning from milk containing phenobarbital, methemoglobinemia (one case)
Primidone	Sedation, feeding problems
Salicylazosulfapyridine (sulfasalazine)	Bloody diarrhea in one infant

*Measure blood concentration in the infant when possible.

tions in the nursing infant. (4) Drug exposure to the nursing infant may be minimized by having the mother take the medication just after completing a breast-feeding and/or just before the infant has his or her lengthy sleep periods.

Data have been obtained from a search of the medical literature. Because methodologies used to quantitate drugs in milk continue to improve, this current information will require continuous updating. Brand names are listed in Table 8 in accordance with the current *AMA Drug Evaluation,* the *USAN* and *USP Dictionary of Drug Names.* The reference list does not include all articles published.

Physicians who encounter adverse effects in infants fed drug-contaminated human milk are urged to document these effects in a communication to the AAP Committee on Drugs and the U.S. Food and Drug Administration. Such communication should include: the generic and brand name of the drug, the maternal dose and mode of administration, the concentration of the drug in milk and maternal and infant blood in relation to time of ingestion, the age of the infant, and the method used for laboratory identification. Such reports may significantly increase the pediatric community's fund of knowledge regarding drug transfer into human milk and the potential or actual risk to the infant.

TABLE 6
Maternal Medication Usually Compatible with Breast-Feeding*

Drug	Reported sign or symptom in infant or effect on lactation
Anesthetics, Sedatives	
Alcohol	Drowsiness, diaphoresis, deep sleep, weakness, decrease in linear growth, and abnormal weight gain; maternal ingestion of 1 g/kg daily decreases milk ejection reflex
Barbiturate	See Table 5
Bromide	Rash, weakness, absence of cry with maternal intake of 5.4 g/day
Chloral hydrate	Sleepiness
Chloroform	None
Halothane	None
Lidocaine	None
Magnesium sulfate	None
Methyprylon	Drowsiness
Secobarbital	None
Thiopental	None
Anticoagulants	
Bishydroxycoumarin	None
Warfarin	None
Antiepileptics	
Carbamazepine	None
Ethosuximide	None; drug appears in infant serum
Phenobarbital	See Table 5
Phenytoin	Methemoglobinemia (one case)
Primidone	See Table 5
Thiopental	None
Valproic acid	None
Antihistamines, decongestants, and bronchodilators	
Dexbrompheniramine maleate with *d*-isoephedrine	Crying, poor sleep patterns, irritability
Dyphylline†	None
Iodides	May affect thyroid activity; see Miscellaneous, iodine
Pseudoephedrine†	None
Terbutaline	None
Theophylline	Irritability
Triprolidine	None
Antihypertensive and cardiovascular drugs	
Acebutolol	None
Atenolol	None
Captopril	None
Digoxin	None
Diltiazem	None
Disopyramide	None
Hydralazine	None
Labetalol	None
Lidocaine	None
Methyldopa	None

*Drugs listed have been reported in the literature as having the effects listed or no effect. The word "none" means that no observable change was seen in the nursing infant while the mother was ingesting the compound. It is emphasized that most of the literature citations concern single case reports or small series of infants.
†Drug is concentrated in human milk.

TABLE 6
Maternal Medication Usually Compatible with Breast-Feeding—cont'd

Drug	Reported sign or symptom in infant or effect on lactation
Metoprolol†	None
Mexiletine	None
Minoxidil	None
Nadolol†	None
Oxprenolol	None
Procainamide	None
Propranolol	None
Quinidine	None
Timolol	None
Verapamil	None
Antiinfective Drugs (all antibiotics transfer into breast milk in limited amounts)	
Acyclovir†	None
Amoxicillin	None
Aztreonam	None
Cefadroxil	None
Cefazolin	None
Cefotaxime	None
Cefoxitin	None
Ceftazidime	None
Ceftriaxone	None
Chloroquine	None
Clindamycin	None
Cycloserine	None
Dapsone	None; sulfonamide detected in infant's urine
Erythromycin†	None
Ethambutol	None
Hydroxychloroquine†	None
Isoniazid	None; acetyl metabolite also secreted; ? hepatoxicity
Kanamycin	None
Moxalactam	None
Nalidixic acid	Hemolysis in infant with glucose-6-phosphate deficiency (G-6-PD)
Nitrofurantoin	Hemolysis in infant with G-6-PD
Pyrimethamine	None
Quinine	None
Rifampin	None
Salicylazosulfapyridine (sulfasalazine)	See Table 5
Streptomycin	None
Sulbactam	None
Sulfapyridine	Caution in infant with jaundice or G-6-PD, and in ill, stressed, or premature infant; appears in infant's urine
Sulfisoxazole	Caution in infant with jaundice or G-6-PD and in ill, stressed, or premature infant; appears in infant's urine
Tetracycline	None; negligible absorption by infant
Ticarcillin	None
Trimethoprim/sulfamethoxazole	None
Antithyroid Drugs	
Carbimazole	Goiter
Methimazole (active metabolite or carbimazole)	None
Propylthiouracil	None
Thiouracil	None mentioned; drug not used in USA

†Drug is concentrated in human milk. *Continued.*

TABLE 6
Maternal Medication Usually Compatible with Breast-Feeding—cont'd

Drug	Reported sign or symptom in infant or effect on lactation
Cathartics	
Cascara	None
Danthron	Increased bowel activity
Senna	None
Diagnostic Agents	
Iodine	Goiter; see Miscellaneous, iodine
Iopanoic acid	None
Metrizamide	None
Diuretic Agents	
Bendroflumethiazide	Suppresses lactation
Chlorothiazide, hydrochlorothiazide	None
Chlorthalidone	Excreted slowly
Spironolactone	None
Hormones	
^{3}H-norethynodrel	None
19-norsteroids	None
Clogestone	None
Contraceptive pill with estrogen/progesterone	Rare breast enlargement; decrease in milk production and protein content (not confirmed in several studies)
Estradiol	Withdrawal, vaginal bleeding
Medroxyprogesterone	None
Prednisolone	None
Prednisone	None
Progesterone	None
Muscle Relaxants	
Baclofen	None
Methocarbamol	None
Narcotics, nonnarcotic analgesics, antiinflammatory agents	None
Acetaminophen	None
Butorphanol	None
Codeine	None
Dipyrone	None
Flufenamic acid	None
Gold salts	None
Hydroxychloroquine	None
Ibuprofen	None
Indomethacin	Seizure (one case)
Mefenamic acid	None
Methadone	None if mother receiving ≤20 mg/24 hrs
Morphine	None
Nefopam	None
Phenylbutazone	None
Piroxicam	None
Prednisolone, prednisone	None
Propoxyphene	None
Salicylates	See Table 5
Suprofen	None
Tolmetin	None

TABLE 6
Maternal Medication Usually Compatible with Breast-Feeding—cont'd

Drug	Reported sign or symptom in infant or effect on lactation
Stimulants	
Caffeine	Irritability, poor sleep pattern, excreted slowly; no effect with usual amount of caffeine beverages
Vitamins	
B_1 (thiamin)	None
B_6 (pyridoxine)	None
B_{12} (cyanocobalamin)	None
D (calciferol)	None; follow infant's serum calcium if mother receives pharmacological doses
Folic acid	None
K_1, Aqua MEPHYTON	None
Riboflavin	None
Miscellaneous	
Acetazolamide	None
Atropine, scopolamine	None
Cimetidine†	None
Cisapride	None
Cisplatin	Not found in milk
Domperidone	None
Iodine (povidone-iodine/vaginal douche)	Elevated iodine levels in breast milk, odor of iodine on infant's skin
Metoclopramide	See Table 4
Noscapine	None
Pyridostigmine	None
Tolbutamide	? Jaundice

†Drug is concentrated in human milk.

TABLE 7
Food and Environmental Agents and Their Effect on Breast-Feeding

Agent	Reported sign or symptom in infant or effect on lactation
Aflatoxin	None
Aspartame	Caution if mother or infant has phenylketonuria
Bromide (photographic laboratory)	Potential absorption and bromide transfer into milk; see Table 6, Anesthetics, sedatives
Cadmium	None reported
Chlordane	None reported
Chocolate (theobromine)	Irritability or increased bowel activity if excess amounts (16 oz/day) consumed by mother
DDT, benzene hexachlorides, dieldrin, aldrin, hepatachlorepoxide	None
Fava beans	Hemolysis in patient with glucose-6-phosphate deficiency (G-6-PD)
Fluorides	None
Hexachlorobenzene	Skin rash, diarrhea, vomiting, dark urine, neurotoxicity, death
Hexachlorophene	None; possible contamination of milk from nipple washing
Lead	Possible neurotoxicity
Methylmercury, mercury	May affect neurodevelopment
Monosodium glutamate (MSG)	None
Polychlorinated biphenyls and polybrominated biphenyls	Lack of endurance; hypotonia; sullen, expressionless face
Tetrachlorethylene-cleaning fluid (perchloroethylene)	Obstructive jaundice, dark urine
Vegetarian diet	Signs of B_{12} deficiency

TABLE 8
Trade Names of Generic Drugs*

Generic	Trade	Generic	Trade
acebutolol	Sectral	desipramine	Norpramin, Pertofrane
acetaminophen	Tylenol, Anacin-3, Panadol, Tempra, Phenaphen	dexbrompheniramine maleate with d-isoephedrine	as Disophrol, as Drixoral
acetazolamide	Diamox	dextroamphetamine	Dexedrine
acitretin	Soriatane	diazepam	Valium
acyclovir	Zovirax	digoxin	Lanoxin, Lanoxicaps
allupurinol	Zyloprim	diltiazem	Cardizem
aminosalicylic acid	Rowasa	dipyrone	Diprofarn, Novaldin (unavailable in United States)
amitriptyline	Elavil, Endep		
amoxapine	Asendin		
amoxicillin	Amoxil	disopyramide	Norpace
amphetamine (dextroamphetamine)	Dexedrine	domperidone	Motilium (unavailable in United States)
aspartame	NutraSweet	dothiepin	Prothiaden (unavailable in United States)
atenolol	Tenormin		
azapropazone (apazone)	Not available in the United States	doxepin	Sinequan
		doxorubicin	Adriamycin
aztreonam	Azactam	dyphylline	Dilor
baclofen	Lioresal	enalapril	Vasotec
bendroflumethiazide	Naturetin	ergotamine tartrate with caffeine	as Cafergot
bishydroxycoumarin	Dicumarol		
bromocriptine	Parlodel	estradiol	Estrace
butorphanol	Stadol	ethambutol	Myambutol
captopril	Capoten	ethosuximide	Zarontin
carbamazepine	Tegretol	fentanyl	Sublimaze
carbimazole	Neo-mecazole (foreign)	flecainide	Tambocor
cefadroxil	Duricef	flufenamic acid	Arlef (foreign)
cefazolin	Ancef, Kefzol	fluoxetine	Prozac
cefotaxime	Claforan	fluvoxamine	. . .
cefprozil	Cefzil	gold sodium thiomalate	Myochrysine
ceftazidime	Fortaz		
ceftriaxone	Rocephin	haloperidol	Haldol
chloramphenicol	Chloromycetin	hydralazine	Apresoline
chloroquine	Aralen	hydrochlorothiazide	HydroDIURIL
chlorothiazide	Diuril, Chlotride (foreign)	hydroxychloroquine	Plaquenil
chlorpromazine	Thorazine	ibuprofen	Advil, Motrin
chlorprothixene	Taractan	imipramine	Tofranil, Janimine
chlorthalidone	Hygroton, as Cambipres	indomethacin	Indocin
cimetidine	Tagamet	iopanoic acid	Telepaque
cisapride	Benzamide (foreign)	isoniazid	INH
cisplatin	Platinol	kanamycin	Kantrex
clemastine	Tavegil (foreign), Tavist	ketorolac	Toradol
clindamycin	Cleocin	labetalol	Normodyne, Trandate
clomipramine	Anafranil	levonorgestrel	as Levlen, as Nordette, as Norplant, as Tri-Levien, as Triphasil
colchicine	(Generic only)		
cyclophosphamide	Cytoxan		
cycloserine	Seromycin		
danthron	Dorbane, Istizin	lidocaine	Xylocaine
dapsone	(Generic only)	loperamide	Imodium

*For convenience, one or more examples of the trade name are given.
Reprinted with permission from *Pediatrics,* 1989; Copyright American Academy of Pediatrics 1984-1985.

TABLE 8
Trade Names of Generic Drugs—cont'd

Generic	Trade	Generic	Trade
lorazepam	Ativan	propoxyphene	Darvon, Dolene, SK65
medroxyprogesterone	Provera, Depo-Provera	propranolol	Inderal
mefenamic acid	Ponstel	propylthiouracil	(Generic only)
mesoridazine	Serentil	pseudoephedrine	as Actified, Novafed, as Sudafed
methadone	Dolophine		
methimazole	Tapazole	pyridostigmin	Mestinon
methocarbamol	Robaxin	pyrimethamine	Daraprim
methotrexate (amethopterin)	Folex, Rheumatrex	quazepam	Dormalin
		quinine	as Quinamm
methyprylon	Noludar	rifampin	Rifadin, Rimactane
metoclopramide	Reglan		
metoprolol	Lopressor	secobarbital	Seconal
metrizamide	Amipaque	senna	Senokot
metronidazole	Flagyl, Protostat	sotalol	(Investigational)
mexiletine	Mexitil	spironolactone	Aldactone
midazolam	Versed	sulbactam	as Unasyn
minoxidil	Loniten, Rogaine	sulfasalazine (salicylazosulfapyridine)	Azulfidine
monosodium glutamate	MSG, Accent		
moxalactam	Moxam	sulfisoxazole	Gantrisin
		suprofen	Suprol
nadolol	Corgard		
nalidixic acid	NegGram	temazepam	Restoril
naproxen	Naprosyn	terbutaline	Bricanyl, Brethine
nefopam	Acupan (unavailable in United States)	tetracycline	Achromycin
		theophylline	Bronkodyl, Elixophyllin, Slo-Phyllin, Theo-Dur
nifedipine	Procardia		
nitrofurantoin	Furadantin, Macrodantin	thiopental	Pentothal
[3H]Norethynodrel	as Enovid	thiouracil	Thiouracil (no longer marketed in United States)
noscapine	Tusscapine		
oxprenolol	Trasicor (foreign)		
perphenazine	Trilafon, as Etrafon, as Triavil	ticarcillin	as Timentin
		timolol	Blocadren, Timoptic
phenindione	Hedulin, Indon (unavailable in United States)	tinidazole	Fasigyn, Simplotan (unavailable in United States)
phenylbutazone	Azolid, Butazolidin	tolbutamide	Orinase
phenytoin	Dilantin	tolmetin	Tolectin
piroxicam	Feldene	trazodone	Desyrel
prazepam	Centrax	trimethoprim with sulfamethoxazole	Bactrim, Septra
prednisolone	Delta-Cortef, Meti-Derm, Prelone	triprolidine	Actidil, as Actifed
		valproic acid	Depakene
prednisone	Deltasone, Meticorten, Sterapred	verapamil	Calan
		warfarin	Coumadin, Panwarfin
primidone	Mysoline	zolpidem	Ambien
procainamide	Pronestyl		

APPENDIX E

Audiovisual Resources

Films, videocassettes, slide-tape packages

CHAPTER 1

The Bonding Birth Experience (16 mm film)
Parenting Pictures
121 NW Crystal Street
Crystal River, FL 32629

Knowing the Unborn (video)
ICEA Bookcenter
PO Box 20048
Minneapolis, MN 55420
(800) 624-4934

Pregnancy after 35 (16 mm film)
Polymorph Films
118 South Street
Boston, MA 02111
(617) 542-2004

I Didn't Think It Would Happen to Me (video)
Centre Productions
1800 30th Street, Suite 207
Boulder, CO 80301

Not Yet, Baby! (16 mm film, video)
Phoenix/BFA Films & Video
468 Park Avenue South
New York, NY 10016

Childbirth . . . the Changing Sounds (16 mm film, video)
The Canadian Institute of Child Health
17 York Street
Ottawa, Ontario K1N 5S7
(613) 238-8425

The Expectant Father (video)
Conmar Publishing, Inc
1176 Angela Court, Suite 106
Minden, NV 89423
(702) 267-4246

When Teens Get Pregnant (16 mm film, video)
Polymorph Films
118 South Street
Boston, MA 02111
(617) 542-2004

Growing into Parenthood (video)
Educational Graphic Aids
1695 East Long Lane
Littleton, CO 80121
(303) 796-0088

Being a Single Parent (video) and *Newfathers* (video)
Films for the Humanities and Sciences
PO Box 2053
Princeton, NJ 08543
(609) 452-1128

Pregnant, Single and Prepared (video)
ICEA Bookcenter
PO Box 20048
Minneapolis, MN 55420
(800) 624-4934

The Road (Frontier Nursing Service) (16 mm film)
ANA-NLN Film Library
267 W 25th Street
New York, NY 10001

Midwife: With Woman (16 mm film, video)
Fanlight Productions
47 Halifax Street
Boston, MA 02130
(617) 524-0980

Labor & Delivery for Teens (video)
Churchill Media
12210 Nebraska Avenue
Los Angeles, CA 90025-3600
(800) 334-7930

CHAPTER 2

The Menstrual Cycle (16 mm film)
Eli Lilly Company
Audio Visual Film Library, Dept MC-340
Indianapolis, IN 46206

About Conception and Contraception (16 mm film)
Canadian Film Institute
303 Richmond Road
Ottawa Ontario, Canada

Placental Circulation (16 mm film, video)
   Film Service ACOG
   PO Box 299
   Wheaton, IL 60187
Inner Woman (16 mm film)
   Merrell Dow Pharmaceuticals, Inc
   Subsidiary of the Dow Chemical Co
   Cincinnati, OH 45215
Miracle of Life (video)
   Crown Publication, Inc
   225 Park Avenue South
   New York, NY 10003

CHAPTER 3

Our Genetic Heritage (video)
   March of Dimes
   1275 Mamaroneck Avenue
   White Plains, NY 10605
   (914) 428-7100
Fetal Development: A Nine Month Journey (16 mm film,
      video)
   AIMS Media
   6901 Woodley Avenue
   Van Nuys, CA 91406-4878
Life Before Birth (film strips)
   Time Education Program
   Time & Life Building
   Rockefeller Center
   New York, NY 10020
The Technological Stork (16 mm film, video)
   National Film Board of Canada
   1251 Avenue of the Americas, 16th Floor
   New York, NY 10020
Trying Times: Crisis in Fertility (16 mm film)
   Fanlight Productions
   P.O. Box 226
   Cambridge, MA 02238
Alcohol: Crisis for the Unborn (16 mm film)
   Film Distribution Division
   March of Dimes
   1275 Mamaroneck Avenue
   White Plains, NY 10605
Laparoscopy: The View Within (16 mm film)
   Merrell Dow Pharmaceuticals, Inc
   Subsidiary of the Dow Chemical Co
   Cincinnati, OH 45215
Born Drunk: The Fetal Alcohol Syndrome (16 mm film, video)
   ABC Learning Resources, Inc
   1330 Avenue of the Americas
   New York, NY 10019
   (212) 887-5000
Gifts of Love (video)
   National Down's Syndrome Society
   70 West 40th Street
   New York, NY 10018
The ABCs of STDs (video) and *Infertility in Women* (video)
   Polymorph Films
   118 South Street
   Boston, MA 02111
   (617) 542-2004

CHAPTER 4

Breastfeeding (video)
   Professional Research
   930 Pitner
   Evanston, IL 60202
The ABCs of Breastfeeding (video)
   Lifecircle
   2378 Cornell Drive
   Costa Mesa, CA 92626
   (714) 546-1427
   FAX: (714) 546-0138
Breastfeeding: Better Beginnings (video)
   Lifecycle Productions
   PO Box 183
   Newton, MA 02165
The Biological Aspects of Sexuality (slide/tape)
   Harper and Row
   Media Department
   10 East 53rd Street
   New York, NY 10022
The Case Against Rubella (16 mm film)
   March of Dimes
   1275 Mamaroneck Avenue
   White Plains, NY 10605
   (914) 428-7100
Eating Right for Two (16 mm film, video)
   Churchill Films
   12210 Nebraska Avenue
   Los Angeles, CA 90025
A Study in Maternal Attitudes (16 mm film)
   American Journal of Nursing
   ANA-NLN Film Library
   267 West 25th Street
   New York, NY 10001
Nutritional Management of High-Risk Pregnancy (16 mm
      film, video)
   Films, Society for Nutrition Education
   1736 Franklin Street
   Oakland, CA 94612
Helpful Hints: Some Ideas to Prevent Preterm Labor (video)
   March of Dimes
   1275 Mamaroneck Avenue
   White Plains, NY 10605
   (914) 428-7100
Feeding Your Baby—From Birth through the First Year (16 mm
      film, video)
   Fairview General Hospital
   Audio Visual Communication
   18101 Lorain Avenue
   Cleveland, OH 44107
Sex and Pregnancy (video)
   Centre Films, Inc
   1103 N El Centro Avenue
   Hollywood, CA 90038
Born Hooked (16 mm film)
   Film Distribution Division
   March of Dimes
   1275 Mamaroneck Avenue
   White Plains, NY 10605
   (914) 428-7100

Prenatal Care (video)
 Polymorph Films
 118 South Street
 Boston, MA 02111
 (617) 542-2004
Pregnancy Exercise Program (video)
 ACOG Exercise Programs
 3575 Cahuenga Blvd West, Suite 440
 Los Angeles, CA 90068
From Conception to Birth (video)
 Lifecircle
 2378 Cornell Drive
 Costa Mesa, CA 92626
 (714) 546-1427
 FAX: (714) 546-0138
Maternal Changes and Prenatal Care (video)
 Medcom/Trainex
 PO Box 3225
 Garden Grove, CA 92642
 (800) 877-1443
 (800) 472-2479 (CA)
Growing into Parenthood (video)
 Educational Graphic Aids
 1695 East Long Lane
 Littleton, CO 80121
 (303) 796-0088

CHAPTER 5

Diagnosis Before Birth (16 mm film)
 March of Dimes
 1275 Mamaroneck Avenue
 White Plains, NY 10605
 (914) 428-7100
Hydatidiform Mole (slide/cassette)
 Oxford Tape-Slide Series in Obstetrics and Gynecology
 Pretest Service, Inc
 71 South Turnpike
 Wallingford, CT 06492
Nursing Management of Hypertension of Pregnancy (video)
 American Journal of Nursing Company
 Educational Services Division
 555 West 57th Street
 New York, NY 10019-2961
 (800) 223-2282
Intrauterine Fetal Transfusion (16 mm film)
 Abbott Laboratories
 Public Relations Department
 Film Service D-384
 North Chicago, IL 60064
Diabetes in Pregnancy, Caring for the Childbearing Woman
 (video)
 Polymorph Films
 118 South Street
 Boston, MA 02111
 (617) 542-2004

CHAPTER 6

Hello Baby: The Childbirth Film in Three Parts (16 mm film, video)
 VIDA (Video Health Communications)
 6 Bigelow Street
 Cambridge, MA 02139
 (617) 864-4334
Magical Moments of Birth (video)
 Childbirth Graphics
 PO Box 21207
 Waco, TX 76702-1207
 (800) 299-3366, ext 287
Saturday's Children (video)
 Childbirth Graphics
 PO Box 21207
 Waco, TX 76702-1207
 (800) 299-3366, ext 287
Labors of Love (16 mm film, video)
 Polymorph Films
 118 South Street
 Boston, MA 02111
 (617) 542-2004
Childbirth Preparation Program (video)
 ACOG Exercise Programs
 3575 Cahuenga Blvd West, Suite 440
 Los Angeles, CA 90068
Welcome to the World: Three Birth Stories
 Injoy Productions, Inc
 1490 Riverside Avenue
 Boulder, CO 80304
 (303) 447-2082
Hey, What about Me? (video on sibling adjustment)
 Childbirth Graphics
 PO Box 21207
 Waco, TX 76702-1207
 (800) 299-3366, ext 287

Films on childbirth education in a cultural context

Tamika's Birth
 English with a black cast
 (11-minute, color 16 mm film, video)
Maternidad (Motherhood)
 Spanish with Latino cast
 (10-minute, color 16 mm film, video)
Childbirth Education Films
 Videograph
 2833 25th Street
 San Francisco, CA 94110

CHAPTER 7

Birth Atlas Slide Series (with guide)
 Maternity Center Association
 48 East 92nd Street
 New York, NY 10028
Special Delivery, Creating the Birth You Want For You and Your Baby (video)
 ICEA Bookcenter
 PO Box 20048
 Minneapolis, MN 55420
 (800) 624-4934

CHAPTER 8

Birth in the Squatting Position (16 mm film, video)
Polymorph Films
118 South Street
Boston, MA 02111
(617) 542-2004

All Together Now: A Birth Plan
Family Centered Childbirth Education Association
4635 NW 50th Street
Des Moines, IA 50323

Essentials of Electronic Fetal Monitoring (3 part
  video/workbook/competency evaluation guide)
NAACOG/EFM
P.O. Box 71437
Washington, DC 20024-1437
(800) 533-8822
(202) 638-0026

CHAPTER 9

Epidural Anesthesia for Vaginal Delivery (16 mm film)
Winthrop Laboratories
90 Park Avenue
New York, NY 10016

Having a Section Is Having a Baby (slide/tape, video)
Polymorph Films
118 South Street
Boston, MA 02111
(617) 542-2004

Once a Cesarean (video)
Nicholas J Kaufman Productions
14 Clyde Street
Newtonville, MA 02160
(617) 964-4466

Another Look at Cesarean (video)
Lifecircle
2378 Cornell Drive
Costa Mesa, CA 92626
(714) 546-1427

Deliverance: A Family's Cesarean Experience (16 mm film,
  video)
Polymorph Films
118 South Street
Boston, MA 02111
(617) 542-2004

Critical-Care Obstetrics, Vol I (video)
NAACOG
409 12th Street SW
Washington, DC 20024-2191

Vaginal Birth After Cesarean: What You Should Know (video)
Video Branching Corp.
3721 S Westridge Ave, Suite 128
Kalamazoo, MI 49008-9990

CHAPTER 10

Adapting to Parenthood (16 mm film)
Polymorph Films
118 South Street
Boston, MA 02111
(617) 542-2004

Are You Ready for the Postpartum Experience? (16 mm film)
Parenting Pictures
121 NW Crystal Street
Crystal River, FL 32629

2 AM Feeding (16 mm film)
New Day Films
PO Box 315
Franklin Lakes, NJ 07417

Caring and Coping: The New Parent Experience (16 mm film,
  video)
Parenting Pictures
121 NW Crystal Street
Crystal River, FL 32629

Sex, Love, and Babies: How Babies Change Your Marriage
  (video)
Childbirth Graphics
PO Box 21207
Waco, TX 76702-1207
(800) 299-3366, ext 287

Conception and Contraception: Family Planning
  (slides/cassette, video)
Career Aids
20417 Nordoff St, Dept HA
Chatsworth, CA 91311
(818) 341-2535

Breast-Feeding: Better Beginnings (video)
Customer Fulfillment Service
Wyeth-Ayerst
350 N Pennsylvania Avenue
PO Box 7600
Wilkes-Barre, PA 18773-7600

Norplant Insertion and Removal Procedures (video)
Customer Fulfillment Service
Wyeth-Ayerst
350 N Pennsylvania Avenue
PO Box 7600
Wilkes-Barre, PA 18773-7600

Now That You're Postpartum (16 mm film, video)
Polymorph Films
118 South Street
Boston, MA 02111
(617) 542-2004

Postpartum: A Bittersweet Experience (video) and *Fragile
  Beginnings: Postpartum Mood and Anxiety Disorders*
  (video)
Lifecycle Productions
PO Box 183
Newton, MA 02165
(617) 964-0047

Hello Parents! (video)
Vida Health Communications
6 Bigelow Street
Cambridge, MA 02139
(617) 864-4334

CHAPTER 11

Modern Obstetrics: Postpartum Hemorrhage (16 mm film)
American Medical Association
535 N Dearborn Street
Chicago, IL 60610

Death of a Newborn (16 mm film)
Ross Laboratories
585 Cleveland Avenue
Columbus, OH 43216

Death of a Wished-For Child
OGR Service Corporation
PO Box 3586
Springfield, IL 62708

To Pick Up the Pieces (video)
Twenty-Twenty Media
Springfield, IL 62705

To Touch Today
Creative Marketing
PO Box 2432
Springfield, IL 62705

We Were Sad, Remember
IFDA
1045 Outer Park Drive, Suite 120
Springfield, IL 62704

To Have and Not to Hold (slide/cassette, video)
Polymorph Films
118 South Street
Boston, MA 02111
(617) 542-2004

Stillbirth, Miscarriage, and Beyond . . . (16 mm film, video)
Audio Visual Communication
Fairview General Hospital
18101 Lorain Avenue
Cleveland, OH 44111-5656

CHAPTER 12

The Amazing Newborn (16 mm film)
Polymorph Films
118 South Street
Boston, MA 02111
(617) 542-2004

Physical Assessment of the Normal Newborn (video and study guide)
Self-Directed Learning Programs
116 Stewart Center
Purdue University
West Lafayette, IN 47907

Infants and Their Families (video)
March of Dimes
1275 Mamaroneck Avenue
White Plains, NY 10605
(914) 428-7100

Babies (and Special Considerations) (140 slides/cassette)
Lifecircle
Marjorie M Pyle, RNC
2378 Cornell Drive
Costa Mesa, CA 92626

The Working Mom's Survival Guide (video)
Childbirth Graphics
PO Box 20540
Rochester, NY 14606-0540
(716) 272-0300

Jonah Has a Rainbow (16 mm film)
Centre Productions, Inc
1800 30th Street, #207
Boulder, CO 80301

Prematurely Yours: Premature Infant Behavior and Personality (slides/cassette, video)
Polymorph Films
118 South Street
Boston, MA 02111
(617) 542-2004

Baby Basics (video)
Audio Visual Communication
Fairview General Hospital
18101 Lorain Avenue
Cleveland, OH 44111-5656

Newborn Care (video)
Childbirth Graphics
PO Box 20540
Rochester, NY 14606-0540
(716) 272-0300

Fetal Sensory Development—The Sensational Baby (16 mm film, slides/cassette, video)
Polymorph Films
118 South Street
Boston, MA 02111
(617) 542-2004

Falling in Love with Your Baby (16 mm film, video) *Early Infant Care* (video)
Johnson & Johnson Baby Products Co
199 Grandview Road
Skillman, NJ 05558
(908) 874-2682

CHAPTER 13

PKU-Preventable Mental Retardation (16 mm film)
Mead Johnson Laboratories
Evansville, IN 47221

Hypoglycemia (slides/cassette)
March of Dimes
1275 Mamaroneck Avenue
White Plains, NY 10605
(914) 428-7100

Resuscitation of the Newborn (16 mm film, video)
ACOG Distribution Center
409 12th Street, SW
Washington, DC 20024

Death of the High Risk Infant (video)
AJN Company Educational Services Division
555 W 57th Street
New York, NY 10019-2961
(800) 223-2282

Memories (video)
CARE Video Productions
1650 Crossings Parkway
Westlake, OH 44145
(216) 835-5872

Thermoregulation in Newborns (video)
March of Dimes
1275 Mamaroneck Avenue
White Plains, NY 10605
(914) 428-7100

Stillbirth, Miscarriage, and Beyond . . . (16 mm film, video)
Audio Visual Communication
Fairview General Hospital
18101 Lorain Avenue
Cleveland, OH 44111-5656

Born Dying (16 mm film, video)
Carle Medical Communications
510 W Main, Dept A
Urbana, IL 61801
(217) 384-4838

Caring for the Premature Infant (series of films and videos)
Mead Johnson & Company
Evansville, IN 47721

Death of a Newborn (video)
Polymorph Films
118 South Street
Boston, MA 02111
(617) 542-2004

APPENDIX F

Organizations Involved in Maternity Care

American Academy of Family Physicians
8880 Ward Parkway
Kansas City, MO 64114
(816) 333-9700

American Academy of Pediatrics
141 Northwest Point Road
PO Box 927
Elk Grove Village, IL 60009-0927
(708) 228-5005

American College of Nurse Midwives (ACNM)
1522 K Street, NW, Suite 1000
Washington, DC 20005
(202) 289-0171
FAX: (202) 289-4395

American College of Obstetricians and Gynecologists
(ACOG)
409 12th Street, SW
Washington, DC 20024
(202) 638-5577

American Nurses Association
1101 14th Street, NW, Suite 200
Washington, DC 20005
(202) 789-1800

American Red Cross
17th and D Streets, NW
Washington, DC 20006
(202) 737-8300

American Public Health Association
1015 15th Street, NW
Washington, DC 20005
(202) 789-5600

Association for Childbirth at Home, International (ACHI)
PO Box 39498
Los Angeles, CA 90039
(213) 667-0839

CDC National AIDS Clearinghouse
PO Box 6003
Rockville, MD 20849-6003
(301) 251-5730

Clearinghouse on Infant Feeding and Maternal Nutrition
American Public Health Association
1015 15th St, NW
Washington, DC 20005
(202) 789-5600

Healthy Mothers, Healthy Babies, National Office
409 12th Street, SW
Washington, DC 20024
(202) 863-2458

Home Oriented Maternity Experience (HOME)
511 New York Avenue
Takoma Park, MD 20012

International Cesarean Awareness Network
PO Box 152
Syracuse, NY 13210
(315) 424-1942

International Lactation Consultants Association (ILCA)
201 Brown Avenue
Evanston, IL 60202-3601
(708) 260-8874

La Leche League International (LLLI)
1400 N Meacham Road
Schaumburg, IL 60173-4840
(800) LA-LECHE
(708) 455-7730

March of Dimes Birth Defects Foundation
  1275 Mamaroneck Avenue
  White Plains, NY 10605
  (914) 428-07100

Maternity Center Association
  448 E 92nd Street
  New York, NY 10128
  (212) 369-7300

Midwives Alliances of North America
  PO Box 175
  Newton, KS 67114
  (316) 283-4543

NAACOG: The Organization for Obstetric, Gynecologic,
  and Neonatal Nurses
  Name Change: The Association of Women's Health,
  Obstetric, and Neonatal Nurses (AWHONN)
  700 14th St, NW, Suite 600
  Washington, DC 20024
  (202) 662-1600

National Association of Childbearing Centers (NACC)
  3123 Gottschall Road
  RR 1, Box 1
  Perkiomenville, PA 18074
  (215) 234-8068

National Association of Parents and Professionals for Safe
  Alternatives in Childbirth (NAPSAC)
  PO Box 535, Route 1
  Marble Hill, MO 63764
  (314) 238-2010

National Association for Perinatal Addiction Research &
  Education (NAPARE)
  11 E Hubbard St, Suite 200
  Chicago, IL 60611
  (312) 329-2512

National Association of Postpartum Care Services (NAPCS)
  PO Box 1020
  Edmonds, WA 98020

National Genetics Foundation
  555 West 57th Street
  New York, NY 10019
  (212) 586-5800

National League for Nursing (NLN)
  10 Columbus Circle
  New York, NY 10019
  (212) 582-1022

National Maternal & Child Health Clearinghouse
  8201 Greensboro Drive, Suite 600
  McLean, VA 22102
  (703) 821-8955, ext 254 or 265

National Organization for Mothers of Twins Clubs, Inc
  PO Box 23188
  Albuquerque, NM 87192-1188
  (505) 275-0955

National Perinatal Association
  3500 E Fletcher Ave, Suite 525
  Tampa, FL 33613
  (813) 971-1008

Planned Parenthood Federation of America
  810 7th Avenue
  New York, NY 10019
  (212) 541-7800

Sex Information & Education Council of the U.S.
  (SIECUS)
  130 W 42nd Street, Suite 2500
  New York, NY 10036
  (212) 819-9770

The Triplet Connection
  Box 99571
  Stockton, CA 95209
  (209) 474-0885 or (209) 474-3073

APPENDIX G

Groups for Grief Help

AMEND
(Aiding a Mother Experiencing Neonatal Death)
4324 Berrywick Terrace
St. Louis, MO 63141
(314) 487-7582

Back to Sleep
PO Box 29111
Washington, DC 20040
(800) 505-CRIB

Compassionate Friends
(Following death of an infant)
PO Box 1347
Oak Brook, IL 60522-3696
(312) 990-0010

National Sudden Infant Death Syndrome Clearinghouse
Health & Human Services Dept
8201 Greensboro Drive, Suite 600
McLean, VA 22102
(703) 821-8955

RTS Bereavement Services
(formerly Resolve through Sharing)
1910 South Avenue
La Crosse, WI 54601
(608) 791-4747

SHARE
St. Joseph's Hospital
300 1st Capitol Drive
St. Charles, MO 63301
(314) 947-6164

SHARE
St. John's Hospital
700 East Carpenter
Springfield, IL 62769
(217) 544-6464, ext 5275

The Sudden Infant Death Syndrome Alliance
10500 Little Patuxent Parkway, #420
Columbia, MD 21044
(800) 221-SIDS

Preparation for Childbirth Organizations

American Academy of Husband-Coached Childbirth
   (AAHCC) (the Bradley method)
   PO Box 5224
   Sherman Oaks, CA 91413
   (800) 423-2397
   (818) 788-6662

American Society for Psychoprophylaxis in Obstetrics, Inc
   (ASPO/Lamaze)
   1200 19th St, NW, #300
   Washington, DC 20036
   (202) 857-1128
   (800) 368-4404

Childbirth Education Foundation
   PO Box 5
   Richboro, PA 18954
   (215) 357-2792

Council of Childbirth Education Specialists
   8 Sylvan Glen
   East Lyme, CT 06333
   (914) 234-7131

C/SEC, Inc (Cesarean/Support, Education, and Concern)
   22 Forest Road
   Farmingham, MA 01701
   (508) 877-8266

International Childbirth Education Association
   PO Box 20048
   Minneapolis, MN 55420
   (612) 854-8660

LaLeche League International, Inc.
   9616 Minneapolis Avenue
   Box 1209
   Franklin Park, IL 60131-8209
   (708) 455-7730

Maternity Center Association (MCA)
   45 E 92nd Street
   New York, NY 10128
   (212) 369-7300

Midwest Parentcraft Center
   627 Beaver Road
   Glenview, IL 60025
   (312) 998-6547

Read Natural Childbirth Foundation, Inc
   1300 S Eliseo Drive, Suite 102
   Greenbrae, CA 94904
   or
   PO Box 956
   San Rafael, CA 94915
   (415) 456-8462

APPENDIX I

Obstetric Admission Record and Obstetric Evaluation Record

The Obstetric Admission and Evaluation Records that follow are intended to be used together.

These forms were developed by a practicing maternity nurse.

For more information about the complete series of forms for use throughout the childbearing experience, write or call:

CSW Forms
PO Box 87
Timberon, NM 88350
1-800-284-2815

Obstetric Admission Record

Maternal / Fetal Risks / Problems*
based on prenatal record, patient interview, current assessment, other

Prenatal Labs	Results	Pending	Not Applicable
Blood type & Rh			
Antibody screen	− / +		
Rubella *immune*	− / +*		
Serology	− / +		
HBsAg	− / +		
HIV	− / +		
β strep	− / +		
Chlamydia	− / +		
GC	− / +		

Prenatal care: ☐ yes ☐ no   Began at approx. ___ wks gestation

Prenatal record available at admit: ☐ yes   ☐ see notes

Prenatal classes attended: ☐ none ☐ Lamaze ☐ C-Section
☐ infant care ☐ _____

Infant care provider: ☐ N/A

Plans for anesthesia/analgesia: ☐ none   ☐ IV analgesia   ☐ local
☐ spinal ☐ epidural ☐ general ☐ _____   ☐ N/A

Feeding preference: ☐ breast   ☐ bottle   ☐ undecided   ☐ N/A

Patient/family requests: ☐ none ☐ _____
_____
_____

Substance abuse *(smoking, alcohol, street drugs)*: ☐ none
☐ smokes _____ ppd   last _____   ☐ other, see notes

Current medications ☐ none	last taken	w/ patient	disposition
_____		Y / N	
_____		Y / N	
_____		Y / N	
_____		Y / N	

Recent illness or exposure to communicable disease: ☐ none
☐ _____

Est. sleep past 24 hrs _____   **Est. fluid intake past 12 hrs** _____

Last oral intake: fluids mo /day time   **solids** mo /day time

Prostheses: ☐ none ☐ contacts ☐ dentures ☐ _____

Ht _____ **Wt** _____ **Fundal ht** _____ **Est fetal wt** _____

Maternal Physical/Psychosocial Assessment

✓ - yes   N - see notes   N/A - not applicable   — - not assessed

Misc Prenatal record reviewed	
Labs reviewed, normal for pregnancy	
Neuro Alert, oriented X 3, appropriate behavior, speech clear	
No weakness or c/o dizziness	
Denies headache or visual disturbances	
Cardiovascular/Skin SBP is within 30mm Hg, and DBP is within 15mm Hg of early/ pre-pregnancy value. If early value is unavailable, BP < 140/90	
Skin warm and dry	
Skin pink	
Mucous membranes moist	
Heart rate regular with no irregularities	
No edema	
Skin intact, no lesions or bruises	
Resp Breathing easily. Respirations regular, normal depth	
Lungs clear bilaterally with good breath sounds to bases	
No rhinitis, nasal stuffiness or cough	
GI No nausea or vomiting	
No epigastric pain resistant to antacids	
No diarrhea or constipation. Last BM _____	
GU Voiding without c/o difficulty or discomfort	
Urine clear, not dark. No strong odor	
Psychosocial Understands, accepts situation, coping well with minimal anxiety	
Significant other is present, supportive	
Denies significant life stress (job, finances, social, loss, other)	
Basic needs (housing, food, clothing) met	
Pt. feels hospitalization will not cause child care or other problems	
No evidence of physical/emotional abuse	
Able to care for self without assistance	
No communication barriers (cultural, cognitive, sensory, language)	

Primary language: ☐ English ☐ Spanish ☐ _____

Significant other (S.O.): Name _____
Relationship _____   tel. no. _____
Comments: _____
Other support: _____

NOTES
_____
_____
_____
_____
_____

Admission information obtained from: ☐ prenatal record ☐ patient ☐ S.O. ☐ MD/CNM ☐ clinic ☐ _____

☐ **ID band on**   ☐ **Allergy band on** ☐ N/A   **Valuables to safe:** ☐ yes ☐ no ☐ N/A

MD/CNM:	**notified by:**	**Date:** / /	**time:**
Admitting nurse signature:		**Date:** / /	**time:**

©1993 *CSW* Forms Timberon, NM   **Obstetric Admission Record**   Form #5100-2

Note: The Obstetric Admission Record is intended for use with Obstetric Evaluation Record

Obstetric Admission Record

Form #5100-2 *(2 part carbonless)*

Use the Obstetric Admission Record with the Obstetric Evaluation Record for complete admission documentation. The Evaluation Record contains essential information not on the Admission Record, such as arrival information, reason patient came to the hospital, pregnancy history, due date, vital signs, allergies, and obstetric evaluation.

An important part of the admission process is the initiation of discharge planning. If you use our Obstetric Discharge Record, complete the middle part of the discharge form at the time of admission. If you do not use our discharge form, you may choose to document initial discharge planning in the "notes" section of the admit record.

If the patient is admitted for delivery, copies of the Admission and Evaluation Records can be sent to the nursery.

Completing the Admission Record

Maternal/Fetal Risks. Perform and document a current risk assessment based on review of the prenatal record, patient interview, current assessment and any other source of information available.

Prenatal labs. Complete as indicated. Use the three blank spaces as necessary for additional lab information—either different labs or repeats of earlier lab tests. For instance, if a chlamydia test is positive and then repeated with a negative result, write the first date in the preprinted chlamydia space and circle the "+" code. Then, in one of the blank spaces, write *chlamydia* and the second date followed by "−" or *neg*.

Prenatal care • Prenatal classes • Infant care provider • Plans for anesthesia or analgesia • Feeding preference. Complete as indicated.

Patient/family requests. Document any special requests, e.g., *no visitors except husband*. If patient has a written birth plan, you might refer to it by writing *see attached birth plan*.

Substance abuse. Complete as indicated. Document when the fetus was last exposed.

Current medications. Complete as indicated.

Recent illness or exposure to communicable disease. Complete as indicated. Include treatment if appropriate.

Estimated sleep past 24 hrs • Estimated fluid intake past 12 hrs. • Last oral intake • Prostheses • Ht • Wt • Fundal ht. Complete as indicated.

Maternal Physical/Psychosocial Assessment. Document maternal assessment using the assessment codes given.

If you are unable to do a complete assessment on admission (e.g., patient presents in advanced labor), follow your unit guidelines regarding documentation. One option would be to complete the assessment as soon as possible, and document in the Assessment Summary using the codes provided. A narrative note might read: *1700 Patient presented @ 1500, 8 cm dilated. Basic maternal/fetal evaluation and risk assessment completed on arrival. Remainder of admission assessment completed at this time.* Whatever you do, remember that no one expects you to do the impossible—the goal is to deliver safe care, which means setting priorities. Just document what you have done, and if there is no convenient box to check or code that tells the story, write it out in plain language.

Primary language • Significant Other • Notes • Admission information obtained from • ID band on • Allergy band on • Valuables to safe • MD/CNM • MD/CNM notified by • Admitting nurse signature. Complete as indicated. The date and time following the admitting nurse signature should reflect the time the admission was completed, unless otherwise indicated in written unit policy.

Obstetric Evaluation Record

Date: ___/___/___ To:_____ by: ☐ walk ☐ w/c ☐ gurney

Time in:_____ From: ☐ home ☐ clinic ☐ _____

Evaluation, procedure(s): ☐ **scheduled** ☐ **unscheduled**

☐ NST ☐ Observation ☐ Direct admit* Other

Indication(s)

☐ Patient oriented to unit and call system. Clinical condition, proce- **Initials**
dures, plan of care explained. Patient verbalizes understanding.

☐ Patient familiar with unit and procedures, denies questions.

NURSE'S NOTES ☐ see OB Evaluation Continuation Sheet

_____
_____
_____
_____
_____
_____
_____
_____
_____
_____
_____
_____

MD/CNM NOTES ☐ see separate progress note

_____
_____
_____
_____
_____
_____
_____
_____
_____
_____
_____
_____
_____
_____
_____
_____
_____
_____

Final Assessment

_____

Plan

_____

                                        MD/CNM

Disposition: ☐ N/A (direct admit) ☐ Admitted* ☐ Discharged

Time discharged or admit decision made:

To: home /   Condition:

By: ☐ walk ☐ w/c ☐ gurney   ☐ Alone With:

*See Obstetric Admission Record

Age	Grav	Term	Preterm	AB	Liv	EDD dates	EDD sono	Est. gest. age (wks)
								dates sono

TIME	BP	T	P	R	ALLERGIES ☐None	Reaction

DTR's: R   L   ☐ N/A

Urine albumin   ☐ N/A

MISCELLANEOUS

Initial Assessment

Fetal Heart Rate	Uterine activity	Membranes	Other
Baseline:	☐ none	☐ intact by hx	☐ no vaginal bleeding
	☐ irritability	☐ ruptured:	
Variability: ☐N/A	☐ contractions	MO / DAY	☐ normal show
	q _____ min	TIME	
Accelerations?	X _____ sec	fluid:	☐ fetus active
☐ yes ☐ no		☐ clear	☐ see notes
Decelerations?	mild / mod / firm		**Assessment**
☐ yes ☐ no	onset:	☐ no foul odor	**Time:**
☐ see notes	MO / DAY TIME	☐ see notes	**Initials:**

Vaginal exam ☐ not done

CERVIX		CERVIX	
☐ soft ☐ anterior	dilated:_____	☐ soft ☐ anterior	dilated:_____
☐ med. ☐ midpos.	effaced:_____	☐ med. ☐ midpos.	effaced:_____
☐ firm ☐ posterior		☐ firm ☐ posterior	
PRESENTING PART station:_____		PRESENTING PART station:_____	
☐ vtx (or)		☐ vtx (or)	
COMMENTS		COMMENTS	
Time: Initials:		Time: Initials:	

NST

☐ **Reactive** Parameters: ≥ _____ FHR accels in _____ minutes
(accelerations ≥15 seconds duration, ≥ 15 BPM amplitude)

☐ **Nonreactive** (not supine, no recent cigarette)

☐ Unsatisfactory   *Describe in notes*

☐ Decelerations present

Interpreted by:

Contraction Stress Test

☐ **Negative**   ☐ Spontaneous

☐ **Positive**   ☐ Nipple stimulation

☐ Suspicious   ☐ Oxytocin challenge

☐ Hyperstimulation   *Describe in notes*

☐ Variable Decels   ☐ Reactive

☐ Unsatisfactory   ☐ Nonreactive

Interpreted by:

ORDERS ☐ see separate order sheet

_____
_____
_____
_____
_____
_____
_____
_____

Short stay discharge instructions ☐N/A ☐See copy attached

_____

☐ Patient verbalizes understanding   Instructor Initials:

INIT	SIGNATURE	INIT	SIGNATURE	INIT	SIGNATURE

©1994 *CSW* Forms Timberon, NM   **Obstetric Evaluation Record**   **Form #5100-1**

Obstetric Evaluation
Continuation Sheet

Date ___ / ___ / ___

Init.	Signature	Init.	Signature

Time	Vital Signs					Fetal Heart Rate					Contractions				Cervix			Optional	Init.
	Blood Pressure	Pulse	Temperature	Respiration	Monitor Mode	Baseline	Variability	Accels	Decels	Frequency (minutes)	Duration (seconds)	Intensity	Dilation (cm)	Effacement (%)	Station			

Assessment Codes

N - see notes
— - not applicable, or not assessed

FHR Monitor Mode
US - ultrasound (*EFM*)
US - ultrasound (*auscultation*)
fts - fetoscope

Variability (long term)
(*electronic fetal monitoring*)
ø - absent (*0–2 BPM*)
↓ - minimal (*3–5 BPM*)
nl - moderate (*6–25 BPM*)
↑ - marked (*>25 BPM*)

Acceleration   Deceleration
ø - absent   **ø** - absent
+ - present   **+** - present
                        (*see notes*)

Contraction intensity
(*tocodynamometer/palpation*)
+ - mild
++ - moderate
+++ - firm

IV Device:	time inserted:	device size/type:	☐ heparin lock site:	Init.	IV pump?
☐ N/A (no IV)	time removed:	device intact: yes / no	☐ site not red, puffy or tender ☐ see notes	Init.	yes / no

	Time ↑	solution	additive	rate	Time ↓	cc infused	Init.		Time	Medication	Init.
IV								MEDS			

_____

_____

_____

_____

_____

_____

_____

_____

_____

_____

_____

_____

_____

_____

_____

_____

_____

_____

_____

Obstetric Evaluation *Continuation Sheet*   Form #5100-CS

©1993 *CSW* Forms   Timberon, NM

Obstetric Evaluation *Continuation Sheet*
Form #5100-CS *(2 part carbonless)*

The Obstetric Evaluation Continuation Sheet is intended for use with the Obstetric Evaluation Record when additional documentation space is needed.

Completing the Evaluation Record

Date/Initials. Note the date. Identify any initials used on the form.

Flowsheet. Make flowsheet entries as indicated, using the Assessment Codes given.

A code for a fetal electrode has not been included, since the Obstetric Evaluation form was designed for outpatient or preadmission monitoring. If a fetal electrode is placed, document on the flow sheet using an abbreviation acceptable to your hospital, or refer to the notes.

Also, since internal monitoring is unusual in an outpatient or observation setting, short term variability (STV) has not been addressed in the assessment codes. However, you may want to document STV and you can do so using the "optional" space or the notes section. (See page 24 for a discussion of STV documentation during external electronic fetal monitoring).

If a patient is on an observation status and goes quickly to delivery, you may (depending on unit guidelines) choose to remain with the Continuation Sheet.

IV/Medications. Complete as indicated.

Notes. Make narrative notes as necessary, keeping repetitive documentation to a minimum.

GLOSSARY

ABO incompatibility A condition that may lead to neonatal hemolytic disease.

Abortion Termination of pregnancy before the fetus is viable, that is, less than 20 to 24 weeks of gestation.

Abruptio placentae Premature separation of a normally implanted placenta.

Acidosis A pathological condition resulting from accumulation of acid in, or loss of base from, the body.

Acini cells Milk-producing cells in the breast.

Acinus A small saclike dilation, particularly one found in various glands.

Acme The highest point of a uterine contraction.

Adolescent A teenager or young adult.

AGA Average for gestational age.

Albumin The major protein in blood.

Alleles One or two or more alternative states of a gene.

Alkalosis The opposite of acidosis.

Alveoli Terminal pulmonary sacs that in fetal life are filled with fluid.

Amniocentesis Procedure to remove amniotic fluid from the uterine cavity by inserting a needle through the abdominal and uterine walls and into the amniotic sac.

Amnion The inner of the two fetal membranes forming the sac that encloses the fetus in the uterus.

Amnionitis Inflammation of the amnion.

Amniotomy Artificial rupture of the amniotic sac (AROM).

Ampulla Saclike dilation of a tube or duct.

Analgesia Relief of pain without loss of consciousness.

Anemia Abnormally low number of red blood cells.

Anesthesia Loss of feeling or sensation, with or without loss of consciousness.

Anomaly An abnormal occurrence or malformation.

Anovulation Lack or absence of ovulation.

Anteflexed The normal forward bending of the uterus.

Antepartum The period of pregnancy before delivery.

Anteverted The bending forward of an organ.

Anticipatory guidance Anticipating the needs of a family and thus providing teaching in advance of these needs.

Apgar score Numerical rating of an infant's condition at 1 and 5 minutes after birth, based on heart rate, respiratory effort, muscle tone, reflex irritability, and color. Developed by Dr. Virginia Apgar.

Apnea Temporary cessation of respiration.

Areola Pigmented ring around the nipple of the breast.

AROM Artificial rupture of membranes.

Artifact Random marks on the fetal heart rate tracing.

Asphyxia A condition in which there is a deficiency of oxygen in the blood and an increase in carbon dioxide in the blood and tissues.

Aspiration pneumonitis Pneumonia secondary to the neonate inhaling mucus, stomach contents, or meconium into the lungs.

Atelectasis Incomplete expansion or collapse of the lungs.

Atony A lack of normal muscle tone or tension.

Augmentation of labor Artificial stimulation of uterine contractions after labor has started but is not progressing.

Axis A line about which any revolving body turns.

Bactericide Agent that destroys bacteria.

Ballottement A term used when, in examining the pregnant woman, the fetus can be pushed about in the uterus.

Barr body Material in the inactivated one of the two female (X) chromosomes in each body cell of normal females.

Bartholin's glands The vulvovaginal glands.

Baseline fetal heart rate The range of a normal fetal heart rate; 120 to 160 beats per minute.

Bicornate uterus Anomalous uterus that may be either a double or a single organ having two horns.

Bilirubin Yellow or orange pigment produced by the breakdown of hemoglobin in cell elements and in the red blood cells.

Bilirubinemia Presence of an abnormal amount of bilirubin in the blood.

Biophysical profile Antepartum surveillance of the fetus at risk by use of tests for fetal well-being; nonstress test, contraction stress test, and fetal movement.

Biparietal diameter Largest transverse diameter of the fetal head; measured from one parietal bone to the other.

Blastoderm The germinal membrane of the ovum.

Bradycardia (fetal) Fetal heart rate below 120 beats per minute.

Bradley method Preparation for labor and birth with active involvement of father; also known as "husband-coached childbirth."

Braxton Hicks contractions Light, irregular, painless contractions of the uterus during pregnancy.

Breast pump Electric or manual pump used to extract milk from the lactating breast.

Breech The buttocks present for delivery instead of the head.

Brown fat Source of heat unique to newborns that is capable of greater thermogenic activity than ordinary fat.

Bulbourethral Two small glands located below the prostate gland on either side of the urethra.

Candidiasis Fungal infection; moniliasis.

Caput succedaneum Swelling produced on the presenting part of the fetal head during labor.

Caudal Local anesthetic injected into the caudal space in the sacrum resulting in caudal anesthesia.

Cephalic Pertaining to the head.

Cephalocaudal Development that progresses from the head to the feet.

Cephalopelvic disproportion (CPD) When the size of the fetal head is too large to pass through the maternal pelvis.

Cephalhematoma An accumulation of blood under the periosteum of any one cranial bone.

Cerclage Encircling an incompetent cervix with a ring or loop of suture.

Cervix Lowest and narrow end of the uterus; "the neck."

Cesarean birth Delivery of the fetus through a surgical incision into the abdominal and uterine walls.

Chadwick's sign Violet color of the vaginal mucous membrane during pregnancy.

Chignon Caput that forms underneath the vacuum cup of a vacuum extractor.

Chloasma A discoloration of the skin of the face occurring in yellowish-brown patches and spots; called "mask of pregnancy."

Chorioamnionitis Inflammation of the chorion and amnion.

Chorion The outer of the two membranes forming the sac that encloses the fetus in the uterus.

Chromosomes Structures in the nuclei of cells that carry the genes or hereditary factors.

Cilia Minute hairlike processes.

Circumcision The surgical removal of the end of the prepuce or foreskin of the penis.

Cleansing breath A deep breath taken by the woman at both the beginning and the end of each uterine contraction.

Cleavage The early, successive splitting of a fertilized ovum into smaller cells (blastomere).

Clitoris Structure of the female genitalia analogous to the penis in the male.

Clonus Spasmodic contraction and relaxation.

Coitus Sexual intercourse, copulation.

Colostrum Yellowish-white fluid expressed from the breasts during pregnancy and preceding the development of milk.

Colposcopy The examination of the cervix, vagina, and vulva with a low power scope introduced through the vagina. It is used in the diagnosis of cervical conditions.

Conduction The transfer of body heat to a cooler solid object in contact with a newborn.

Congenital Existing at or before birth.

Congenital anomaly Abnormality present at birth.

Convection The flow of heat from the body surface to cooler surrounding air.

Convoluted A tortuous irregularity caused by the unfolding of a structure upon itself.

Coombs' test Indirect: determination of Rh-positive antibodies in maternal blood; direct: determination of maternal Rh-positive antibodies in fetal cord blood.

Copulation Coitus; sexual intercourse.

Cornu Horn; a hornlike projection.

Corpus luteum The yellow mass found in the Graafian follicle after the ovum has been expelled.

Cotyledon Segment or subdivision of the uterine surface of the placenta.

CPAP (continuous positive airway pressure) Often used in treating respiratory distress syndrome in the newborn.

Crowning Stage in delivery when the widest part of the fetal head appears at the vulva.

Cul-de-sac of Douglas Pouch formed by a fold of the peritoneum dipping down between the anterior wall of the rectum and the posterior wall of the uterus.

Culdocentesis Puncture of Douglas's cul-de-sac through the vagina for aspiration of fluid.

Cystitis Infection in the urinary bladder.

Cytomegalovirus (CMV) A group of highly host-specific herpes viruses causing cytomegalic inclusion disease in man.

Deceleration A decrease in speed.

Decidua The endometrium during pregnancy.

Decidua basalis The portion of the decidua directly under the implanted zygote.

Decrement Decrease in intrauterine pressure after the acme of a uterine contraction.

Dehiscence Bursting open of a surgical scar.

Descent Passage of the presenting part of the fetus into and through the birth canal.

Dextro stix The brand name for a small strip of plastic with a chemically reactive tip. A color change caused by a drop of blood placed on the tip provides an estimate of the blood sugar level.

Diabetes mellitus A metabolic disorder in which the body's ability to use sugar is impaired owing to a disturbance in normal insulin activity.

Diabetogenic state Producing diabetes-like symptoms.

Diagonal conjugate The distance between the sacral promontory and the lower margin of the symphysis pubis.

Diaphoresis Profuse perspiration.

Dick-Read method An approach to childbirth based on the premise that fear of pain produces muscular tension, producing pain and greater fear.

Dilation (dilatation) Enlargement of an organ or orifice.

Dilation and curettage (D & C) A surgical procedure involving dilation of the cervix and removal of uterine contents.

Disassociation Lessening the perception of pain by focusing attention away from the pain.

Diuresis Increased secretion of urine.

Diuretics Drugs that cause an increased excretion of urine.

Dizygotic Derived from two fertilized cells.

Dominant Capable of expression when carried by only one of a pair of homologous chromosomes.

Doppler instrument A device used to detect changes in blood flow through a blood vessel. Doppler instruments may be used to measure blood pressure in an arm or leg or to detect fetal heart beats.

Doula A lay person who provides support during labor.

Ductus arteriosus A communicating channel between the aorta and the pulmonary artery of the fetus.

Ductus venosus A fetal vessel that establishes a direct communication between the umbilical veins, through the liver, to the inferior vena cava.

Dura (dura mater) Outermost, toughest of the three meninges covering the brain and spinal cord.

Dyspnea Difficult or labored breathing.

Dystocia Difficult labor or delivery.

Early deceleration A decrease in fetal heart rate early in a contraction, suggesting fetal head compression.

Eclampsia Abnormal reaction of the body to pregnancy resulting in convulsions; preceded by preeclampsia.

Ectopic pregnancy Implantation of the fertilized ovum outside the cavity of the uterus.

Edema Swelling due to an excessive amount of fluid in the tissues.

Effacement A thinning and shortening of the cervix that occurs during late pregnancy and/or labor.

Effleurage Gentle stroking of the abdomen used during labor in some childbirth preparation methods.

EFM Electronic fetal monitoring.

Ejaculation A sudden expulsion of semen.

Embolism The sudden blocking of an artery or vein by a clot or foreign material that has been brought to its site of lodgment by the blood current.

Embryo Products of conception from the second to the eighth weeks of gestation.

Emesis Vomiting.

Endometriosis Presence of endometrial tissue in the fallopian tube, peritoneum, or bladder, usually leading to infertility with signs of dysmenorrhea.

Endometritis Inflammation of the endometrium.

Endometrium The membrane lining the cavity of the uterus.

Endothelium The layer of epithelial cells that lines the cavities of the heart and of the blood and lymph vessels and the serous cavities of the body.

Endotracheal tube A tube inserted within the trachea.

Engagement In obstetrics engagement has occurred when the widest diameter of the fetal head has passed through the inlet of the pelvis.

Engorgement Lymph and venous stasis occurring in the breasts before the flow of milk.

Epididymis Coiled tube located on the testes; the storehouse for sperm.

Epidural External to the dura mater.

Episiotomy Surgical incision of the perineum as the fetal head crowns to facilitate delivery.

Erythema Redness of the skin produced by congestion of the smallest blood vessels.

Erythema toxicum A rash of unknown cause occurring on the newborn. It goes away spontaneously without treatment.

Erythroblastosis fetalis Blood disorder in the fetus or newborn in which maternal anti-Rh antibodies destroy fetal blood cells, causing jaundice and other symptoms.

Estriol A relatively weak human estrogen that is the oxidized end product of estradiol and estrone.

Estrogen Female sex hormone manufactured in the ovaries.

Ethnic Pertaining to a social group who share cultural bonds or physical (racial) characteristics.

Exchange transfusion Replacement of 75% to 85% of circulating blood by withdrawing the recipient's blood and injecting a donor's blood in equal amounts.

External cephalic version (ECV) Turning the fetus to a vertex position by exerting pressure on the fetus externally.

Fallopian tubes The two oviducts extending from the sides of the uterine fundus.

Familial Used to describe a disease or defect that affects more members of a family than would be expected by chance.

Ferning Fernlike pattern seen microscopically when cervical mucus is thinly applied to a glass slide and allowed to dry.

Fertilization Union of the male sperm and the female ovum to form a zygote, from which the embryo develops.

Fetal Pertaining to the fetus.

Fetal advocate A person who recognizes the health and well-being of the fetus as top priority.

Fetal bradycardia A slowing down of the fetal heart rate below 100 beats per minute.

Fetal heart rate (FHR) Number of fetal heart beats in a given time; normal FHR is 120 to 160 beats per minute.

Fetal heart rate variability The beat-to-beat changes that occur in the baseline fetal heart rate.

Fetal heart tones (FHT) Beat of the fetal heart that can be heard through the maternal abdomen.

Fetal tachycardia Fetal heart rate over 160 beats per minute for 10 minutes or more.

Fetopelvic disproportion Inability of the fetus to pass through the maternal pelvis.

Fetoscope A scope used to visualize the fetus in its sac. A specially designed stethoscope for listening to fetal heart tones.

Fetus Products of conception from the eighth week of gestation until birth.

Fibrin An insoluble protein that is essential to clotting of blood, formed from fibrinogen by action of thrombin.

Fibrinogen A normal blood constituent necessary for the formation of clots.

Fimbriae Fringelike opening (end) of the fallopian tubes.

Flexion The act of bending or the condition of being bent.

Floating Term used to describe presenting part of fetus that is freely movable above the pelvic inlet.

Focal point A point to focus on during the uterine contractions of labor.

Follicle Secretory cavity or sac.

Follicle stimulating hormone (FSH) Hormone that stimulates the maturation of the graafian follicle.

Follicular phase Early phase of the menstrual cycle where follicles enlarge and migrate toward the surface of the ovary.

Fontanel An unossified space or "soft spot" lying between the cranial bones of the skull of a fetus.

Foramen ovale Opening between the right and left atria of the fetal heart.

Fourchette The posterior junction of the labia majora.

FSE Fetal scalp electrode.

Fundus Upper portion of the uterus.

Gamete Mature male or female germ cell; a spermatozoon or ovum.

Gavage Feeding by a stomach tube.

Genes The factors that transmit hereditary characteristics to offspring.

Genetic counseling Process of determining the risk of occurrence or actual occurrence of a genetic disorder within a family and of providing appropriate information and advice about the choices available.

Gestation Length of time a pregnancy is carried.

Gestational age Estimated age of fetus using the first day of the last normal menstrual period, expressed in completed weeks.

Glottis The vocal cords and opening between them that leads to the trachea.

Glucosuria Presence of glucose in the urine.

Gonad Gamete-producing or sex gland; the ovary or testes.

Goodell's sign Softening of the cervix.

Graafian follicle Fluid-filled sac in the ovary containing the maturing ovum.

Gravida The number of times a woman has been pregnant.

Grunting A sign of respiratory distress in the neonate.

Gynecoid Typical female pelvis; heart shaped.

Hegar's sign Softening of the lower segment of the uterus that is classified as a probable sign of pregnancy.

Hemangioma A benign tumor made up of newly formed blood vessels.

Hematocrit A blood test signifying the percentage of red blood cells in whole blood; it is abbreviated Hct.

Hematoma A collection of blood in tissue.

Hemolysis Destruction of red blood cells.

Hemostasis The arrest of bleeding.

Heterozygous Having different alleles in regard to a given characteristic on each gene of a pair.

Homans' sign Pain in the calf on dorsiflexion of the foot; an indicator of thrombosis.

Homozygous Having identical alleles for a characteristic on each gene of a pair.

Human chorionic gonadotropin (HCG) A hormone produced by the trophoblast.

Hydramnios Excessive amniotic fluid inside the uterus leading to overdistention.

Hydrocephalus An excess of cerebrospinal fluid within the ventricular system.

Hymen Membranous fold that partially closes the vaginal orifice.

Hyperbilirubinemia Elevation of unconjugated serum bilirubin concentrations.

Hyperplasia Increase in the number of normal cells in normal arrangement in an organ or tissue.

Hyperthermia High body temperature; fever.

Hypertonic Increased tonicity or tension.

Hypoglycemia Low level of sugar (glucose) in the blood.

Hypotonic Weak and ineffective.

Hypovolemic shock Shock caused by abnormally decreased volume of circulating fluid (plasma) in the body.

Hypoxemia Deficiency of oxygen in the blood.

Hypoxia Reduction to below physiological levels in the supply of oxygen to the tissues.

Icterus neonatorum Jaundice in a newborn.

Incompetent cervix A cervix that is prone to dilate before the normal period of gestation. Frequently this happens between the sixteenth and twenty-eighth weeks of gestation.

Increment Increasing intrauterine pressure as a uterine contraction begins.

Incubator Equipment that maintains a premature infant in an environment of appropriate temperature and humidity.

Induction Labor brought on by artificial means.

Inertia A sluggishness or inactivity of uterine contractions during labor.

Infant mortality rate (IMR) The number of deaths of liveborn infants per 1000 live births either within the first 28 days (neonatal) or from 28 days to 1 year (postneonatal) in a specified geographic area or institution.

Infertility Decreased capacity to conceive.

Infusion pump A machine used to push fluid at a controlled, preset rate into an artery or vein.

Innominate bone One of the two pelvic bones.

In situ In position.

Intensity Usually expressed as mild, moderate, or strong in relation to uterine contractions of the uterine muscle.

International unit (IU) Internationally accepted amount of a substance.

Intrauterine growth retardation (IUGR) Fetal condition characterized by failure to grow at the expected rate.

Intubation The insertion of a tube.

Intertuberous diameter Distance between ischial tuberosities. Measured to determine dimension of pelvic outlet.

Inversion A turning inward, inside out, or upside down.

Involution The return of the reproductive organs to the nonpregnant state when pregnancy is over.

Ischial spines Bony prominence; one on each side of the ischium at about the midlevel of the true pelvis.

Ischium The lower part of the innominate bone.

Isoimmunization Development of antibodies in response to isoantigens (e.g., development of anti-Rh antibodies in an Rh-negative person).

IUPC Intrauterine pressure catheter.

Jaundice Yellow discoloration of the body tissues caused by the deposit of bile pigments (unconjugated bilirubin).

Kegel exercise An exercise to strengthen the perineal muscles; first described by Dr. Kegel.

Kernicterus Erythroblastosis fetalis with brain damage.

Ketoacidosis Acidosis resulting from accumulation of ketone bodies.

Ketones End products of fat metabolism.

Ketosis Accumulation of abnormal amounts of ketones in the body, resulting from inadequate ingestion of carbohydrates.

Labia majora The large, outer lips of the vulva.

Labia minora The folds of delicate skin inside the labia majora.

Laceration Irregular tear of wound tissue.

Lactation The secretion of milk.

Lactose Milk sugar.

Lamaze (PPM) method Psychoprophylactic method of prepared childbirth.

Lanugo Fine downy hair growing over the body of the fetus.

Laparoscopy Examination of the abdominal cavity by the introduction of a laparoscope through a small abdominal incision.

Laryngoscope An endoscope for examining the larynx.

Late deceleration Decreased fetal heart rate after a contraction ends, suggesting uteroplacental insufficiency.

Latent phase Early labor; cervical dilation from 0 to 3 cm.

LDR Labor-delivery-recovery room.

LDRP Labor-delivery-recovery-postpartum room.

Lecithin One of the surfactant substances produced in the lung. The amount of lecithin produced increases with increasing gestational age of the fetus.

Lecithin/sphingomyelin (L/S) ratio Ratio of lecithin to sphingomyelin in the amniotic fluid. A ratio of 2:1 is used as an indicator of fetal lung maturity.

Leopold's maneuvers Abdominal inspection and palpation to determine how the fetus is positioned in utero.

Let-down reflex A new mother's body's response to oxytocin that allows milk in the breast alveoli to flow into the milk ducts.

Leukocytosis Abnormally high white blood cell numbers in the blood.

Levator ani muscle Powerful muscle that helps support the organs in the pelvis.

LGA (large for gestational age) An infant whose birth weight falls above the 90th percentile.

Lie In obstetrics the relationship of the long axis of the fetus to the long axis of the mother.

Lightening Descent of the uterus into the pelvic cavity before or during labor.

Linea nigra A dark line appearing longitudinally on the abdomen of pregnant women.

Linea terminalis Line dividing the upper (false) pelvis from the lower (true) pelvis.

Lobule A small segment or lobe, especially one of the smaller divisions making up a lobe.

Lochia The vaginal discharge during the puerperium, consisting of blood, mucus, and tissue.

Lochia alba The final yellowish-white vaginal discharge after childbirth.

Lochia rubra The red, sanguinous vaginal discharge of the first 2 to 4 days postpartum.

Lochia serosa The serous vaginal discharge occurring 4 to 5 days after birth.

Lunar month 28 days.

Luteal phase Phase of the menstrual cycle after the mature follicle ruptures and the corpus luteum stimulates production of the hormone progesterone.

Macrosomia Unusually large body. Infants of diabetic mothers are often macrosomic.

Mastitis Inflammation or infection of the breast.

Meconium The dark green or black, sticky, tarry substance in the large intestine of the fetus or newly born baby.

Meiosis Process by which germ cells divide and decrease their chromosomal number by one half.

Menarche First menstrual flow.

Meningocele Congenital malformation of the spine in which the meninges protrude through a defect in the cranium or vertebral column.

Menopause Cessation of menses during middle age as part of the climacteric.

Menstruation Periodic vaginal discharge of bloody fluid from the nonpregnant uterus that occurs from the age of puberty to menopause.

Metabolic acidosis A disturbance affecting the bicarbonate element of the bicarbonate-carbonic acid buffer pair; bicarbonate deficit.

Metrorrhagia Vaginal bleeding or spotting between normal menstrual cycles.

Micturition Urination, voiding.

Milia Distended sebaceous glands commonly found over the bridge of the nose, chin, and cheeks of newborn infants; appear like tiny "whiteheads."

Mitosis Indirect cell division.

Molding Temporary changes in the shape of the newborn's head as it accommodates to the birth canal during labor and birth.

Mongolian spots Areas of dark blue pigmentation over the lumbar, sacral, and gluteal regions.

Moniliasis Infection of the mucous membranes of the skin caused by a yeastlike fungus.

Monitrice Labor coach especially trained in the psychoprophylactic (Lamaze) method of childbirth.

Monozygotic Derived from one fertilized cell, such as identical twins.

Montgomery's tubercles Sebaceous glands of the areola of the breast.

Morbidity State of being sick or diseased.

Moro's reflex A startle reflex with stimulation in which the infant's arms are suddenly thrown out in an embrace attitude.

Mortality Death.

Morula Solid mass of cells formed by division and redivision of the fertilized ovum.

Mother-baby nursing A nursing model in which one nurse provides care to the mother-baby dyad.

Myometrium Muscle coat of the uterus.

Nägele's rule Method of estimating the expected date of confinement (EDC), or due date. Count back 3 months from the first day of the last menstrual period and add 1 year and 7 days.

Nasal flaring A sign of respiratory distress. The edges of the nostrils fan outward as the baby inhales.

Natural childbirth Concept introduced by Grantley Dick-Read of England that posed that childbirth was a natural physiological process not meant to be painful.

Neonatal From birth to 28 days of life.

Neonatologist A physician who specializes in caring for newborn infants.

Neutral thermal environment The grouping of environmental conditions in which the neonate's oxygen consumption is at a minimum and the temperature is within normal limits.

Nonshivering thermogenis Infant's method of producing heat by increasing metabolic rate.

Occiput The back part of the head.

Oligohydramnios An abnormally small amount of amniotic fluid.

Organogenesis Formation of body organs from embryonic tissue.

Oscilloscope An instrument that displays a visual representation of electrical variations on the fluorescent screen of a cathode ray tube.

Ovaries Two glands in the female situated on either side of the pelvic cavity. Each ovary produces the female reproductive cell, the ovum, and the hormones estrogen and progesterone.

Ovulate Release of the ovum from the graafian follicle.

Ovulation Rupture of the graafian follicle and discharge of the ovum.

Ovum Female reproductive cell.

Oxytocin Pharmaceutical agent that stimulates uterine contractions. Also, a naturally-produced posterior pituitary hormone that causes contraction of uterine myometrial cells and myoepithelial cells of the breast.

Papanicolaou's test (Pap) Microscopic examination of scrapings from the cervix, endocervix, or other mucous membranes that will reveal the presence of premalignant or malignant cells.

Para Past pregnancies continued to period of viability; refers to pregnancies, not fetuses.

Paracervical block A regional anesthetic injected into the area around the cervix to reduce the pain caused by cervical dilatation.

Parturient Woman in labor.

Parturition Act of giving birth.

Passage The internal pelvic rim through which a fetus must pass in order to be born.

Passenger The fetus during labor and delivery.

Pelvic floor The soft tissues closing the pelvic outlet.

Perfusion The passage of a fluid through the vessels of a specific organ.

Perimetrium The serous membrane enveloping the uterus.

Perinatal period Period from the 28th week of gestation to the 28th day after birth.

Perinatologist Obstetrician who cares for high-risk mothers in the perinatal period.

Perineum In obstetrics the area between the lower end of the vagina and the anus.

Periodic rate changes Fetal heart rate accelerations and decelerations that occur intermittently in response to uterine contractions.

Peristaltic action Wavelike, rhythmical contractions.

Pessary Device placed inside the vagina to function as a supportive structure for the uterus or a contraceptive device.

Phenylketonuria (PKU) An inborn error in metabolism in which the infant lacks the enzyme necessary to metabolize phenylalanine (an essential amino acid).

Phototherapy Use of fluorescent lights to treat hyperbilirubinemia in neonates by breaking down bilirubin accumulated in the skin.

Physiological jaundice Mild yellowing of the newborn's skin and eyes occurring the first few days after birth and self-resolving.

PID Pelvic inflammatory disease.

Pitocin A synthetic oxytocin that stimulates uterine contractions.

Placenta The organ attached to the wall of the uterus through which the fetus derives its nourishment and oxygen.

Placenta accreta A placenta abnormally adherent to the uterine wall.

Placenta previa A placenta that is implanted in the lower uterine segment so that it partially covers the internal os of the cervix.

Plasma The liquid part of the blood.

Polyhydramnios Abnormally large amount of amniotic fluid.

Position Relation of the fetal presenting part to the maternal pelvis.

Posterior Situated behind.

Postmaturity syndrome An infant born after 42 weeks of pregnancy with nutritional deficiencies.

Postpartum blues A temporary period after childbirth that is characterized by periods of crying and depression alternating with joy and happiness.

Postpartum period The time after delivery to 6 weeks after birth.

Postterm Refers to a fetus or baby whose gestation has been longer than 42 weeks.

Powers A process that causes cervical dilatation and expulsion of the fetus. The powers of labor are supplied by the fundus of the uterus and implemented by uterine contractions.

Precipitous delivery A rapid, uncontrolled delivery.

Preeclampsia A disorder that can be present during pregnancy or early in postpartum period, characterized by hypertension, edema, and albuminuria.

Premature rupture of membranes Rupture of the membranes ("bag of waters") before the onset of labor.

Prepuce The fold of skin that covers the glans penis of the male and clitoris of the female.

Presentation Relationship of the long axis of the fetus to the long axis of the mother.

Presentation The part of the fetus that enters the pelvis first.

Presumptive signs Manifestations that suggest pregnancy but are not absolutely positive. These include cessation of menses, Chadwick's sign, morning sickness, and quickening.

Preterm labor Labor that begins before 37 weeks of gestation.

Primary infertility Inability to conceive or carry a pregnancy to viability with no previous history of pregnancy carried to live birth.

Probable signs Manifestations or evidence that indicates there is a definite likelihood of pregnancy. These include Goodell's sign, Hegar's sign, enlargement of the abdomen, and positive pregnancy tests.

Progesterone Hormone produced by the corpus luteum.

Prolactin Hormone that stimulates lactation.

Prolapsed cord The umbilical cord presenting beside or ahead of the presenting part.

Proliferative phase Preovulatory, follicular, or estrogen phase of the menstrual cycle.

Prostaglandins Biological substances naturally occurring in semen, menstrual fluid, and various tissues of the body; stimulate contractility of the uterine and other smooth muscle.

Prostate Gland that surrounds the urethra at the base of the male bladder.

Proteinuria Presence of protein (albumin) in the urine.

Psychoprophylaxis Mental and physical education of the parents in preparation for childbirth.

Pudendal block Anesthesia produced by injection of a regional anesthetic into the pudendal nerves, numbing the perineum and vagina.

Puerperal sepsis Infection during the puerperium (postpartum period).

Puerperium 42 days after birth.

Pulmonary Refers to the lungs.

Quickening The first time fetal movements definitely can be felt by the mother; usually occurs near the 20th week of gestation.

Radiant warmer A servo-controlled heating device that is placed over the baby and provides radiant heat to keep body temperature normal.

Radiation Loss of heat to a distant cold surface.

Recessive Inheritance requiring genes from both mother and father.

Reflex Automatic response built into the nervous system.

Reflux Backward flow of undigested food or fluid from the stomach.

Regimen A strictly regulated scheme of diet, exercise, or other activity.

Respiratory distress syndrome (RDS) A disease resulting from immaturity of the lungs and a lack of surfactant; mainly affects preterm infants.

Respite To provide rest and/or relief to the family or caretaker(s) of the dying patient.

Restitution Spontaneous turning of fetal head to right or left after it has extended through the vulva thus assuming a normal alignment with the baby's shoulders.

Retrolental fibroplasia A formation of fibrous tissue behind the lens of the eye, resulting in blindness. One cause of this condition is administration of oxygen in concentrations too high for premature infants.

Retroverted A condition in which the normally anteflexed uterus is tipped posteriorly.

Retroverted (uterus) Displaced uterus with the body of the uterus tipped backward.

Ripening The softening of the cervix before labor.

Rooming-in Newborn remains at the mother's bedside instead of in the newborn nursery.

Rooting reflex Newborn's head turns toward direction of touch on the cheek in search of the nipple.

Rubella German measles.

Rugae Transverse folds of the vaginal mucous membranes.

Saddle block A form of low spinal anesthesia.

Secondary infertility Inability to conceive or carry a pregnancy to a live birth after one or more successful pregnancies.

Secretory phase (of menstrual cycle) Postovulatory, luteal, progestational, and premenstrual phase of menstrual cycle.

Sedative A drug that allays irritability or excitement.

Semen Thick, white, viscid secretion discharged from the urethra of the male at orgasm; the transporting medium of the sperm.

Sepsis Infection of the blood; also referred to as *septicemia.*

Septate Divided by a septum.

Septicemia Severe generalized illness caused by bacteria in the blood stream.

Servo-control A system that automatically maintains a baby's temperature at a preset temperature.

SGA (small for gestational age) An infant who falls below the 10th percentile for weight.

Show Blood-tinged mucous discharge occurring during labor as the cervix dilates. Also known as bloody show.

Sibling Any of two or more offspring of the same parents; a brother or sister.

Skene's glands Ducts found on each side of the urethral meatus.

Small for gestational age (SGA) An infant whose weight is lower than the 10th percentile for infants of that gestational age.

Spermatozoa The male generative cells.

Spina bifida Defect in closure of the bony spinal canal.

Station The location of the presenting part of the fetus in relation to the ischial spines of the pelvis.

Striae gravidarum Reddish-purple, irregular depressions that appear in the skin of the abdomen, thighs, and buttocks of pregnant women.

Subinvolution Failure of the uterus to return to its normal size following pregnancy.

Supine Position of a person who is flat on the back.

Supine hypotensive syndrome Hypotension resulting from the pressure of the enlarged uterus on the vena cava, blocking venus return.

Surfactant A surface-active agent secreted by type II cells in the alveoli of the lungs. It reduces the surface tension of the pulmonary fluids and thus prevents the alveoli from collapsing.

Surrogacy To put in another's place as a substitute.

Sutures (of the fetal skull) Line of cartilage separating the bony plates of the skull.

Symphysis pubis Thick mass of fibrocartilage formed at the union of the pubic bones.

Synchronous Happening at the same time.

Syphilis A sexually transmitted disease that is transmitted by the spirochete *Treponema pallidum.*

Systemic Refers to the whole body.

Tachycardia Rapid heart rate. Fetal tachycardia is a fetal heart rate of 160 beats or more per minute.

Tachypnea Rapid respiration.

Telemetry Using an electronic device to measure pressure and transmitting the information to a central receiver.

Teratogen Substance that causes abnormal development of embryonic structures.

Term Normal end period of pregnancy, occurring between 38 and 42 weeks.

Testes The two glands contained in the male scrotum.

Testosterone Male sex hormone produced by the interstitial cells in the testes.

Tetanic contraction Abnormally long uterine contraction, lasting more than 70 seconds; usually occurs in response to hyperstimulation from oxytocin infusion.

Therapeutic touch Serving to cure or heal through touch.

Thermogenesis Heat production.

Thermogenic activity Activity that creates or produces heat, especially in the body.

Thrombophlebitis Inflammatory process along the walls of the blood vessels.

Thrush A fungus infection of the oral membranes, usually caused by *Candida albicans*. White patches on a red, moist, inflamed surface are apparent in the mouth.

Titer The quantity of a substance required to react with or to correspond to a given amount of another substance.

Tocolytic agent Drug that alters the force of uterine contractions.

Tonic neck reflex Postural reflex of newborn.

Tonus Tone or contraction of skeletal muscles.

Toxoplasmosis Disease caused by a type of protozoa (a tiny animal made up of one cell and seen only with a microscope).

Transition The last part of the active phase of labor (from 8- to 10-centimeter dilation).

Transitional Between phases.

Trichomonas vaginalis Protozoan infection of the vagina.

Trimester Three-month period.

Trisomy The presence of three chromosomes rather than the usual two.

Trophoblast Cells that form outer layer of the blastula.

Tuboplasty Plastic surgery to repair severed or damaged fallopian tubes.

Ultrasonography A technique by which high-frequency sound waves are beamed into the body and then reflect back, enabling the deep structures of the body to be visualized on a screen.

Umbilicus The navel.

Urethra The passage through which urine is discharged from the bladder to outside the body.

Uterine souffle Soft, blowing sound made by the blood in the arteries of the pregnant uterus and synchronous with the fetal heart sounds.

Uteroplacental insufficiency Refers to the uterus and the placenta *not* working well together as a functioning unit.

Uterus The womb; a hollow muscular organ in which the embryo and fetus develop.

Vagina A tubelike passage leading from the vulva to the uterus in the female.

Vaginitis An infection in the vagina.

Variability Degree of deviation from the baseline fetal heart rate.

Variable deceleration Fetal heart rate drops below baseline at various times with no consistent relationship to contractions. Usually due to umbilical cord compression.

Varicocele Varicose vein of the spermatic cord, more often the left; a common cause of male infertility.

Vas deferens A thick, smooth, muscular tube that allows sperm to exit from the epididymis and pass from the scrotal sac into the abdominal cavity; also known as the ductus deferens.

VBAC Vaginal birth after a cesarean.

Vernix A white cheeselike substance that covers the skin of the fetus.

Version Manual turning of the fetus.

Vertex The crown of the head.

Vestibule The space below the clitoris and between the labia minora.

Viable Able to live.

Villi A small vascular process or protrusion on a membranous surface.

Vitamin K A vitamin used to promote blood clotting and thus prevent hemorrhage by aiding in the synthesis of prothrombin by the liver.

Vulva The external genitals of the female.

Zygote The fertilized ovum.

INDEX